CLINICAL EPIDEMIOLOGY

Hanna Shevchuk and
Yevhen Tarasov

ALLIED
HEALTH
PRESS

Clinical Epidemiology

Authors: **Hanna Shevchuk and Yevhen Tarasov**

Allied Health Press
4164 Lakeshore Road
Burlington ON L7L 1A4
Canada
www.alliedhealthpress.com
Email: orders@arclereducation.com

ISBN: 978-1-77956-821-2

ABOUT THE AUTHORS

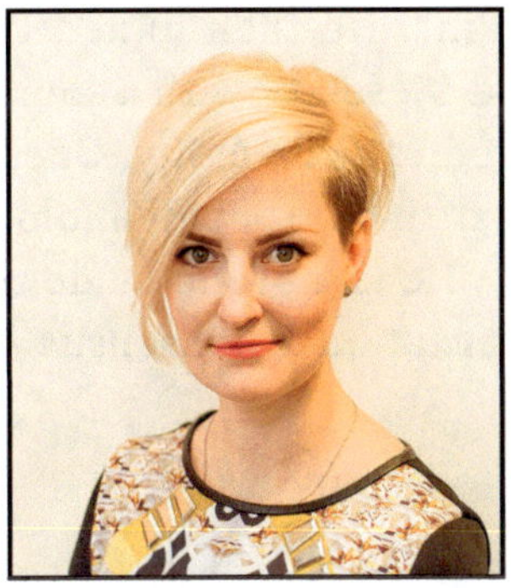

Hanna Shevchuk, PhD, is an Associate Professor and Head of Study at the Department of General and Clinical Epidemiology and Biosafety with a course in Microbiology and Virology at Odessa National Medical University (ONMedU), Ukraine. She also serves as a visiting lecturer at the International European University, Malta Campus.

As. Prof. Shevchuk received her Master's degree in Microbiology and Virology from Odessa I.I. Mechnikov National University in 2005 and earned her PhD in Biological Sciences (specialty: molecular genetics) from the Institute of Food Biotechnology and Genomics of the National Academy of Sciences of Ukraine in 2012. Her academic journey includes positions ranging from laboratory assistant to researcher and faculty member at leading Ukrainian research institutes and universities.

Her research interests focus on molecular genetics, microbiology, immunology, virology, epidemiology and innovative pedagogical practices in medical education. As. Prof. Shevchuk is an active member of the Society of Microbiologists of Ukraine named after S.M. Vynogradskyi, the Vavilov Society of Geneticists and Breeders of Ukraine and the Association of Clinical Chemistry and Laboratory Medicine of Ukraine. She has participated in international internships and seminars dedicated to modern challenges in higher medical education and is the author and co-author of scientific publications in microbiology, immunology, and pedagogy.

As. Prof. Shevchuk is recognized for her contributions to the development of educational programs and the implementation of advanced teaching methods, aiming to enhance the quality of training for specialists in medicine. In 2024, she was awarded the academic title of Associate Professor at Odessa National Medical University.

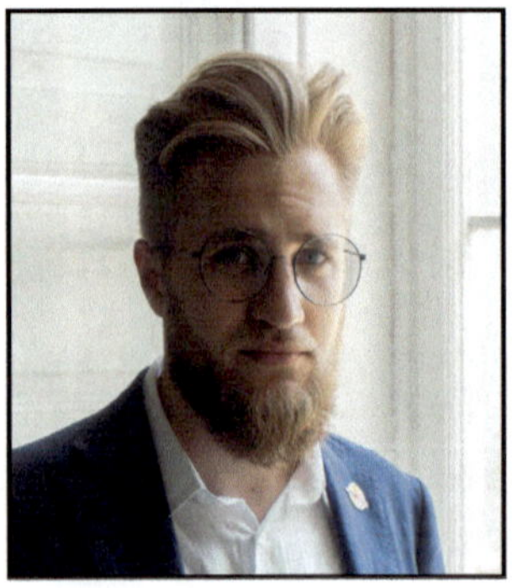

Yevhen Tarasov, MD, EuSpLM is a Senior Lecturer at the Department of General and Clinical Epidemiology and Biosafety with a course on Microbiology and Virology at Odesa National Medical University. Yevhen Tarasov received his MD in 2018 and got specialization in Medical Laboratory Science in 2019 with residency at The Filatov Institute of Eye Diseases and Tissue Therapy of the National Acadeny if Medical Science of Ukraine. He then joined the Department of General and Clinical Epidemiology and Biosafety with a course on Microbiology and Virology at Odesa National Medical University, Odesa, Ukraine as an assistant professor. His research interests include epidemiology and diagnostics of autoimmune diseases and allergy. He is a group leader of work group on Ukrainian adaptation of the the International Consensus on Antinuclear Antibody (ANA) Patterns (ICAP).

Brief Table of Contents

Detailed Table of Contents

CHAPTER 3

Study Designs in Clinical Research 59

CHAPTER 4

Diagnostic Test Evaluation 95

CHAPTER 5

Screening in Epidemiology 119

CHAPTER 9

CHAPTER 10

LIST OF FIGURES

PREFACE

Clinical decision-making relies on far more than experience and intuition. It requires a formal process of recognizing disease patterns, evaluating interventions, and interpreting information so that it can have a useful bearing on patient care. Decisions affecting diagnostics, therapy, and prevention in medicine today tend to rely more on empirical analysis. Such a basis guarantees that medical decisions are not just biologically sound but also evidence-based. That systematic, data-based structure is a product of a field of research bridging clinical practice and population-based science to enable healthcare providers to make better-informed decisions with improved outcomes.

Across the globe, health care systems have never had a greater demand for accountability, efficiency, and precision in diagnosis and treatment. With shifting infectious and chronic disease burdens, health practitioners must risk assess, validity-test clinical instruments, and critically appraise scientific evidence. Those responsibilities require disciplined comprehension of the measurement of disease patterns, the detection of risk and outcome associations, and the interpretation of findings in the face of real-world realities such as confounding variables and bias. That disciplined methodology is provided by clinical epidemiology—a field that equips clinicians with tools for asking the right questions, gathering relevant data, and making conclusions within a clinically meaningful context.

Clinical Epidemiology has been made an all-embracing and accessible overview of this important discipline. The book contains a logical and progressive structure, beginning with fundamental principles and extending through to more specialized areas of study. The work introduces readers to the basis and applications of epidemiology in clinical practice. Throughout the chapters, emphasis is placed on practical usefulness, critical judgment, and evaluation of evidence used in day-to-day patient care. The purpose of this book is not only to transmit information but to build competence in the application of epidemiologic principles to real clinical investigation. This resource enables the acquisition of fundamental competencies on the part of medical students, clinicians, researchers, and public health professionals who are expected to integrate evidence into clinical decision-making.

Chapter 1 provides the context for the topic of clinical epidemiology, outlining its purpose, scope, and relevance to healthcare practice. Chapter 1 establishes the argument for applying epidemiological principles to clinical decision-making.

Chapter 2 covers disease frequency measures, including incidence, prevalence, and rates that are used to quantify health issues in specific populations. Chapter 2 further addresses concepts like person-time and cumulative incidence.

Chapter 3 outlines the major study designs used in clinical trials, including cohort studies, case-control studies, cross-sectional studies, and randomized controlled trials, and addresses their advantages and disadvantages in clinical environments.

Chapter 4 covers the evaluation of diagnostic tests, such as terms of sensitivity, specificity, likelihood ratios, and predictive values. Chapter 4 teaches the reader how to estimate the clinical applicability and drawbacks of diagnostic tests.

Chapter 5 introduces a discussion of epidemiological screening methods, such as early detection concepts, requirements for effective screening programs, and statistical techniques used in evaluating the performance of screening.

Chapter 6 describes different types of bias in clinical trials, such as selection bias, information bias, and confounding. Readers learn about how to avoid or control for bias when designing and analyzing studies.

Chapter 7 describes causation in epidemiology, outlining frameworks like the Bradford Hill criteria and techniques for establishing causal associations between exposures and health outcomes.

Chapter 8 introduces significant statistical methods often used in epidemiology, such as measures of association, confidence intervals, hypothesis testing, regression analysis, and risk estimation techniques.

Chapter 9 covers prognosis studies by pointing out the importance of follow-up, outcome measurement, survival analysis, and prognostic modeling to predict disease course.

Chapter 10 addresses clinical trials, in the form of randomized controlled trials, and issues related to design, randomization techniques, blinding, outcome measurement, and results analysis.

Chapter 11 defines evidence-based medicine (EBM), including how to critically appraise clinical literature, integrate research and clinical experience, and apply patient values to decision-making.

Chapter 12 describes the epidemiology of infectious diseases, including modes of transmission, investigation of outbreaks, reproductive numbers, and control measures.

Chapter 13 continues with chronic disease epidemiology with the focus on study methods for non-communicable diseases such as cardiovascular disease, diabetes, and cancer, focusing on long-term risk and cohort studies.

Chapter 14 introduces genetic epidemiology, which examines the role of heredity in disease causation and ways of estimating genetic contribution by means of linkage studies, association studies, and twin studies.

Chapter 15 discusses nutritional epidemiology, such as dietary assessment techniques, the interface of nutrition and disease, and the challenge in accurately measuring food intake and nutritional exposure.

This book is designed for a broad spectrum of readers, including medical students who need basic information, practicing physicians who wish to have greater confidence in interpreting research, public health workers who conduct applied health research, and novice researchers planning or evaluating clinical studies. It is suitable for learning at both an academic and professional level. For instructors, it offers a structured framework that can be applied to curriculum planning. For practicing clinicians and postgraduate students, it offers a theoretical framework that bridges between theory and practice in real clinical settings.

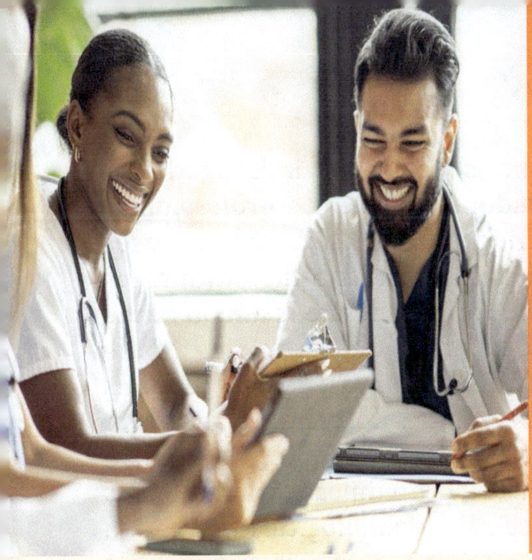

Chapter 1

INTRODUCTION TO CLINICAL EPIDEMIOLOGY

Contents

Introduction

Clinical epidemiology is a central science that cuts across biomedical clinical practice and epidemiologic principles. It translates facts into effective health interventions through a logical examination of the determinants and distribution of disease among populations of patients. Clinical epidemiology allows health providers to establish risk factors contributing to the incidence and prevalence of disease. Such factors are particularly important in shaping evidence-based practice aimed at enhancing patient outcomes. Clinical epidemiology plays a crucial role not only in improving care for individual patients but also feeds into health policy at the level of public health regarding disease prevention and health promotion. Due to this, it is a central support mechanism in clinical as well as public health, guiding practitioners' practice in solving health issues through a framework that operates on the basis of good research procedures and evidence. Armed with critical thinking skills, clinical epidemiologists investigate and assess the efficacy of medical interventions, extending beyond simple counting of diseases to an examination of causation mechanisms. An important aspect of this investigation is the organization of a Journal Club, which provides a forum for students and health professionals to critically appraise current research. Such collaborative learning exercise not only exposes students to the newest developments but also compel them to critically examine the advantages and disadvantages of empirical studies (Caron et al., 2019). By promoting discussions aimed at the rigor and applicability of research findings, such exercises promote better understanding of the peer-review process and its impact on clinical decision-making. The inclusion of practical sessions like the Journal Club in clinical epidemiology training is, therefore, central to creating an astute and thoughtful health care workforce. An adequate overview of clinical epidemiology is marked by emphasizing how epidemiological measures must be harmonized with clinical evidence. This process of learning enables professionals to appreciate the importance of epidemiological information in informing clinical practice. For example, the comprehension of incidence and prevalence rates can have far-reaching consequences for public health planning and resource allocation. Further, deconstruction and interpretation of results of epidemiological research assist in the development of best practice in clinical settings (Phelps et al., 2004). The ongoing process of situating new knowledge within clinical models reflects how research and practice are reciprocally dynamic. Overall, an introductory clinical epidemiology course equips health professionals with the essential skills to evaluate health interventions and consequently encourage an engaged response to managing health, which is ever-sensitive to new trends and evidence in treating patients (Figure 1.1).

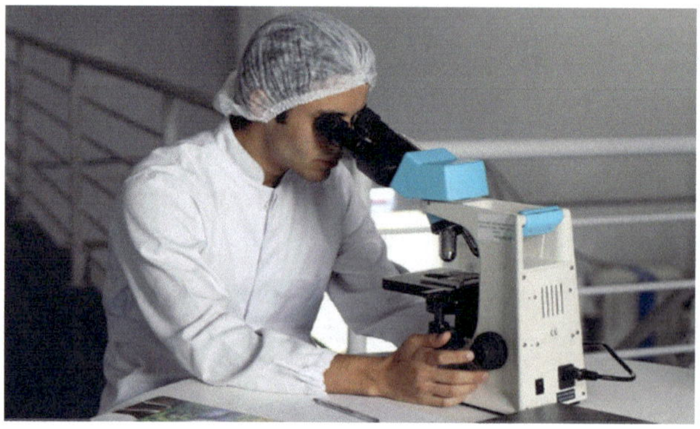

Figure 1.1. Clinical epidemiology.

Source: https://www-s3-live.kent.edu/s3fs-root/s3fs-public/jobs.jpg?VersionId=RwOZPv1a_oxW9IK90G2c2su17NazG7Sf.

1.1. Key Concepts in Clinical Epidemiology

One of the most important concepts within the science of clinical epidemiology is the explanation and application of epidemiologic data for health care quality improvement. Epidemiology is the foundation of clinical and public health by providing data regarding disease patterns, cause, and treatment outcomes. Recognize the incidence and prevalence of disease, as well as the techniques used in data collection and analysis, in order to enable practitioners to become sensitive to trends that may foretell health issues among some populations. Also, ongoing debates bring forward the importance of health administrators in filling the gap of data and insights with policy and practice, and eventually leading to improved community health outcomes. This critical exchange not only fosters informed decision-making but also fosters cooperation among health care providers, ultimately an improved health care delivery system consistent with contemporary public health objectives (Phelps et al., 2004). A second key precept of clinical epidemiology is the distinction between observational and experimental study designs. Observational studies, such as cohort and case-control studies, enable scientists to examine the associations between exposures and outcomes without using specific interventions. These studies are particularly valuable in identifying potential risk factors and establishing correlations that can inform future studies or policy interventions. In contrast, experimental studies, such as randomized controlled trials (RCTs), are required to test causality by establishing the effects of interventions under controlled conditions. With regard to these approaches, education advances the ability of a clinician to evaluate studies critically and apply outcomes wisely in practice. As science advances, integrating developments in statistical techniques and technological innovations into such designs makes conclusions from epidemiological studies more credible (Carmalt et al., 2018). Finally, the concept of population health has come to represent a prominent theme within clinical epidemiology, indicating the shift of focus from patient-level care to more general attention to health outcomes at the level of community and population. This paradigm places a premium on addressing social determinants of health and advancing health equity in practice. Good health administration must engage with population health concepts to maintain that healthcare organizations stay abreast of the requirements of value-based care. This is not only a matter of healthcare delivery knowledge but also understanding how public health systems engage with clinical environments. Integration of population health content in health administration instruction is essential to the learning of future health care leaders, as these leaders will need to maneuver the nuances of the interconnectedness of public health programs and medical practice in achieving sustainable health outcomes for heterogeneous populations (Carmalt et al., 2018) (Figure 1.2).

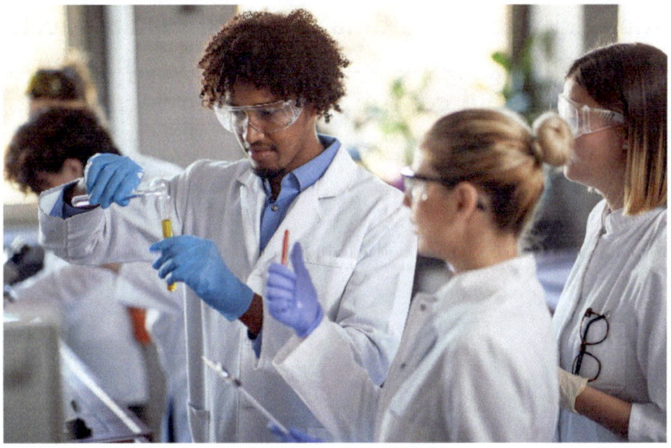

Figure 1.2. Science students conducting an experiment in a laboratory setting.

Source: https://www.bestdegreeprograms.org/wp-content/uploads/2023/06/shutterstock_1962097666-scaled.jpg.

1.1.1. Incidence and Prevalence

The words incidence and prevalence are central to clinical epidemiology because they are critical measures for ascertaining the distribution and dynamics of disease within populations. Incidence refers to the rate at which new cases of a disease occur within a specified period, usually per 100,000 persons annually. This is the key to establishing the risk of falling sick, hence guiding public health interventions and resource planning. For instance, the amyotrophic lateral sclerosis (ALS) documented in the Tuscany region had a standardized incidence rate of 0.81 per 100,000 individuals, demonstrating that monitoring such rates could be valuable in learning about disease incidence and health trends over time (Bianchi et al., 2025).

This data aids epidemiologists in determining potential risk factors and environmental factors, which will aid in preventive interventions. Prevalence, however, measures the total number of a disease's cases present in a population at a specific point in time and denotes a total disease burden. Prevalence encompasses both new and prevalent cases and is crucial to employ in valuing the health requirements of a population. For ALS, the prevalence was estimated in the Tuscany region at 5.36 per 100,000, and it shows the chronic character of this disease because of its long duration and large morbidity burden associated with it (Bianchi et al., 2025).

Prevalence rates can be utilized by healthcare planners and policymakers to better focus resources, plan interventions, and phase public health campaigns on high-prevalence groups by examining prevalence rates. These results enable a consolidated understanding of disease impact, enabling increased patient care and health outcomes. The incidence-prevalence relation underscores the use of data collection and statistical analysis within clinical epidemiology. As a case in point, in canine atopic dermatitis (CAD), epidemiologic studies documented an incidence of 1.7 cases per 1,000 dog years at risk, identifying breed and geographical factors in susceptibility to disease. These studies not only indicate directions of disease pattern occurrence but also underscore the necessity of longitudinal data to examine how incidence and prevalence patterns over a period. Furthermore, collaborating with big databases, such as in CAD studies, is able to unveil patterns of association and potential risk factors, ultimately resulting in successful intervention plans. With the development of epidemiology, understanding of these measures will remain vital to the improvement of disease prevention and control measures in various populations (Figure 1.3).

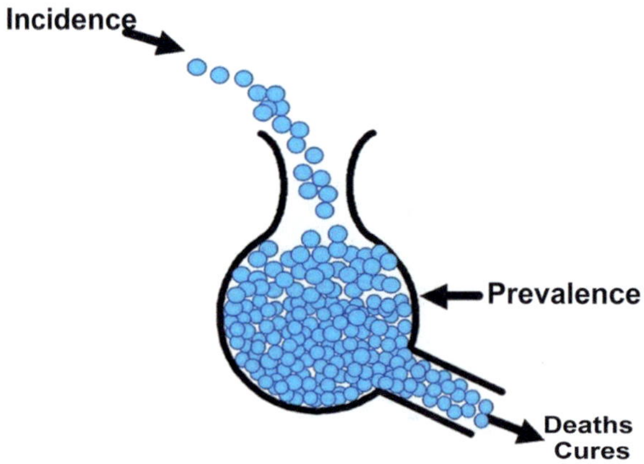

Figure 1.3. This illustration demonstrates the relationship between incidence and prevalence.

Source: https://upload.medbullets.com/topic/101004/images/incidence.jpg.

1.1.2. Risk Factors and Causation

Understanding the concepts of risk factors and causation is significant in clinical epidemiology since it will allow scientists to identify and manage factors causing diseases and illnesses. Risk factors are typically divided into modifiable and non-modifiable risk factors. Modifiable risk factors, for example, lifestyle factors, are amenable to change through environmental setting and personal behavior, whereas non-modifiable risk factors, including genetics and age, are personal. The epidemiologic dilemma is one of correlation versus causation, and this requires rigorous methodology. Classification and understanding of such factors in a correct manner enable public health practitioners to formulate and apply interventions to reduce incidence rates of diseases, ultimately improving population health outcomes through policy and practice informed by evidence. The exploration of causation extends beyond the recognition of risk factors; it attempts to ascertain if exposure to a certain risk factor actually increases the risk of developing a certain outcome. Various frameworks exist for the assessment of causation in an epidemiological context, and one of them is the Bradford Hill criteria, which is a well-established framework. It emphasizes the existence of certain properties, such as strength, consistency, and plausibility of associations to infer causation. Furthermore, the legal definition of causation, particularly in cases involving negligence and harm, adds yet another layer of complexity. Legal causation often hinges on whether or not an exposure was a significant cause of adverse health effects, and as seen in Mengersen et al. (2007), understanding the nuances of statistical terminology is critical in making defensible causative inferences in both science and the law. Successful management of health outcomes requires an integrated framework that considers both biomedical and psychosocial determinants. For instance, in managing upper limb disorders (ULDs), solely biomedical interventions have proven insufficient. A biopsychosocial approach, which embraces both biological functions along with psychological and social determinants, has proven to be central, as seen in Burton et al. (2008). This multifaceted strategy not only addresses physical treatment but also emphasizes the role of psychosocial determinants in return-to-work and rehabilitation outcomes. By coordinated, multifactorial interventions, public health programs are capable of addressing the intricacies of risk factors as well as causal relationships in order to enhance individual and community health in an integrated manner (Figure 1.4).

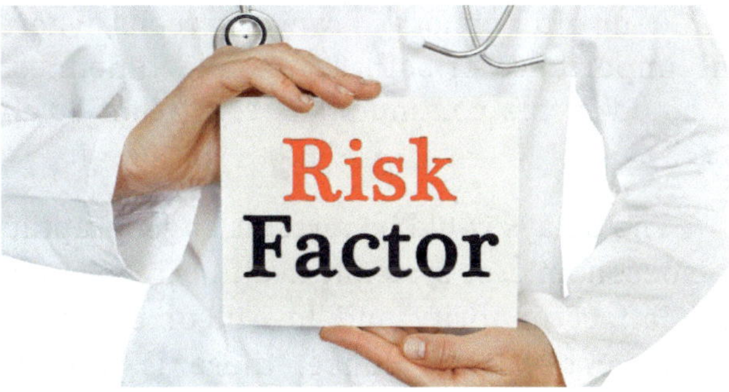

Figure 1.4. Risk factor.

Source: https://cdn.cancercenter.com/-/media/ctca/images/others/blogs/2020/03-march/blog-risk-factor-l.jpg.

1.1.3. Screening and Diagnostic Tests

In clinical epidemiology, the role of screening and diagnostic tests is important in disease prevention and control. Screening tests are only for the detection of potential health disorders before symptoms appear, and this is crucial for diseases such as cancers, sexually transmitted diseases, and chronic conditions. Such tests allow intervention at the early stages, which significantly improves the prognostic outcome. For instance, the integration of point-of-care testing (POCT) for sexually transmitted infections, as highlighted by Blondeel et al. (2017), has a substantial effect on reducing

STI control through instant diagnosis and treatment. Detection of infection at an early stage via POCT enables providers to provide treatment for health complications on a single visit, thereby curbing the risk of transmission as well as improving public health outcomes. The effectiveness of screening tests can be threatened by numerous factors, including accessibility, cost, and the ability of a population to receive healthcare services. For low-income urban dwellers, the obstacles might transcend access to screening tests. Research found that the women referred from community health centers to specialty hospitals often face significant delays in resolution of diagnostic follow-up after abnormal cancer screens, where the importance of both access and timeliness is noted in the continuum of care (Han et al., 2013).

The delays could be a result of geographic, socioeconomic, or systemic health care barriers that affect minority and low-income groups disproportionately. Hence, there is a need to understand and address these challenges in order to optimize the effectiveness of screening programs. Moreover, the design and implementation of screening and diagnostic tests should be evidence-based medicine-driven. Target product profiles (TPPs) defined for point-of-care tests play a vital role in ensuring diagnostic innovation will be aligned with the actual requirements of heterogeneous populations (Blondeel et al., 2017).

These TPPs include functional aspects necessary for proper implementation, hence acting as a reference point for developers and healthcare professionals. However, to ensure that such tests meet patients' diversified needs, there should be constant evaluation and enhancement of the healthcare system. This will include strengthening diagnostic validation infrastructure and making low-cost tests accessible, particularly in low- and middle-income nations, to foster health equity among different population groups (Figure 1.5).

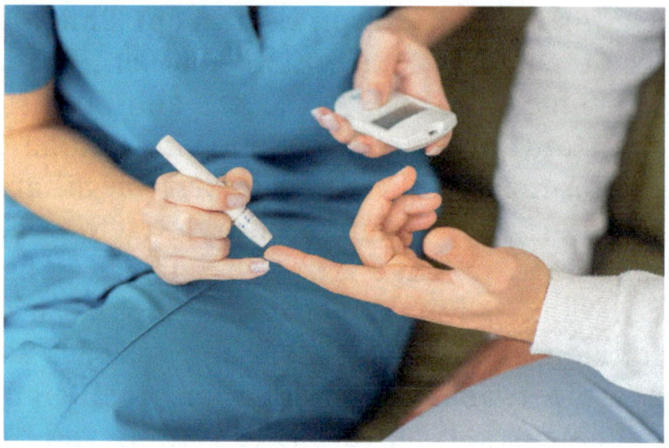

Figure 1.5. Point-of-Care Testing.

Source: https://etimg.etb2bimg.com/photo/112777616.cms

1.2. Study Designs in Clinical Epidemiology

Study designs are important in clinical epidemiology for the determination of disease patterns and the effectiveness of health interventions. Observational studies, such as cohort and case-control designs allow data from populations to be gathered without changing the environment, hence informing about natural disease courses and etiology. For instance, cohort studies can track long-term health outcomes in groups that have been exposed to particular risk factors, and case-control studies are useful in determining likely causes through comparison between individuals with and without a specific condition. These research designs contribute importantly to the body of literature surrounding health disparities and guide public health interventions aimed at preventing and controlling disease. Randomized controlled trials (RCTs) are an integral part of clinical epidemiology due to their rigorous methodology, generating high-level evidence on how well interventions work. Randomization of study participants into an experimental group or a control group by investigators enables them to minimize biases and adjust for confounders, thereby making causal relationships between the treatment and outcomes. RCTs are strongest in their capacity to regulate outside influences, which makes them best suited to try new drugs or treatments. Their application, though, can be resource-hungry and ethically complex in cases involving vulnerable groups. Additionally, RCTs cannot always reproduce real-life situations, so it is necessary to couple the outcomes with those of observational studies to gain a complete insight into therapeutic effectiveness .

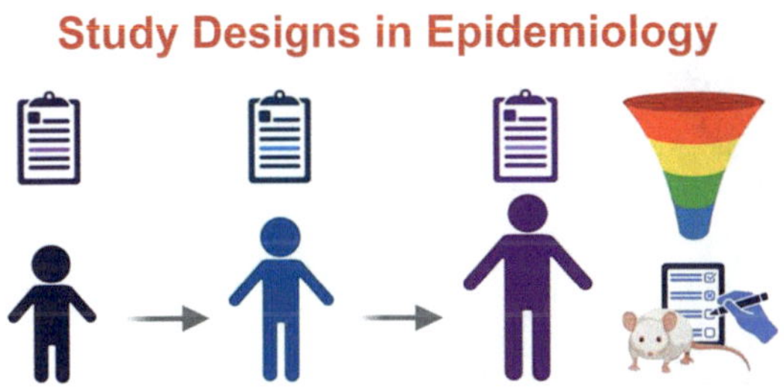

Figure 1.6. Study designs in epidemiology.

Source: https://microbenotes.com/wp-content/uploads/2024/10/Study-Designs-in-Epidemiology.jpeg.

In addition, the integration of omics technologies in clinical epidemiology is revolutionizing the manner in which scientists carry out disease research. Omics-genomics, proteomics, and metabolomics allow the collection and analysis of vast volumes of data that can be informative about the biological processes operating in states of health. Multi-omics enhances the capacity to identify stable biomarkers and contributes to personalized medicine, designing interventions based on individualized biological profiles. As underscored by recent discussions, the incorporation of omics content into epidemiological investigation enables the improved understanding of complex diseases, including cardiometabolic diseases, which involve multi-factorial biological activities and require advanced management schemes. Aging research leveraging these advanced approaches not only ennobles the data world but also aligns research with emerging trends in healthcare, ultimately delivering innovation in clinical practice and public health interventions (Cindy et al., 2015; Argano et al., 2019) (Figure 1.6).

1.2.1. Cohort Studies

Cohort studies are an important methodological instrument for clinical epidemiology by which researchers may study systematically the association between exposure to certain risk factors and subsequent disease. Observing a particular group of individuals—a cohort—over time, cohort studies allow the incidence and natural history of various health states to be studied. This longitudinal design is precious in establishing temporal relationships and hence in aiding the determination of causality. For instance, analysis of individual participant data can shed light on complex associations, such as the impact of birth size on breast cancer risk, emphasizing the importance of well-designed cohort studies in revealing hidden health risks and informing public health interventions (Collaborative et al., 2008). The strengths of cohort studies are not only that they are capable of detecting risk factors but also that they are relatively resistant to recall bias, as exposure information will typically be determined prior to the development of disease. Cohort studies are therefore particularly valuable in chronic disease, where a diagnosis early in the course of the disease is significant. For example, biomarker analysis of B-type natriuretic peptide (BNP) in the blood shows how this type of research can be employed to estimate predictive relationships for diseases such as type 2 diabetes. Controlling for several confounding factors, scientists can derive data on the independent effects of particular exposures and thereby guide specific prevention regimes and therapeutic interventions in clinical epidemiology (Meirhaeghe et al., 2011). While cohort study advantages are clear, practical challenges in their implementation must not be downplayed. The need for large numbers of study participants and long follow-up times may pose issues such as participant loss to follow-up and costs. Loss to follow-up can also potentially generate biases that can impact the inference made from results. Researchers must bear these in mind when interpreting outcomes and designing studies. Despite these limitations, cohort studies are indispensable tools in clinical epidemiology and contribute significantly to the understanding of disease causation as well as to the process of creating evidence-based public health policy. Reducing methodological limitations with innovative study designs and statistical analyses will make results arising from these valuable research investigations more robust (Figure 1.7).

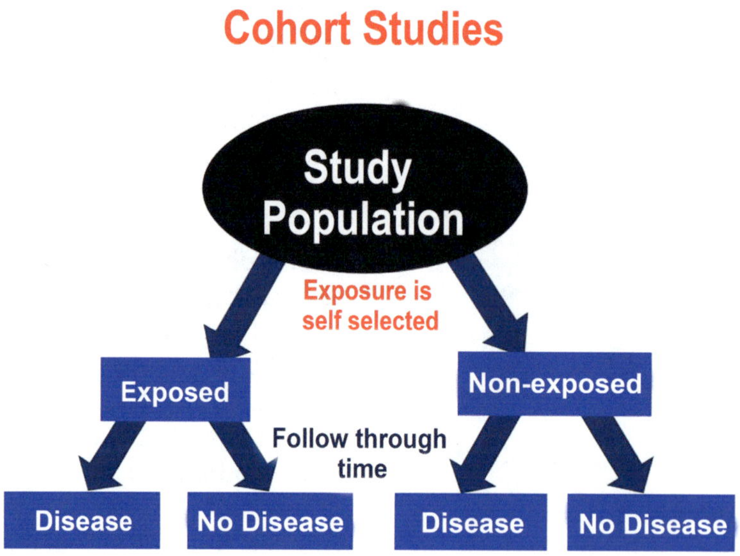

Figure 1.7. Cohort studies.

Source: https://howmed.net/wp-content/uploads/2013/07/Cohort-studies.jpg.

1.2.2. Case-Control Studies

Case-control studies are an important methodology in the field of clinical epidemiology, providing insight into the relationship between exposures and health events. The design of case-control studies is especially useful where rare diseases are being studied, since it enables researchers to compare cases easily. The primary objective is to find out if the cases received greater exposure to a particular exposure than the controls. Unlike cohort studies, however, the groups are not followed over time. With retrospective analysis of history among participants, case-control studies enable the identification of risk factors and possibly causal factors and provide useful insights regarding public health intervention and prevention strategies. Case-control studies have limitations, however. One of the significant issues is the potential for selection bias, particularly in the control selection. If controls are poorly matched to cases with regard to significant demographic or health characteristics, the findings will be biased and therefore provide false interpretations of the exposure-outcome relation. Furthermore, self-reported exposure data can be subject to validity influenced by recall bias, so cases will recall their exposures differently than controls. To reduce these reservations, researchers often use strict selection criteria and validate exposure histories using multiple sources where possible. Despite all these issues, when performed carefully, case-control studies can yield strong and actionable epidemiological evidence. Aggregation of evidence from case-control studies can significantly enhance public health action, especially in the detection and intervention of epidemiological threats. For instance, analysis of the hospital excess length of stay due to nosocomial infection employing case-control techniques can illustrate the immediate need for improved infection control. As suggested in the research specific to intensive care unit (ICU) facilities, use of advanced analytical techniques, such as inverse probability–weighted survival curves, can account for confounding factors, leading to improved estimation of the effect of infection on patient outcomes (Batra et al., 2020). Furthermore, incorporation of cutting-edge genomics techniques into the epidemiological framework may enhance new approaches for outbreak identification and control, underscoring the utility of cross-disciplinary work in maximizing disease surveillance and control (Boon et al., 2019) (Figure 1.8).

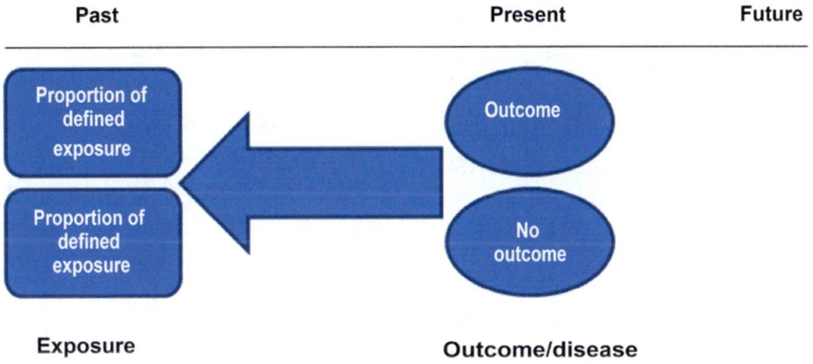

Figure 1.8. Case-control study design.

Source: https://s4be.cochrane.org/app/uploads/2017/12/Screenshot-2017-12-05-16.50.03.png.

1.2.3. Randomized Controlled Trials

Randomized controlled trials (RCTs) are the clinical epidemiological gold standard, with a formal system of ascertaining whether medical interventions work. Random assignment to treatment and control groups, RCTs minimize the risk of bias and confounders and guarantee that effects can be causally attributed to the intervention. This is the solution to causal inference between health outcomes and treatments. The rigorous study design of RCTs allows researchers to critically evaluate not only the efficacy of interventions but also their safety profiles, facilitating evidence-based clinical practice. The implications of RCT evidence can have a powerful impact on guidelines and policies within healthcare, ensuring that treatment advice is guided by scientifically sound evidence. RCTs are not without difficulty, however, despite their significance. Such a major issue is the risk of missing data, which can impair the validity and power of trial results. As seen in systematic reviews, the occurrence of missing data can be large and may affect the reliability of the conclusions made based on these studies. In a given systematic review of RCTs evaluating palliative interventions, a weighted estimate reported a 23.1% rate of missing data at primary endpoints, with increasing proportions associated with more assessments and longer studies. Missing data in such cases can introduce biases that distort conclusions, particularly if lost participants differ systematically from trial completers. Missing data needs to be managed in order to maintain the validity of RCTs and ensure that their results are reliable and actionable.

Furthermore, the effect of vitamin D supplementation on health outcomes, as studied using RCTs, illustrates the intricacies of interpreting trial results. Systematic review of vitamin D influence on the incidence of breast cancer revealed that though the global risk ratio showed no significant association, treatment benefit appeared to increase with higher dose and combined therapy. This points towards the need for rigorous analysis and subgroup analysis within RCTs despite initial results demonstrating no discernible benefits. Demonstrating the importance of such research within clinical epidemiology, these findings underscore the need for ongoing studies and developing modifications of treatment practices according to accruals of new evidence. The continuous refinement of RCT methodology is needed to improve the quality of scientific investigation and the relevance of results to clinical practice (Figure 1.9).

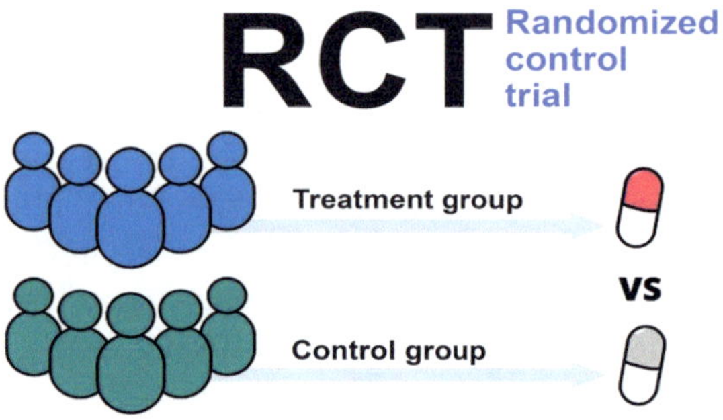

Figure 1.9. Randomized controlled trials.

Source: https://i.ytimg.com/vi/mWfjbmRZowM/maxresdefault.jpg.

1.3. Data Collection Methods

In clinical epidemiology, the validity of data collection methods has a direct impact on the reliability of research results. Among them, cohort studies, which collect data over time in a fixed group, facilitate better assessment of disease progression and treatment impact. For instance, longitudinal cohort data clarify dynamics of infection in dual-disease contexts, i.e., HIV-hepatitis C virus (HCV) coinfection. A study of post-highly active antiretroviral therapy (HAART) dynamics that might involve regular but well-planned data collection is a good case in point for how longitudinal methodologies can make more significant contributions to our understanding of viral suppression mechanisms. With Bayesian analysis and interval-censored data-friendly models, researchers are better positioned to investigate complex interactions and correlations in cohort studies and, ultimately, improve clinical interventions as attested from existing literature (Hogan et al., 2011). One of the helpful data collection methods in clinical epidemiology is cross-sectional studies, which assess disease prevalence at a single moment in time. It allows researchers to have a snapshot of health and risk factors among populations and is very helpful to identify patterns and associations. For example, researchers can analyze data regarding lifestyle determinants of chronic diseases or infectious diseases to inform public health policies. Compared to longitudinal studies, cross-sectional designs can measure large demographic variables and stratify data according to factors such as age and sex, which facilitates targeted interventions. However, despite their advantages, the studies are usually marred by limitations in terms of the inability to ascertain causality. Therefore, although cross-sectional studies are helpful for generating hypotheses and formulating future research questions, they must be complemented with more robust methodologies in clinical epidemiology

(Cortey et al., 2016). Case-control studies are also an important data collection technique in the field of clinical epidemiology. With case-control studies, patients having a specific condition may be looked at retrospectively with their controls who do not have the condition, providing important information on potential risk factors as well as outcomes. By comparing exposures among cases and controls, researchers can identify associations that are potentially valuable to study or intervene upon. Although case-control studies are extremely useful in populations where diseases are uncommon or take many years to develop, case-control studies also possess inherent biases like recall bias or selection bias that researchers must be aware of and counteract. Secondly, the application of sophisticated data gathering equipment, like genetic and bioinformatic tools, complements the traditional method of approaches by ensuring broader coverage of disease epidemiology. Researchers continue to uncover technological advancements that improve data gathering procedures, such that results are able to incorporate the complexities of health matters today (Hogan et al., 2011).

1.3.1. Surveys and Questionnaires

Surveys and questionnaires are essential tools in clinical epidemiology, which give researchers the capacity to acquire and analyze data significant in health patterns understanding, treatment efficiency, and patient status. Through the use of formal questions, researchers can offer quantitative and qualitative data from various populations and thus determine the correlation between factors. The appearance and design of the instruments affect response rates and the validity of the information collected, making proper adherence to strict methodologies appropriate. Effective surveying has to consider the nature of the target populations, accessibility, and mode of administration, paper or electronic, to secure maximum participation and reduce response bias. Recent literature has indicated that survey distribution mode has had a significant impact on response rates. For instance, one study contrasted response rates among surgeons and found that Internet questionnaires yielded much lower participation than mail questionnaires, despite the notion that electronic means would be more efficient and more convenient.

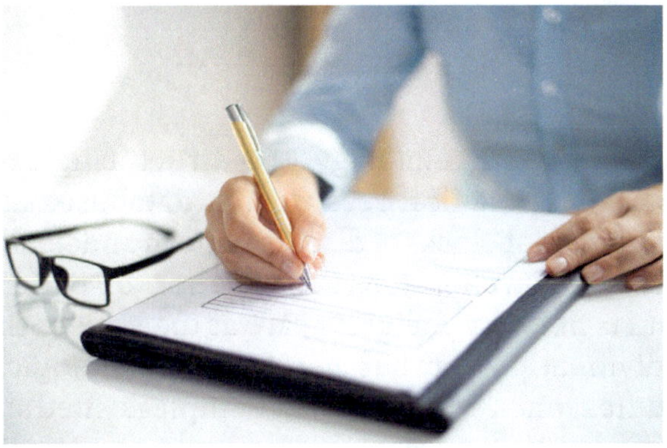

Figure 1.10. Surveys and questionnaires.

Source: https://www.fullsession.io/wp-content/uploads/2024/01/closeup-business-woman-making-notes-document-1-1.jpg.

The results indicated that the Internet arm had only a 45% response rate compared to 58% for the mail questionnaire, with an absolute difference of 13% ($P<0.01$) (Bhandari et al., 2004). These findings refute the thesis that more technology use can only replace conventional practice, and stress careful consideration in choosing ways of distribution in clinical research settings. In addition, innovations in data collection techniques, e.g., via the use of Personal Digital Assistants (PDAs), contain meaningful improvements in survey practice. Such technologies permit real-time collection of data and provide patients with a convenient means of recording their experiences, notably pain relief. The ability to capture pain data spatially and temporally enhances the richness of the information gained and enables one to comprehend better patient response to treatment

(Ghinea et al., 2005). This approach not only facilitates greater accessibility for patients with mobility problems but also contributes to the prevailing trend of placing technology within health studies, demonstrating how the evolution of tools can produce more efficient surveys and questionnaires in clinical epidemiology (Figure 1.10).

1.3.2. Medical Records and Databases

In clinical epidemiology, the structuring and analysis of medical records and databases are fundamental blocks of disease pattern and health trend comprehension. Organization of patient data is not only useful for care at the level of the individual patient but also for epidemiological studies on a wider scale. Complete medical records allow health professionals to identify prevalent health conditions, monitor treatment outcomes, and determine the efficacy of interventions. Also, aggregation of several data sources is able to enhance validity since different types of clinical data, ranging from demographic to coding diagnoses, contribute to a better understanding of population health processes. The most significant factor in employing medical records within clinical epidemiology is the inherent challenge of overcoming data quality and representation challenges. Issues such as selection bias and misclassification can have the ability to skew findings and hinder the generalizability of results. For instance, insurance claims, as comprehensive as they are, typically capture just a fraction of the population due to coverage limitations and claims submitted. Such a limitation underscores the importance of rendering data collection mechanisms representative and sustainable. To this end, active surveillance efforts based on secondary healthcare data may end up being the most viable means of providing good insight into healthcare trends in settings that will have limited systems of passive reporting (Brodbelt et al., 2014). Furthermore, the advent of technology has also paved the way for new means in managing medical records, ultimately leading to an enhancement in research capacity in healthcare settings. The creation of easy-to-use computerized databases, e.g., PsyCase, illustrates the manner in which customized solutions enhance data analysis and retrieval, thereby maximizing research in particular areas of science such as psychiatry (Karakkamandapam et al., 2010). These databases not only facilitate the management of large volumes of data but also encourage collaboration among departments, resulting in more comprehensive epidemiological studies. Through the power of technological innovations, healthcare professionals can use more advanced analyses, thus providing great insights to inform decision-making as well as policy formulation in clinical epidemiology (Figure 1.11).

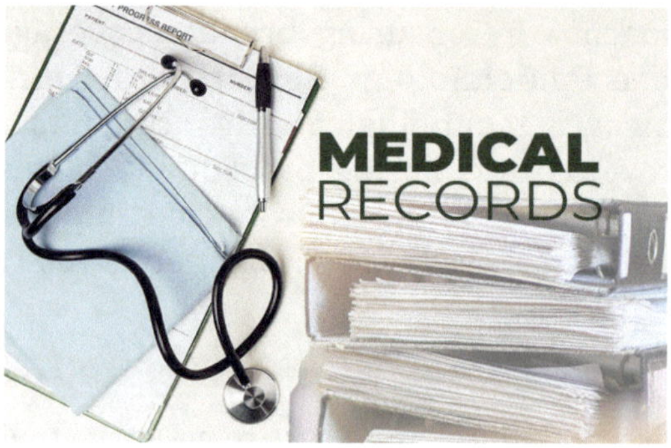

Figure 1.11. Medical records.

Source: https://www.managedoutsource.com/wp-content/uploads/2022/04/medical-records-scanning-a-brief-guide.jpg.

1.3.3. Clinical Trials and Observational Studies

Clinical trials and observational studies are two fundamental cornerstones in clinical epidemiology, offering distinct approaches to extend medical understanding and improve patient outcomes. Clinical trials are characterized by their formal format, with a degree of randomization and controlled environment employed to ascertain the efficacy of interventions. These studies have the direct responsibility of establishing causal links between treatments and health outcomes, primarily by means of randomized controlled trials (RCTs). In comparison, observational studies, without the controlled variables of clinical trials, are nonetheless treasure troves of information regarding real-world scenarios, capturing data on populations as they occur naturally. This comparison underscores the two-way nature of these two methods, allowing scientists to validate clinical findings against trends in the general population and gain a more comprehensive picture of disease distributions. The integration of cutting-edge methods into observational studies is being viewed increasingly as a new paradigm for clinical epidemiology. Hybrid studies that use elements of both clinical trials and observational approaches hold promise for enhancing research efficiency and validity. For example, making use of existing cohort registries and studies coupled with trial data enables researchers to effectively assess the effects of treatment and inform clinical decision-making while being practical, cost-effective, and feasible, as well as patient-centered. Embedding big data analytics further facilitates this capacity through the utilization of large sets of data to analyze intricate relationships and establish pertinent factors influencing health outcomes. Importantly, stakeholder buy-in and participation are essential to the viability of such innovative design, which ensures research is consistent with the demands and aspirations of the target populations, and therefore extending the shelf life of clinical findings beyond the boundaries of highly constrained trial settings (Anderson et al., 2016). Notably, observational studies such as the NordiNet® International Outcome Study (IOS) and the American Norditropin® Studies (ANSWER Program®) demonstrate the advantages of this study methodology in clinical epidemiology. Collecting long-term data on the safety and effectiveness of growth hormone therapy, these studies provide insight into patient outcomes in routine clinical practice, not under the strict conditions of clinical trials. The research design of these observational studies meets rigorous pharmacoepidemiological criteria for allowing for a proper evaluation of treatment outcomes in different populations receiving treatment under actual clinical practice conditions. This not only enhances the generalizability of findings but also responds to the complexities of heterogeneity of treatment outcomes received by heterogeneous patients. As evidenced by their adherence to established guidelines, such studies contribute vital knowledge that can influence clinical decision-making and further refine therapeutic strategies, ultimately fostering improved patient outcomes in everyday practice (Christesen et al., 2013) (Figure 1.12).

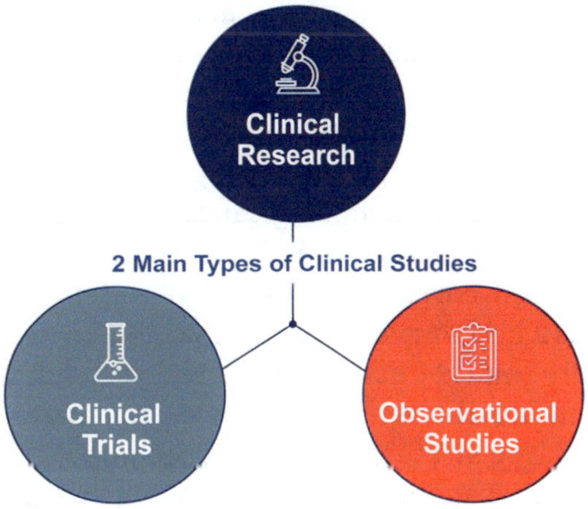

Figure 1.12. Clinical trials.

Source: https://elearning.wfh.org/wp-content/uploads/2022/04/01.clinical-study-graphic.png.

1.4. Statistical Analysis in Clinical Epidemiology

Statistical analysis forms the foundation of clinical epidemiology in its role as a primary tool for explaining the interassociations between health outcomes and several risk factors. By utilizing proper statistical methods, researchers can conduct an analysis of data acquired from clinical trials or observational studies. With such analysis, patterns, correlations, and causative risk factors that affect public health can be identified. As seen in the early work of clinical intervention research, advanced statistical approaches can inform treatment safety and efficacy mechanisms, and their findings can powerfully influence future treatments. Particularly in drug intervention trials targeting cardiometabolic disorders, the use of advanced statistical approaches enhances the evidential strength and therefore reliability of risk estimations and treatment responses as discussed in Preiss et al. (2016). In addition to improving the understanding of treatment effects, statistical analysis in clinical epidemiology also facilitates the measurement of disease outbreaks and their epidemiological characteristics. This is particularly evident with the study of infectious diseases, where the establishment of incidence, prevalence, morbidity, and mortality rates is imperative to public health responses. Statistical processing of epidemiological data, as in the case of sheep pox epidemics in Morocco, suggests significant correlations between endemicity of disease and various factors that affect it, such as rural market activity. Such analyses not only illuminate the epidemiological landscape but also shape strategic action to curb and mitigate disease transmission, resonating with the need for extensive information collection and sophisticated analytic tools to maximize disease surveillance systems, highlighted in Clercq et al. (2019). Moreover, advancements in statistical techniques, particularly in biostatistics and bioinformatics, enable scientists to effectively use big data. Techniques such as predictive modeling and machine learning are becoming more integrated into clinical epidemiology to help us better understand more sophisticated health data. As researchers adopt new methodologies, the potential for personalizing medicine and improving outcomes is rising exponentially. For instance, the application of metabolomics data alongside longitudinal clinical endpoints can be applied to the identification of predictive biomarkers of drug response, resetting paradigms in patient care. The journey of harnessing advanced analytics in clinical epidemiology has the promise to refine health interventions, offer better resource distribution, and ultimately improve the quality of services being delivered to different populations.

1.4.1. Descriptive Statistics

Descriptive statistics form an integral component of clinical epidemiology because they offer fundamental information about the distribution, central point, and spread of health data. Descriptive statistics utilizes numeric summaries such as means, medians, modes, standard deviations, and frequency distributions to aggregate complex datasets into digestible information. For instance, in the study of disease-related health consequences, researchers can immediately identify prevailing characteristics in a population and assist public health authorities in the identification of vulnerable groups. Descriptive statistics is also important when a retrospective descriptive study is undertaken, such as the analysis of anisakiasis cases in Italy, as it is necessary to portray the demographic and clinical patterns of patients involved, identifying significant patterns, such as geographical differences and the evolution of allergic symptoms in different populations (Cavallero et al., 2018). In the clinical epidemiological environment, descriptive statistics are not number-crunching per se; they are also a basis for further statistical analysis. By reducing data to a manageable level, researchers can then go on to make hypotheses about potential associations and causal connections that may be explored further. For instance, in anisakiasis studies, descriptive statistics provided important information on the spatial and temporal distribution of allergic symptoms due to the infection, which guided multivariate analyses. These analytic methods allow researchers to gain a clearer understanding of the effect on health outcomes of specific variables—such as demographic variables like age and sex—so that the explanatory value of the findings can be enhanced for guiding public health interventions (Cavallero et al., 2018). In addition, descriptive statistics also allow for easy communication of epidemiological results to various stakeholders, such as policymakers and health care workers. The presentation of information through graphs, charts, and tables, all derived from descriptive statistical analysis, can easily communicate intricate information in a readable format. This is crucial to public health surveillance and intervention planning. As recorded by the STROBE initiative, which aims to enhance the reporting quality of observational studies, the essence of research findings' validity and utility in clinical epidemiology is a transparent account of data grounded in sound statistical methodology. With the application of properly arranged descriptive statistics, researchers present an evidence base that informs clinical practice and public health policy with a view to promoting better health outcomes (Figure 1.13).

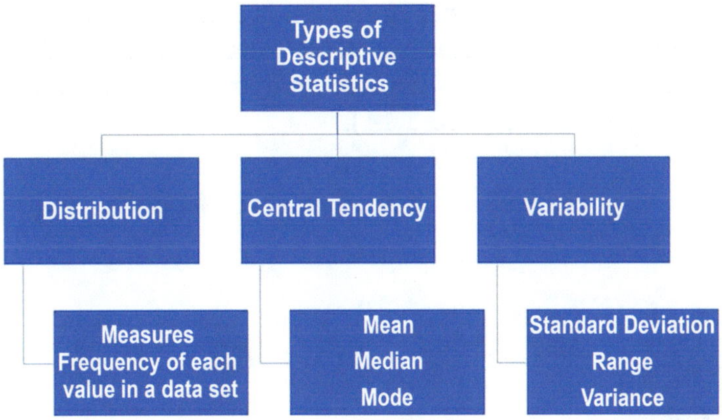

Figure 1.13. Types of descriptive statistics.

Source: https://www.bachelorprint.com/wp-content/uploads/2023/07/Descriptive-statistics-types.jpg.

1.4.2. Inferential Statistics

Inferential statistics play a key role in clinical epidemiology because they help researchers draw inferences about a population from a sample that is representative of the population. This is particularly important in medical sciences because ethical considerations most often do not permit direct observations on entire populations. By applying inferential techniques, researchers are able to estimate parameters in a population, test hypotheses, and make predictions from sample data. The value of statistical skills is underscored by evidence prioritizing the necessity for medical researchers to be competent in these techniques. Research demonstrates that even the fundamental skills are identifying sources of variation and bias, accepting limitations of one's statistical expertise, and assessing the strengths and limitations of different study designs. Acquisition of inferential statistics not only enhances the quality of research outcomes but also encourages evidence-based decision-making in clinical practice (Benn et al., 2017). Application of inferential statistics transcends simple numerical calculations; it serves as a cornerstone for research studies and intervention planning. Clinical epidemiology practitioners utilize methods such as confidence intervals and significance testing to ensure that conclusions drawn from a sample are extendable to the population at large. This process is especially important when carrying out health outcome and treatment effectiveness studies, as exemplified through enormous surveys like the NAHMS Dairy 96 Study, whose aim was to acquire in-depth information on dairy animals in America. Utilizing a statistically valid sampling procedure, the study was able to procure important information without compromise to scientific integrity. Such robust statistical frameworks enable scientists to quantify uncertainty and validate results, leading finally to more reliable health policies and advice within the field (Ott et al., 2025). Furthermore, the relevance of inferential statistics in clinical epidemiology does not only lie in the examination of data but also in presenting the results. Robust statistical proficiency is critical in the reporting of results to different stakeholders, including policymakers, other researchers, and members of the public. With clinical guidelines and population health efforts being driven more and more by medical research, the ability to convey and interpret statistical findings takes on a pivotal role. The ability to communicate complex statistical concepts in understandable terms helps create increased public awareness and trust in medical research. Incorporating education in inferential statistics into curricula for medical education is consequently essential. Developing skills in these competencies equips emerging medical professionals to be involved contributors to and active participants in the evolving world of clinical epidemiology, ultimately leading to improved health outcomes (Benn et al., 2017) (Figure 1.14).

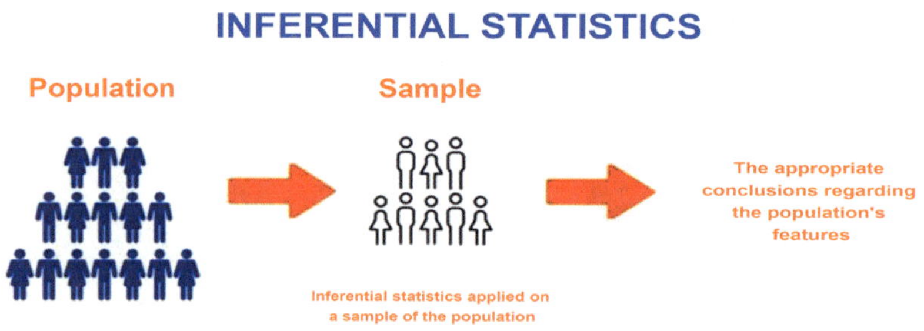

Figure 1.14. Inferential statistics.

Source: https://brainalyst.in/wp-content/uploads/2023/02/inferential-Statistics-1024x394.jpg.

1.4.3. Interpretation of Statistical Results

Statistical interpretation of results is a significant aspect of clinical epidemiology since it forms the basis of understanding how results can affect public health. Researchers apply various statistical techniques to conclude what the data implies, but there is a need to understand that statistical significance does not always imply clinical significance. The two are distinguished; an effect may be statistically significant and yet have minimal implications for patient care or health outcomes more broadly. The interpretation, therefore, must account not only for the figures but for their practical significance, so conclusions are of value to the clinical setting. This complex interaction highlights the importance of epidemiologists having a proficiency not only in statistical techniques but also in the implications of their interpretations for healthcare policy and practice, ultimately affecting sound decision-making and intervention in a clinical setting (Abrahams et al., 2009). Furthermore, the temporal dynamics used in epidemiological studies are also important in the interpretation of outcomes. The contrast between cross-sectional and cohort studies, for instance, affects the ability to infer causation from correlation. Cross-sectional studies give snapshots of data at one point in time, while cohort studies track data over time and enable improved understanding of the interaction between risk factors and outcomes. Misinterpretation results if scientists fail to consider these differences and draw unjustified conclusions that have the power to shape health outcomes. Additionally, synergistic risk factors must be taken into account when results are interpreted accurately, since collective risks could enhance public health significance beyond what separate factors may suggest.

This elaborate method emphasizes the importance of time-related matters in statistical interpretation, which in turn demonstrates how they indeed can make a real difference in clinical research findings (Abrahams et al., 2009). Recent advances in genetic epidemiology, including those from studies of the outcome of investigations of the QT interval, serve to demonstrate the challenge of statistical analysis in clinical science. Identification of common variant loci involved in the QT interval serves to underscore the multicausal nature of factors of risk for diseases like long-QT syndrome (LQTS). The challenge lies in translating such statistical correlations to a biological context, particularly for both frequent and infrequent genetic variants that might play a role in disease phenotypes. Statistical calculations reveal correlations that need to be carefully scrutinized for relevance and causality, particularly as coding variants have unclear implications. This identifies the need for integrated analyses that integrate genetic data into other biological knowledge, creating a solid foundation to comprehend risks associated with arrhythmias and sudden cardiac death. This is a classic example of the demand for rigorous system interpretations that are employed in order to properly direct clinical practice and research.

1.5. Applications of Clinical Epidemiology

The application of clinical epidemiology is widespread and priceless in addressing contemporary health challenges with evidence-based measures. Clinical epidemiology informs policy for health and clinical decisions by emphasizing systematic approaches to analyzing the distribution and determinants of health states. One of the best examples of its application is the establishment of the Patient-Centered Clinical Research Network (PCORnet) by the Patient-Centered Outcomes Research Institute (PCORI). This initiative, implemented in 2013, aims to grow faster and cheaper clinical studies aligned with the needs of patients and healthcare providers. The network promotes collaboration across institutions and the establishment of research agendas, focusing on a wide array of areas such as cardiovascular disease and cancer. Lastly, the continuous emergence of collaborative study networks in PCORnet demonstrates the importance of clinical epidemiology in enhancing the quality and stakeholder relevance of health research activities that lead to improved patient outcomes and resource allocation (Carton et al., 2018). In regions with high rates of health disparities, clinical epidemiology has critical applications in minimizing the burden of NCDs. For example, in Latin America, anticipated increases in cardiovascular disease (CVD) deaths present significant challenges to the public health infrastructure. Clinical epidemiology is central to assessing risk factors and creating targeted interventions in this region. Interestingly, mobile health (mHealth) initiatives have been seen as a viable intervention, taking advantage of the high coverage of mobile phones in the region to boost the capability of disease prevention and control, especially for cardiometabolic diseases. This strategy integrates fresh solutions in solutions specifically targeting NCDs' diverse social and health environments in low- and middle-income countries. By evaluating mHealth interventions in Argentina, Guatemala, and Peru, researchers have highlighted the importance of bringing epidemiological knowledge into the local context to address and manage NCDs effectively, thereby demonstrating the capability of clinical epidemiology to inform diverse environments (Beratarrechea et al., 2016). In addition, the landscape of clinical epidemiology is continually shaped by emerging technologies and techniques, broadening its field of application.

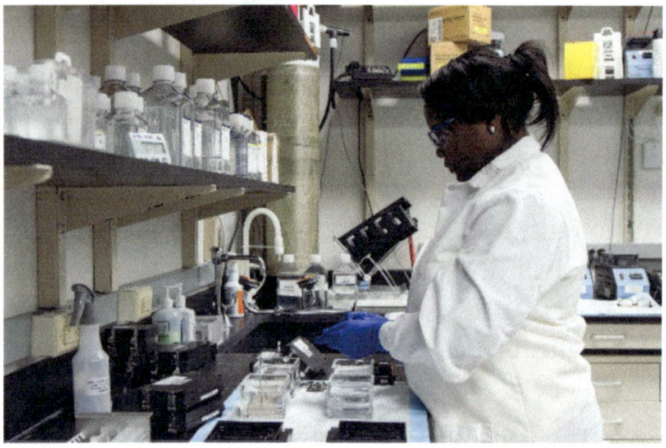

Figure 1.15. Researcher preparing samples in an advanced epigenetics laboratory.

Source: https://images.unsplash.com/photo-1579154204449-47c454770447?crop=entropy&cs=tinysrgb&fit=max&fm=jpg&ixid=M3w3MDgyMDR8MHwxfHNlYXJjaHwxfHxhZHZhbmNlZCUyMGVwaWRlbWlvbG9ieXxlbnwwfHx8fDE3NDUwMTY5MDZ8MA&ixlib=rb-4.0.3&q=80&w=1080?utm_source=numberanalytics&utm_medium=referral.

The integration of big data analysis, machine learning, and new designs, such as randomized controlled trials and observational studies, enhances the capacity of researchers to make valuable inferences regarding health interventions. This paradigm shift is extremely valuable in the context of chronic disease management, where information-based insights can inform preventive measures and therapeutic interventions. Second, the interplay between researchers and clinicians encourages effective implementation of results in clinical practice, which bridges the gap between research and practice. Thus, clinical epidemiology not only powers scientific inquiry but also is increasingly providing health care professionals with knowledge that is practically applicable, ultimately resulting in an evidence-based response to fulfilling public health agendas and improving patient care in diverse populations (Figure 1.15).

1.5.1. Disease Prevention Strategies

Effective disease prevention strategies are essential in decreasing all types of health conditions and enhancing the health status of the population. In clinical epidemiology, disease prevention strategies are categorized into three categories: primary, secondary, and tertiary prevention. Primary prevention aims to avoid the onset of disease through the implementation of interventions like vaccination and lifestyle modifications that address the risk factors before the disease develops. As an example, public health programs' promotion of healthy eating and exercise plans made available to the community have been shown to significantly reduce the incidence of chronic illnesses like diabetes and cardiovascular disease. Through early action on risk factors, primary prevention activities are not only cost-effective but also improve the quality of societal life overall. Early intervention guarantees that investment in healthcare education and universal healthcare benefits are part of an effective disease prevention policy. Secondary prevention targets the early detection and control of diseases to prevent progression and reduce morbidity. Screening programs are a traditional example of secondary prevention strategies, allowing for the detection of diseases such as breast cancer or hypertension among asymptomatic individuals. Successful screening can lead to timely intervention, thereby enhancing survival rates and reducing the long-term burden of such conditions. Furthermore, secondary prevention is critical in managing illnesses that cannot be prevented entirely, as evidenced by the increasing prevalence of acute diverticulitis (AD). Although therapeutic maneuvers such as modulating gut microbiota and reducing mucosal inflammation offer limited efficacy in AD prevention, identifying risk factors is critical in developing more effective screening techniques and treatment protocols.

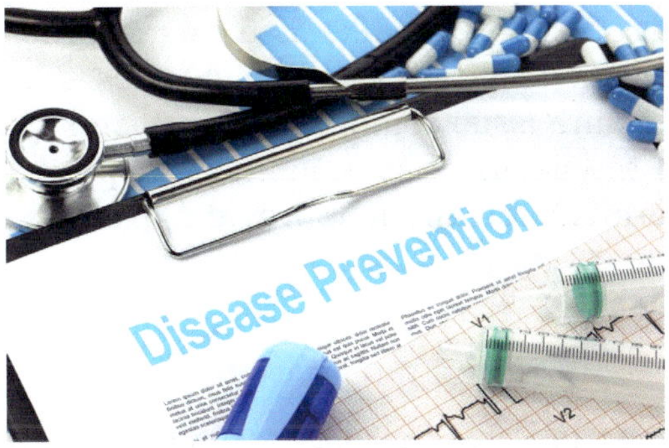

Figure 1.16. Disease prevention strategies.

Source: https://microbiotics.com.ng/wp-content/uploads/2021/05/disease-prevention.jpg.

This ongoing inquiry underscores the necessity of extensive clinical studies in informing preventive interventions, particularly for specific populations and their specific health concerns (Annibale et al., 2018). Tertiary prevention encompasses actions that are intended to curtail the impact of a diagnosed illness, aiming to increase the quality of life and functional capacity of those afflicted. This also includes rehabilitation services and chronic disease management programs that navigate people through their health process. For infection prevention, when it comes to infection control, the relationship between infection prevention and antimicrobial stewardship (AS) emphasizes the necessity of collaborative practice among healthcare facilities to avert the development of multidrug-resistant organisms (MDROs). By promoting appropriate use of antibiotics and implementing strict infection control measures, healthcare systems can reduce the incidence of healthcare-associated infections. IPC and AS program leaders must adopt a cooperative approach to safeguard patient safety while maintaining the efficacy of antibiotics for future generations. Last but not least, the successful application of such disease prevention methods into clinical practice justifies the central role of clinical epidemiology within public health programs (Ashley et al., 2018) (Figure 1.16).

1.5.2. Health Policy Formulation

Health policy formulation is a critical role of clinical epidemiology, whereby evidence-based guidelines and approaches are formulated to make an impact on health outcomes at different levels of society. It usually begins with the identification of health issues that require tackling using rigorous epidemiologic data. The role of evidence in the formulation of health policy cannot be overlooked; policymakers utilize credible data to understand the burden and prevalence of diseases. Furthermore, the integration of health equity thinking into policy development is important to guarantee that the needs of disadvantaged populations are met. Research has shown that assessing the impact on equity of expected interventions has been proven to enhance the relevance of health policies to vulnerable populations, thereby promoting inclusivity in healthcare systems (Akl et al., 2017). Therefore, a proper policy-making process grounded in epidemiological principles is significant in the development of successful health interventions. In practice, translating epidemiological evidence into policy involves traversing a sequence of complex barriers. For example, guidelines to control surgical site infections (SSIs) illustrate tremendous barriers for healthcare workers. A recent professional conference highlighted such issues as poor compliance with evidence-based care and the absence of proper local policies (Gallagher et al., 2015). These barriers occur most frequently due to the lack of leadership and clear roles among healthcare professionals, which makes it difficult to put health policies in place. It is therefore crucial for policymakers to promote a culture that facilitates active engagement and training among healthcare professionals. By surmounting these obstacles, health policy formulation can be made better, ultimately to bear better health outcomes. Best practice emphasis is not a process requirement but a duty to reduce morbidity and mortality among patient groups. Additionally, the cyclical nature of health policy formulation requires ongoing monitoring and adaptation to respond to new health problems effectively. Policy makers should employ instruments that can adapt to new information and knowledge through time. For instance, instruments like the GRADE (Grading Recommendations Assessment and Development Evidence) EtD have guidelines for systematic assessment of health interventions, including their potential impact on health equity (Akl et al., 2017). Interactive participation among various stakeholders, like medical practitioners, researchers, and community members, is also important in facilitating policy changes that are applicable. Promoting dialogue spaces can improve local health issue comprehension, foster shared accountability, and render health policies a reflection of the needs of communities. By promoting progress and recurrence, health policies can be evidence-informed and fair, providing solutions to the complex dimensions of public health.

1.5.3. Clinical Practice Guidelines

The creation and implementation of clinical practice guidelines (CPGs) play a significant role in clinical epidemiology practice, as CPGs provide evidence-based recommendations to healthcare practitioners. CPGs are deliberately created from high-quality research and serve the purpose of improving patient outcomes by making the practice of medicine uniform. By compiling information from various studies, CPGs guide clinicians in navigating the complexity of treatment options, especially for diseases where there is uncertainty in clinical practice. It is necessary that these guidelines are in line with the latest scientific data and emerging trends in medicine to be up to date and useful. Further, as suggested by the review of dental healthcare providers' risk of Legionella infection, the dissemination of new infection control guidelines is critical to maintaining safe health facilities and enhancing patient safety against preventable diseases (Petti et al., 2017). In addition to impacting clinical guidelines, CPGs also move public health interventions forward by addressing particular health concerns prevalent among various groups. For instance, the ICON: Anaphylaxis project points out the importance of the establishment of widely accepted global guidelines for anaphylaxis treatment, a condition of severe allergic reaction that can prove lethal. These guidelines offer useful guidelines regarding instant intervention and point towards the importance of having complete emergency plans in place, incorporating access to epinephrine auto-injectors. Furthermore, they suggest ongoing patient education and follow-up to avoid recurrence risk (Alvarez-Twose et al., 2014). By the integration of specialist consensus and evidence-based research, guidelines such as these are a valuable resource that assists healthcare professionals in their management of acute medical conditions, ultimately resulting in better individual patient outcomes. However, clinical practice guidelines' effectiveness in practice largely depends upon whether they are accepted and adhered to by healthcare professionals. Variability in clinical judgment, availability of resources, and different interpretations of guidelines can hinder their effective use. Moreover, inequities in access to healthcare can exist across differing healthcare systems, which eventually impact patient outcomes. To overcome such problems, ongoing research and monitoring of compliance with

CPGs are essential regarding the identification of barriers and integration into routine clinical practice. As was evident from the various research studies on occupational hazards among dental professionals, continued observation and revision of the guidelines are necessary to ensure high-quality care that is responsive to the shifting context of public health and clinical practices (Petti et al., 2017) (Figure 1.17).

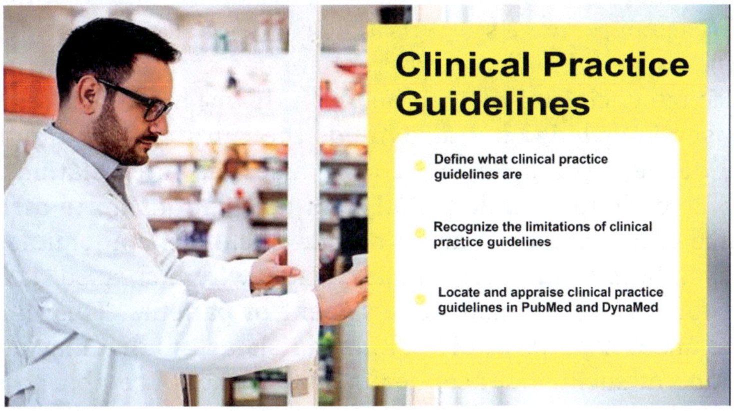

Figure 1.17. Clinical practice guidelines.

Source: https://i.ytimg.com/vi/v9eU5Sp3Rnw/maxresdefault.jpg?sqp=-oaymwEmCIAKENAF8quKqQMa8AEB-AH-CYAC0AWKAgwIABABGGUgZShlMA8=&rs=AOn4CLCh6iR-Kxl-TxfXBVbGFxyYOwSOhw.

Summary

In synthesizing the results of various studies, it becomes apparent that clinical epidemiology is an evidence-based practice in health. Through thorough evaluation of the quality and applicability of the studies, practitioners establish well-informed decisions whose impacts are direct on public health outcomes. The Journal Club activity best demonstrates the practice since it enhances critical thinking and analytical reasoning among students and professionals. Through peer-reviewed research, participants gain an understanding of how different studies find their way into clinical guidelines and health policies, ultimately closing the gap between theory and practice. The exercise not only enhances discipline-based knowledge but also builds the culture of continuous learning required in efficient healthcare delivery (Caron et al., 2019). Also, the interrelationship between various indices of health, such as body mass index (BMI) and its relationship to atrial fibrillation, says it all about the importance of meticulous analysis of data in clinical epidemiology. Experiments have established that various indices of adiposity are associated with increased risks of atrial fibrillation, emphasizing the need for a comprehensive assessment of patients. This illustrates the ability of clinical epidemiology to uncover patterns of health and risk factors that may otherwise be obscured. Knowing the implications of such evidence, healthcare workers are able to implement evidence-based, focused interventions that are tailored to reduce the prevalence of conditions linked with obesity and other risk factors. This underscores the value of conducting epidemiologic research in the clinical environment (Aune et al., 2017). Overall, the role of clinical epidemiology cannot be overemphasized; it informs evidence-based healthcare practice that rewards both professionals and patients with better health outcomes. The integration of systematic review results and meta-analyses offers a robust platform for understanding complex health issues. With health care continuously evolving in response to new evidence, the importance of analytical training, such as the Journal Club, cannot be overstated. Not only do they equip future healthcare professionals with the necessary skills, but they also instill a culture of critically examining research. Through intense scrutiny and evidence-based practice devotion, eventually, the healthcare community can continue to move forward toward its objective of improving population health and addressing ongoing public health challenges (Caron et al., 2019; Aune et al., 2017).

One of the core lessons of clinical epidemiology is the need for robust surveillance systems to identify and control disease. Initiatives such as innovative joint projects conducted by the FAO in Southeast Asia indicate the successful influence that epidemiological frameworks are able to make towards increasing responses to emerging diseases. These efforts emphasized the multidisciplinary character of work, recognizing that an interdisciplinary partnership among various stakeholders—veterinary services, diagnostic labs, and epidemiological centers—is critical to efficient disease surveillance and control. By closing gaps in current processes of surveillance, these efforts contribute not just to immediate public health action but also readiness in the long term against future zoonotic challenges, demonstrating the essential role of coordinated epidemiological effort towards global health. Another important area that arises in clinical epidemiology is the practice of evidence-based reporting guidelines, for instance, the STROBE statement. Initially developed to improve transparency and quality of observational study reporting, STROBE has been modified for veterinary medicine to cover special features inherent in this discipline. By converting the original STROBE guidelines into veterinary language, investigators can more clearly describe and appreciate their findings, and hence improve the quality of data reported in observational studies. This adaptation represents an acknowledgement of the specific challenges of veterinary epidemiology and the necessity for maintaining high reporting standards in order to inform more efficient health policies and interventions. Besides, the ongoing exchange of knowledge and experience among countries, as captured in the FAO training workshops, highlights the necessity of international collaboration in clinical epidemiology. The workshops facilitate shared learning opportunities and the exchange of best practices among participants from varied backgrounds. Through participation and concerted efforts, countries can work together towards building their respective epidemiological strengths while forging a collective action against international health challenges. Although engaging different degrees of surveillance quality, the obtained data can identify and settle system weaknesses. In the long term, such interactions not only set the level of epidemiological services higher but also contribute to the international disease prevention and health promotion program, encapsulating the essence of an interdependent approach in clinical epidemiology.

CLOSER LOOK

THE ROLE OF CLINICAL EPIDEMIOLOGY IN IMPROVING HEALTH OUTCOMES

Clinical epidemiology plays a vital role in shaping healthcare practices and policies to improve health outcomes. By highlighting the determinants and distribution of states or occurrences of interest in designated populations, clinical epidemiologists provide decision-makers in clinical practice with important information. Clinical epidemiology not only detects risk factors for diseases but also examines the effectiveness of interventions aimed at controlling them. With healthcare focusing on a value-based framework, understanding population health and its intricacies has become more important than ever before. Clinical epidemiology, through advanced research, generates evidence that equips healthcare practitioners and managers to make informed decisions regarding disease prevention as well as strategies for promoting health. This transformation is essential because it guides resource investment and determines intervention priorities that impact population health outcomes the most (Carmalt et al., 2018).

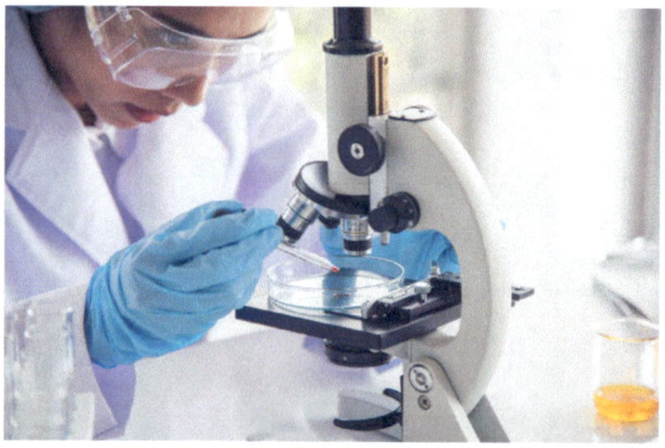

Figure 1.18. A scientist examining a specimen under a microscope in an epidemiology laboratory.

Source: https://online.arizona.edu/sites/default/files/styles/az_large/public/2025-03/Epidemiologyarticle.jpeg.webp?itok=jtyxdwsy.

Moreover, clinical epidemiology is central in training healthcare practitioners by shaping curricula to address real health issues. With the rising demand for good healthcare leaders, integrating clinical epidemiology into health administration curricula is imperative. Educators have a responsibility to equip future health administrators with knowledge and skills to meaningfully grasp the complexity of population health. A robust curriculum that incorporates best practices equips a health care workforce with the capacity to tackle health disparities and optimize health outcomes in communities. Salient findings from qualitative analysis of focus group feedback at conferences, such as the 2017 AUPHA meeting, have identified predominant content areas and learning strategies that can enhance health administration curricula (Carmalt et al., 2018). This points to the necessity of continuous discussion among teachers on best practice in reading students for achievement in an increasingly dynamic healthcare system. Moreover, emphasis on clinical epidemiology within health systems points to the necessity of coordination between healthcare and public health systems. As models of healthcare evolve, the intersection of the two promotes the overall efficiency of health programs working towards improving population health outcomes. Clinical epidemiologists are prone to partner with public health professionals in conducting research to inform policy and its application. The annual reports from institutions of learning provide evidence of activities and achievements of such collaborative activity and successful initiatives demonstrating the viability of collaborative solutions to health issues. By fostering partnerships between disciplines, clinical epidemiology can drive the way in projects that are innovative as well as science-based, and therefore ultimately produce enhanced health gains for diverse populations (Figure 1.18).

References

1. Abecasis, G. R., Ackerman, M. J., Adamkova, V., Alonso, A., et al. (2013). Genetic association study of QT interval highlight's role for calcium signaling pathways in myocardial repolarization. https://core.ac.uk/download/29469527.pdf (accessed on 25th June 2025).
2. Abrahams, E., Acion, L., Altman, R., Altman, D., Altman, J., Bogarty, S., Boyce, A., et al. (2009). *Epidemiological Methods: About Time.* https://core.ac.uk/download/pdf/8376923.pdf (accessed on 25th June 2025).
3. Akl, E. A., Alonso-Coello, P., Briel, M., Eslava-Schmalbach, J., et al. (2017). GRADE equity guidelines 4: Guidance on how to assess and address health equity within the evidence to decision process. https://core.ac.uk/download/96882593.pdf (accessed on 25th June 2025).
4. Alvarez-Twose, R., Muraro, A., Arga, M., Armstrong, K., Arroabarren, E., Sheikh, A., Barnett, T., et al. (2014). International consensus on (ICON) anaphylaxis. https://core.ac.uk/download/28978204.pdf (accessed on 25th June 2025).
5. Ambayo, H., Bouwman, J., Bronselaer, A., De Baets, B., et al. (2019). An ontology to standardize research output of nutritional epidemiology: From paper-based standards to linked content. https://core.ac.uk/download/222452585.pdf (accessed on 25th June 2025).
6. Anderson, C. M., Lyon, D. E., McCarthy, D., Corwin, E. J., Taylor, J. Y., Voss, J., Gregory, K. E., et al. (2015). Educating future nursing scientists: Recommendations for integrating omics content in PhD programs. https://core.ac.uk/download/213074828.pdf (accessed on 25th June 2025).
7. Anderson, G., Avilés-Santa, M. L., Heiss, G., Howard, B. V., et al. (2016). Embedding clinical interventions into observational studies. https://core.ac.uk/download/304662993.pdf (accessed on 25th June 2025).
8. Annibale, B., Carabotti, M., Cicenia, A., Pallotta, N., et al. (2018). Recent advances in understanding and managing diverticulitis. https://core.ac.uk/download/160052854.pdf (accessed on 25th June 2025).
9. Argano, V., Balistreri, C. R., Giarratana, R. M., Lio, D., et al. (2019). On the road to accurate biomarkers for cardiometabolic diseases by integrating precision and gender medicine approaches. https://core.ac.uk/download/268910274.pdf (accessed on 25th June 2025).
10. Ashley, E. S. D., Cosgrove, S. E., Fakih, M. G., Manning, M. L., et al. (2018). Antimicrobial stewardship and infection prevention—leveraging the synergy: A position paper update. https://core.ac.uk/download/155271805.pdf (accessed on 25th June 2025).
11. Aune, D., Janszky, I., Norat, T., Riboli, E., et al. (2017). Body mass index, abdominal fatness, fat mass and the risk of atrial fibrillation: A systematic review and dose–response meta-analysis of prospective studies. https://core.ac.uk/download/78075183.pdf (accessed on 25th June 2025).
12. Avenell, A., Harstrick, A., Inanir, A., Kerst, A., Zittermann, A., Millen, A. E., Eliassen, A. H., et al. (2013). Vitamin D supplementation and breast cancer prevention: A systematic review and meta-analysis of randomized clinical trials. https://core.ac.uk/download/16664256.pdf (accessed on 25th June 2025).
13. Babcock, S., Beverley, J., Cowell, L. G., Smith, B., et al. (2021). The infectious disease ontology

in the age of COVID-19. https://core.ac.uk/download/305120399.pdf (accessed on 25th June 2025).

14. Barnholtz-Sloan, J. S., Basu, A., Borowsky, A. D., Bui, M. M., et al. (2020). Cancer Informatics for Cancer Centers (CI4CC): Building a community focused on sharing ideas and best practices to improve cancer care and patient outcomes. https://core.ac.uk/download/288432567.pdf (accessed on 25th June 2025).
15. Bashinskaya, B. (2016). *Effects of Obesity on Walking Patterns and Adaptability During Obstacle Crossing*. https://open.bu.edu/bitstream/2144/16125/1/Bashinskaya_bu_0017N_11114.pdf (accessed on 25th June 2025).
16. Batra, R., Edgeworth, J., Pouwels, K. B., Robotham, J. V., et al. (2020). Estimating the effect of healthcare-associated infections on excess length of hospital stay using inverse probability-weighted survival curves. https://core.ac.uk/download/322827632.pdf (accessed on 25th June 2025).
17. Bauer, R., Duez, P., Fan, T. P., Guo, D. A., et al. (2013). The quest for modernization of traditional Chinese medicine. https://core.ac.uk/download/42337105.pdf (accessed on 25th June 2025).
18. Benn, E. K. T., Carter, R. E., Enders, F. T., Grambow, S. C., et al. (2017). Statistical competencies for medical research learners: What is fundamental? https://core.ac.uk/download/323070500.pdf (accessed on 25th June 2025).
19. Beratarrechea, A. G., Diez Canseco, F., Irazola, V., Miranda, J. J., et al. (2016). Use of m-Health technology for preventive interventions to tackle cardiometabolic conditions and other non-communicable diseases in Latin America—Challenges and opportunities. https://core.ac.uk/download/159285900.pdf (accessed on 25th June 2025).
20. Bhandari, M., Devereaux, P. J., Guyatt, G. H., Leece, P., et al. (2004). Internet versus mailed questionnaires: A randomized comparison (2). https://open.bu.edu/bitstream/2144/3420/1/pmc1550617.pdf (accessed on 25th June 2025).
21. Bianchi, F., Minichilli, F., Pierini, A., Pieroni, L., et al. (2025). Amyotrophic lateral sclerosis: Results from Tuscany Registry of Rare Diseases. https://core.ac.uk/download/pdf/37831063.pdf (accessed on 25th June 2025).
22. Bland, M., Currow, D. C., Hussain, J. A., Johnson, M. J., et al. (2016). Missing data in randomized controlled trials testing palliative interventions pose a significant risk of bias and loss of power: A systematic review and meta-analyses. https://core.ac.uk/download/151157324.pdf (accessed on 25th June 2025).
23. Blondeel, K., Cordero, J., Kiarie, J., Murtagh, M., et al. (2017). Advancing prevention of sexually transmitted infections through point-of-care testing: Target product profiles and landscape analysis. https://core.ac.uk/download/147056121.pdf (accessed on 25th June 2025).
24. Bonilla-Velez, J., Lomberk, G., Small, M., Urrutia, R., et al. (2017). The enduring value of research in medical education. https://core.ac.uk/download/270177626.pdf (accessed on 25th June 2025).
25. Boon, N. A. M., Descamps, T., Devleesschauwer, B., Robert, A., et al. (2019). Status and potential of bacterial genomics for public health practice: A scoping review. https://core.ac.uk/download/227041617.pdf (accessed on 25th June 2025).
26. Brodbelt, D. C., Church, D. B., McGreevy, P. D., O'Neill, D. G., et al. (2014). Approaches to canine health surveillance. https://core.ac.uk/download/36777547.pdf (accessed on 25th June 2025).

27. Burton, A. K., Abasolo, M., Alizadehkhaiyat, O., Pearce, B. G., Baldwin, M., Beaton, D. E., Bonde, J. P., et al. (2008). Management of work-relevant upper limb disorders: A review. https://core.ac.uk/download/1649687.pdf (accessed on 25th June 2025).

28. Carmalt, J. H., Caron, R. M., Hewitt, A. M., Hooker, R. S., et al. (2018). Teaching population health: Innovations in the integration of the healthcare and public health systems. https://core.ac.uk/download/286641618.pdf (accessed on 25th June 2025).

29. Caron, R. M. (2019). Journal club revisited: Teaching evidence-based research and practice to graduate students in a professional degree program. https://core.ac.uk/download/286641622.pdf (accessed on 25th June 2025).

30. Carton, T. W., Forrest, C. B., & Pletcher, M. J. (2018). PCORnet's collaborative research groups. https://core.ac.uk/download/323072044.pdf (accessed on 25th June 2025).

31. Cavallero, S., De Vito, C., D'Amelio, S., Iavicoli, S., et al. (2018). Anisakiasis in Italy: Analysis of hospital discharge records in the years 2005–2015. https://core.ac.uk/download/195776795.pdf (accessed on 25th June 2025).

32. Cevallos, M., Dohoo, I., Egger, M., Erb, H., et al. (2016). Explanation and elaboration document for the STROBE-Vet statement: Strengthening the reporting of observational studies in epidemiology—Veterinary extension. https://core.ac.uk/download/76980915.pdf (accessed on 25th June 2025).

33. Christesen, H. T., Germak, J., Höybye, C., Lee, P., et al. (2013). The NordiNet® International Outcome Study and NovoNet® ANSWER Program®: Rationale, design, and methodology of two international pharmacoepidemiologic registry-based studies monitoring long-term clinical and safety outcomes of growth hormone therapy (Norditropin®). https://core.ac.uk/download/46972310.pdf (accessed on 25th June 2025).

34. COHERE Expert Review Group, Cole, S., Conti, L., Davis, M. F., et al. (2017). Checklist for One Health Epidemiological Reporting of Evidence (COHERE). https://core.ac.uk/download/323070004.pdf (accessed on 25th June 2025).

35. Collaborative, GOP-NRFASROBC, De Stavola, B., Dos Santos Silva, I., McCormack, V., et al. (2008). Birth size and breast cancer risk: Re-analysis of individual participant data from 32 studies. https://core.ac.uk/download/1719695.pdf (accessed on 25th June 2025).

36. Cortey, M., Drigo, M., Franzo, G., Hughes, J., et al. (2016). Phylodynamic analysis of porcine circovirus type 2: Methodological approach and datasets. https://core.ac.uk/download/46558715.pdf (accessed on 25th June 2025).

37. Clercq, K., Ennaji, M., Haegeman, A., Khayli, I., et al. (2019). Clinical and epidemiological evolution of sheep pox in Morocco. https://core.ac.uk/download/286072988.pdf (accessed on 25th June 2025).

38. Desvaux, S., Goutard, F., & Roger, F. (2005). Workshop to deliver epidemiology and laboratory training for HPAI diagnostic network. http://agritrop.cirad.fr/529308/1/ID529308.pdf (accessed on 25th June 2025).

39. Dixon, B. E., Kharrazi, H., & Lehmann, H. P. (2015). Public health and epidemiology informatics: Recent research and trends in the United States. https://core.ac.uk/download/299808964.pdf (accessed on 25th June 2025).

40. Facey, K., Granados, A., Guyatt, G., Kent, A., et al. (2014). Generating health technology

assessment evidence for rare diseases. https://core.ac.uk/download/42361346.pdf (accessed on 25th June 2025).

41. Gallagher, R., Neachell, J., Stott, D., Topley, N., et al. (2015). The One Together collaborative approach to reduce the risk of surgical site infection: Identifying the challenges to assuring best practice. https://core.ac.uk/download/46597998.pdf (accessed on 25th June 2025).

42. Ghinea, G., & Serif, T. (2005). Visualizing pain data for wheelchair users: A ubiquitous approach. https://core.ac.uk/download/337669.pdf (accessed on 25th June 2025).

43. Gomez, S. L., Keegan, T. H. M., Kroenke, C. H., Kushi, L. H., et al. (2015). Representativeness of breast cancer cases in an integrated health care delivery system. https://core.ac.uk/download/323063518.pdf (accessed on 25th June 2025).

44. Han, A. M. (2013). *Proximity to Clinical Care and Time to Resolution Following an Abnormal Cancer Screening in An Urban Setting*. https://open.bu.edu/bitstream/2144/12113/12/Han_Ann_2013_nosig_nocv.pdf (accessed on 25th June 2025).

45. Hogan, J. W., & Su, L. (2011). HIV dynamics and natural history studies: Joint modeling with doubly interval-censored event time and infrequent longitudinal data. http://arxiv.org/abs/1105.0543 (accessed on 25th June 2025).

46. Hulstine, A. (2017). *Vaccine Implementation: Alaska 2017*. https://core.ac.uk/download/286607590.pdf (accessed on 25th June 2025).

47. Iversen, A., Vahratian, A., American Statistical Association, Briesacher, B., Woodward, B., Junghans, C., Verity, C., et al. (2008). Ethical issues in implementation research: A discussion of the problems in achieving informed consent. https://core.ac.uk/download/48972.pdf (accessed on 25th June 2025).

48. Johnson, A., Ippolito, A., Zimolzak, A., Moses, C., Stone, D. J., Moody, G., Celi, L. A., et al. (2014). Making big data useful for health care: A summary of the inaugural MIT Critical Data Conference. https://core.ac.uk/download/78058114.pdf (accessed on 25th June 2025).

49. Karakkamandapam, S., Nair, N. S. K., Sharma, P. S. V. N. (2010). Development of a cost-effective database software for psychiatric research: A study from tertiary care teaching hospital. https://core.ac.uk/download/pdf/14946.pdf (accessed on 25th June 2025).

50. London School of Hygiene & Tropical Medicine. (2013). *Annual Report 2013*. https://core.ac.uk/download/19452766.pdf (accessed on 25th June 2025).

51. Meirhaeghe, A., Ropero, A. B., Tabak, A. G., Meirhaeghe, A., Voight, B. F., Newton-Cheh, C., Sengenes, C., et al. (2011). Mendelian randomization study of B-type natriuretic peptide and type 2 diabetes: Evidence of causal association from population studies. https://core.ac.uk/download/1437139.pdf (accessed on 25th June 2025).

52. Mengersen, K., Moynihan, S. A., & Tweedie, R. L. (2007). Causality and association: The statistical and legal approaches. https://core.ac.uk/download/10883828.pdf (accessed on 25th June 2025).

53. Ministry of Health and Social Welfare (MoHSW). (2025). *Proposal to Strengthen Health Information System [HIS]*. https://core.ac.uk/download/pdf/11307107.pdf (accessed on 25th June 2025).

54. Nødtvedt, A. (2007). *Epidemiology of Canine Atopic Dermatitis*. https://core.ac.uk/download/11695161.pdf (accessed on 25th June 2025).

55. Ott, S. L. (2025). *Digital Dermatitis on U.S. Dairy Operations.* https://core.ac.uk/download/pdf/6813887.pdf (accessed on 25th June 2025).

56. Petti, S., Y Vitali, M. (2017). Occupational risk for *Legionella* infection among dental healthcare workers: Meta-analysis in occupational epidemiology. https://core.ac.uk/download/141696035.pdf (accessed on 25th June 2025).

57. Phelps, C. L. (2004). *Advances in Teaching & Learning Day Abstracts 2005.* https://core.ac.uk/download/46714715.pdf (accessed on 25th June 2025).

58. Preiss, D., Rankin, N. J., Sattar, N., Welsh, P., et al. (2016). Applying metabolomics to cardiometabolic intervention studies and trials: Past experiences and a roadmap for the future. https://core.ac.uk/download/46567783.pdf (accessed on 25th June 2025).

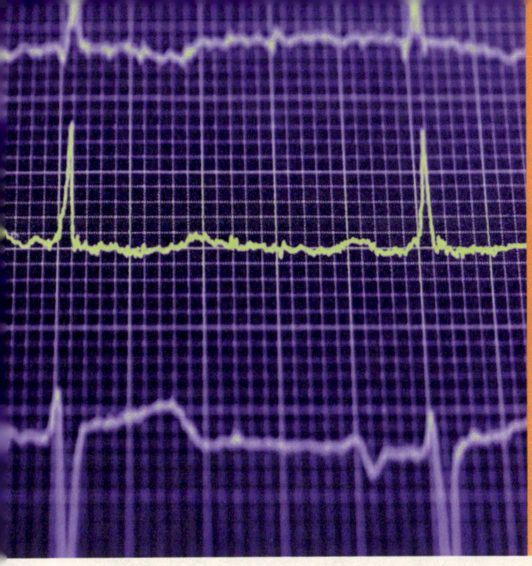

Chapter 2

MEASUREMENT OF DISEASE FREQUENCY

Contents

Introduction

Measurement of the frequency of disease in human beings is one of the central roles of epidemiology since it tells us about the determinants and distribution of health status in populations. Understanding how diseases manifest within specific populations will allow researchers and public health practitioners to determine the at-risk populations, allocate resources in proportion, and implement interventions. The worth of these measurements extends beyond the measurement of health effects, for they are also charged with underlying environmental and social determinants that cause disease burden. As we explore the variety of methods employed in measuring disease frequency, it is imperative to have a complete understanding of both incidence and prevalence rates in order to plan public health policies and programs. Over the past few years, advances in diagnostic technologies have further enhanced the capacity to quantify disease accurately. Emerging technologies, such as optical non-invasive diagnostics in the literature, have demonstrated the potential to detect early microcirculatory conditions associated with certain medical conditions. Such techniques have proved highly sensitive and specific, with the capacity to offer interventions in a timely fashion that have a significant capability to change the outcomes of disease. As noted by epidemiological studies, the integration of new diagnostic tools with traditional measures of disease frequency will be in a position to provide multi-faceted insight into health trends. Through these developments, researchers are better placed to understand and combat chronic diseases, thereby improving population health statistics in general. However, with all that progress, the complexities involved in capturing disease frequency cannot be overlooked. Factors such as heterogeneity of the population, health inequality at the underlying level, and environmental factors complicate data interpretation. Variation in the incidence of disease across different subpopulations of the population can yield insights into genetic susceptibility, income status, and access to healthcare resources. It is necessary to interpret such data in relation to higher-level social determinants of health to frame proper public health policies. Resolving these intricacies not only streamlines our efforts toward disease pattern understanding but also illuminates the possible paths of intervention, emphasizing the need for ongoing research in this pressing area of public health (Figure 2.1).

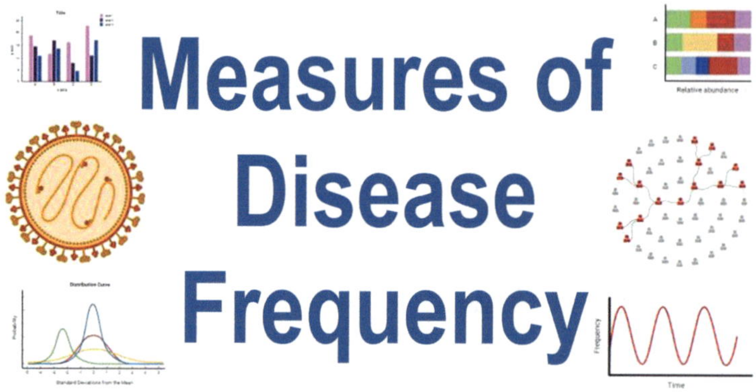

Figure 2.1. Measures of disease frequency.

Source: https://microbenotes.com/wp-content/uploads/2024/09/Measures-of-Disease-Frequency.jpeg.

2.1. Types of Disease Frequency Measures

Disease frequency measures are the fundamentals of public health issues and research, as well as of epidemiology. Frequency measures enable researchers to quantify the incidence and prevalence of disease within populations. Incidence can be employed to quantify the number of new cases of a disease arising in some specified time within a clearly defined population, and it is key when it comes to the measurement of the acute impact of diseases. For example, incidence measurement of a spreading disease can help determine if an intervention is immediately needed. Alternatively, prevalence will measure new and existing cases of disease within a population at one point in time, which may provide insight into the disease burden. This is important since high prevalence might be used to make decisions regarding the distribution of health resources, while incidence might detect future health risks. A valuable aspect of disease frequency measures is the application of rate calculations to gain a more advanced analysis of disease patterns. Rates, typically in terms of per some number of individuals (e.g., per 1,000 or 100,000), enable comparisons among different populations or geographic locations. This statistical technique allows examination of variables like age, sex, and socioeconomic status that can influence health outcomes. For example, for cardiovascular disease rates, the data must be stratified according to age groups so that an understanding can be gained of how it impacts different populations. Furthermore, these calculations assist in identifying groups at risk and consequently guide interventions where the interventions are needed most. With the knowledge of these differences in measurement, public health practitioners can develop measures to minimize disease transmission and improve overall health outcomes. Besides, the inferences that arise from disease frequency measures also apply to evaluating the effect of public health interventions. Tracking changes in incidence and prevalence rates before and after an intervention provides empirical evidence for its efficiency. For instance, in case a vaccination program effectively reduces the incidence rates for a contagious disease, then the evidence can warrant additional funding for this kind of program. Additionally, the influence of genetics and disease frequency is an interesting field of study. Research has emphasized how genetic variation, for example, in the major histocompatibility complex (MHC), might be connected to health and disease resistance within a society (Borghans et al., 2025). Therefore, the incorporation of genetic components into measures of disease frequency not only deepens our knowledge about the dynamics of disease but also introduces a more holistic strategy for public health management (Borghans et al., 2025). The integrated vision of this could open doors to focused, efficient health intervention programs based on the particular needs of the community.

2.1.1. Prevalence

Prevalence knowledge is useful in quantifying the frequency of the disease among human populations. Prevalence refers to cases present at a point in time in relation to the population and provides information on the general amount of disease burden. Prevalence is not just a way of measuring health at a specific time, but also useful in public health planning and the provision of resources. For instance, a high prevalence of certain conditions, such as diabetes, demands certain interventions and health care services to manage and limit their impact. Quantifying prevalence allows researchers and public health practitioners to determine temporal trends, assess the effect of public health interventions, and identify areas needing intervention. The prevalence of certain genetic variants for resultant diseases explains the role played by population studies in unraveling health outcomes. For example, the transthyretin (TTR) pV142I variant is associated with high rates of systemic amyloidosis cases, notably prevalent in African American populations at the allele frequency rate of 0.0173. This shows genetic prevalence can vary drastically between different demographic populations, affecting disease expression and progression. Identifying these differences not only facilitates population at risk identification for targeted screening but also provides insights into the genetic determinants of disease susceptibility. In this case, prevalence is pivotal in guiding clinical practice and intervention. Further, investigating infectious disease-related practices determines prevalence complexity in settings. A review of avian influenza infection systematically illustrated the effects of direct and indirect exposure to poultry on rates of prevalence. The study revealed that high-risk behavior prevalence differences were immense, with stronger associations being observed in live markets compared to homes. This emphasizes the importance of situational determinants of disease prevalence. Better understanding of the prevalence of infection-related behavior—and the reasoning behind it—can be used to strengthen public health intervention planning. Coupling epidemiological data with an understanding of behavior can assist in making interventions more successfully targeted towards not just the disease itself but also to the cultural and social behavior that facilitates its persistence (Ahad et al., 2017) (Figure 2.2).

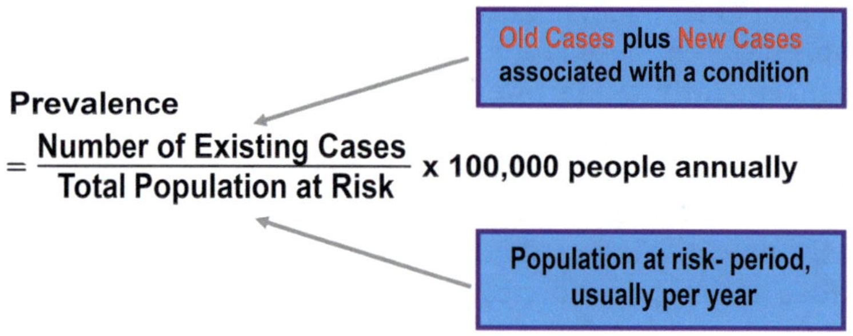

Figure 2.2. Prevalence.

Source: https://i0.wp.com/immersionconcept.com/wp-content/uploads/2023/09/Screenshot-2023-09-18-220726.png?w=926&ssl=1.

2.1.2. Incidence

Incidence is a key epidemiological measure, expressing the frequency of new cases within a specified population within a given period of time. It provides measures of disease transmission dynamics, such that researchers and health administrations can identify trends and predict epidemics. Through the calculation of incidence, epidemiologists can differentiate between the efficiency of interventions, track the impact of determinants of social health on well-being, and allocate resources more optimally. This measurement can be in one of two broad forms, that is, incidence proportion (ratio of a population that is coming down with the disease over a specified period of time) or incidence rate (new cases per unit at risk population over a defined interval), and this allows for the appreciation of disease prevalence in various demographic groups to be more nuanced. Incidence is extremely significant in interpreting the implications of epidemiological findings on a larger scale. For instance, differences in incidence rates can be indicative of health outcome differences among populations, which normally reflect social, economic, and environmental determinants. These differences can be utilized by researchers to advocate for certain health policies and programs among specific groups of people. As in epidemic response research, attention to how the incidence rate varies over the progression of an epidemic has been found to guide health interventions that will stem its spread and ease its recovery. This incidence of targeted health intervention relationship indicates the importance of precise measurement and recording, as noted in initiatives like the STROBE statement to enhance transparency and completeness of observational studies (Cevallos et al., 2016). Besides, the complexity of measuring incidence demands cautious examination of disease susceptibility patterns by socio-economic status and genetics. Empirical data have confirmed genetic heterogeneity between populations, particularly concerning the major histocompatibility complex (MHC), to have far-reaching implications on health and productivity outcomes. Greater MHC diversity in populations can illustrate improved resistance to disease, further impacting infectious disease incidence rates (Borghans et al., 2025). Therefore, it is required to use an interdisciplinary approach considering biological, environmental, and socio-economic variables in order to correctly interpret and make sense of incidence data. By incorporating these various factors, public health practitioners can develop more integrated interventions to address the disease causes on the individual and population level and thus eventually attain improved general health outcomes across populations (Figure 2.3).

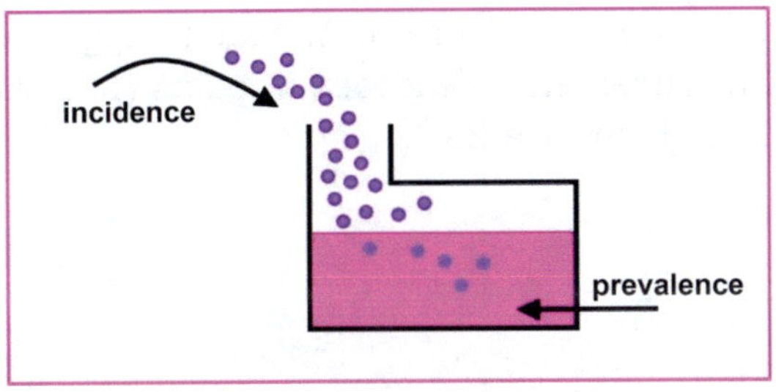

Figure 2.3. Incidence and prevalence.

Source: https://www.sltinfo.com/wp-content/uploads/2016/02/incidence-and-prevalence-1200x600-c-default.jpg.

2.1.3. Mortality Rates

The assessment of mortality rates is a critical indicator of the' health of populations across the world. Mortality rates identify not only the frequency of death but also discern health disparities that may exist between different population groups. For instance, within sub-Saharan Africa, high mortality rates among children and women continue to be common, pointing to significant public health concerns. New advances in genomic technologies are facilitating the undertaking of studies with a view to disentangling the causation entanglements of disease in such risk groups. This focus on mortality rates not just assists in the estimation of the direct health effects but also brings attention to the larger implications of measures of disease frequencies, which can be utilized to develop intervention and resource allocation policies for high-risk populations (Campbell et al., 2011). A second tier of mortality rates is their association with circumstances such as maternal health and the environment. According to one study, maternal lifestyles play a significant role in influencing birth, and that consequently leads to modifications of overall mortality rates. One such study examined the effect of glycyrrhizin, a chemical found in licorice, on birth weight and gestational age. Findings indicated that extensive application of glycyrrhizin did not significantly affect birth weight but was linked to increased chances of preterm births, thereby complicating infant mortality history. With a 2.5 odds ratio for giving birth at less than 38 weeks of gestation, the above result goes to uncover how food choice in pregnancy contributes to newborn mortality hazards." These results underscore the necessity for the inclusion of several factors in the determination of mortality rate, supplementing the value of precise data collection in the measurement of frequency of disease (Järvenpää et al., 2001). Mortality rates impact far beyond patient health outcomes and are an impetus for policy development and public health action. By examining mortality data, policy-makers can more effectively identify vulnerable groups and apply preventative measures to reduce deaths. Women's and children's mortality rates in sub-Saharan Africa reflect systematic issues with restricted health care access and the prevalence of avoidable diseases. By disaggregating mortality statistics along the lines of variables such as age, sex, and socioeconomic status, interventions can more effectively be crafted. Moreover, longitudinal surveillance of long-term changes in mortality could deliver extremely useful data, allowing measurement of the effectiveness of health programs and the overall success of public health interventions. Finally, a more detailed understanding of mortality rates will contribute more effectively to disease frequency measurement activities and to disease prevention campaigns globally (Campbell et al., 2011).

2.2. Prevalence: Understanding the Concept

Knowledge of the concept of prevalence is very important in measuring disease frequency among human populations. Prevalence refers to the total number of both new and existing cases of a specific disease in a given population over a certain period of time. The measure is an important one for both public health practitioners and researchers to be in a position to estimate the size of health issues in communities. Through the determination of how prevalent a certain disease is, stakeholders can better allocate resources and create specialized interventions. In addition, prevalence can play an important role in informing policy-making activities through highlighting the importance of a subtle analysis in creating efficient health strategies. Prevalence can be measured as point prevalence and period prevalence, both of which offer special information regarding disease dynamics. Point prevalence quantifies the cases at a moment in time, while period prevalence counts all the cases arising over a set time frame and therefore shows a broader snapshot of disease burden. This distinction is important for epidemiological research because it will influence the way data are interpreted and utilized. For instance, variations in prevalence rates between groups may reflect the underlying socio-economic and environmental determinants favoring disease propagation. Such analyses may allow for the design of more targeted public health interventions to address community-specific needs. Furthermore, prevalence data interpretation needs to correct for confounding factors like demographic characteristics, socio-economic status, and health care access. For example, higher prevalence rates of some diseases in marginalized populations can uncover systemic injustices that must be addressed to enhance overall public health returns. At the same time, continued biological explanations of race in health research, as reported in recent studies, can shape how prevalence is theorized and expressed. The results indicate that these theories, instead of being totally rejected, continue to influence contemporary scholarship, maybe even leading to the misinterpretation of race and health interactions in society (Darling et al., 2015). Therefore, complete comprehension of prevalence is not merely a matter of statistical accuracy but also an essential consideration in addressing broader social determinants of health inequities, such as in the nuanced suggestions for measurement of disease impacts (Ionova et al., 2018) (Figure 2.4).

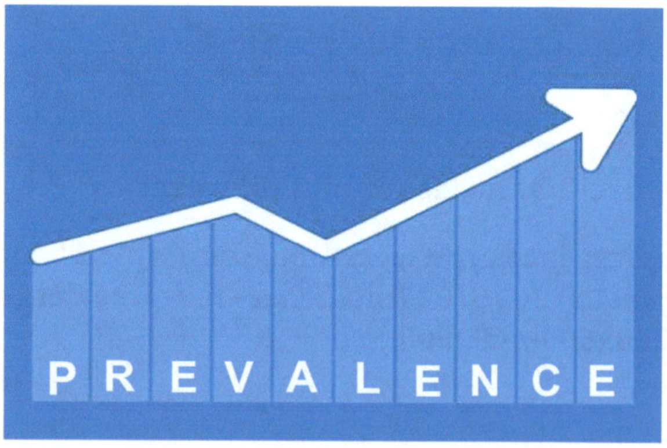

Figure 2.4. The prevalence of autism in adults is increasing rapidly in the U.S.

Source: https://autism.org/wp-content/uploads/2019/01/prevalence.jpg.

2.2.1. Definition and Calculation of Prevalence

Prevalence, an important epidemiologic measure, is defined as the total number of cases of a specific disease in a given population at a specific time. Both existing and new cases are included in this measurement, giving a full picture of disease burden among the population. Public health officials and researchers need to know the prevalence since it will guide resource utilization, healthcare planning, and disease prevention. By calculating prevalence, stakeholders can quantify the influence of public health interventions and verify targeted approaches with various populations. This kind of insight feeds into the broader goal of improved health outcomes and disease burden reduction for communities. Calculating prevalence is a straightforward calculation: the number of present cases of disease divided by the total at-risk population across a specific time period.

This figure can be given as a proportion or a percentage, which makes it that much easier to compare between various populations or geographic regions. Precautions must be taken to properly define the at-risk population so that bias in findings is avoided. Variations in prevalence rates may be attributed to numerous factors, including socio-economic status, access to healthcare, and risky behavior. Hence, disaggregated data are invaluable in understanding the multiple factors responsible for disease prevalence, which allows for targeted public health intervention and policy action. In addition, the consequences of prevalence data extend beyond immediate healthcare concerns; they also have significant economic and social implications. High rates of prevalence, for instance, suggest a mounting public health crisis, prompting government agencies to allocate additional resources towards disease control and prevention. The relationship between chronic conditions and health-related quality of life also points to the importance of prevalence knowledge. Studies have established that a higher prevalence of chronic disease is linked with decreasing measures of health, which underscores the need for effective intervention efforts (Alwan et al., 2013). In addition, assessment of the central accumulation of body fat associated with particular diseases like non-alcoholic fatty liver disease can also be guided by prevalence data, highlighting its multi-dimensional utility in health assessments (Cortez-Pinto et al., 2016) (Figure 2.5).

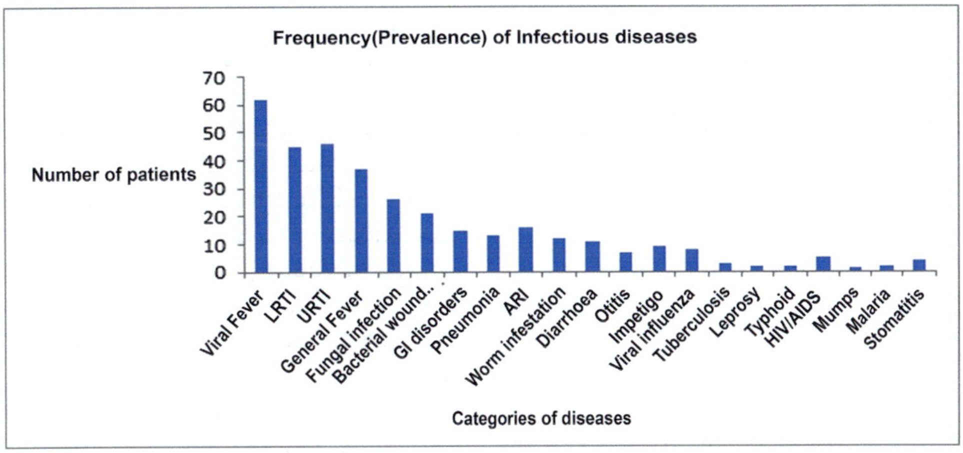

Figure 2.5. Frequency (prevalence) of Infectious diseases II.

Source: https://www.researchgate.net/profile/Vijay-Kumar-Panthi/publication/316605226/figure/fig3/AS:667868823818243@1536243744376/FrequencyPrevalence-of-Infectious-diseases-II-Distribution-of-infectious-diseases-Out.ppm.

2.2.2. Point Prevalence vs. Period Prevalence

In epidemiology, point prevalence and period prevalence differ in small yet significant ways in assessing how frequently diseases occur in a population. Point prevalence refers to the number of individuals in a specified population who have a particular disease at a specific point in time. This is a snapshot that can be very useful in quantifying the immediate disease burden in a community. For instance, in one study that measured community viral load among men who have sex with men (MSM) in San Francisco, a point prevalence estimate yielded valuable data on the viral kinetics of HIV in specific years (Das et al., 2013). By reporting the size of the disease at one moment in time, point prevalence is useful for planning and resource allocation in public health during emergencies.

On the other hand, period prevalence measures the proportion of a population diseased at any time point during a given time period, perhaps between days and years. It encompasses both new and prevalent cases, thus providing more room for disease experience over a period. For instance, investigating period prevalence could reveal trends in HIV incidence among the same MSM cohort according to longitudinal surveys. It encompasses fluctuations that might not be evident in point prevalence, including seasonal epidemics or changes in treatment effectiveness (Aprili, 2008). Period prevalence is, therefore, essential for capturing long-term patterns and the efficacy of interventions to prevent disease spread. This situation can inform healthcare policies and interventions against disease prevention. Although both point and period prevalence have their advantages, the choice of which to employ may well depend on the specific research question, as well as on the nature of the disease being inquired about.

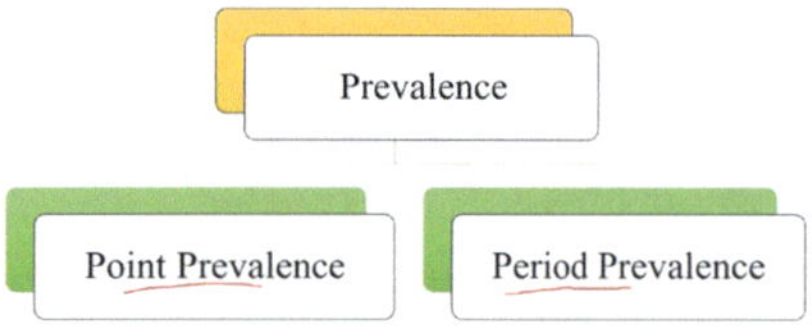

Figure 2.6. Point prevalence and period prevalence.

Source: https://i.ytimg.com/vi/LONQQVrBdwk/maxresdefault.jpg.

Point prevalence may be employed where immediate assessments are needed, whereas period prevalence might be employed where chronic disease requires long-term assessment. Moreover, methodological concerns such as population dynamics and variations in health-seeking behaviors can influence prevalence measurement choice. Population health policymakers and researchers can build a comprehensive view of disease burdens as indicated by the determination of HIV transmission capacity within the community through an integration of comprehension of both prevalence types (Das et al., 2013; Aprili, 2008). This general structure finally assists in the formulation of effective public health policies tailored for specific populations (Figure 2.6).

2.2.3. Factors Influencing Prevalence Rates

The prevalence rate of disease in human populations is determined by a range of environmental and biological variables. Geographical variation is significant; for instance, diseases that thrive in specific climates can be more prevalent in such areas. Socio-economic status also greatly determines access to healthcare, health education, and lifestyle, which can assist in the prevention or enhancement of disease prevalence. Urban populations may differ in their health status from their rural equivalents, typically due to differences in lifestyle and access to healthcare. Public health practitioners must be aware of these geographic and socio-economic disparities in order to prioritize and allocate resources and plan interventions that will appropriately address different populations with the aim of determining the level of disease presence among such communities. Besides, genetic predispositions are also a significant determinant in the incidence of some diseases. Certain populations carry genetic variants that predispose them to certain illnesses and thereby have a higher incidence of these diseases. For example, certain genetic disorders are largely present in isolated populations due to negligible gene flow. Lifestyle determinants such as diet, exercise, and use of drugs also interact extensively with genetics to modify individual health profiles. The cross-action between the environmental and genetic determinants has the ability to create complex health landscapes in which disease prevalence rates change continually. With increasing evidence emphasizing the involvement of genetics in disease causation, it becomes increasingly important that physicians and epidemiologists consider these determinants in their prevalence investigations and health interventions. Public health policy also significantly influences prevalence rates because it defines the conditions under which health interventions are implemented. Effective vaccination campaigns, screening operations, and health education can minimize the prevalence of infectious as well as chronic diseases in populations. For example, the use of universal immunization programs has helped decrease outbreaks of diseases such as measles and polio in various regions of the globe. Conversely, ineffective public health interventions can lead to rising incidence rates, such as in regions with low rates of vaccine coverage and healthcare facilities. Therefore, the evaluation of the efficacy and accessibility of public health policy is essential to establish its impact on the prevalence of disease. Analyzing these policies against demographic and genetic variables allows a better understanding of the myriad factors driving the prevalence of disease, and subsequently towards improved outcomes for populations as a whole.

2.3. Incidence: A Closer Look

It is of cardinal significance that epidemiologists comprehend the concept of incidence in quantifying disease frequency within a population. Incidence is the extremely precise quantification of the number of new cases of a disease during a specific time period, relative to the at-risk population. By measuring it, it is possible to assess disease dynamics and intervention effectiveness. By following new cases, researchers are able to establish trends over time, quantify the impact of health policy, and redistribute resources. Additionally, rates of incidence tell us something about the etiological factors behind disease occurrence, and that it is possible to prevent disease occurrence. A more critical examination of incidence is therefore not only contributing value to the understanding of disease transmission but also enhancing public health response capability so that intervention is possible and can significantly minimize disease occurrence. When looking at incidence, it is important to make a difference between cumulative incidence and incidence rate since both of these present different views of the frequency of disease. Cumulative incidence determines the proportion of a population that develops a disease over a given time period, expressed as a percentage. In contrast, the incidence rate looks at the number of new cases per unit of time in those who are at risk, typically expressed per person-time. This is a significant distinction in interpreting epidemiologic data, as it affects the capacity for interpreting the disease burden and the public health consequences. For example, cumulative incidence can suggest an explosive outbreak, while the incidence rate can reflect steady, chronic transmission. These levels of analysis provide increased insight into trends in disease, ultimately affecting programmatic responses to public health issues. Incidence evaluation also requires attention to methodological challenges that influence measurement accuracy. These include population migration, diagnostic characteristics, and varying reporting patterns, which can distort data and thus inform public health inference. For instance, studies on gastroesophageal reflux (GER) in anesthetized cats demonstrated how specific interventions, like omeprazole therapy, can yield significant differences in disease prevalence in the controlled setting, with around 33.3% of cats showing GER events during anesthesia (Belafsky et al., 2017). Such findings highlight the need for study designs that are stringent in minimizing bias and yielding unbiased prevalence estimation. In addition, adequate training for individuals responsible for gathering and analyzing data is necessary, as the accuracy of incidence measurement depends on sound and consistent reporting systems by different health facilities (Curtis et al., 2014) (Figure 2.7).

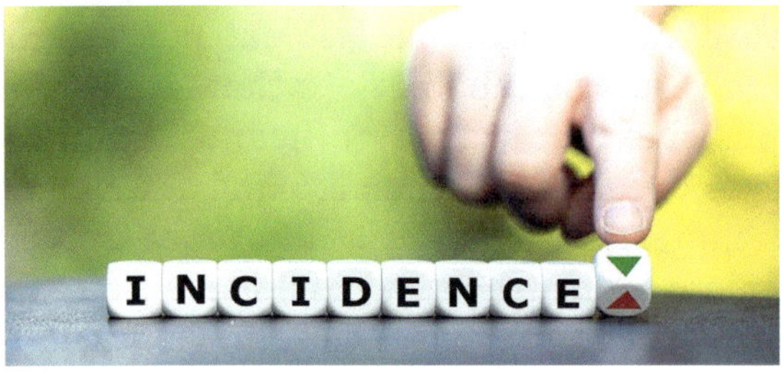

Figure 2.7. Incidence.

Source: https://cdn.corporatefinanceinstitute.com/assets/incidence-rate-1024x479.jpeg.

2.3.1. Definition and Calculation of Incidence

It is essential to understand the definition and measurement of incidence in public health, as it indicates the number of new cases of a disease that exist in a population over a period. Incidence is numerically defined as the number of new cases occurring in a population at risk divided by the number of individuals in the said group, typically multiplied by a specific constant like 1,000 in order to facilitate easier interpretation of rates. It measures the dynamic aspect of disease occurrence because it specifically counts new cases, not including all cases, as seen in the case of prevalence, both new and long-standing. By highlighting new cases, incidence calls attention to risk factors and potential changes in patterns of disease transmission, ultimately assisting public health administrators to identify urgent health needs and allocate resources, thus highlighting its rudimentary role of disease frequency measurement in human populations. For increasing the validity and reliability of incidence calculations, certain data collection methods have to be employed. There has to be a clear definition of the at-risk group, which involves individuals who are still being exposed to the disease throughout the study. In the case of a communicable disease, for instance, only those who are not infected are counted in the numerator. The period over which new cases are contracted is also significant because it provides the denominator for at-risk individuals. On top of that, the ability to readily observe new events with monitoring and reporting systems cannot be overstated. As cited in the literature at hand, especially in research regarding effective public health interventions, an understanding of incidence calculation subtleties and context can play a vital role in deciding upon health policy and preventive interventions (John et al., 2004). In addition, incidence data use is not merely a calculation; it plays a critical role in guiding interventions and evaluating public health interventions. In antimicrobial use studies, incidence rates can be used to elucidate the correlation between trends in drug consumption and disease events. A sound measurement system for antimicrobial exposure has the potential to offer valuable comparisons over time and across populations (Hémonic et al., 2017). Understanding incidence allows health practitioners to recognize patterns regarding many factors, including demographic changes, environmental influences, and accessibility to healthcare. Finally, accurate incidence calculation promotes wise decision-making in health interventions, which ultimately results in improved health outcomes and disease control measures within populations (Figure 2.8).

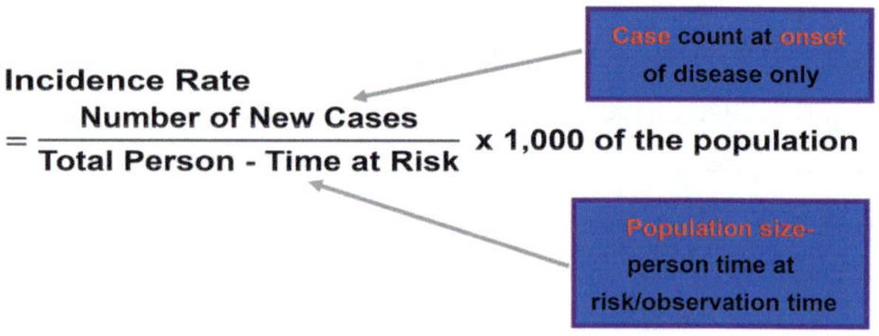

Figure 2.8. Incidence rate/density.

Source: https://i0.wp.com/immersionconcept.com/wp-content/uploads/2023/09/Screenshot-2023-09-18-214052.png?w=901&ssl=1.

2.3.2. Cumulative Incidence vs. Incidence Rate

In the measurement of disease frequency, it is of utmost significance within the area of research to distinguish between incidence rate and cumulative incidence so that disease occurrence dynamics among populations can be measured effectively. Cumulative incidence provides the proportion of a population that develops a disease within a specified time period and is very useful in describing the risk of disease within a specified cohort. This estimate is based on the premise that all members of the population are at risk for the entire duration of the study, thus giving a straightforward expression of risk that is routinely applied in public health surveillance. However, one should point out that the cumulative incidence does not take into account the duration for which each member is in the risk pool and may thereby result in oversimplification of the risk of disease, especially in studies with varying follow-up times or population loss to follow-up. Incidence rate, on the other hand, describes a more specific measurement of disease frequency in terms of accounting for the time at risk for each individual and providing a rate that represents the new occurrences in a specified unit of person-time. This type of measurement allows researchers to quantify alterations in the occurrence of disease over time while accounting for the exact time period when each participant is at risk. Through the employment of person-time, the incidence rate is able to indicate the speed with which a disease advances in a population, a particularly beneficial practice when researching rapidly evolving health crises or illnesses with fluctuating exposure duration. This differentiation points toward the importance of selecting appropriate measures on the basis of the question one seeks to answer in the research, for example, understanding long-term diseases or evaluating the effect of interventions on outcomes in health. Both cumulative incidence and incidence rate are eventually combined, thus complementing epidemiologic studies in terms of relaying risk patterns and disease burden. Cumulative incidence is often preferred where the outcome takes precedence, especially when screening, as is evident in studies assessing the impact of screening mammography on overdiagnosis of breast cancer by age group (Barratt et al., 2018). On the other hand, the incidence rate is crucial to measure environmental determinants on health conditions, as studies evaluating the effect of air pollutants on pregnancy outcomes demonstrate how differences in exposure can affect disease occurrence over time (Carman et al., 2009). By strategically deploying such interventions, researchers can provide comprehensive accounts of trends in disease that inform public health responses and interventions aimed at minimizing the risk of disease in populations.

2.3.3. Importance of Incidence in Public Health

Incidence, the rate of new or newly diagnosed cases of disease in a specified group within a fixed period of time, is a building block for public health activities. Incidence rates are crucial to know in order to identify and track trends in health occurrences so that public health practitioners can systematically allocate resources. For example, rising incidence rates of certain cancers can stimulate targeted screening programs or prevention interventions in certain groups. Incidence monitoring also allows for early detection of outbreaks, including infectious disease surveillance, where new cases are quickly reported and addressed. In this way, the strategic use of incidence data not only informs policy but maximizes overall health intervention efficiency aimed at reducing disease prevalence and maximizing health outcomes in populations. Second, incidence measurement can have a dramatic influence on research and education activities within public health. By analyzing changing incidence patterns, investigators are best equipped to identify the causal risk factors responsible for disease emergence or expansion. For instance, studies on sexually transmitted disease prevalence among some groups, i.e., men who have sex with men, can identify health behaviors and social determinants influencing health outcomes. Such insight is then used to inform public education campaigns and curricula designed to cut risk, such as in the KABaSTI study, which measured knowledge and behavior towards sexually transmitted diseases among men who have sex with men in Germany (Velasco et al., 2025). Thus, the meaning of incidence extends beyond mere statistical computation; it underpins a proactive policy towards public health education and intervention. Besides its role in guiding effective health policy and education, incidence measurement is also helpful in providing information on the contrasts between health outcomes among various subpopulations. Understanding who gets affected and to what extent assists public health practitioners in the application of targeted interventions directed to address specific needs. For example, religious health in cancer survivors, as determined in a study comparing breast and cervical cancer patients, indicates dramatic variation according to religious activity and uncertainty (Sari et al., 2019). This evidence emphasizes the importance of a thorough understanding of incidence across various cohorts. By addressing the unique requirements of diverse groups in a population, public health interventions can be better planned to incorporate and address disparities in health. Therefore, the value of incidence measurement lies in its capacity to guide fair, relevant, and effective health measures.

2.4. Mortality Rates: Measuring Deaths

Death rates are quantified as a focal point in understanding public health as well as assessing the impact of diseases on populations. Death rates are important in portraying the common condition of a population's well-being and can indicate the severity of health crises. Through focusing on specific populations and applying varied measurements such as crude mortality rates, age-specific mortality rates, and cause-specific mortality rates, researchers and health practitioners are able to identify temporal trends and comparisons among groups. Such measures guide health policy, resource allocation, and the development of targeted interventions for reducing preventable mortality. Also, the understanding of mortality rates helps in evaluating healthcare systems and their capacity for disease control, thereby encouraging healthcare improvement in delivery and outcome. The determinants for mortality rates are numerous and diverse, with environmental, social, and biological influences. For instance, socioeconomic status, access to healthcare, and lifestyle play a monumental role in health status and, consequently, mortality rates. The impact of specific diseases, i.e., non-communicable or infectious diseases, can be explained more adequately with detailed mortality information. The study of populations afflicted by a given disease can yield insights into a complete picture of its burden and the effectiveness of existing interventions. In addition, the evidence of maternal health contribution, as evidenced by studies on glycyrrhizin consumption during pregnancy, illustrates how certain behaviors influence elements such as birth weight and gestational age, affecting infant and newborn mortality. These observations underscore the relevance of integrative approaches to public health research. Further, it is important to understand the immune response to disease based on mortality rates, especially for extremely infectious diseases like those caused by *Trypanosoma cruzi*. From scientific research on the immune response of such pathogens, it is reported that the protective immunity is in a complicated interaction with potential immunopathological consequences, which may influence mortality rates. The role of single immune cells, i.e., CD8+ T cells, highlights the importance of immune competence in clinical outcome and prediction of mortality. Increased frequencies of T. cruzi-specific T-cell responses are linked to enhanced survival, which highlights how the qualities of immune response can have a direct impact on infectious disease-related mortality. As we collaborate towards improving health conditions and interventions, understanding these underlying mechanisms will enhance our measurement potential and ultimately decrease mortality rates in intended populations, which will continue to bring about further public health progress (Figure 2.9).

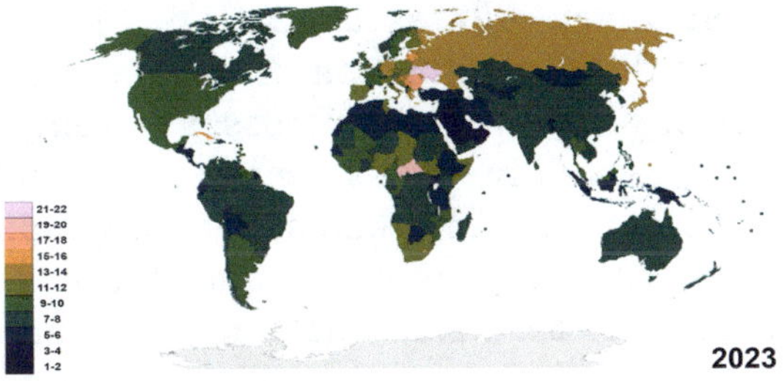

Figure 2.9. Mortality rate of countries, deaths per thousand.

Source: https://upload.wikimedia.org/wikipedia/commons/7/7f/Mortality_Rate_Map_by_Country.svg.

2.4.1. Definition and Calculation of Mortality Rates

The mortality rates are crucial in the description of disease frequency and how it relates to public health. The mortality rate, which refers to the number of deaths in a population over a specific time period, is a critical measure of the population's health. It is typically expressed per 1,000 individuals to facilitate standardized comparison of populations from various groups. Crude mortality rate focuses on overall causes of death in their undifferentiated form, but age-specific and cause-specific mortality rates retain more information regarding the risk of mortality in various populations. The ability to differentiate between these rates not only facilitates easier identification of health disparities but also enables policymakers to allocate resources best in areas of higher risk of mortality. Epidemiological study developments generally rely on precise mortality measures in an effort to evaluate the effectiveness of health interventions and identify the disease burdens (Basombrío et al., 2009). The estimation of mortality rates calls for meticulous aggregation and processing of data based on established epidemiological criteria. Data collected by public health researchers and policymakers tend to be from registries of vital statistics, which provide data on mortality and births, as well as population data. Once data are gathered, statistical formulas are applied by researchers to determine various types of mortality rates. Crude mortality rate, for instance, is determined through the formula of total deaths divided by mid-year population multiplied by 1,000. Further stratification by age or cause makes it more informative about specific patterns of mortality that the crude rate could not detect. Trend analysis of mortality gives the basis to assess interventions and public health programs, such as vaccination programs aimed at reducing disease-related mortality, hence overall population health (Järvenpää et al., 2001). Mortality rate calculations have more than mere statistical interest; they are fundamental in guiding health policies and interpreting epidemiological trends. For instance, a rising mortality rate may trigger urgent public health intervention, highlighting the need for effective disease prevention or health change. On top of that, certain populations may experience greater mortality rates due to certain socio-economic status, access to healthcare services, or cultural practices. Detailed analysis of mortality rates thus identifies vulnerable groups, which assists in alleviating health inequities with targeted interventions. By analyzing mortality rates with other health measures, researchers are able to create a wide-ranging picture of community health to inform governmental and organizational policy that results in healthier populations and improved quality of life (Basombrío et al., 2009) (Figure 2.10).

$$\text{Mortality Rate} = \frac{\text{Number of Deaths Recorded}}{\text{Number of People in the Population}}$$

Figure 2.10. Formula to calculate mortality rate.

Source: https://www.learntocalculate.com/wp-content/uploads/2020/08/mortality-rate.png.

2.4.2. Crude vs. Age-Specific Mortality Rates

In an epidemiological study, the difference between crude and age-specific mortality is vital for accurately assessing disease frequency within populations. Crude mortality rate is a basic measure of deaths within a population over a specified period relative to the total population. However, it does not account for variations in mortality between different age groups, which can result in misleading interpretations. For instance, a population with a high proportion of older individuals can potentially experience an increased crude death rate solely due to aging impacts, but not necessarily due to overall health conditions. Thus, the application of crude rates alone can conceal the concealed health dynamics and lead to possibly wrong conclusions about the effectiveness of public health interventions or the true disease burden among different demographic groups. Alternatively, age-specific mortality rates focus this estimate by presenting a more precise picture of mortality risk within delineated age groups. The division of data by age enables researchers to identify trends and differences that could be masked in crude mortality rates. For example, in one recent retrospective study, the percentage of transmissible infections in blood donors was evaluated, and it was indicated that younger first-time donors were characterized by different levels of infection compared to older ones (Dulaimi, 2016). These results highlight the importance of taking age-related risk into account, which is very relevant in disease prevention and health promotion programs. Moreover, age-specific information provides for efficient resource allocation, targeting interventions to those who are most at risk—potentially reducing total mortality within those specific age brackets and enhancing public health. In addition to simple recognition of mortality inequality, the implication of comparing crude to age-specific rates extends beyond descriptive purposes to policy and research uses. Policy-makers would prefer crude rates due to ease when presenting health statistics to the public, but in the absence of cautionary contextualization, this can result in the dissemination of misinformation concerning health risks across different age groups. Secondly, age-specific death rates are a very useful instrument for longitudinal analysis, such that one can quantify change over time. For example, a meta-analysis pointed out that systemic therapies for some illnesses experienced mixed effectiveness depending on the age of patients, further emphasizing the necessity of sophisticated data analysis (Ballin et al., 1994). This means that, for a complete understanding of disease frequency among human beings, a comparison of both crude and age-standardized mortality rates is necessary to enable informed decision-making and specific health measures that suitably meet the specific needs of various age groups.

2.4.3. Implications of Mortality Data in Health Policy

Mortality data analysis is important in guiding health policy decisions since it provides a perspective on disease burden among populations. Through the analysis of mortality rates, health authorities can distinctly identify prevalent conditions that cause mortality, which in turn guides resource planning and focused intervention. For instance, information regarding the disease burden of conditions such as anemia, cited in a study conducted in Kazakhstani data, allows policymakers to direct their action against some health issues that disproportionately affect specific groups, such as adult non-pregnant women who show significant levels of iron deficiency anemia (Dangour et al., 2001).

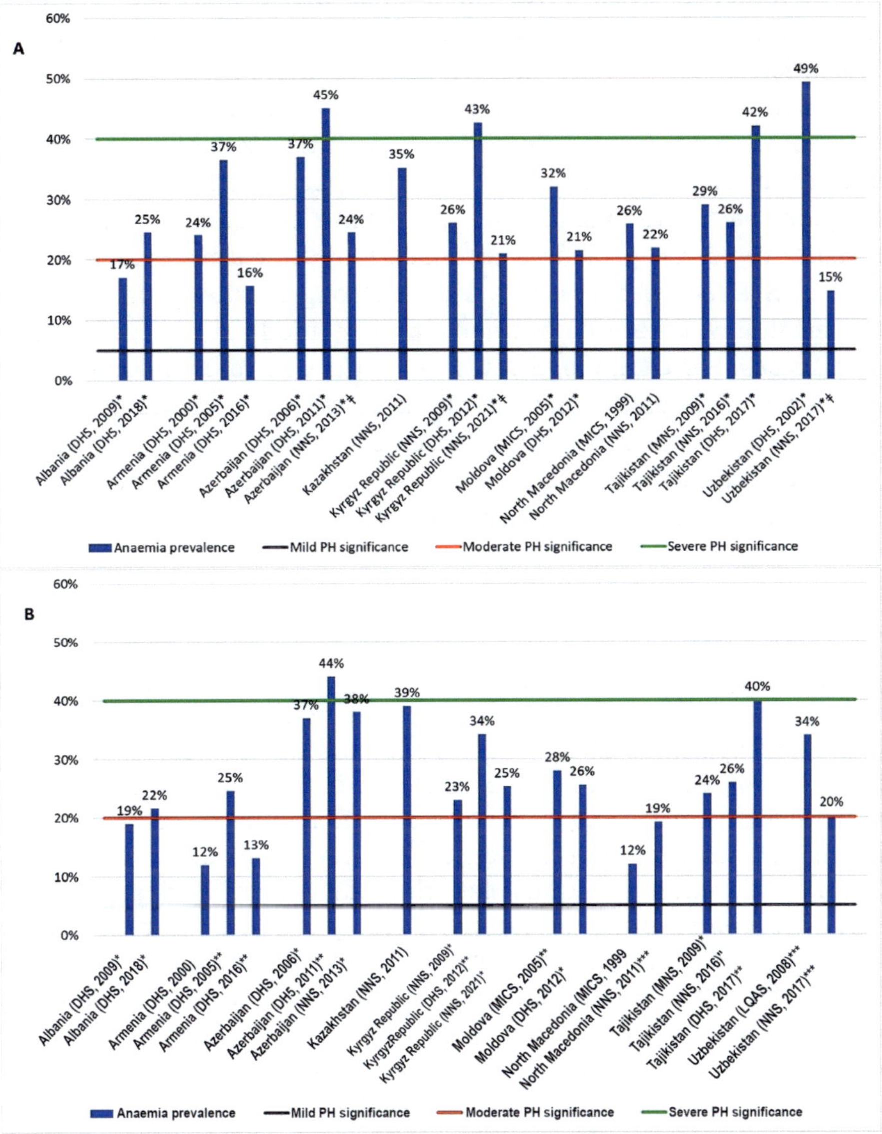

Figure 2.11. Prevalence of anemia among preschool children (PSC) (A); and women of reproductive age (WRA) (B); latest available data and change over time since 1999, for ECA countries with national survey data. Cut-offs shown for WHO categorization of public health (PH) significance of anemia based on prevalence estimated from blood hemoglobin.

Source: https://ars.els-cdn.com/content/image/1-s2.0-S2475299124024119-gr1_lrg.jpg.

Targeted interventions of this sort can yield more effective public health initiatives that not only lower death rates but also improve the overall health of the general population. Furthermore, beyond the determination of imminent health problems, the implications of mortality data also elucidate systemic inequalities in the delivery of health care. In developing countries, as an example, research has established extreme disparities within the availability of health care personnel, which have a tendency to be linked to death rates among marginalized groups (Wagstaff et al., 2009). Research that controls for a variety of health care needs indicators indicates that death rates can uncover hidden inequities, directing policymakers towards interventions that are critically needed. Such disparities are identifiable, allowing health policies to be substantively developed in a way that addresses differences in access and quality of care, ultimately aiming to improve the health status of marginalized populations and public health impact. Lastly, using mortality numbers in health policymaking also serves to evaluate existing health programs and interventions. Ongoing monitoring of mortality rates can provide a feedback loop that can be used to tell public health strategies over time how effective they are. Without strong mortality data, health policymakers will be unable to determine whether interventions implemented have succeeded in lowering death rates from certain diseases. For example, if rates of deaths due to communicable diseases reduce following a series of immunization campaigns, this is an effective public health intervention that should continue to receive investment and reinforcement (Dangour et al., 2001). Rather, stagnant or rising mortality rates may necessitate a review of policies and interventions to ensure that resources are being used well to resist diseases with the greatest impact on health (Figure 2.11).

2.5. Data Sources for Disease Frequency

Estimation of the frequency of disease among human populations is largely reliant on diverse and reliable sources of data. One of the principal sources is epidemiologic studies, which can be broadly categorized into experimental and observational studies. Observational studies, such as cross-sectional, case-control, and cohort studies, allow scientists to quantify disease incidence and prevalence under real-world conditions, collecting data that reflects actual-world exposures and outcomes. Such studies are invaluable in the sense that they tell us about the causes and trends of health outcomes within different populations. Experimental designs such as randomized controlled trials, however, offer strict control of variables, and causality can be determined. Through combining findings from both study designs, scientists can generate an elaborate and detailed image of disease frequency that can guide public health interventions and policies to mitigate the causes of ill health. Apart from traditional epidemiological studies, databases and registries of health are fundamental sources of information to understand disease frequency. National and regional cancer registries, for instance, gather detailed information on cancer incidence and survival, and allow for the examination of trends over time and geographic variation. These registries gather information from a number of health care facilities, and give a comprehensive view of disease patterns that can be stratified by demographic criteria like age and sex. Furthermore, administrative health databases used to track healthcare use and outcomes offer a wealth of information regarding the burden of chronic disease in populations. Such advanced methods of data collection enable real-time tracking of patterns of disease and contribute significantly to the development of targeted public health interventions to improve health outcomes. Lastly, integration of data from multiple sources enhances the analysis of the frequency of disease. New tools and techniques make it possible for researchers to incorporate environmental, genetic, and lifestyle information into epidemiological studies. As has been described in Burke et al. (2011), for example, the new fields of genomics and biomonitoring provide the promise of integrating chemical exposures with health impacts, thus giving a broader view of the etiology of disease. In addition, predictive models that merge food intake data with eating patterns can establish how diet contributes to disease frequency, as outlined in Dekker et al. (2002). With these dynamic data sources, epidemiologists can develop improved frameworks that more comprehensively outline disease risk factors, and interventions can be performed more efficiently. The dynamics between these heterogeneous sources offer enriching disease frequency analysis, eventually yielding improved public health outcomes and reactions (Figure 2.12).

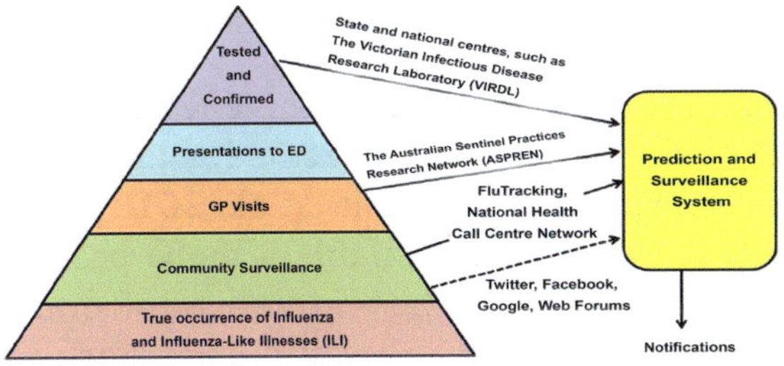

Figure 2.12. Disease prevalence pyramid and notification data sources; dotted line is proposed.

Source: https://www.researchgate.net/profile/Anthony-Nguyen-16/publication/274965027/figure/fig3/AS:267485983277098@1440785036937/Disease-prevalence-pyramid-and-notification-data-sources-dotted-line-is-proposed.png.

2.5.1. Surveillance Systems

Surveillance systems are valuable instruments in the quantification of disease frequency among human populations and are valuable for efficient infectious disease monitoring and control. Active and passive surveillance can be broadly classified as surveillance systems. Active surveillance involves active collection of data by continuous outreach and testing, while passive surveillance relies on health workers' reporting of health events. The functioning of these systems has direct implications for public health interventions. For instance, studies have established that passive surveillance can be highly sensitive using a full dataset, thus suggesting that even low-cost approaches may be able to generate very insightful information on patterns of disease. This is most relevant in resource-poor environments where the use of sophisticated active systems is normally out of reach (Barbara et al., 2015). Developing robust surveillance networks is, therefore, key to knowing and being able to react to public health crises. Reliability in surveillance systems can influence the course of disease control interventions. Relying on the Swedish experience with bovine tuberculosis, applying a tuberculin testing control program highlighted the complexities in human health surveillance (Wahlström et al., 2004). The challenges that veterinarians face, particularly with regard to providing reliable tests due to variation in skill and experience, illustrate how similar issues can be experienced in human health delivery contexts. Quality indicators, for instance, baseline information and training to health staff, may facilitate surveillance activity efficiency by minimizing variation in reporting and measurement of disease. It is thus essential to have funding for capacity building and training in surveillance systems since it can render collected data more accurate and, therefore, improve disease frequency measures. Additionally, improvements in technology are increasingly affecting what disease surveillance systems are like. The intersection of technology and data analysis has increased the capacity to collect, analyze, and transmit information regarding health in a timely manner. Such technologies facilitate real-time monitoring of disease outbreaks and the improvement in the timeliness of public health interventions.

For instance, during disease outbreaks, mobile technology in reporting and tracing can offer real-time information about transmission and patterns of infections, which is essential for initiating a response quickly. With increasing evidence mounting regarding the benefits of these technologies, understanding their potential in the construction of effective surveillance systems is essential. Lastly, developing a culture of relentless evolution and resilience in surveillance designs ensures that disease frequency measurement is both practical and actionable, paving the way for improved public health outcomes (Figure 2.13).

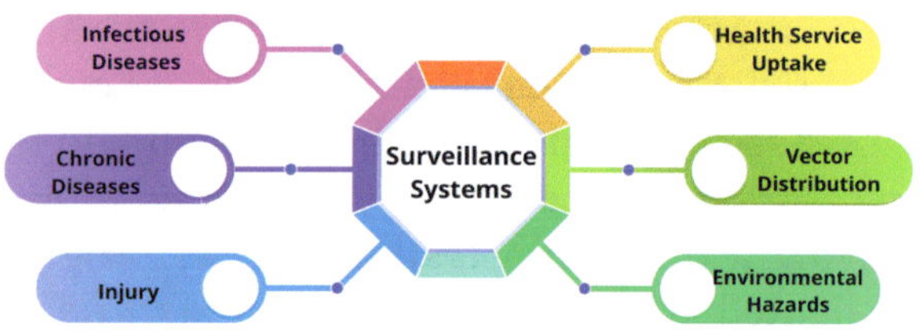

Figure 2.13. Indicators of useful surveillance systems.

Source: https://publichealthprepared.org/wp-content/uploads/2022/09/Evaluating-Surv-System-Image-1080x675.png.

2.5.2. Health Surveys

Surveys of health are crucial in disease frequency estimation in human populations and represent an exhaustive way of accumulating data on determinants, conditions, and behaviors for health. Surveys of health can adopt various methodologies, like cross-sectional, longitudinal, and case-control studies, depending on the research question. Information from health surveys not only facilitates comprehension of the incidence and prevalence of conditions but also informs public health interventions and policies. For instance, surveys that provide evidence of exposure to potential risk factors facilitate explaining associations between behaviors, for instance, handling practices for poultry and diseases, avian influenza, and thus inform prevention interventions among at-risk populations (Ahad et al., 2017). With the increasing depth and breadth of health surveys, they can generate more specific information needed to quantify disease frequency in a broad context and create public health programs targeted towards specified goals. Further, the use of more advanced methods of survey adds validity and utility to the results of health surveys. Techniques such as matched surveys enable scientists to connect human activities with specific environmental exposure, for instance, in studies concerning the malaria vectors and human relationships. By examining how frequently individuals are exposed to vectors indoors and outdoors, health surveys have the capability to provide essential measures that guide vector control interventions, for instance, the effectiveness of bed nets treated with insecticides and indoor residual spraying (Abdulla et al., 2013). These quantitative analyses enable a more profound understanding of the influence of human behavior on disease transmission patterns. On this account, health surveys that adopt new approaches are pivotal to evidence-informed decision-making in epidemiology and public health and ultimately contribute to improved health outcomes through disease prevalence reduction. Lastly, potential pitfalls in health surveys should be handled with utmost care to ensure the collection of high-quality, actionable data. Difficulties such as respondent bias, error in sampling, and the complexity of measuring practice behavior can complicate the interpretation of survey results. For instance, studies on poultry handling practices within markets and households revealed heterogeneity in prevalence that complicates how to translate results to effective public health interventions (Ahad et al., 2017). Additionally, understanding the determinants of some health behaviors necessitates combining epidemiological surveys with qualitative research techniques. This holistic viewpoint can explain the intrinsic incentives that guide health-related decisions, thus enhancing the efficacy of interventions aimed at reducing disease frequency among human populations. By acknowledging and addressing these problems, health surveys can further evolve as key tools towards measurement and prevention of the disease burden (Figure 2.14).

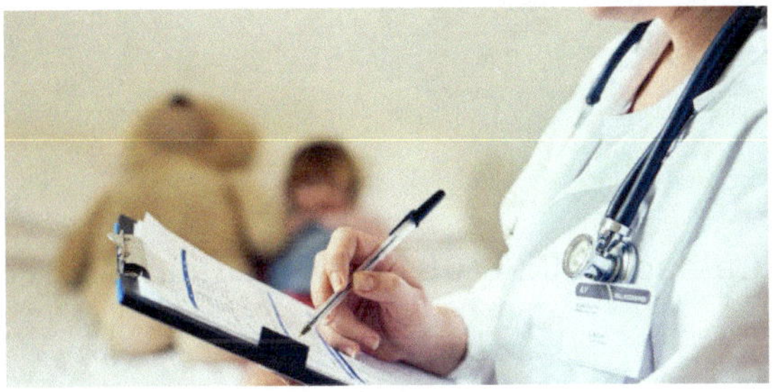

Figure 2.14. Health surveys.

Source: https://www.surveycrest.com/blog/wp-content/uploads/2022/07/Healthcare-Surveys.jpg.

2.5.3. Hospital and Clinical Records

Utilization of hospital and clinical records is a built-in component of the measurement of disease frequency in human beings and generates a plethora of data for application in bolstering epidemiologic research. The records yield a diverse collection of patient information, such as demographics, history of disease, treatment regimen, and outcomes, all of which are critical in defining trends of disease in patients. Through systematic analysis of such records, researchers are able to quantify the incidence and prevalence of various diseases, which allows for the identification of high-risk groups and the implementation of targeted interventions. For example, longitudinal studies tracing the health of patients over time can determine trends in disease incidence, which will contribute to improved understanding of diseases such as COPD. This integrated approach emphasizes the supervisory role of accurate and complete record-keeping in clinical settings. Additionally, the advancement in electronic health records (EHRs) has revolutionized the collection and evaluation of clinical information, so that electronic measures of quality of care are constructed from clinical and hospital records. As illustrated through a number of provider organizations, merging EHR data into models of quality assessment has been challenging and rewarding. Among the key benefits is the provision for easy extraction and analysis of huge amounts of data, which is helpful in monitoring health patterns and measuring the efficacy of treatments. The application of the indicators is, however, not without challenges, particularly with respect to standardizing and combining data from various healthcare systems. Such problems can undermine the accuracy of disease frequency estimates, and the need to further improve EHRs to maximize their utility for monitoring population health cannot be overstated.

Moreover, the relation between objective clinical-record-based measurements and self-reported measures cannot be overestimated. In studies of diseases like COPD, objective data from continuous monitors can be aligned with subjective patient reports, providing an overall view of disease impact. For instance, a recent study employing systems for cough monitoring demonstrated the significant decrease in the frequency of cough after acute exacerbation of COPD, and such patterns were recognizable through continuous monitoring systems (Crooks et al., 2017). Such results can optimize clinicians' potential for quantifying the severity of the disease and the patterns of recovery, in turn affecting clinical practice. The synergy between hospital records and advanced data gathering methods illustrates the significant role that diligent record-keeping has in enhancing the measurement of disease frequency and overall patient care in contemporary healthcare facilities (Brian et al., 2008) (Figure 2.15).

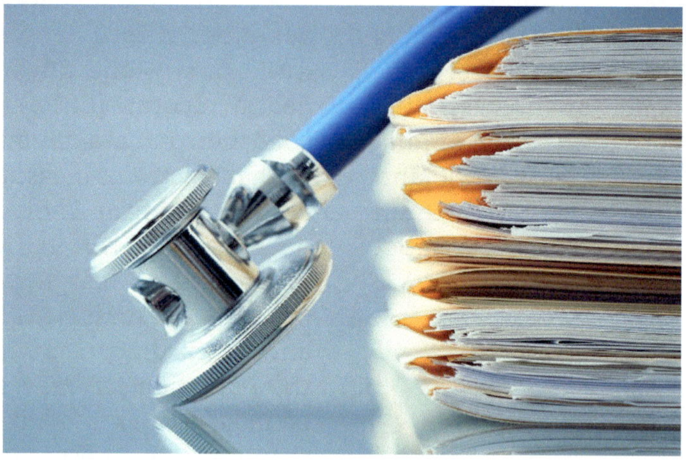

Figure 2.15. Clinical records.

Source: https://www.247digitize.com/wp-content/uploads/2021/08/Why-Medical-Records-Management-Is-Essential-for-Healthcare-Providers.jpg.

Summary

In short, measurement of disease frequency in humans is a significant component of public health surveillance and epidemiological research. By measuring the frequency of occurrence of diseases in specific populations, scientists can identify trends, detect susceptible groups, and efficiently allocate resources. For instance, understanding the population genetics of diseases such as trypanosomiasis, specifically *Trypanosoma brucei* rhodesiense, is crucial in managing the disease. Studies suggest that the T. b. rhodesiense gene pool varies geographically, demonstrating patterns consistent with the complexity of host relationships and environment (MacLeod et al., 2013). Such identification not only adds to our understanding of transmission disease but also to intervention, slowing outbreaks and improving health outcomes on a larger scale as well. In addition, the methodology for measuring disease frequency is crucial to arriving at significant summations from epidemiological data. Traditional methods, like prevalence and incidence rates, constitute fundamental measures that guide healthcare policy and research initiatives. The growing application of microsatellite markers in measuring genetic differences in pathogens is a key advancement in the field. These exacting analyses help to inform a greater understanding of how genetic transmission among disease-causing pathogens might affect transmission and virulence (Mansour et al., 2011). Eventually, improved measurement tools will help us to predict improvements in tracing the epidemiology of disease as well as designing targeted public health responses. Lastly, the consequences of measuring disease frequency accurately extend beyond individual health measures; they have implications for more general societal policy. With enhanced data, public health practitioners can plan more effective educational campaigns, enhance surveillance networks, and model healthcare delivery to suit the needs of diverse populations. This is particularly critical in regions where pathogens such as those caused by *Trypanosoma brucei* rhodesiense remain endemic. Through an acceptance of the complexities and difficulties in measuring the frequency of disease, all stakeholders are capable of facilitating collaboration that transcends traditional silos, ultimately producing a healthier world population. Hence, continued investment in research and innovation in disease measurement methods is necessary to propel public health programs forward and attain effective disease control.

Measurement of disease frequency is crucial in establishing disease prevalence and incidence rates in human populations. The measurements are necessary to provide public health officials with the required information to effectively use resources and form evidence-based interventions. Prevalence is employed to quantify the rate of disease in the population at any particular time, while incidence quantifies the number of new cases that develop within a specific time period. Understanding these differences is significant to correctly interpreting epidemiological data. These true measurements serve as the foundation for informing policy related to health and guiding research aimed at decreasing disease burden. Without measurement, thus, public health programs would lack empirical support to make substantial changes in disease control efforts. With the prevalence and incidence definitions, these need to be discussed regarding varying methodologies for their data collection. Registries and surveys are utilized most frequently to obtain disease occurrence data; however, bias in data collection can obscure the reliability of results. Cohort, case-control, and cross-sectional studies offer different strengths of measurement of disease frequency, and with varying impacts on results. For instance, longitudinal cohort studies are able to track over time, but may require considerable resources and effort to keep participants. The choice of methodology impacts not only the validity of the data but also its applicability to real health scenarios. Practitioners consequently must critically assess their methods to present accurate representations of disease prevalence among human populations. Furthermore, disease frequency measurement is important beyond its statistical application, influencing policy, funding, and health communication. Accurate disease incidence and prevalence measurements guide health education programs and disease awareness campaigns, specifically in addressing community needs. For instance, knowledge about the elevated rates of disease occurrence among specific groups may offer improved screening programs for such groups. Besides that, reporting such findings in the arena of social determinants of health and health equity enhances public understanding about disease risks and disparities. To improve health outcomes effectively, stakeholders must be provided with data on the frequency of disease in ways that transcend statistical calculation to create actionable strategies that address the root causes of disease occurrence and facilitate preventive health interventions.

CLOSER LOOK

THE ROLE OF DISEASE FREQUENCY MEASUREMENT IN PUBLIC HEALTH

In public health, disease frequency is quantified to identify the patterns of population health and to map newly emerging conditions. Through systematic estimation of incidence and prevalence of diseases, health officials can map patterns on which resource allocation, policy, and intervention can be planned. Measurement is the cornerstone of epidemiological research, enabling researchers to identify high-risk groups and measure the effectiveness of public health interventions. For instance, if the prevalence of chronic disease in a given population is found to be on the rise, particular interventions in health may be designed to address lifestyle factors behind the trend. Therefore, precise measurement of disease frequency is an important tool in advancing health equity and optimizing public health interventions.

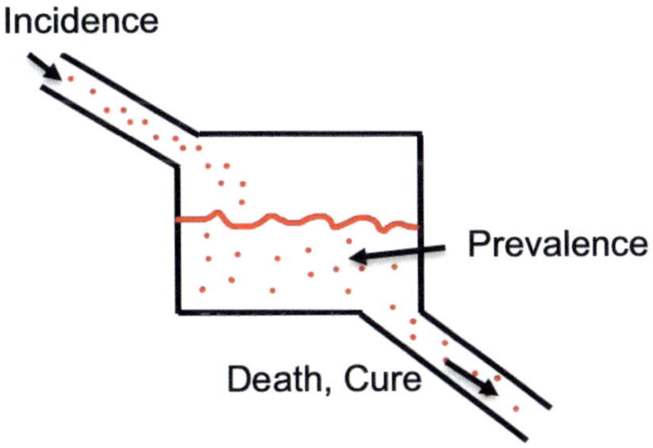

Figure 2.16. Conceptual diagram illustrating the relationship between incidence, prevalence, and outcomes such as death or cure in epidemiology.

Source: https://upload.medbullets.com/topic/101004/images/incidence_prevalence.jpg.

Besides, understanding disease frequency dynamics offers the foundation for using evidence-based prevention and harm reduction strategies. Culturally based education and community participation, according to research, are essential ingredients of effective public health interventions. Motivational interviewing (MI)-based programs have the potential to facilitate behavior change by resolving ambivalence to the uptake of healthier ways of living (N/A, 2020). On recognizing the specific barriers to various populations, public health organizations can thus adjust their strategies such that disease incidence is brought down effectively, most significantly cardiovascular disorders, which are key healthcare burdens. The aim here is not only to quantify how often the disease occurs but also to interpret the findings as a proper action plan that may lead to concrete improvement in the population's health outcomes. Measurement of disease frequency becomes all the more significant in the context of containing infectious diseases such as HIV. Public health officials can identify clusters of people with higher transmission levels using molecular epidemiology, highlighting the role viral loads can play in guiding infection dynamics. The synergy between viral load and transmission underlines the need for ongoing follow-up and adaptive public health interventions targeted at high-risk populations. Data indicate that individuals in larger transmission networks are more likely to have greater viral loads, and therefore, there is a pressing need to act in targeted prevention in those places (Campbell et al., 2019). This sophisticated understanding of disease frequency measurement is important for effective combat against infectious diseases and for ensuring timely as well as scientifically founded public health interventions (Figure 2.16).

References

1. Abdulla, S., Bayoh, N., Briët, O., Diallo, D., et al. (2013). Consistently high estimates for the proportion of human exposure to malaria vector populations occurring indoors in rural Africa. https://core.ac.uk/download/13116593.pdf (accessed on 25th June 2025).
2. Abel, P., Ahmed, H. U., Akehurst, G., Almquist, H., et al. (2017). A core outcome set for localized prostate cancer effectiveness trials. https://core.ac.uk/download/80698016.pdf (accessed on 25th June 2025).
3. Adams, C., Briggs, J., Fallahkhair, S., Iluyemi, A., et al. (2012). M-health review: Joining up healthcare in a wireless world. https://core.ac.uk/download/29582923.pdf (accessed on 25th June 2025).
4. Agresti, A., Egenvall, A., Gough, A., Kathrani, A., Kyriazis, A., Peiravan, A., German, A. J., et al. (2017). Demography and disorders of German Shepherd Dogs under primary veterinary care in the UK. https://core.ac.uk/download/84659839.pdf (accessed on 25th June 2025).
5. Ahad, A., Allen, H., Areechokchai, D., Aunger, R., Barennes, H., Barennes, H., et al. (2017). A systematic review and meta-analysis of practices exposing humans to avian influenza viruses, their prevalence, and rationale. https://core.ac.uk/download/82968871.pdf (accessed on 25th June 2025).
6. Alexander, A. A., Buxbaum, J. N., Garvey, W. T., Jacobson, D. R., et al. (2016). The prevalence and distribution of the amyloidogenic transthyretin (TTR) V122I allele in Africa. https://core.ac.uk/download/98337502.pdf (accessed on 25th June 2025).
7. Alwan, A., Yeung, A., Supina, A. L., Pickard, A. S., Lam, C. L. K., Dowdy, D. W., Pappa, E., et al. (2013). Health-related quality of life as measured with EQ-5D among populations with and without specific chronic conditions: A population-based survey in Shaanxi province, China. https://core.ac.uk/download/18488584.pdf (accessed on 25th June 2025).
8. Ambayo, H., Bouwman, J., Bronselaer, A., De Baets, B., et al. (2019). An ontology to standardize research output of nutritional epidemiology: From paper-based standards to linked content. https://core.ac.uk/download/222452585.pdf (accessed on 25th June 2025).
9. Antonopoulos, D. A., Armitage, G., AVA Singapore, Azad, M. B., Bäckhed, F., Schneeman, B. O., et al. (2019). Establishing what constitutes a healthy human gut microbiome: State of the science, regulatory considerations, and future directions. https://core.ac.uk/download/323068488.pdf (accessed on 25th June 2025).
10. Aprili, G. (2008). Safety in transfusion medicine. *Blood Transfusion = Trasfusione del Sangue, 6*(3), 121–126. https://www.semanticscholar.org/paper/2b352a67f2d6d11887ec0d9ee5cd7a12568c11f1 (accessed on 25th June 2025).
11. Ballin, S., Antman, E., Neuhaus, K., Essen, R., Tebbe, U., Jessel, A., Heinrichs, H., et al. (1994). The role of cardiovascular research and clinical training in health care reform. *Circulation, 90*(4), 1611–1612. https://www.semanticscholar.org/paper/a506d419ef54d136057e00ad521bc61066572d39 (accessed on 25th June 2025).
12. Barratt, A., Bell, K., Glasziou, P. P., Houssami, N., et al. (2018). Overdiagnosis due to screening mammography for women aged 40 years and over. https://core.ac.uk/download/196606884.pdf (accessed on 25th June 2025).

13. Basombrío, M. Á. M., Padilla, Á. M., & Ramoneda, C. M. P. (2009). Protective immunity against *Trypanosoma cruzi*. https://core.ac.uk/download/159300953.pdf (accessed on 25th June 2025).

14. Bassett, A. (2019). *Evaluating the Epidemiology and Management of Bovine Congestive Heart Failure*. https://core.ac.uk/download/288431601.pdf (accessed on 25th June 2025).

15. Belafsky, P. C., Della Maggiore, A., Fulton, A., Garcia, K., et al. (2017). Prevalence of gastroesophageal reflux in cats during anesthesia and effect of omeprazole on gastric pH. https://core.ac.uk/download/323069592.pdf (accessed on 25th June 2025).

16. Borghans, J. A. M., Borghans, L., & Weel, B. (2025). Is there a link between economic outcomes and genetic evolution? Cross-country evidence from the major histocompatibility complex. https://core.ac.uk/download/pdf/6936921.pdf (accessed on 25th June 2025).

17. Boston, J. R., Durrant, J., & Huang, E. (2011). On the mechanism of response latencies in auditory nerve fibers. https://core.ac.uk/download/12210392.pdf (accessed on 25th June 2025).

18. Bowman, A., Dowell, F. J., Evans, N. P., Scottish SPCA, et al. (2017). The effect of different genres of music on the stress levels of kennelled dogs. https://core.ac.uk/download/80696791.pdf (accessed on 25th June 2025).

19. Burke, T. A., Fox, M. A., Nachman, K. E., Rodricks, D., et al. (2011). Leveraging epidemiology to improve risk assessment. https://core.ac.uk/download/323074701.pdf (accessed on 25th June 2025).

20. Campbell, A., & Rudan, I. (2011). Systematic review of birth cohort studies in Africa. https://core.ac.uk/download/28973487.pdf (accessed on 25th June 2025).

21. Campbell, E., Heneine, W., Johnson, J. A., Oster, A. M., et al. (2019). Natural selection favoring more transmissible HIV detected in United States molecular transmission network. https://core.ac.uk/download/323065212.pdf (accessed on 25th June 2025).

22. Carman, A. E. (2009). *Ambient Air Toxic Releases and Adverse Pregnancy Outcomes in Allegheny County, Pennsylvania*. https://core.ac.uk/download/12206720.pdf (accessed on 25th June 2025).

23. Cevallos, M., Dohoo, I., Egger, M., Erb, H., et al. (2016). Explanation and elaboration document for the STROBE-Vet statement: Strengthening the reporting of observational studies in epidemiology—Veterinary extension. https://core.ac.uk/download/76980915.pdf (accessed on 25th June 2025).

24. Coleman, T. P., Gharibans, A. A., Kriegsfeld, L. J., Kunkel, D., et al. (2018). Artifact rejection methodology enables continuous, noninvasive measurement of gastric myoelectric activity in ambulatory subjects. https://core.ac.uk/download/323082131.pdf (accessed on 25th June 2025).

25. Colford, J. M., & Fewtrell, L. (2004). Water, sanitation and hygiene: Interventions and diarrhea–A systematic review and meta-analysis. https://core.ac.uk/download/71360183.pdf (accessed on 25th June 2025).

26. Cortez-Pinto, H., Melo, X., Pimenta, N., Santa-Clara, H., et al. (2016). Waist-to-hip ratio is related to body fat content and distribution regardless of the waist circumference measurement protocol, in non-alcoholic fatty liver disease patients. https://core.ac.uk/download/153231073.pdf (accessed on 25th June 2025).

27. Crooks, M. G., den Brinker, A., Hayman, Y., Hill, S. L., et al. (2017). Continuous cough monitoring using ambient sound recording during convalescence from a COPD exacerbation. https://core.ac.uk/download/151161835.pdf (accessed on 25th June 2025).

28. Curtis, K. M., Hannaford, P., Phillips, S. J., Polis, C. B., et al. (2014). Hormonal contraceptive methods and risk of HIV acquisition in women: A systematic review of epidemiological evidence. https://core.ac.uk/download/29151052.pdf (accessed on 25th June 2025).

29. Dangour, A. D., Hill, H. L., & Ismail, S. J. (2001). Hemoglobin status of adult non-pregnant Kazakh women living in Kzyl-Orda region, Kazakhstan.

30. Darling, K., Harris-Wai, J. N., Keagy, C., Obasogie, O. K., et al. (2015). Race in the life sciences: An empirical assessment, 1950–2000. https://core.ac.uk/download/144230409.pdf (accessed on 25th June 2025).

31. Das, M., Raymond, H., Chu, P., Nieves-Rivera, I., Pandori, M., Louie, B., Rauch, L., et al. (2013). Measuring the unknown: Calculating community viral load among HIV-infected MSM unaware of their HIV status in San Francisco from National HIV Behavioral Surveillance, 2004–2011. *Journal of Acquired Immune Deficiency Syndromes, 63*(2), e84–e86. https://www.semanticscholar.org/paper/c19492793b78f37bedf75c433a59c3915e552af0 (accessed on 25th June 2025).

32. Dekker, M., Jongen, W. M. F., & Plaami, S. P. (2002). Functional foods: A conceptual model for assessing their safety and effectiveness. https://core.ac.uk/download/pdf/29295489.pdf (accessed on 25th June 2025).

33. Dremin, V. V., Dunaev, A. V., Goltsov, A., Makovik, A., et al. (2019). Multimodal optical diagnostics of the microhemodynamics in upper and lower limbs. https://core.ac.uk/download/228178569.pdf (accessed on 25th June 2025).

34. Drove, B., Gifford, K. L., Gonzalez-Meijome, J. M., Gray, L., et al. (2019). IMI–Industry guidelines and ethical considerations for myopia control report. https://core.ac.uk/download/293867276.pdf (accessed on 25th June 2025).

35. Dueñas Rodríguez, M. Á., Failde Martínez, I., Ojeda, B., Salazar Couso, M. Á., et al. (2010). Health related quality of life in coronary patients. https://core.ac.uk/download/161360213.pdf (accessed on 25th June 2025).

36. Dulaimi, D. A. (2016). Recent advances in liver disease. *Gastroenterology and Hepatology from Bed to Bench, 9*, 150–152. https://www.semanticscholar.org/paper/97a3c6aabf626a89f163949da5ecf070c097d249 (accessed on 25th June 2025).

37. Gilhooly, K., Gilhooly, M., & Jones, R. B. (2008). Quality of life: Conceptual challenges in exploring the role of ICT in active ageing. https://core.ac.uk/download/336247.pdf (accessed on 25th June 2025).

38. Goll, A., & Meng, H. (2014). A smart tool for the diagnosis of Parkinsonian syndrome using wireless watches. https://core.ac.uk/download/29139347.pdf (accessed on 25th June 2025).

39. Häsler, B., Corner, L., Doherr, M. G., Subasinghe, D., Gilbert, W., Gongal, G., Hadorn, D., et al. (2015). Reconciling surveillance systems with limited resources: An evaluation of passive surveillance for rabies in an endemic setting. https://core.ac.uk/download/36778661.pdf (accessed on 25th June 2025).

40. Hazlehurst, B. L., Sittig, D. F., Kind, E. A., Krizak, J. T., Fowles, J. B., Weiner, J. P., Chan, K. S., et al. (2008). Performance measures using electronic health records: Five case studies. https://core.ac.uk/download/71353765.pdf (accessed on 25th June 2025).

41. Hémonic, A., Aarestrup, F., Achermann, Y., Adriaenssens, N., Agata, N., Agga, G. E., Akwar, H., et al. (2017). Guidance on the selection of appropriate indicators for quantification of antimicrobial usage in humans and animals. https://core.ac.uk/download/76980840.pdf (accessed on 25th June 2025).

42. Höglund, K. (2007). *Systolic Ejection Murmurs and The Left Ventricular Outflow Tract in Boxer Dogs*. https://core.ac.uk/download/11695170.pdf (accessed on 25th June 2025).

43. Ionova, T., Johns, J., Oliva, E. N., Salek, S., et al. (2018). Appraisal of patient-reported outcome measures in analogous diseases and recommendations for use in phase II and III clinical trials of pyruvate kinase deficiency. https://core.ac.uk/download/287581341.pdf (accessed on 25th June 2025).

44. Jansson Mörk, M. (2009). *Validation of Disease Recordings in Swedish Dairy Cattle*. https://core.ac.uk/download/11695440.pdf (accessed on 25th June 2025).

45. Järvenpää, A. L., McKeigue, P. M., Strandberg, T. E., & Vanhanen, H., et al. (2001). Birth outcome in relation to licorice consumption during pregnancy.

46. Kakkar, M., Shah, N. K., Sekar, N., & Abbas, S. S. (2011). Research options for controlling zoonotic disease in India, 2010–2015. https://core.ac.uk/download/19765602.pdf (accessed on 25th June 2025).

47. MacLeod, A., MacLeod, A., MacLeod, A., Tait, A., Tait, A., Tait, A., Tait, A., et al. (2013). Population genetics of *Trypanosoma brucei rhodesiense*: Clonality and diversity within and between foci. https://core.ac.uk/download/18492337.pdf (accessed on 25th June 2025).

48. Mansour, S. F. (2011). *Corporation Robots*. https://core.ac.uk/download/12007787.pdf (accessed on 25th June 2025).

49. N/A. (2010). *Criteria for the Diploma Qualifications in Science at Advanced Level: Principal Learning*. https://core.ac.uk/download/4151080.pdf (accessed on 25th June 2025).

50. Powell, D., & Schlotz, W. (2014). Ambulatory assessment in neuropsychology: Applications in multiple sclerosis research. https://core.ac.uk/download/80685934.pdf (accessed on 25th June 2025).

51. Sari, N. P. (Ni). (2019). Spiritual wellbeing in breast and cervical cancer survivors: Differences in each stage of survivorship. https://media.neliti.com/media/publications/300527-spiritual-wellbeing-in-breast-and-cervic-70b6122c.pdf (accessed on 25th June 2025).

52. Velasco, E. (2025). *Behavioural Surveillance and HIV Prevention in Men Who Have Sex with Men: Reports from Australia, Belgium, Canada, France, Germany, Switzerland, the United Kingdom, and the United States*. https://core.ac.uk/download/pdf/6628131.pdf (accessed on 25th June 2025).

53. Wagstaff, A., Marchal, B., Wilkinson, D., Cutler, D. M., Madigan, E., Muhondwa, E., Kessy, F., et al. (2009). Measuring inequalities in the distribution of health workers: The case of Tanzania. https://core.ac.uk/download/pdf/17181066.pdf (accessed on 25th June 2025).

54. Wahlström, H. (2004). *Bovine Tuberculosis in Swedish Farmed Deer*. https://core.ac.uk/download/11694788.pdf (accessed on 25th June 2025).

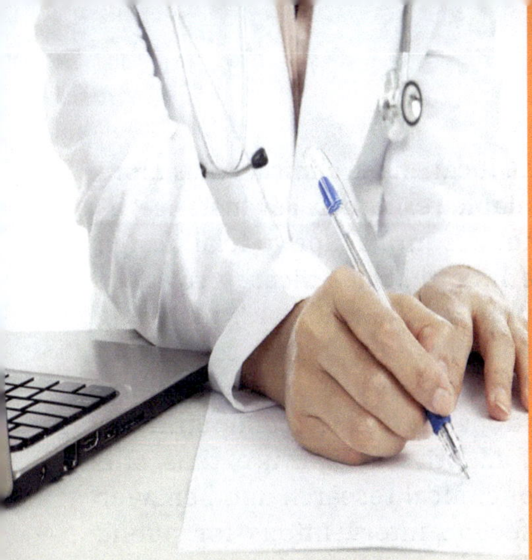

Chapter 3

STUDY DESIGNS IN CLINICAL RESEARCH

Contents

Introduction

Clinical research is a key component of the development of medical practice and knowledge. In this domain, study designs dictate the manner in which questions are formulated and investigated, eventually with implications for the validity and reliability of findings. Knowledge of clinical research begins with the recognition of the types of study design, categorized broadly under observational studies and interventional studies. Observational studies, such as cohort and case-control studies, enable researchers to investigate the relationship between exposure and outcome while not interfering with the study setting. However, interventional studies, such as randomized controlled trials (RCTs), involve active intervention to ascertain the relative efficiency of different treatments. These two designs add uniquely to the evolution of the evidence base on which clinical guidelines and healthcare practice are based and therefore require selecting an appropriate design based on the research question under investigation. Adaptive designs represent a new generation in clinical research because they allow for the modification of study protocols based on analyses of interim data. It can make clinical trials more effective, and also more reactive to emerging trends in data and available resources. For instance, as elaborated in Brennan et al. (2020), the integration of health economics into adaptive trial design is able to maximize health gains compared to research cost, something that healthcare providers globally are prioritizing more and more. Adaptive trials are favored by stakeholders, including decision-makers and researchers, due to the potential to shorten decision-making processes and improve outcomes. It is difficult to utilize these designs due to challenges such as the handling of the dynamic nature of cost data and ensuring that trial adaptations are clearly communicated and well executed by all concerned. The potential and relevance of adaptive designs are, thus, still significant areas of concern in clinical research. The convergence of clinical research and behavior change theory is essential in the transition of research into effective interventions for public health. Systematic reviews that yield evidence-based recommendations highlight the imperative of customization of interventions to facilitate better compliance from health professionals, as evident in Boyce et al. (2018). While various strategies have been tested, such as social influence strategies and education strategies, the effectiveness is not unequivocal without strict behavioral models that guide the execution processes. Systematic reviews, therefore, point to the necessity for future research to employ strong methods of defining the intervention components that are targeted as well as modes of delivery. By aligning clinical study design with theory of behavioral change, scientists maximize the likelihood that their findings will be applicable and, in the long run, contribute to better health outcomes and further develop the field overall (Figure 3.1).

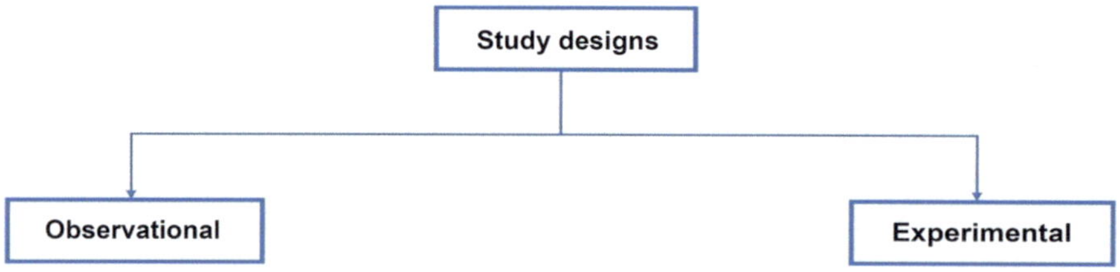

Figure 3.1. Overview of clinical research study designs.

Source: https://onlinelibrary.wiley.com/cms/asset/6ac34883-5984-4701-9adf-ccd41b459d66/ped412166-fig-0001-m.jpg.

Definition of Clinical Research

The definition of clinical research is important to understanding the breadth of study designs within the field. Basically, clinical research aims to create new knowledge on the causes, consequences, and treatments for health conditions through research that includes human subjects. Clinical research involves a variety of methodologies from observational studies to controlled trials to address specific questions about the effects of health interventions and patient outcomes. By proper identification of the objectives of a study, scientists can make an informed choice about the most suitable design, descriptive, analytical, or experimental. This precision in design not only optimizes the validity of the outcomes but also ensures the guarantee that the lessons that are gained can be meaningfully transferred to practice and to health policy, bridging the constantly-mooted gap between studies and application. In a rapidly evolving health care climate, the definition of clinical research becomes increasingly crucial because it informs the approaches utilized to study disease and treatment.

Systematic review of definitions within particular contexts, such as acute flare of knee osteoarthritis, underlines the importance of clear definitions in clinical research. This review demonstrates the necessity of concord on words and study design, emphasizing the manner in which definitions agreed upon can make research activity easier and enhance collaboration among researchers and healthcare providers (Parry et al., 2018). Understanding these nuances in the definitions of clinical research not only assists in the design of effective treatments but also plays an important role in the regulatory sphere, aiding trials to be ethical and yielding valid results that can be translated across various patient groups. Further, examining the definition of clinical research may assist in bringing out its interdisciplinary nature involving aspects of medicine, psychology, and social sciences. For instance, ongoing research in psychotherapy illustrates how embodied processes influence therapeutic practices by emphasizing the impact of interpersonal dynamics on clinical practice (Gennaro et al., 2019). Interconnectedness in this way facilitates an integrated perspective of understanding health issues such that diverse methodologies may be applied to reflect on the multidimensionality of human health. Clinical research, thus, is an essential avenue through which hypotheses may be tested and customized to produce richer treatment models and more favorable patient outcomes. The dynamic interaction of clinical research not only enhances the depth of data collected but also renders it still more clinically relevant, exemplifying the beauty of a well-defined scope that seeks to address various dimensions of health and treatment paradigms (Figure 3.2).

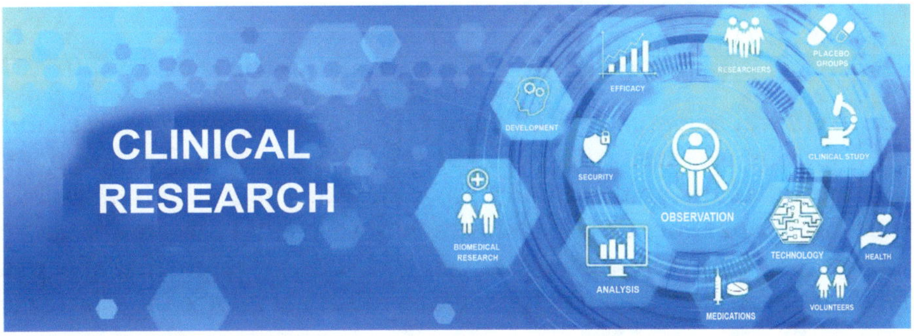

Figure 3.2. Clinical research.

Source: https://bioresscientia.com//uploads/journals/1686814533CC.png.

Importance of Study Designs

The value of clinical research study designs cannot be overemphasized as they provide the foundation for the investigation's validity, credibility, and relevance. Adequate study design enables investigators to carefully address specific research questions and minimize biases and confounding factors. Various study designs, such as randomized controlled trials (RCTs), cohort studies, and case-control studies, each have varying strengths and weaknesses that may have a significant bearing on the outcome of clinical research. For instance, RCTs are the best because they are able to establish causality, while observational studies may be more cost-effective and ethical in certain contexts. The awareness of the nuances between these strategies matters for clinicians and researchers in that it translates directly to results interpretation and application translation, which eventually affects patient care and public health interventions. Maximizing study designs, by extension, works to significantly improve the formulation of clinical research results with limited resources. With the growing demands for efficient treatment modalities, researchers are being forced to create innovative study designs that boost the efficiency and efficacy of drug development processes. As noted in recent studies, methods of optimal clinical trial designs have been plentiful, where researchers can solve vexing issues at all phases of clinical drug evaluation. For example, phase I dose–toxicity studies and phase III multi-arm studies are increasingly complex, necessitating robust design methodologies to manage effectively a high number of treatment arms and outcome measures. Incorporating well-thought-out design elements, researchers are better able to navigate the challenges associated with clinical trials, ultimately resulting in faster approval of effective therapy and better patient outcomes (Ryeznik et al., 2019). Within the context of substance abuse treatment, the importance of well-planned studies is also hastened by the need for evidence-based practice. Policymakers, practitioners, and researchers are increasingly engaged in debates aimed at integrating evidence-based practice into clinics. The model of the empirical-analytical subtype based on evidence-based practice relies in significant part on randomized controlled trials to inform the effectiveness of treatment. However, even as methodological rigor of this sort cannot be challenged, it is important to respond to its implications and limitations critically. It supports an improved, more inclusive understanding of how different paradigms may engage and reciprocate to support one another, ultimately in enhancing quality care. Adopting a varied array of study designs frees the clinical research community to address the complex nature of human behavior and needs, fostering a whole-systems approach to patient care that balances evidence, humanism, and social justice (Autrique et al., 2010).

Overview of Various Study Designs

Study designs used in clinical research vary across a range of methodologies, each uniquely designed to properly answer specific research questions. Of the numerous designs, randomized controlled trials (RCTs) are regarded as the gold standard since they are able to minimize bias and establish causality. RCTs use randomization to allocate subjects to treatment groups and control groups to ensure that the group characteristics are equal. This design is particularly convenient in the assessment of novel interventions because it provides robust evidence on efficacy and safety. RCTs are, however, resource-intensive and not always feasible, particularly where follow-up is long-term. The researchers thus typically turn to observational studies, which, although less stringent, can provide insightful information regarding the effect of interventions in practice. Another basic study design employed in clinical research is the cohort study, which examines the association between exposure and outcome over time. In this design, researchers follow a group of people who share something in common and see what happens to their health in an effort to find out the effect of specific exposures. Cohort studies are particularly useful when examining rare diseases or long-term outcomes due to the fact that they allow sufficient data to be collected over extended periods of time. However, they also have drawbacks, like the possibility of confounding variables distorting results. Furthermore, the temporal nature of cohort studies can complicate the identification of direct causal relationships. Despite these limitations, cohort studies have a significant role to play in hypothesis generation and disease patterns in chronic disease. Cross-sectional studies provide a snapshot of a population at a single moment and allow researchers to examine relationships between variables uninfluenced by the confound of time. This approach is best for establishing the prevalence of outcomes and risk factors in a population. With concurrent data collection on outcome and exposure, cross-sectional surveys can account for patterns but lack the ability to establish causality. The correlation that is noted can be made susceptible to confounding, and the lack of temporal information does not provide insight into disease trajectories. Yet, cost-effectiveness and efficiency are features of cross-sectional surveys that make them appealing for pilot studies and public health surveillance. In summary, while each study design possesses inherent strengths and limitations, as a whole they form an essential set of tools for promoting knowledge in clinical research, health outcome advances, and clinical practice guidance (Figure 3.3).

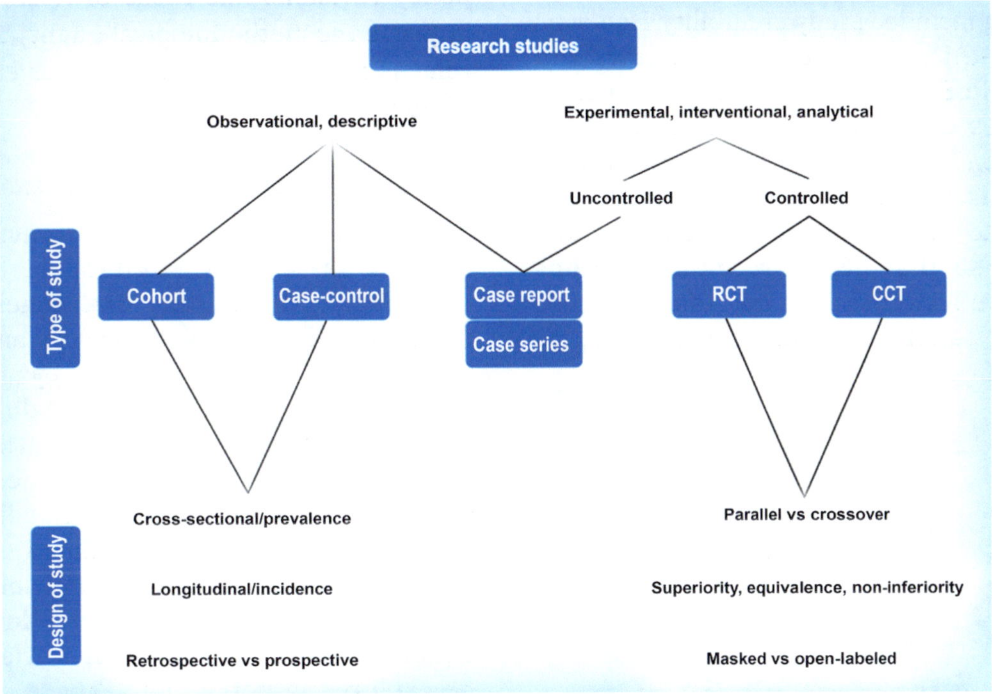

Figure 3.3. Summary of clinical research types and designs.

Source: https://www.researchgate.net/profile/Paul-Varner/publication/277902025/figure/fig1/AS:673024353267714@1537472918788/Summary-of-clinical-research-types-and-designs-CCT-Controlled-clinical-trial-RCT.png.

3.1. Observational Study Designs

Observational study designs are significant in clinical research due to the fact that they allow researchers to examine health outcomes and behavior under natural conditions without the experimenter's influence. Non-experimental designs consist of several methods, including cohort studies, case-control studies, and cross-sectional studies. These methods enable researchers to discover relationships between exposures and outcomes in varied populations that can be especially beneficial where randomized controlled trials are not feasible. While observational studies can introduce biases, they remain a staple of the study of public health and epidemiology, providing insight into the natural history of disease and the effects of interventions in the population as a whole. Thus, an understanding of the strengths and limitations of such designs is required to determine their value in evidence-based practice and clinical guidelines. Critical appraisal of observational studies is very important to interpret their findings and deriving accurate recommendations. There needs to be an evaluation of risk of bias (RoB) for every study from a systematic review of observational studies, which has been reported in the findings of a large-scale systematic review of systematic reviews published in leading medical journals. Evidence synthesis is more in favor of enhanced decision-making by balancing included study credibility. However, nearly one-third of systematic reviews did not report RoB analyses in their conclusions, which raises concerns about the robustness of recommendations that originate from such studies. It is important for researchers and physicians to be vigilant in ascertaining such limitations so that health recommendations genuinely reflect the best possible evidence to improve patient care and clinical practice outcomes (Egan et al., 2014).

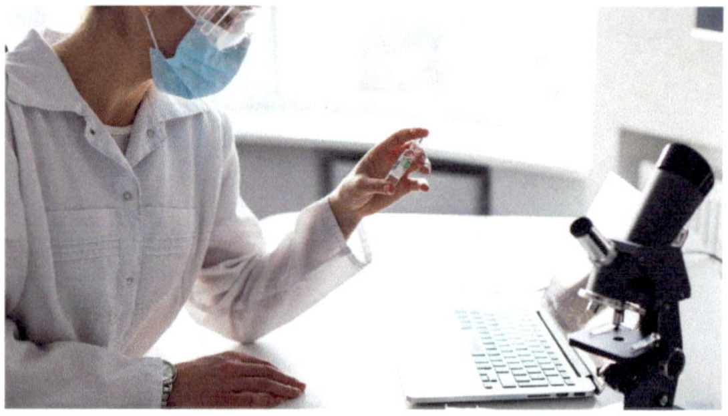

Figure 3.4. Observational study design.

Source: https://scientific-publishing.webshop.elsevier.com/wp-content/uploads/2021/09/2020-30-Observational-Study-1200x675.jpg.

Integrating different sources of evidence is essential to developing integrated clinical guidelines to address the multifaceted health issues. As seen from the example of depression counseling, integrating quantitative evidence from randomized controlled trials and qualitative information from patient experience can make more effective treatment guidelines. Evidence quality should no longer be reliant on randomized studies but rather the employment of large routine datasets and qualitative research enhances the understanding of multiple interventions effectiveness and acceptability. Knowing the deficits of solely relying on RCTs, evidence-based guidelines are enhanced to enhance overall patient care. Finally, generating more inclusion of evidence types, as seen in policy revisions like those of NICE, can richly improve the methodological quality and clinical relevance of the research (Barber et al., 2017) (Figure 3.4).

3.1.1. Definition and Characteristics

The definition and characteristics of study designs in clinical studies are crucial in establishing the validity and generalizability of findings. Study designs are systematic plans in which researchers collect, analyze, and make meaning of the data. They may be differentiated into experimental and observational frameworks on a large scale. Experimental designs have controlled interventions, often in clinical trials, with variables being manipulated to measure their effect on outcomes. Observational designs record events or states without intervention, enabling associations and real-world actions to be explored in populations. These distinctions are essential when evaluating the validity of research conclusions within the medical literature. Features inherent in different study designs profoundly shape the evidence generated by quality. Key attributes include randomization, blinding, and control groups, which strengthen experimental designs and minimize bias. For example, randomized controlled trials (RCTs) are at times regarded as being the gold standard since their study design allows causal inferences to be made, in effect isolating the intervention's effect from confounding variables. Conversely, observational studies may lack such attributes, with issues emerging in determining causality. Study validity also relies on sample size, selection bias, and compliance with intervention protocols, illustrating how factors of methodology determine research results' validity (Chan et al., 2020). Additionally, the refinement of standards and guidelines of study design has immensely changed in order to address the complexities of modern clinical research. As biomedical publications grow exponentially, there is a critical need for clarity and consistency in reporting study designs. This is precipitated by the prospect of knowledge representation standards supporting data mining and collaborative research (Burke et al., 2009). As researchers strive to make sense of a growing pool of literature, the potential to synthesize outcomes across multiple studies relies on well-defined methodologies. Therefore, enhancing the replicability and transparency of study designs benefits researchers as well as underpins the broader objectives of evidence-based healthcare practice.

3.1.2. Types of Observational Studies

Observational research is a critical component of clinical studies that allows researchers to investigate the interdependencies between variables without intervening or manipulating them. Cross-sectional, cohort, and case-control studies are three significant types of observational research. Cross-sectional studies take a snapshot of the population at a single point in time and allow the measurement of the prevalence of conditions or characteristics. This type of study works particularly well in establishing risk factors' associations with health outcomes. Its limitation is that causality cannot be established because temporal relationships cannot be established. Hence, researchers must be careful while selecting observational designs to meet their purposes in conducting research in order to derive meaningful insights and practice implications. Cohort studies are another potent type of observational research design. These investigations track cohorts of individuals over time, often comparing exposed and unexposed groups to particular risk factors. Through tracking the development of outcomes within those cohorts, researchers can make estimates of incidence rates and assess potential causal relationships between exposures and health outcomes. Cohort studies may be prospective, where individuals are tracked forward over time, or retrospective, where already existing data are utilized. While cohort studies are robust in the imposition of temporal ordering and presumptively causal variables, they will also be expensive and susceptible to such factors as attrition and confounders. Familiarity with this study's strengths and weaknesses is important to researchers who wish to provide evidence-based recommendations (Eloise et al., 2024). Case-control studies compare individuals with an outcome of interest with a control group without the outcome. This retrospective study has a particular strength in the study of rare diseases because it allows for efficient sampling of cases with minimal lost effort. Researchers screen and study retrospective exposures to determine potential risk factors for the outcome. As much as case-control studies yield valuable information on disease etiology, they too have some major challenges, such as recall bias and difficulties in establishing temporal associations. Hence, participant selection of study subjects and selection of control groups are crucial in minimizing biases and making valid as well as relevant observations. Altogether, the understanding of every type of observational study is critical for the execution of high-caliber clinical research that can effectively impact health interventions as well as policy (Figure 3.5).

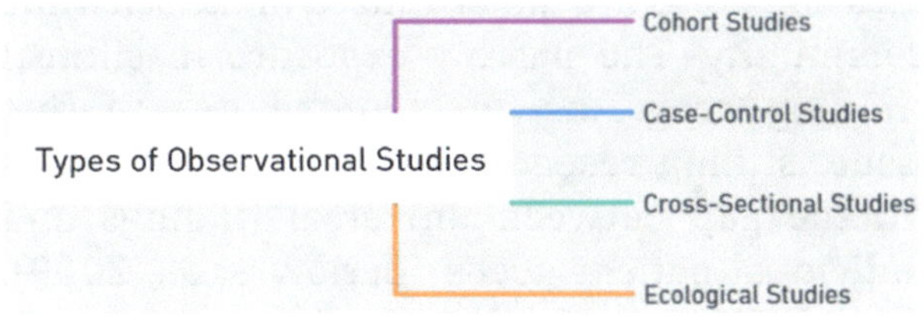

Figure 3.5. Types of observational studies.

Source: https://static.wixstatic.com/media/bd93cb_8a4cc1bbbb8a4501a160d8d1be9f14f3~mv2.webp/v1/fill/w_568,h_192,al_c,q_80,usm_0.66_1.00_0.01,enc_avif,quality_auto/bd93cb_8a4cc1bbbb8a4501a160d8d1be9f14f3~mv2.webp.

3.1.3. Strengths and Limitations

The revelation of study design strengths and limitations in clinical research unveils important information on their effectiveness. One of the inherent strengths of classical group comparison designs manifests itself in the form of their capacity to yield results that can be generalized across populations. Because of their focus on aggregated data, statistical associations can be identified and conclusions for use in larger populations drawn. This methodology is typically constrained when it comes to flexibility as well as context-based findings. It tends to overlook individual variability and nuances that can significantly influence outcomes. Thus, although group designs play a central role in establishing general trends, they sometimes fail to reflect the richness of human behavior and experience, ultimately limiting their applicability in clinical practice (Barlow et al., 2009). In contrast, idiographic research strategies, which concentrate on the in-depth study of single cases over time, offer a balanced perspective. These methods allow for a more nuanced understanding of the difference between persons and can uncover new results that group designs standardized by statistically adjusting for group differences may miss. The flexibility built into idiographic methods can be extremely valuable in clinical work where individualized approaches are essential. Nevertheless, despite their potential, these methods are underutilized in the scientific community. The narrow exposure in clinical training programs only contributes to this issue, stifling research development that can fill the gap between universal findings and individual patient needs (Barlow et al., 2009). Therefore, though idiographic methods are well-supported strengths, their integration within clinical research is an issue that needs to be addressed. Future randomized controlled trials are also a cornerstone of clinical research, renowned for their rigor and ability to establish cause-and-effect relationships. Future trials enable researchers to closely control variables, providing robust evidence on the effectiveness of interventions. However, prospective studies also have inherent limitations, primarily regarding their practicability and applicability. They can be data-hungry and may not reflect real events, most likely creating problems with the external validity of the research. But retrospective studies from administrative data give a different picture and enable scientists to handle large sets of data to observe patterns and outcomes. Although this strategy brings with it biases and the limitation of depth of inference, it is valuable as an add-on design to randomized trials and allows for a more comprehensive understanding of outcomes and practice over diverse populations.

3.2. Experimental Study Designs

Experimental study designs are at the core of clinical research, particularly for evaluating intervention effectiveness. Experimental designs are all about stringent methodologies to establish cause-and-effect relationships between dependent and independent variables. Standard experimental designs are RCTs, which stringently control confounding variables by randomly allocating subjects into treatment or control groups. By controlling for these variables, researchers are able to more accurately attribute effects that are observed to the interventions at hand, maximizing the internal validity of the findings. The advantages of RCTs, including minimizing bias, are key in the development of evidence-based medical care that can directly influence clinical practice. Quasi-experimental designs offer a less intense option in cases where randomization is not feasible, in addition to randomized controlled trials. These designs hold on to elements of experimental techniques, such as independent variable manipulation, with the potential to observe impacts in naturally occurring groups. Such studies can be helpful, especially in real-life situations where ethical reasons might preclude randomization. But lack of control over extraneous variables presents a significant stumbling block to establishing clear cause-and-effect relationships. This is evident in considering the impact of mutual help groups on psychological functioning, where quasi-experimental evidence has suggested potential beneficial effects but also suggests the necessity of rigorous controls in establishing findings, as was delivered in a review of empirical studies into mutual help groups and mental health issues (Barker et al., 2008). In addition, varied methodologies like process research complete experimental paradigms with investigations of the complexity of change in therapy. Process research determines how particular interventions result in certain outcomes, thus gaining a more nuanced comprehension of mechanisms at work. Among these procedures, the Significant Events framework connects qualitative and quantitative approaches to shed light on significant events that drive therapeutic change. This pluralism in methods is required in clinical research as it acknowledges that human conduct is too intricate to be explained through similar perspectives. By employing a broad spectrum of experimental designs and adjunctive procedures, researchers can build a comprehensive picture of therapeutic efficacy and foster theory and practice in clinical psychology (Elliott et al., 2009) (Figure 3.6).

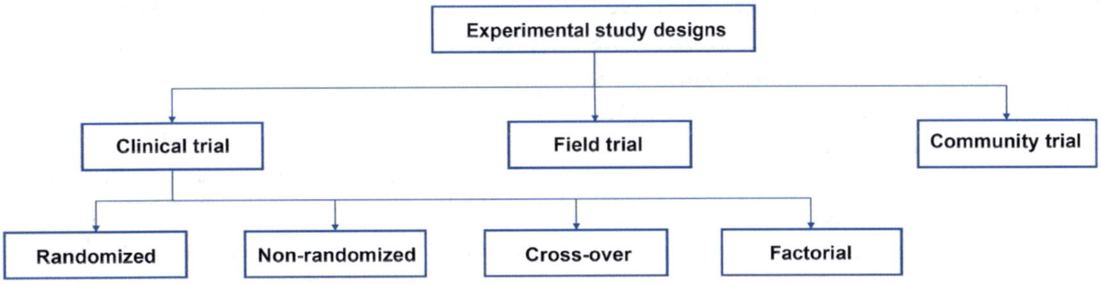

Figure 3.6. Experimental study designs.

Source: https://onlinelibrary.wiley.com/cms/asset/2f98cf3b-8b5a-47b4-9505-e84e0ed30f4d/ped412166-fig-0005-m.jpg.

3.2.1. Definition and Characteristics

Clinical research study designs are the templates that form the backbone for conducting experiments to evaluate medical interventions. The definition of the study designs typically involves experimental and observational approaches, which are selected based on the questions being investigated. Experimental designs, such as RCTs, allow for the provision of variable control, hence defining causal relationships between interventions and outcomes. Conversely, observational studies highlight the observation of outcomes without intervention, and they provide data on real-world circumstances but less accuracy than experimental designs. It is vital to appreciate these categorizations because each design possesses unique strengths and limitations, greatly influencing the validity and applicability of research findings in clinical practice (Amendoeira et al., 2018). Among the characteristics that mark study designs is their methodological rigor, such as factors of randomization, blinding, and control groups in experimental research. These features are required for minimizing bias and ensuring that the results are attributable to the intervention being studied. Further, the choice of study design also carries implications for the generalizability of findings; for instance, RCTs yield high internal validity but are bound to have problems with issues of external validity by virtue of often strict inclusion criteria. Observational studies, and their valuable reflective estimates of health in populations, however, are likely to bring in confounding variables that confound causal interpretation. The intersection of methodological rigor and the study's objectives significantly determines the clinical research scene, providing researchers with needed tools for making sound conclusions about their studies (Babb et al., 2018). The evolution of clinical research study design has been driven by the need for more effective and efficient mechanisms for assessing emerging treatments and therapies. With the advancement of science, adaptive trial designs have become a priority, where the trial protocol can be changed based on interim analysis of the information. This adaptability will improve patient safety and make the entire drug development process more efficient. Moreover, elements such as Bayesian adaptive designs, that utilize prior information and update predictions based on further data availability, reflect the ongoing development in clinical study designs. By understanding the definition and characteristics of various study designs, researchers can better cope with the complexities of clinical research and eventually contribute to bettering medical science (Amendoeira et al., 2018; Babb et al., 2018).

3.2.2. Randomized Controlled Trials (RCTs)

The RCT is invariably hailed as the gold standard of clinical trials due to its rigorous design, ensuring a maximum level of bias avoidance and allowing causal inferences about the effectiveness of treatment. Its core is the randomization process that allocates subjects into intervention or control groups, negating confounding forces that would otherwise affect outcomes. This rigorous approach ensures that any effects noted can more confidently be attributed to the intervention under investigation. However, even though RCTs are renowned for their internal validity, they have been criticized on the grounds of their lack of external validity, or the potential to generalize results to larger groups. This casts doubt on their use in real-world contexts, which, by design, entail more diverse populations and complex variables not controlled in the laboratory settings typical of RCTs. The use of RCTs within the broader context of clinical research generates questions regarding the interpretation of their findings and use in health policy. Evidence has been established through studies that the sole use of RCTs is lacking, particularly for knowledge on the effects of multifaceted interventions like microcredit in public health environments. This sole utilization may be insensitive to the nuance needed for realizing the polyvalent effects of these interventions.

In investigating the evidence of microcredit effects, for instance, Biosca et al. (2017) argue that a narrow focus on RCT-based evidence threatens to stifle the production of relevant data on public health impacts. Therefore, there exists a pressing need to synthesize diverse study types other than RCTs in advancing an extensive knowledge base on the effectiveness, cost-effectiveness, and acceptability of interventions. Moreover, the limitations of RCTs to capture the complexity of treatment efficacy further uphold the need for a broader methodological outlook in clinical research. The NICE guidelines reinforce that sole reliance on RCTs may not be adequate to address the complexity associated with health interventions like counseling for depression. Evidence presented in Barber et al. (2017) depicts that while RCTs provide positive outcomes for counseling, other sources of data, such as large routine outcome datasets and qualitative work, provide valuable information about treatment acceptability and effectiveness in routine practice. This many-faceted approach enriches the evidence base, thereby facilitating more evidence-informed clinical guidelines that account for patient experience and contextual data, thereby enhancing both the quality and utility of health care delivery (Figure 3.7).

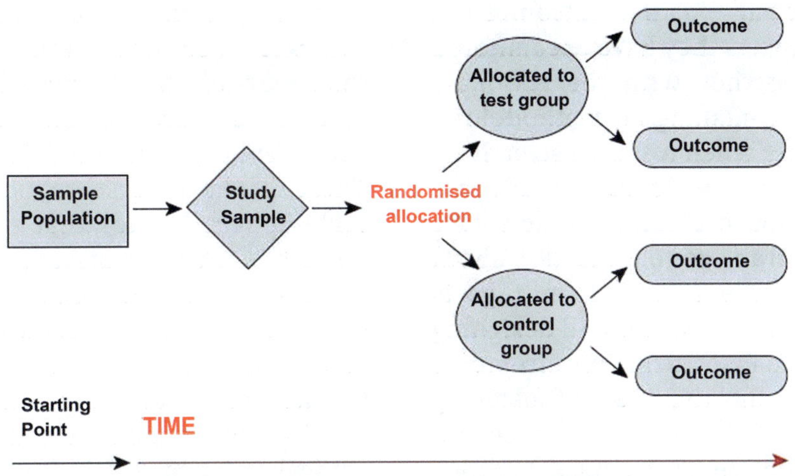

Figure 3.7. Diagrammatic representation of a randomized controlled trial.

Source: https://media.springernature.com/full/springer-static/image/art%3A10.1038%2Fsj.ebd.6400473/MediaObjects/41432_2007_Article_BF6400473_Fig1_HTML.jpg?as=webp.

3.2.3. Ethical Considerations in Experimental Designs

The ethical standards in experimental research are crucial to the validity and authenticity of clinical research. The researchers must consider the well-being of participants, informed consent having been obtained, and participants being knowledgeable about the risks and benefits of their involvement. Ethical considerations also involve the research itself, where scientific excellence and safety of the participants must be balanced. For instance, when conducting research on novel drug therapies, the study design should aim to minimize harm and apply maximum benefit potential. With emerging methodologies, the use of optimal designs is instrumental, as highlighted in the literature that continues to assert optimal design methodologies play an important role in improving drug development efficiency (Ryeznik et al., 2019). Addressing ethical issues at the design stage can have the aim of deepening the relevance of research findings, ultimately leading towards an ethically sensitive research culture. A second imperative area for ethical reflection is responding to socio-demographic diversity among participants. Representative samples are often the source of worry in clinical trials, leading to skewed findings and loss of applicability to broader contexts. Combining stratification and covariate-adaptive randomization during study design can aid in the guaranteed balanced representation, promoting fairness across different socio-economic groups. However, one should consider that balance, as ideal as it may be ethically, does not necessarily imply efficiency; the two variables may be contrasting in the course of executing the study. Research has highlighted the importance of covariate-adjusted response-adaptive (CARA) randomization methods, which seek to promote ethical considerations alongside maximum data efficiency at the same time (Rosenberger et al., 2011). This subtle approach plays a significant role in weighing the objectives of equitable participant representation against the international objectives of clinical research. Lastly, experimental design ethics also encompass researchers' responsibility in the reporting and dissemination of results. Transparency is central to the maintenance of public trust in scientific investigation. Scientists ought to report not only positive outcomes but also any adverse impacts they have encountered in experiments, together with the rationale behind their decision-making on methodology. Ethical concerns arise when research selectively publishes results or fails to report adverse data, jeopardizing the credibility of scientific journals. Moreover, frank communication about the implications of the research findings is crucial in guiding clinical practice and designing subsequent research. Prioritizing requirements for ethical reporting has the effect of fostering a culture of accountability in clinical research and supports the notion that ethical practice and scientific advancement are complementary, rather than contradictory, to each other.

3.3. Cohort Studies

Cohort studies are a mainstay of clinical research, providing valuable data regarding the associations between exposures and outcomes over time. Cohort studies track a cohort of persons who all share some common factor, usually their exposure to some risk factor or intervention. Unlike case-control studies that often look back at outcomes retrospectively, cohort studies are prospective or retrospective, allowing researchers to analyze data from various time points. The benefit of cohort studies is that they can establish temporal associations, which are crucial in disease causation. For instance, cohort studies can clarify how environmental or lifestyle factors cause chronic diseases and thereby inform public health preventative strategies. In clinical practice, cohort studies have also enlightened us about the complexity of comorbid conditions, such as how diabetes and tuberculosis interact with each other. According to research, diabetes greatly increases susceptibility to active tuberculosis and indicates the interconnectedness of these diseases in various populations. Epidemiological evidence from research conducted in other areas, such as sub-Saharan Africa, has shown diabetic patients to be much more likely to contract tuberculosis, and odds ratios for more than four-fold higher prevalence among those patients compared to non-diabetic controls have been reported (Faurholt-Jepsen et al., 2013). These results underscore the necessity for large-scale cohort studies that not only assess the impact of chronic disease on acute infection but also investigate treatment responses and survival in dual-diagnosed individuals. Cohort studies also provide access to large amounts of longitudinal data, which can be instrumental in informing guidelines and risk assessment in clinical practice.

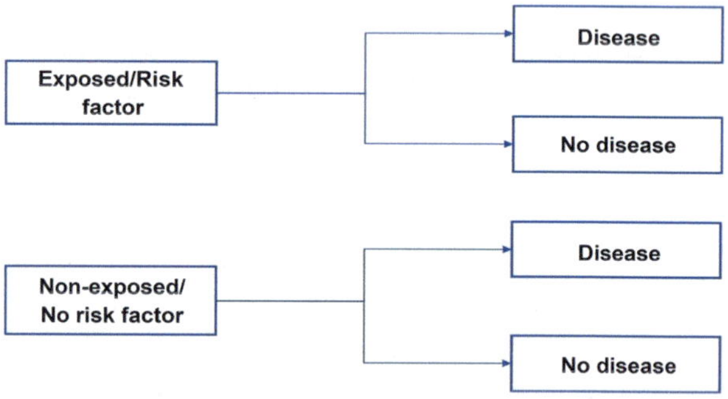

Figure 3.8. Cohort study design.

Source: https://onlinelibrary.wiley.com/cms/asset/474d3e2b-290a-4d2d-9562-4792f547cae2/ped412166-fig-0004-m.jpg.

For example, analysis of eosinophilic granulomatosis with polyangiitis patient cases in cohort studies by systematic analysis showed significant head and neck presentations, with a significant proportion of patients being responsive to steroid therapy (Basnyat et al., 2016). This shows the critical position that such studies play in clinical decision-making and the necessity for using standardized criteria, such as those provided through the American College of Rheumatology, to inform diagnosis and management. Overall, the various uses of cohort studies in clinical research highlight their potential to not only elucidate disease onset but also improve patient outcomes by informing evidence-based healthcare choices (Figure 3.8).

3.3.1. Definition and Methodology

In clinical research, the study design definition is the basis for which questions are answered and addressed in research. A study design refers to a systematic plan that determines the way data is collected, analyzed, and interpreted. The definition not only encompasses the type of study but also the methodologies employed are specific in the application to address specific hypotheses. For instance, RCTs are highly prized for their ability to minimize bias through randomization. Single-case experimental designs, however, can obtain rich, subtle information quite efficiently, particularly in behavioral interventions. The establishment of standard reporting guidelines, such as the SCRIBE 2016 checklist, enhances the accuracy and readability of single-case study reporting to ensure that all the factors under consideration are addressed in an orderly manner, thereby enhancing the overall integrity of research (Albin et al., 2016).

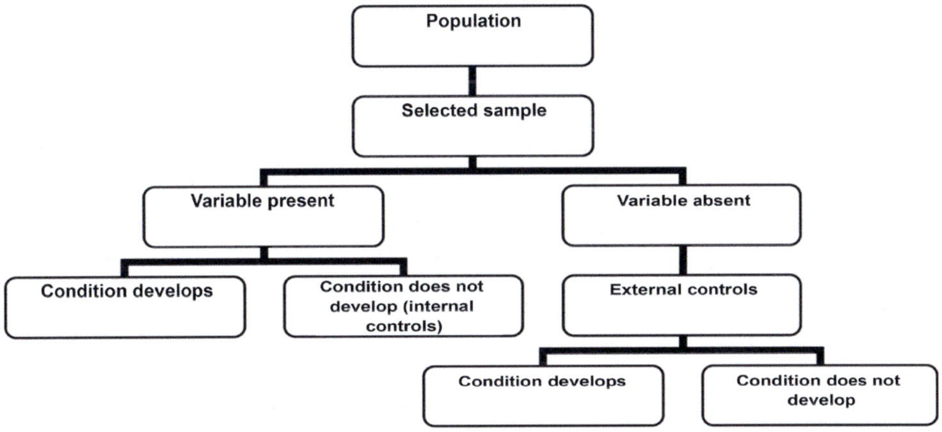

Figure 3.9. Study design for cohort studies.

Source: https://ars.els-cdn.com/content/image/1-s2.0-S2211419X11001637-gr1.jpg.

Clinical research methodology encompasses the orderly and unbiased process used to conduct studies. Selecting a proper methodology is critical because it will determine the validity and reliability of findings. Various methodologies, such as qualitative and quantitative, are applied based on the nature of the research inquiry. Quantitative research generally applies statistical calculations for hypothesis testing, whereas qualitative methodologies focus on identifying underlying motivations and actions. With the progression of technology, new methodologies have emerged; for instance, mobile health technologies currently encompass real-time capture of data through in-device sensors as well as user-sourced logs. The integration allows for convenient measurements of engagement as well as acceptability, which are core components in determining user interaction with health applications. Therefore, methodological innovation contributes to reconsideration of traditional methods and provides avenues to more discriminative analyses in clinical research (Gray et al., 2018). In addition, the introduction of new methodologies alongside traditional practice emphasizes the need for flexible clinical study designs. Rapid research designs, as proposed, offer the potential to keep pace with technological advances, particularly in the evaluation of interventions such as mobile phone applications. With evolving methodologies, researchers increasingly must reconcile calls for good evidence with the demands of efficient study conduct. For instance, while RCTs are now the norm, their relative inflexibility can restrict real-time findings within highly specialist fields like digital health. By favoring the use of various study designs, including quick measures among them, researchers are able to present balanced assessments incorporating both effectiveness and user interaction metrics. Finally, the interplay among definition, methodology, and adaptive strategies highlights the subtlety of developing effective clinical research studies (Gray et al., 2018) (Figure 3.9).

3.3.2. Prospective vs. Retrospective Cohort Studies

Cohort studies provide the basis of clinical studies through the capacity to look at the interrelationship between exposure and outcome. Cohort studies can be categorized into prospective and retrospective designs with their respective methods and data collection implications. Prospective cohort studies involve following a population of individuals over time whose exposures to a given factor are ascertained before outcomes are measured. This temporal relationship is crucial in the determination of causality and is strengthened by its ability to minimize recall bias. Retrospective cohort studies, on the other hand, study already present data, establishing prior exposure status from records and assessing outcomes that have previously been encountered. While this approach is likely to be faster and cheaper, it is more susceptible to data completeness and accuracy biases. Yet both strategies offer enormous promise for the enlargement of clinical knowledge and the direction of practice. Among prospective and retrospective cohort studies, choosing between them depends on different considerations, including study questions, resources available, and time. Prospective studies are typically time- and resource-consuming, requiring systematic follow-up of participant health outcomes over extended periods. This period of time allows researchers to capture data real time, improving the validity of the findings. Retrospective research, however, uses easily accessible data, being cheaper but enabling the examination of larger sample populations.

Retrospective research often struggles with limitations such as missing data and errors due to the lack of randomization. Notably, the validity of results from retrospective analyses relies on the quality of initial data and a clear definition of inclusion and exclusion criteria, with meticulous planning emerging as a top priority in either approach. Implications of some study designs extend beyond direct consequences and need to be balanced against their broader implications in clinical research. Observational studies, for example, those outlined in veterinary pathology, emphasize doing studies that address pertinent gaps in knowledge while being creative and systematic in their methodologies. One of these is balancing the merits and demerits of prospective versus retrospective studies. For example, while prospective studies can directly observe causality, retrospective studies will allow for broader analysis using existing data sets, but with potential bias and confounding variables. Researchers need to exercise caution in making use of good controls and setting clear hypotheses so that their findings will provide value additions to the literature. Such balanced comprehension of study design strengthens the evidence base needed to inform clinical practice and target future research, securing comparative analyses' place in understanding study types (Evans et al., 2019; Amanda et al., 2018) (Figure 3.10).

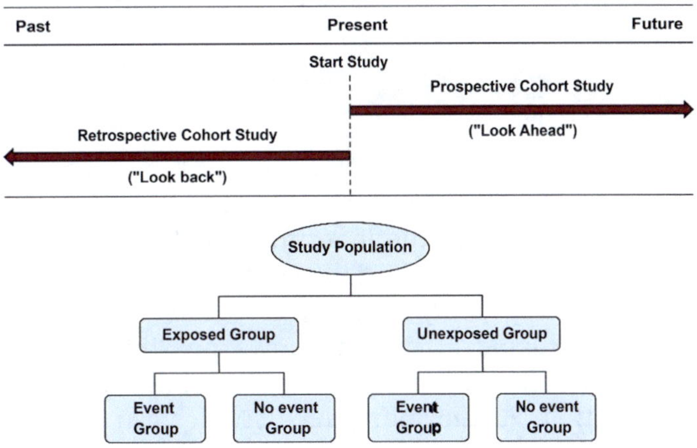

Figure 3.10. Graphical representation of the timeline in a prospective vs a retrospective cohort study design.

Source: https://ars.els-cdn.com/content/image/1-s2.0-S0012369220304645-gr1_lrg.jpg.

3.3.3. Applications in Clinical Research

In clinical trials, the employment of study designs is core to enhancing drug development quality and efficiency. Scientists are now using optimal designs that solve mixed problems encountered in the different stages of clinical trials. These designs encompass phase I dose–toxicity studies and phase I/II trial conduct with simultaneous measurement of early efficacy and toxicity endpoints. With the application of optimal study designs such as modeling strategies and multi-arm trials, clinical researchers can obtain results more accurately at reduced costs. Overall, optimal study designs enable effective drug development as well as address relevant questions of treatment effect and patient safety required to drive medical science and public health forward (Ryeznik et al., 2019). Moreover, making the transition from traditional trial designs to new ways of conducting studies has profound implications for answering complex health-related questions. The abundance of applications of meta-analysis is an ideal example of the transformation of study design. By combining Frequentist and Bayesian principles, meta-analysts are able to synthesize conclusions of different studies effectively, addressing challenges with heterogeneous outcomes and bias prevalent in clinical studies. Notably, meta-analysis permits comparisons across studies of diverse designs, a feature that renders it an invaluable resource for making treatment efficacy determinations and creating clinical practice guidelines. Such methodological flexibility renders meta-analysis irreplaceable in answering vital questions of prevention, diagnosis, and treatment, thus becoming a valuable asset to evidence-based healthcare practice (Vogel et al., 2018). As clinical research evolves, the need to incorporate intricate study designs cannot be overstated. These designs not only improve the solidity of clinical trials but also allow investigators to expand into new frontiers in biostatistics. Merging newer analytical tools in the design of clinical research has provided the possibility for more nuanced comprehension of patient outcomes, either in survival data analysis or in policy-relevant queries in trials. Lastly, the unguided advancement of study designs within clinical research not only enhances our understanding of medical interventions but also keeps scientists at the forefront of the field when it comes to scientific inquiry, thus enabling the general progression of health that is innovative and effective in practice (Ryeznik et al., 2019; Vogel et al., 2018).

3.4. Case-Control Studies

Case-control studies constitute an important study design in the clinical study field, specifically in the investigation of rare diseases or conditions where direct experimentation will be impossible or is unethical. This study design starts with the identification of individuals who have the disease, or cases, and those who do not have the disease, or controls. Researchers then look back at rates of usual exposures within each group to try to discover possible risk factors for the disease. This specific study design is most valuable in that it allows possible dispassionate review of data already in hand, making research more efficient through the utilization of existing cohorts instead of demanding fresh data collection. Furthermore, such studies can give cues towards correlations that can inform future longitudinal studies, in order to further elucidate disease processes and health determinants.

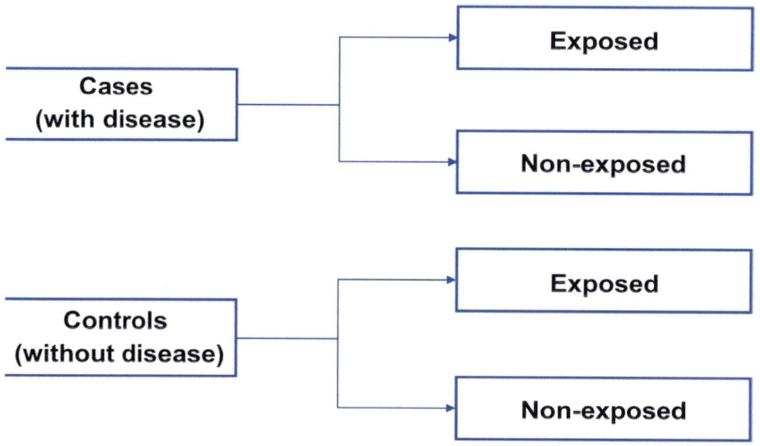

Figure 3.11. Case-control study design.

Source: https://onlinelibrary.wiley.com/cms/asset/696167df-2a87-4c5d-a01b-b7303e009f89/ped412166-fig-0003-m.jpg.

Case-control studies are not only solid by virtue of their economy but are also powerful since they are capable of handling rare or complex diseases. By contrasting the history of exposure among cases and controls, researchers can uncover strong correlations that can lead to the establishment of causal associations between specific risk factors and disease. The design, however, is imperfect; one of the primary drawbacks is that it is prone to recall bias, or subjects lying about prior exposure. This yields biased results that can inaccurately depict the real relationship between exposure and disease. Case-control studies have also been criticized on grounds of these biases, but data thus derived are frequently of considerable clinical importance, especially when supplemented by wider epidemiological findings. As clinical research continues to expand, case-control studies remain pertinent but must be applied in conjunction with methodological innovations that enhance their validity. For instance, the combination of case-control study findings with other types of studies, such as cohort studies or randomized controlled trials, has the potential to balance out each method's methodological limitations. Further, with greater attention to mental health interventions in parenting and family experiences, the application of multiple multidisciplinary sources of information may add depth to case-control analysis. For instance, understanding the interaction of psychosocial factors in the aetiology of conditions may inform prevention and intervention design. Thus, advances in research technology and methodology retain the potential to enhance the validity and usefulness of case-control studies in contemporary clinical investigation as with progress in cancer therapies such as proton and ion beam radiation therapy, emphasizing the imperative for continued investigation and improvement in study designs (Alonso et al., 2013; McMillan et al., 2010) (Figure 3.11).

3.4.1. Definition and Methodology

The principle of study design in clinical research is the foundation because it sets the pattern under which scientific questions are developed. Various definitions of study designs range from simple categorizations to complex approaches involving multiple disciplines. Basically, a study design is a coordinated plan indicating how research objectives will be achieved and what methodology will be employed in data collection and analysis. This organizing principle plays a central role in guaranteeing that the research is both systematic and reproducible. The selection of study design, as a defining feature, is capable of dictating the validity and quality of the subsequent findings, thus compelling researchers to pay special attention to the frameworks used. Additionally, a clear conceptual distinction among various types of educational and research practice enhances stakeholders' ability to identify rigorous studies from weaker alternatives, as outlined in Hernández Fernández et al. (2020). In clinical science, methodologies usually fall under the categories of qualitative and quantitative approaches, each with specific applications and producing various forms of information. Quantitative methods, which are typically experimental and observational designs, allow hypothesis testing and permit statistical analysis, thus providing results that are more generalizable to populations. In contrast, qualitative methodologies give in-depth information about patient experiences, perceptions, and behaviors, allowing for a deeper understanding of health-related phenomena. Awareness of the complex interplay of these methodologies is important in probing clinical questions comprehensively. In addition, the tendency to emphasize quantitative techniques in medical studies tends to marginalize qualitative, which play an essential role in the unfolding of complex patient problems. To gain a complete grasp of health problems, methodological pluralism must be adopted as it enables researchers to triangulate findings and derive more integrative conclusions, as alluded to in Breen et al. (2008). The application and creation of study methods and designs in clinical trials have become increasingly relevant in contemporary health discourse, particularly in augmenting patient outcomes and informing policy development. Clinical trials serve as the benchmark for measuring interventions' efficacy through rigorous processes with controlled environments that eliminate biases. These designs not only facilitate ethical research procedures but also contribute to a growing body of evidence-based medicine. The creation of these methods demonstrates an attempt to enhance the quality of clinical inquiries while addressing practical issues such as access and cultural sensitivity in recruiting participants. Suggestions for improving existing paradigms will be augmented by ongoing discussion throughout the scientific community regarding the proper balance between various methodologies, announcing the hope of an age where differing methods may coexist and exchange learning with one another. With regard to this, the development of a clearly stated experimental design, as identified in Hernández et al. (2020), is crucial in establishing credibility and trust in clinical studies (Figure 3.12).

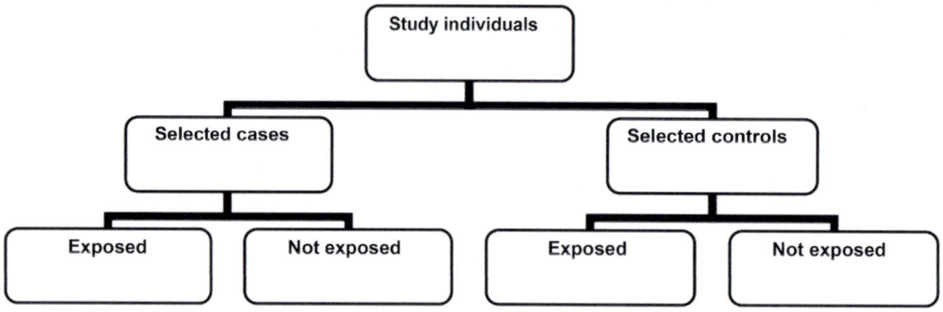

Figure 3.12. Study design for case–control studies.

Source: https://ars.els-cdn.com/content/image/1-s2.0-S2211419X11001637-gr3.jpg.

3.4.2. Selection of Cases and Controls

The selection of cases and controls is a fundamental component in case-control study designs, which are widely used in clinical research to establish the relationships between diseases and exposures. In case-control studies, cases are the patients with the disease or condition of interest, and controls are the non-cases but with comparable characteristics such as age, sex, and other demographic features. The validity of this comparative technique rests upon the judicious selection of both groups such that the relationship under consideration is not dominated by external variables. A recognition of the significance of these choices serves to minimize bias and maximize the validity of the outcome, allowing researchers to have a clearer sense of how particular exposures might produce health outcomes. Last but not least, the eligibility criteria used in case and control selection can profoundly affect a study's outcome. Researchers should emphasize the importance of eligibility criteria, which define the characteristics of cases and controls, so that they become representatives of the populations from which they are chosen. For example, it is necessary to consider the diagnostic time of cases since the selection of those diagnosed over a specific time can bring disease presentation and severity variations. Furthermore, control matching with cases needs caution; unmatched controls may lead to false conclusions of association strength. The careful examination of these factors not only contributes to the internal validity of the study but also allows generalizability of findings to broader clinical situations. In addition to the technical accuracy involved in case and control recruitment, researchers must also consider ethical issues while planning the study. Researchers have an obligation to provide informed consent and assurance regarding confidentiality to all the participants. The fine art of selecting individuals afflicted with a certain disease must be done with utmost care so as not to cause any harm or distress. Also, where vulnerable groups are involved, there is a paramount need to embrace measures that ensure their respect and dignity in the research process. Balancing scientific inquiry with fulfilling ethical obligations is crucial in assisting researchers and participants in establishing confidence in one another, which ultimately helps in ensuring the quality and reliability of the research findings. Through careful consideration of both methodological and ethical considerations of the case and control selection, clinical researchers are able to significantly contribute towards effective interventions and improved health outcomes among different populations (Figure 3.13).

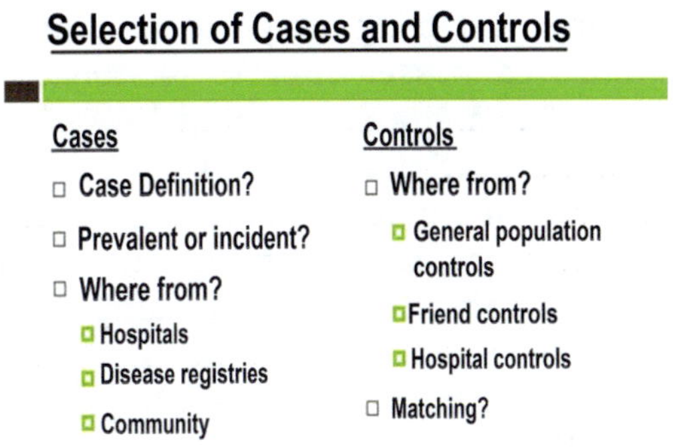

Figure 3.13. Selection of cases and controls.

Source: https://slideplayer.com/slide/13850028/85/images/6/Selection+of+Cases+and+Controls.jpg.

3.4.3. Advantages and Disadvantages

In clinical studies, it is crucial to be aware of the advantages and disadvantages of various study designs so that reliable data can be produced and patient care can be improved. One of the most significant advantages of RCTs is that they help eliminate bias, thereby making the internal validity of the results strong. By random assignment of study participants to control groups and intervention groups, researchers can establish causality more reliably than in observational studies. However, RCTs also present challenges, including ethical problems of blinding and the applicability of experimental conditions to real life. Here, then, while RCTs are widely referred to as the gold standard for clinical research, they are not always the most convenient for all questions or groups; the need for the application of careful thought in the selection of study design is stressed. On the other hand, observational studies, such as cohort and case-control studies, also offer a high return, particularly given ethical constraints and feasibility. They do not necessarily require such stringent control and can be done more in a naturalistic setup to allow for a broader observation of patient behavior and outcomes. They can also permit researchers to observe rare conditions or outcomes that would be impossible to study in RCTs. Due to these strengths, however, observational research is plagued by inherent constraints, essentially the potential for confounding factors that will obscure causal relationships. To this end, while valuable to hypothesis development and understanding associations, researchers must be cautious in making definitive conclusions from observational data, due to the complexity of the interaction involved in health outcomes. Moreover, the choice of study design might have a significant impact on the quality of research findings, and therefore, investigators must carefully weigh their choices. Thoroughly planned studies may yield high-quality outcomes that would make an impact in clinical practice, while poorly selected methodology might yield inaccurate conclusions and lost resources. For instance, although cross-sectional studies provide one with a snapshot of association at a given point, they might not be able to define temporal relationships. In contrast, longitudinal research is able to trace change with the passing of time but is likely to require large amounts of time and cost. Clinicians and investigators ought to take these advantages and disadvantages into consideration when selecting their designs, with the chosen one being appropriate to their research purposes and type of subjects or data at hand (Benson et al., 2008).

3.5. Cross-Sectional Studies

Cross-sectional studies are valuable in clinical research because they present a snapshot of a population at a specific point in time, allowing researchers to compare and analyze health conditions or demographic characteristics at the same point in time. The design is particularly useful to determine the prevalence rates of conditions, determinants of risk, and the association between variables, and can be utilized as a pilot study to pave the way for further longitudinal or experimental research. By utilizing existing data and observations, cross-sectional studies can effectively generate hypotheses and determine important associations that should be further explored. The studies are, however, not ideally suited for making inferences about causation since they measure exposure and outcome simultaneously, thereby obscuring temporal relationships. This nuance is crucial in the evaluation of the strengths and weaknesses of cross-sectional study design in the broader context of clinical study methodologies. The methodological quality of cross-sectional studies is often in doubt, particularly in terms of data collection and sampling procedures. Random sampling will enhance generalizability, but the majority of studies provide limitations due to convenience sampling, which can introduce biases. For instance, the identification of muscle dysmorphia (MD) from cross-sectional investigations might be compromised by a sample that is largely composed of fitness-oriented individuals rather than a representative sample, as in Lavallee et al. (2018). Consequently, homogeneity in samples can lead to false inferences on the prevalence and type of various disorders. Besides, self-report information is typically employed in cross-sectional studies that are susceptible to errors and social desirability biases. Therefore, scientists must pay utmost attention to strong sampling and data verification techniques in order to enhance the validity of their findings in healthcare environments. While constrained, cross-sectional studies are highly valuable, particularly in the research's starting stages on matters related to health. They can efficiently test associations, e.g., in recent meta-analyses of amyloid-linked cognitive impairments in age-normal older adults, where cross-sectional data provided important insights into relationships among amyloid burden and cognitive performance (Baker et al., 2016). These findings explain the capacity of cross-sectional studies to provide insight into possible indicators of cognitive worsening and even more necessitate a longitudinal study. Lastly, while cross-sectional studies cannot establish causation, they remain an invaluable tool for researchers and clinicians desirous of mapping the terrain of health and disease, testing hypotheses, and setting agendas for research in clinical practice in the future (Figure 3.14).

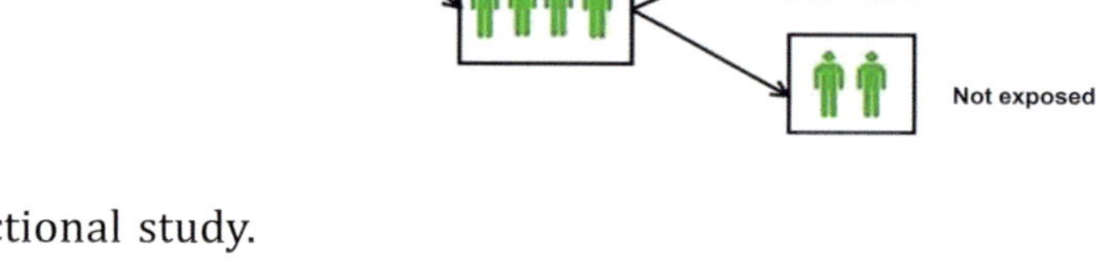

Figure 3.14. Cross-sectional study.

Source: https://microbenotes.com/wp-content/uploads/2021/12/Cross-Sectional-Study-Definition-Types-Applications-Advantages-Limitations.jpg.

3.5.1. Definition and Characteristics

In medical research, study designs are essential elements that define the methodology and findings of research. They are specific plans for the collection, measurement, and quantitative analysis of data, ultimately determining the validity and reliability of outcomes. A clearly articulated study design should encapsulate the technique by which research scholars arrive at conclusions about health interventions, disease incidence, or efficacy of treatment. Various traits, including experimental over observational distinction, the extent of control over variables, and the timing of data collection, further divide these designs. For instance, experimental designs, such as RCTs, allow for genuine hypothesis testing under controlled settings. Observational studies provide valuable information in real settings, though they typically have trouble dealing with confounding variables distorting causal relationships. This general background is essential for comprehending the subtleties of clinical research. Beyond the universal definitions, the nature of study designs also encompasses their design and the type of questions to be answered. A good study design would need to set out the population under study, the sampling methods used, and the type of intervention or exposure to be investigated. Additionally, the expected outcomes should also be clearly stipulated so that the study can establish whether or not the research question has been adequately addressed. For example, when evaluating the efficacy of a new drug, a double-blind randomized trial study would eliminate biases and increase the credibility of findings, therefore addressing criticisms of earlier studies, which failed to translate findings into practice (Amendoeira et al., 2018). Such meticulous design features not only support the study's robustness but also enable its ultimate practicality in clinical practice, where clinical realities usually short-circuit theoretical outcomes. Furthermore, innovative methodologies like Bayesian adaptive designs are indicative of the evolving environment of clinical study designs. These new designs allow researchers to modify elements of the trial according to increasing data, thus increasing participant safety and overall efficiency of the intervention under scrutiny. This is particularly applicable in pharmacology trials of combination drugs, where determination of the highest dose that can be tolerated (MTD) through consideration of toxicity is essential (Babb et al., 2018). High-level statistical methods enable more advanced interaction and modeling of complex interactions between variables, thereby improving data interpretation. As clinical research evolves, study design definition and study design features will remain crucial, guiding researchers in their quest for evidence that has implications in clinical practice and health policy (Figure 3.15).

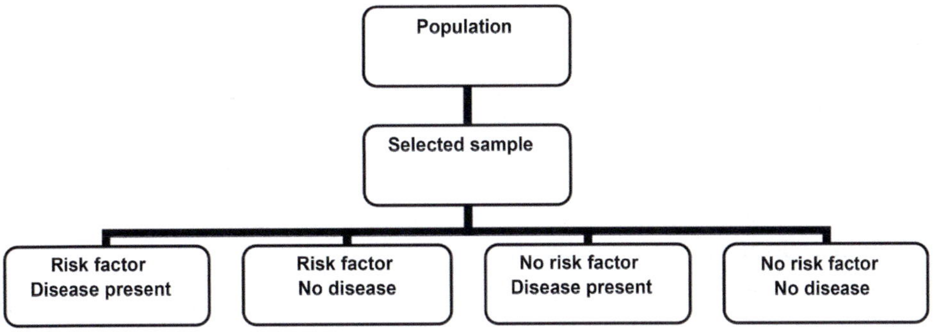

Figure 3.15. Study design for cross-sectional studies.

Source: https://ars.els-cdn.com/content/image/1-s2.0-S2211419X11001637-gr2.jpg.

3.5.2. Data Collection Methods

In clinical trials, proper collection of data is important to the validity and integrity of study findings. Traditional methods for the collection of data involve direct measurement, i.e., clinical evaluation and laboratory examinations; however, with the advancement of science, modern methods have led to more inclusive approaches. One of these new methods is developing national cohorts that collect multidisciplinary data, such as clinical data, tumor tissues, and patient-reported outcomes (PROs). A known example highlights the feasibility of such a strategy using an enriched cohort in gastrointestinal cancer patients, informed consent for ample reuse of information, biobanking, and PRO harvesting. The integration of these disparate points from multiple data sources not only overcomes the drawbacks of conventional designs but also greatly increases the quality and variety of research outcomes (Berbee et al., 2017). Another evolving data collection method is point-of-care clinical trials, which are designed to organically integrate research into the standard care protocol. The trials are also designed to minimize burdens on physicians and participants through minimizing processes such as recruitment and randomization. Utilizing data collected through electronic medical records enhances efficiency and reduces fatigue for participants, hence increasing compliance. The adaptive designs applied in these kinds of studies, for instance, Bayesian designs, support real-time adaptation when receiving data, arguably leading to more precise and effective results. These developments in study designs are a step towards more applied research goals that better match the realities of clinical practice and ultimately lead to more dynamic knowledge of patient responses and treatment success (Leatherman et al., 2016). The adequacy of data collection protocols in clinical studies hinges to a great extent on whether or not they will be able to adapt to new data arising and maintain ethical standards. As highlighted in the gastrointestinal cancer cohort study, longitudinal PRO collection not only adds to the dataset but also allows researchers to understand the patient experience longitudinally. Similarly, a point-of-care trial's adaptive design optimizes the responsiveness of the research to real-world concerns by enabling quick intervention and adjustments. With the rise in the significance of personalized medicine, these data collection methods are significant developments that promote a more patient-centric strategy for clinical studies. Actually, the confluence of such diverse approaches not only strengthens study designs but also builds an environment of innovation towards better clinical outcomes and advancing healthcare research (Berbee et al., 2017; Leatherman et al., 2016).

3.5.3. Use in Public Health Research

In recent years, adaptive designs have been increasingly applied in public health studies due to their inherent flexibility, whereby adjustments could be ascertained in trials as and when data emerge. Adaptive clinical trials are a precious resource for the allocation of resources, as through them, scientists can make informed decisions that can cumulatively enhance the efficiency of health technology appraisals. By incorporating health economics into these designs, researchers are able to balance clinical and cost-effectiveness outcomes so that finite research budgets are invested effectively. Decision-makers, health care professionals, and other stakeholders have been particularly interested in this adaptive design and appreciate its worth in addressing pressing public health questions while alleviating issues of budget and resource limitations (Brennan et al., 2020). This discussion of adaptive trial designs reflects a growing recognition of the necessity for creative approaches to the public health field that prioritize efficiency and usability. Some of the importance of public health research is in discovering consumer interaction with health advice and dietary guidelines. Food-based dietary guidelines (FBDG), which promote healthier food consumption and risk reduction for chronic diseases, have become increasingly applied to public health strategies. However, it has been demonstrated through research that there exists a large gap between the public use of these guidelines. Most current studies point to a knowledge-practice mismatch among consumers, indicating that despite a high level of consumer familiarity with FBDG, knowledge and application to daily life remain poor. This relationship leads to the necessity of selective evaluation processes in public health research to ascertain how far FBDG can go in influencing impactful changes in behavior. In looking at awareness, understanding, and practice as interdependent factors, researchers stand a better opportunity to meet the needs of varied populations (Achterberg et al., 2011). Finally, the nuances of stakeholder engagement in public health studies point to the importance of merging diverse perspectives into study design and analysis in clinical studies. Engaging stakeholders—researchers, clinicians, and members of the public—will more effectively capture the meaning of study findings for practice and translate them into applicability to real-world scenarios. For instance, when concerns are raised by stakeholders over changing trial designs to incorporate health economic outcomes, it opens the way for arguments over facilitation and training needed for successful implementation. Resolving such challenges ensures that final health technology assessments can effectively mimic the complex nature of healthcare decision-making processes. Moreover, the incorporation of varying viewpoints in conceptual models can enhance the reliability and validity of such research, resulting in the creation of effective public health interventions that align with the actual needs and behaviors of populations (Brennan et al., 2020) (Figure 3.16).

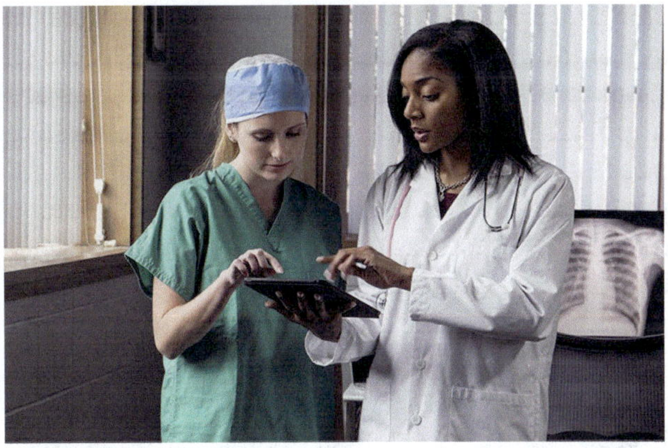

Figure 3.16. Revolutionizing clinical studies with adaptive trial designs.

Source: https://www.medidata.com/wp-content/uploads/2023/04/featured-image-revolutionizing-clinical-studies-with-adaptive-trial-designs-flexibility-mid-study-changes-and-expert-teams-for-optimal-results.jpg.

3.6. Systematic Reviews and Meta-Analyses

Systematic reviews and meta-analyses are the keystone tools in clinical studies by which researchers can combine evidence from multiple studies. By systematic searching, critical appraisal, and synthesis of evidence from research for specific health-related questions, these tools provide more robust evidence than isolated studies. Reproducibility and transparency are secured through the systematic review process, which offers more authentic conclusions of efficacy and effectiveness. For instance, recent systematic reviews in the area of animal-assisted interventions (AAIs) noted the inconsistent quality and unclear terminology used across the field, ultimately restricting comparability of providers' methods and outcomes. The occurrence highlights the necessity for firm operational procedures and universal terminologies that everyone can understand, affirming the significance of systematic reviews in informing future research (Amato et al., 2020). Hence, these methods are important in the formation of robust evidence bases, which inform clinical guidelines and promote health outcomes. Meta-analyses, being a type of systematic review, quantitatively synthesize findings from several studies to provide a more holistic understanding of a given intervention or treatment. Statistical analysis enhances the power and validity of outcomes, thereby improving clinical practice through more knowledgeable decision-making. For instance, within the field of prenatal and postnatal care, systematic reviews have compared the effectiveness of dynamic elastomeric fabric orthoses (DEFO) for the treatment of symptoms linked to pregnancy. With a rigorous review leading to 17 studies that were found eligible, disparities in the terminology and differences in DEFO descriptors made it difficult to compare across studies. These nuances also demonstrate how meta-analyses are able to extract valuable information, uncovering trends that individual studies might overlook. This minute integration not only allows for clinical recommendations to be made practically but also recognizes areas within the present literature that remain unclear and must be investigated further (Hing et al., 2019). The application of systematic reviews and meta-analyses is necessary to advance clinical research methodology. Their role in synthesizing and evaluating research evidence plays a part in constructing a stronger model for explaining the effects of health interventions. Systematic reviews have the potential to resolve methodological problems that have plagued the majority of previous studies in alleviating the variation in results. The findings derived from systematic reviews can influence policy, clinical practice, and research directions. For example, the inconsistent quality of AAIs in the literature calls for additional research and standardization. As systematic reviews and meta-analyses continue to evolve, their position in evidence-based practice remains all the more vital, enabling better patient care and contributing to better medical knowledge (Amato et al., 2020) (Figure 3.17).

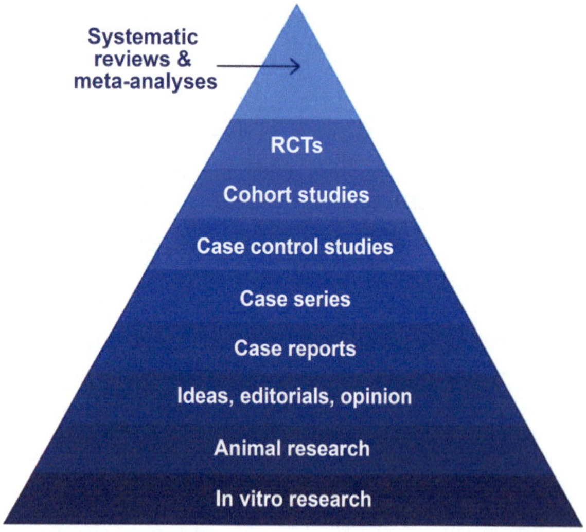

Figure 3.17. Quality of evidence ranking.

Source: https://digitalho.com/wp-content/uploads/2023/03/systematic-review-and-meta-analysis-03.jpg.

3.6.1. Definition and Purpose

In the context of clinical research, study design and objective play crucial foundational elements determining research effectiveness with the aim of elucidating health outcomes. A study design constitutes a research plan involving data collection and analysis to answer specific clinical questions. Its principal function is to make sure that the study design conforms to the objectives of the study so that it is simple to derive valid and credible conclusions. Lack of a properly designed study invites scientists into the trap of producing incorrect conclusions that may mislead clinical practice and guidelines. Thus, having an understanding of the definition of different study designs is a fundamental step in the process of formulating evidence-based health interventions that allow practitioners and policy-makers to make informed decisions that determine patient outcomes and public health outcomes. Aside from the acquisition of data, the significance of study design cannot be overstated because it is central in informing results and their application in clinical practice. For instance, systematic reviews and meta-analyses aggregate evidence from different research studies and offer aggregated insights into treatment efficacy and best practice. Aggregate analyses in this case follow a set methodological approach, which lends greater validity to their evidence (Plumbley et al., 2017). Furthermore, stringency that follows well-designed studies allows for consequent, reliable implementation of findings in practice, helping bridge the gap between practice and theoretical research. Researchers must ensure that the study design they employ is adequate to encompass the richness and complexity of the clinical questions under investigation, thereby fostering an iterative process of refining the delivery of healthcare. Innovative design solutions also emerge from concerted advances in therapeutic interventions and technology, affirming the dynamic nature of clinical research. An example is marker strategy design (MSGD), which has been suggested as a model for the assessment of predictive markers for targeted therapies. This structure allows researchers to randomly allocate patients based on marker status and thus compare treatment outcomes in a more advanced manner (Han et al., 2019). These developments are quintessential instances of how modifying research designs narrows down the identification of impactful interventions without falling into traps associated with less rigorous approaches. As clinical research continues to advance, studies need to adjust their designs to incorporate newer information without forgetting their ultimate purpose: improving patient outcomes through methodologically sound questions (Figure 3.18).

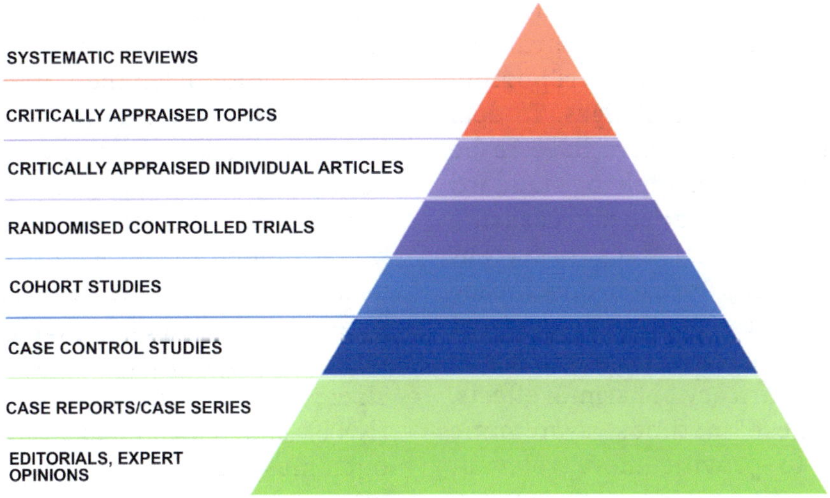

Figure 3.18. Systematic reviews are considered to be the gold standard of scientific evidence.

Source: https://www.covidence.org/wp-content/uploads/2021/05/Screen-Shot-2021-05-04-at-12.14.54-pm.png.

3.6.2. Methodology of Conducting Systematic Reviews

The systematic review process is critical in bringing together research evidence within clinical practice. Systematic reviews attempt to synthesize evidence answering a specific research question, hence impacting clinician decision-making. One of the fundamental steps in this process is the development of a focused and precise research question. The systematic review is subsequently targeted at relevant studies, hence optimizing the utility of results. Various study designs can be incorporated, i.e., randomized controlled trials and observational studies, which bring different pieces of evidence. There must also be good quality assessment techniques to evaluate the study methods of included studies in a proper review. Systematic quality assessment brings illumination regarding the precision of findings, filling gaps within the available literature that otherwise would mislead health care providers and policy makers. The efficacy of systematic reviews thus lies heavily with a systematic approach that focuses on completeness as well as clarity. In practice, researchers are left with numerous challenges in undertaking systematic reviews. In most cases, study inclusion criteria for prospective studies may lead to inconsistencies, particularly in assessing the quality of included studies. As seen in the recent appraisals, variations in study designs and reporting guidelines pose significant challenges. To deal with these challenges, researchers have to be resourceful and adaptable in applying standard methods. Special difficulties arise in measuring harmful effects in clinical trials because current methodologies have only focused on efficacy and not on side effects. Quality assessment techniques, therefore, have to be advanced to better represent the intricacy of harmful effects. By streamlining these methods, systematic reviews are able to provide more relevant information for health care decision-making, which in turn culminates in more informed clinical guidelines and practice (Bagnall et al., 2004). The arrival of scoping studies is a significant milestone in the development of systematic reviews. While traditional systematic reviews focus on the synthesis of quantitative results from curated research, scoping studies engage in a broader search of a topic, attempting to chart overarching concepts and expose knowledge gaps in the literature. This is a key distinction in the development of a complementary relationship between the two approaches. Scoping studies can direct future systematic reviews by identifying areas deserving further investigation. In addition, inclusion of consultation exercises in scoping studies enhances stakeholder engagement, and findings are more relevant to policy makers, practitioners, and service users. However, inclusion of scoping studies in traditional review models triggers a controversy regarding their unique contribution towards research methodology. Overall, such developments ensure that clinical research remains dynamic, flexible, and responsive to the rapidly changing health care demands environment (Antman et al., 2005).

3.6.3. Importance in Evidence-Based Practice

The significance of evidence-based practice (EBP) in clinical research cannot be overstated, as it revolutionizes the patient care paradigm. Drawing on systematic findings of research in guiding clinical practice, practitioners are better placed to implement interventions that are not only effective but also efficient. The process emphasizes the integration of the latest best evidence, clinical expert experience, and patient values, and higher-quality healthcare outcomes. For instance, the usage of effect sizes, such as the number needed to treat (NNT), enables clinicians to interpret research outcomes more appropriately and apply them in a real-world manner (Talley et al., 2019). Emphasis on this kind not only bridges the gap in understanding statistical significance but also bridges the gap in translating research into action, ensuring interventions chosen are indeed effective for patients. In addition, methodical reporting of clinical trial outcomes based on various study designs is a crucial element of EBP. Non-transparency in reporting skews the generalizability of outcomes, and it becomes challenging for practitioners to make valid decisions. The SCRIBE 2016 guidelines are one such resource that focuses on extensive and transparent reporting of single-case experimental designs, further adding transparency and completeness to the literature (Albin et al., 2016). By employing such guidelines, research can be carried out so that its evidence is a solid basis for informing clinical practice. Such methodological emphasis on rigor and transparency specifically challenges the core principles of EBP, which compel clinicians to critically evaluate and put into practice research evidence in their patient care practices. The merit of EBP in clinical research, in the end, lies in its power to foster a culture of continuous improvement in the provision of healthcare. With every increasing pile of evidence from various study designs, practitioners are being encouraged to keep learning and refine their practices by the most current available data. This dynamic of interaction not only enhances individual practice but also contributes to the overall medical knowledge base. For example, understanding and applying measures like NNT has the potential to reshape rehabilitation practitioners' thinking of treatment plans, such that patient-centered care can thrive (Talley et al., 2019). Hence, foundations of EBP are needed so that healthcare is in a position to react to shifting demands of patients, so effective study designs continue to play a key role in clinical research (Figure 3.19).

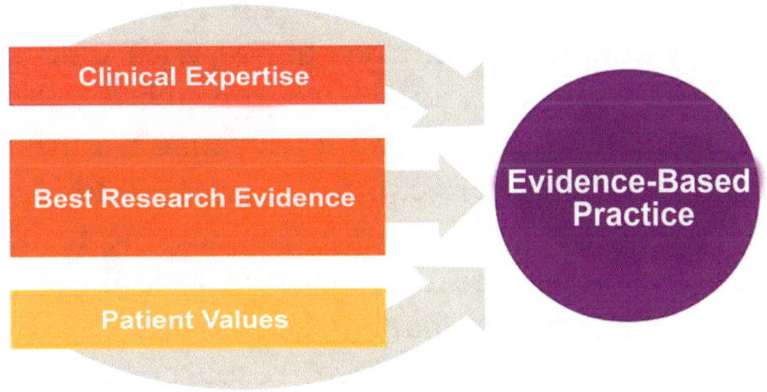

Figure 3.19. Evidence-based practice.

Source: https://uq.pressbooks.pub/app/uploads/sites/125/2023/11/EBP-diagram.jpg.

Summary

The summary of a study is an important element within the larger framework of clinical research, especially when it comes to the effectiveness and use of multiple types of study designs. Summaries based on high-quality research immediately impact clinical guidelines and educational curricula within the health professions. In accordance with the underlined importance of recent studies, evidence-based practice depends on the validity of the research methodology behind it. By the recognition that flawed study designs have the capability of yielding misleading results, it is clear that sound methodology and correct selection of participants are imperative for successful results. In low back pain treatment, for instance, creation of practice guidelines has been guided by systematic reviews critically examining methodological quality, leading to the discarding of certain treatments like traction because of diluted evidence. The implications stretch into the future, predetermining the clinical practice of new graduates to come with an unyielding commitment to methodologically higher-quality clinical research (Plumbley et al., 2017). Furthermore, there is a need to recognize the dynamic nature of clinical trial methodologies, especially with the advent of point-of-care trials that seek to connect research and clinical practice seamlessly. This new approach not only minimizes the burden of traditional research for both patients and clinicians but also optimizes result applicability by aligning closely with practice. Application of Bayesian adaptive methods facilitates adaptive study design adaptation in accordance with data accrual, thereby optimizing chances for obtaining valid conclusions. This adaptive approach is valuable, particularly in studies that involve complex or heterogeneous patient groups, because traditional designs will more likely fail. By refining these approaches, researchers can make it possible for the generation of evidence that is not only scientifically sound but also readily translatable to actual clinical settings so as to improve patient outcomes and inform future practice guidelines (Leatherman et al., 2016). In sum, the validity of clinical research summations depends solely on the validity of the study designs employed. With continued growth in clinical research, emphasis needs to be placed on enhancing methodological strength so that evidence can be valid and useful to clinical practice. The accumulation of evidence should be conducive to actionable recommendations that reflect the intricacies of patient care, bridging the gap between research and practical applicability. This ongoing evolution of research practice, including the application of point-of-care studies, is a paradigm shift towards more pragmatic methods that will better serve practitioners and patients. Through critically conceptualizing the boundaries of historical interventions and continuously refining research methods, the clinical research community can unlock the door to improved health outcomes as well as a deeper appreciation of effective clinical practice in a changing medical landscape (Plumbley et al., 2017; Leatherman et al., 2016).

In clinical trials, the selection of the study design is most important to obtain valid and reliable data. The complexity of healthcare demands a pluralistic strategy involving multiple methodologies, each with its own suitable hypotheses and requirements. For instance, randomized controlled trials (RCTs) are generally considered the gold standard since they have the ability to reduce bias and establish causality. On the other hand, observational studies are of utmost importance in investigating clinical practice and outcomes in real-life contexts, which allows researchers to gain evidence in settings where RCTs would be impractical. This series of designs, such as case studies and qualitative methods, emphasizes how research approaches should be matched with specific questions and the context of the healthcare setting, which makes findings relevant and useful.

Besides, the evaluation of psychotherapy interventions strongly emphasizes the need for a systematic process of outcome assessment. The format provided for assessment of psychotherapy and training in psychotherapy comprises eight distinct measurement domains that guide researchers on what to measure rigorously. The protocol assists not only with collaboration among various centers for training but also in providing consistency in the evaluation of the efficacy of treatment. The systematic approach also facilitates inclusion of both specific treatment outcomes and overall ideas, so researchers can orient their approaches to suit changing therapeutic settings. By encouraging systematic case studies and minimal designs as transferable to private practice, the system encourages the richness and quality of psychotherapy research, thereby benefiting patients through improved clinical care (Elliott et al., 2006). Organizational formats like those established by NHS Quality Improvement Scotland also play a significant role in clinical research quality improvement. By issuing directives on best clinical practice and encouraging the adoption of quality improvement activities, NHSQIS plays an important role in the development of research methods that focus more on patient care. Their focus on setting standards and assessing performance not only enhances the quality of research but also ensures that outcomes are translated into beneficial alterations in clinical practice. This mutual support between research and the measurement of quality helps to provide a solid foundation for creating effective interventions for health. Through the alignment of research designs with quality improvement targets, researchers are in a stronger position to meet the imperatives of healthcare delivery and ensure their activities convert into tangible benefits for patient groups (Bowers et al., 2009).

CLOSER LOOK

FUTURE DIRECTIONS IN CLINICAL RESEARCH

Clinical research development has constantly been directed by scientific knowledge and methodological developments. Future directions as the field progresses must be a more integrated approach commensurate with the complexity of healthcare in modern times. This includes a strong emphasis towards multi-dimensional family preservation programs, for which research questions must revolve around tangible improvements in the lives of children and families. Research must go beyond the common measures to examine organizational conditions' impact on service delivery, building more knowledge about service fidelity and worker performance. Mitigating these overlooked factors will enable subsequent research to enhance the efficiency of therapeutic interventions, resulting in a significant increase in outcomes for those receiving such programs (Meezan et al., 2001).

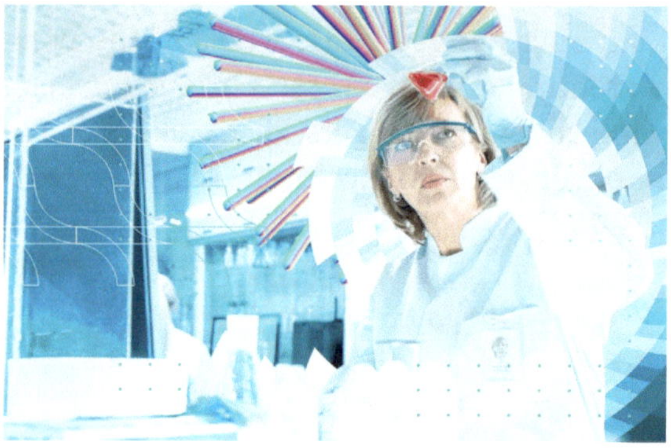

Figure 3.20. Researcher analyzing a sample in a digitally enhanced clinical research environment.

Source: https://www.bgosoftware.com/blog/wp-content/uploads/2023/09/bgo-software-blog_post-size-%CE%93Co-Future-of-Clinical-Research_no_title.png.

This combined strategy in clinical research can lead to increased policy and practice impact, such that solutions, not only theoretically sound but also practically viable , are guaranteed. Another direction for clinical research with possibilities is the merging of novel scientific disciplines such as omics, which include genomics, transcriptomics, and proteomics, among others. These courses of study have the potential to revolutionize our understanding of disease and health by offering insights into the biological mechanisms that give rise to various medical conditions. As nursing education evolves, PhD programs must become integrated with this content so that the next generation of nursing scientists are capable of conducting innovative and interprofessional research that will address current health concerns. This purposeful integration will allow researchers to design studies that are not merely good but highly relevant to patient treatment and care outcomes (Cindy et al., 2015). Secondly, through establishing a culture where new scientific findings are readily incorporated into clinical research design, the field can advance more rapidly in terms of informing improved healthcare practice. Lastly, the future of clinical research must involve theory-guided longitudinal research. Theory can be applied to inform data point collection over the duration of a study in a manner such that changes in the dynamic functioning of families and individuals can be monitored over time. When testing specific interventions, multi-dimensional measures must be employed to capture constructs such as safety and child well-being. A multi-method approach in such work will allow more nuanced insights into the outcomes that are attributed to health interventions and the contextual factors that influence these outcomes. Additionally, using more than one informant in these studies could provide a richer picture of program success, widening the range of information drawn from the study endeavor. Through these approaches, clinical research can build a firm foundation for evidence-based practice that is very sensitive to the needs of patients and communities (Meezan et al., 2001) (Figure 3.20).

References

1. Achterberg, C., Achterberg, J., Achterberg, R., Auld, G., Cameron, A., Campbell, N., Contento, I., et al. (2011). A review of consumer awareness, understanding and use of food-based dietary guidelines. https://core.ac.uk/download/9633232.pdf (accessed on 25th June 2025).
2. Adam, R., Bansal, A., Barnes, H., Barroso, J., Barroso, I., Bay, J., Belza, M., et al. (2013). Unstimulated cortisol secretory activity in everyday life and its relationship with fatigue and chronic fatigue syndrome: A systematic review and subset meta-analysis. https://core.ac.uk/download/20443927.pdf (accessed on 25th June 2025).
3. Albin, R., Backman, C., Barlow, D. H., Douglas, B., et al. (2016). The Single-Case Reporting Guideline In BEhavioural Interventions (SCRIBE) 2016 statement. https://core.ac.uk/download/289166471.pdf (accessed on 25th June 2025).
4. Alonso, J., Holder, D., MacKay, R., Owen, R., et al. (2013). Technologies for delivery of proton and ion beams for radiotherapy. http://arxiv.org/abs/1310.0237 (accessed on 25th June 2025).
5. Amato, A., Carratu, R. C., Dice, F., Fioretti, A., et al. (2020). Methodological and terminological issues in animal-assisted interventions: An umbrella review of systematic reviews. https://core.ac.uk/download/pdf/323188218.pdf (accessed on 25th June 2025).
6. Amendoeira, J., Borglin, G., Hanssen, T. A., Richards, D. A., et al. (2018). The second triennial systematic literature review of European nursing research: Impact on patient outcomes and implications for evidence-based practice. https://core.ac.uk/download/213548053.pdf (accessed on 25th June 2025).
7. Anderson, C. M., Lyon, D. E., McCarthy, D., Corwin, E. J., Taylor, J. Y., Voss, J., Gregory, K. E., et al. (2015). Educating future nursing scientists: Recommendations for integrating omics content in PhD programs. https://core.ac.uk/download/213074828.pdf (accessed on 25th June 2025).
8. Antman, E., Arksey, H., Badger, D., Dixon-Woods, M., Hagell, A., Arksey, H., Jepson, R., et al. (2005). Scoping studies: Towards a methodological framework. https://core.ac.uk/download/56237.pdf (accessed on 25th June 2025).
9. Argano, V., Balistreri, C. R., Giarratana, R. M., Lio, D., et al. (2019). On the road to accurate biomarkers for cardiometabolic diseases by integrating precision and gender medicine approaches. https://core.ac.uk/download/268910274.pdf (accessed on 25th June 2025).
10. Autrique, A., Broekaert, E., Colpaert, K., Vanderplasschen, W., et al. (2010). The human prerogative: A critical analysis of evidence-based and other paradigms of care in substance abuse treatment. https://core.ac.uk/download/55790687.pdf (accessed on 25th June 2025).
11. Babb, J., Braun, M., Gasparini, A., Iasonos, A., Lee, S., Mander, A., Miles, C., et al. (2018). Cancer phase I trial design using drug combinations when a fraction of dose limiting toxicities is attributable to one or more agents. https://core.ac.uk/download/pdf/234924131.pdf (accessed on 25th June 2025).
12. Bagnall, A. M., Aronson, J. K., Bagett, R., Bagnall, A. M., Crombie, I. K., Cuervo, G. L., Deeks, J. J., et al. (2004). Assessing harmful effects in systematic reviews. https://core.ac.uk/download/30267422.pdf (accessed on 25th June 2025).
13. Baker, J. E., Hassenstab, J., Lim, Y. Y., Maruff, P., et al. (2016). Cognitive impairment and decline

in cognitively normal older adults with high amyloid-β: A meta-analysis. https://core.ac.uk/download/80495053.pdf (accessed on 25th June 2025).

14. Barber, M., Barkham, M., Barnes, D., Barth, J., Beattie, D., et al. (2017). How should we evaluate research on counselling and the treatment of depression? A case study on how NICE's draft 2018 guideline considered what counts as best evidence. https://core.ac.uk/download/131316410.pdf (accessed on 25th June 2025).

15. Barker, C., Humphreys, K., & Pistrang, N. (2008). Mutual help groups for mental health problems: A review of effectiveness studies. https://core.ac.uk/download/1673502.pdf (accessed on 25th June 2025).

16. Barlow, D. H., & Nock, M. K. (2009). Why can't we be more idiographic in our research? https://core.ac.uk/download/28933579.pdf (accessed on 25th June 2025).

17. Basnyat, S., Goldfarb, J. M., Nyquist, G. G., Rabinowitz, M. R., et al. (2016). Head and neck manifestations of eosinophilic granulomatosis with polyangiitis: A systematic review. https://core.ac.uk/download/83049399.pdf (accessed on 25th June 2025).

18. Beck, A. P., Gröne, A., Caswell, J. L., Meyerholz, D. K., Dohoo, I. R., LaDouceur, E. E. B., Origgi, F. C., et al. (2018). Observational study design in veterinary pathology, Part 1: Study design. https://core.ac.uk/download/160499856.pdf (accessed on 25th June 2025).

19. Benson, P. E. (2008). *Evaluation of White Spot Lesions on Teeth with Orthodontic Brackets.* https://core.ac.uk/download/42627042.pdf (accessed on 25th June 2025).

20. Berbee, M., Besselink, M. G., Bloemendal, H. J., Bruno, M. J., et al. (2017). Nationwide comprehensive gastro-intestinal cancer cohorts: The 3P initiative. https://core.ac.uk/download/154410641.pdf (accessed on 25th June 2025).

21. Biosca, O., Donaldson, C., & McHugh, N. (2017). From wealth to health: Evaluating microfinance as a complex intervention. https://core.ac.uk/download/293860192.pdf (accessed on 25th June 2025).

22. Bowers, R., NHS Quality Improvement Scotland (Funder), & Ross, K. (2009). *Best Practice Statement: Use of Ankle-Foot Orthoses Following Stroke.* https://core.ac.uk/download/9025419.pdf (accessed on 25th June 2025).

23. Boyce, D., Doronina, O., Gould, D., Reilly, J., MacDonald, J., Price, L., Shepherd, L., et al. (2018). Interventions to improve healthcare workers' hand hygiene compliance: A systematic review of systematic reviews. https://core.ac.uk/download/293885604.pdf (accessed on 25th June 2025).

24. Breen, L., & Darlaston-Jones, D. (2008). Moving beyond the enduring dominance of positivism in psychological research: An Australian perspective. https://core.ac.uk/download/61302010.pdf (accessed on 25th June 2025).

25. Brennan, A., Flight, L., Hind, D., Julious, S. A., et al. (2020). How can health economics be used in the design and analysis of adaptive clinical trials? A qualitative analysis. https://core.ac.uk/download/288346143.pdf (accessed on 25th June 2025).

26. Burke, D., Squires, J., Carl, M., Dahlke, D., Hagler, D., Herb, J., Herb, L., et al. (2009). Ontology-based knowledge representation of experiment metadata in biological data mining. https://core.ac.uk/download/131216239.pdf (accessed on 25th June 2025).

27. Chan, J. C., Chan, N., Dickson, K. S., Stahmer, A. C., et al. (2020). Fidelity assessment in community programs: An approach to validating simplified methodology. https://core.ac.uk/download/287622282.pdf (accessed on 25th June 2025).

28. Compare, A., Griffiths, M. D., Shonin, E., Van Gordon, W., et al. (2014). Buddhist-derived loving-kindness and compassion meditation for the treatment of psychopathology: A systematic review. https://core.ac.uk/download/30650462.pdf (accessed on 25th June 2025).

29. Egan, M., Katikireddi, S. V., & Petticrew, M. (2014). How do systematic reviews incorporate risk of bias assessments into the synthesis of evidence? A methodological study. https://core.ac.uk/download/42356896.pdf (accessed on 25th June 2025).

30. Elliott, R. (2009). Psychotherapy changes process research: Realizing the promise. https://core.ac.uk/download/9025553.pdf (accessed on 25th June 2025).

31. Elliott, R., & Zucconi, A. (2006). Doing research on the effectiveness of psychotherapy and psychotherapy training: A person-centered/experiential perspective. https://core.ac.uk/download/9029991.pdf (accessed on 25th June 2025).

32. Eloise, Q. (2024). The impact of "multiple looks" when performing survival analysis. https://core.ac.uk/download/619599308.pdf (accessed on 25th June 2025).

33. Evans, J. C., Hirani, S. P., & Needle, J. J. (2019). Nutritional and post-transplantation outcomes of enteral versus parenteral nutrition in pediatric hematopoietic stem cell transplantation: A systematic review of randomized and nonrandomized studies. https://core.ac.uk/download/196222605.pdf (accessed on 25th June 2025).

34. Faurholt-Jepsen, D. (2013). *The Double Burden*. https://core.ac.uk/download/pdf/16666765.pdf (accessed on 25th June 2025).

35. Gennaro, A., Kleinbub, J. R., Mannarini, S., Palmieri, A., et al. (2019). Training in psychotherapy: A call for embodied and psychophysiological approaches. https://core.ac.uk/download/288795295.pdf (accessed on 25th June 2025).

36. Gray, C. M., McCallum, C., & Rooksby, J. (2018). Evaluating the impact of physical activity apps and wearables: Interdisciplinary review. https://core.ac.uk/download/150600185.pdf (accessed on 25th June 2025).

37. Guller, U. (2018). Surgical outcomes research based on administrative data: Inferior or complementary to prospective randomized clinical trials? https://core.ac.uk/download/159146296.pdf (accessed on 25th June 2025).

38. Han, Y. (2019). On the use of marker strategy design to detect predictive marker effect in cancer immunotherapy. https://core.ac.uk/download/228066053.pdf (accessed on 25th June 2025).

39. Hernández Fernández, A. (2020). Good practices, innovation or scientific research in education? A conceptual reflection. https://core.ac.uk/download/294829555.pdf (accessed on 25th June 2025).

40. Hing, W. A., Milne, N., Pope, R. R., Szkwara, T., et al. (2019). Effectiveness, feasibility, and acceptability of dynamic elastomeric fabric orthoses (DEFO) for managing pain, functional capacity, and quality of life during prenatal and postnatal care: A systematic review. https://core.ac.uk/download/225011383.pdf (accessed on 25th June 2025).

41. Kaiseler, M., Queirós, C., & Rodrigues, S. (2015). Psychophysiological assessment of stress under ecological settings: A systematic review. https://core.ac.uk/download/29194544.pdf (accessed on 25th June 2025).

42. Lavallee, D., & Sandgren, S. S. (2018). Muscle dysmorphia research neglects DSM-5 diagnostic criteria. https://core.ac.uk/download/228178259.pdf (accessed on 25th June 2025).

43. Leatherman, S. M. (2016). *Adaptive Methods for Bayesian Time-to-Event Point-of-Care Clinical Trials* [Doctoral thesis, Boston University]. https://open.bu.edu/bitstream/2144/14317/9/Leatherman_bu_0017E_10368.pdf (accessed on 25th June 2025).

44. McMillan, A. S., & Stewart-Brown, S. L. (2010). *Home and Community-Based Parenting Support Programmers and Interventions: Report of Work Package 2 of the Data Prev Project.* https://core.ac.uk/download/46468.pdf (accessed on 25th June 2025).

45. Meezan, W., & Yoo, J. (2001). Family preservation research: Where we've been, where we should be going. https://core.ac.uk/download/46715794.pdf (accessed on 25th June 2025).

46. O'Brien, G., Rodriguez-Labajos, L., & Thomson, C. (2018). Performance measurement for the strategic management of healthcare estates. https://core.ac.uk/download/293884853.pdf (accessed on 25th June 2025).

47. Parry, E. L., Peat, G., & Thomas, M. J. (2018). Defining acute flares in knee osteoarthritis: A systematic review. https://core.ac.uk/download/161128902.pdf (accessed on 25th June 2025).

48. Plumbley, G. D. (2017). *Traction for Low Back Pain, The Evidence Is Flawed: A Thesis Presented in Partial Fulfilment of The Requirements for the Masters of Health Science (MHlthSci) in Environmental Health at Massey University Campus, Wellington, New Zealand.* https://core.ac.uk/download/158297899.pdf (accessed on 25th June 2025).

49. Rosenberger, W. F., & Sverdlov, O. (2011). Handling covariates in the design of clinical trials. http://arxiv.org/abs/1102.3773 (accessed on 25th June 2025).

50. Ryeznik, Y., Sverdlov, O., & Wong, W. K. (2019). On optimal designs for clinical trials: An updated review. https://core.ac.uk/download/286729243.pdf (accessed on 25th June 2025).

51. Talley, S. A. (2019). *Reporting Number Needed to Treat in Clinical Trials Published in Physical Therapy Specific Literature 1989–2018.* https://core.ac.uk/download/343749524.pdf (accessed on 25th June 2025).

52. Vogel, R. (2018). *BIOS 9331—Meta Analysis.* https://core.ac.uk/download/229150785.pdf (accessed on 25th June 2025).

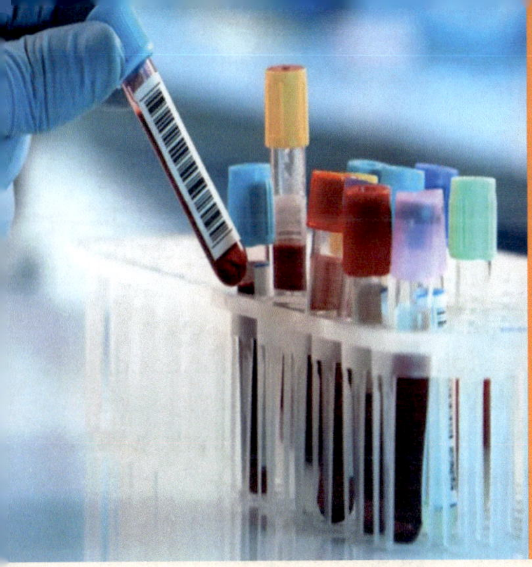

Chapter 4

DIAGNOSTIC TEST EVALUATION

Contents

Introduction

In medical diagnostics, the emergence of advanced test methods has transformed the context of disease recognition and management. Diagnostic tests form the core of clinical decision-making, particularly with difficult conditions like autism spectrum disorder (ASD). With the rising prevalence of ASD, unraveling the subtleties of diagnostic evaluations has become increasingly important. Chromosomal microarray analysis (CMA) is often positioned as a first-line diagnostic test, being capable of identifying copy number variants (CNVs) involved in ASD. However, as studies indicate, not all identified CNVs are of the type that clarify the disorder, with a high proportion constituting variants of unknown significance. This also raises critical issues about the efficacy and interpretation issues associated with such testing methods, which require study to enhance clinical outcomes for ASD-affected patients (Aceti et al., 2023). The rich diversity of ASD also increases the complexity of interpreting the results of diagnostic tests. Not every diagnosis is an indication of a set of symptoms, but also points to the interactions between genes and environment, which result in the manifestation of the condition. Recent studies employing advanced technologies in gene analysis, such as comparative genome hybridization (array-CGH), show that children with ASD have a high incidence of CNVs, which emphasizes the need for developing genetic information. However, clinical evaluations indicate that cognitive abilities and ASD symptoms do not show uniform distinctions among individuals with various CNVs. The outcomes suggest that although diagnostic tests like CMA provide valuable insights, they may also be unconsciously creating confusion in clinical evaluations.

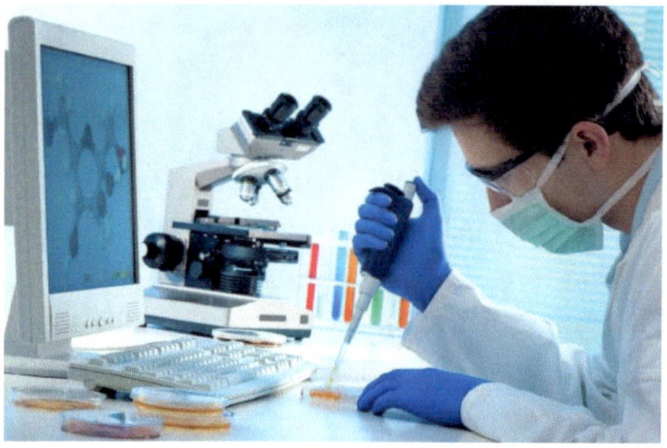

Figure 4.1. Early disease detection through diagnostic testing.

Source: https://www.quantumspecialitydiagnostics.com/web_assets/uploads/5f48c54ed211ca37fbb8416c4e37f968.jpeg.

Therefore, a merged approach with information on genetics and clinical evaluations is essential in order to build more accurate diagnosis profiles (Aceti et al., 2023). Furthermore, the cost implications of diagnostic tests cannot be overlooked, particularly with the capital-intensive nature of healthcare. The added costs of advanced diagnostic services have triggered a timely debate among the medical community regarding the drivers of such costs. Multifaceted analyses of hospital-related data ascertain that various factors, spanning patient characteristics to service sophistication, inexorably affect the cost of diagnostic testing and treatment. With the support of large data sets and sophisticated analysis software, healthcare professionals can infer information about how different parameters, such as age and hospital provider, affect day-to-day operation costs. This intersection of diagnostic efficiency with economic practicability points towards ongoing evaluation of diagnostic strategies in a way that ensures they are not only clinically significant but also economically feasible (Figure 4.1).

Definition of Diagnostic Tests

Diagnostic tests hold a pivotal role in clinical assessment, serving to establish a baseline understanding of a patient's state of health prior to the administration of therapeutic interventions. In the end, the tests are constructed to identify conditions that already exist, providing healthcare professionals with vital information upon which to base individualized patient treatment. By accurately defining the parameters of a patient's health, diagnostic tests not only inform treatment but also aid in monitoring disease state or remission. The effectiveness of these tests lies in their ability to generate reproducible and reliable results, paving the way for a consistent assessment process that can have a critical bearing on patient outcomes. From a wider scope, the development and application of diagnostic tests are a scientific method based on established scientific principles. An appropriately validated diagnostic test measures a certain set of signs or health indicators, which can range from laboratory biomarkers to imaging modalities. All types of diagnostic tests are meant to measure the presence or magnitude of a disease, considering the inherent complexities of patient variability. Furthermore, diagnostic test reliability can also be impacted by various factors, including the respective methodologies employed and the professional standards that accompany their use. Data on the limitations of different diagnostic tests is essential, emphasizing shortcomings in sensitivity, specificity, and clinical utility in practice. Their ultimate value aside, the incorporation of diagnostic tests in learning curricula, including learning environments that accommodate individual learners, appears not to receive its proper rating. A review of various case studies reveals that the majority of educational programs exclude comprehensive diagnostic tests at key points of the learning pathway, i.e., the initial test, ongoing progress monitoring, and the summative assessment. As a result, without robust diagnostic tests, students and teachers can be left without the right information in order to alter learning pathways. Such disparity not only erodes the individualized learning experience but also supports inefficient assessment of learning outcomes, as evidenced by research on the implementation of personalized learning (Berankova et al., 2016). Strengthening the diagnostic function in this respect could thus lead to more learner-focused strategies that respect diversity and support overall performance (Figure 4.2).

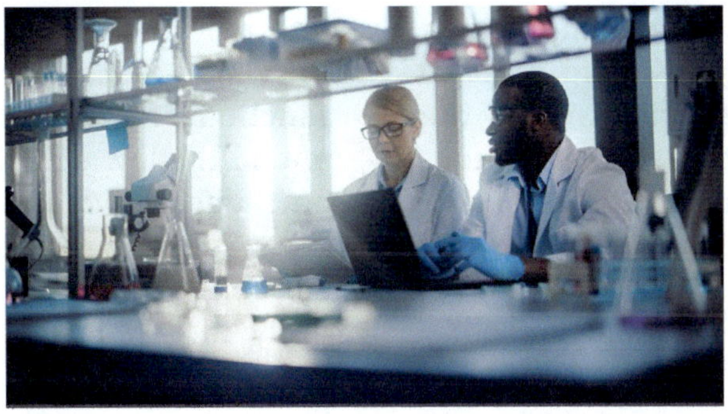

Figure 4.2. The concept of clinical utility for diagnostic tests.

Source: https://www.thermofisher.com/blog/clinical-conversations/wp-content/uploads/sites/18/2023/04/PG2815-PJT10585-COL024660-sh1873353685-1200x675-1.jpg.

Importance of Diagnostic Test Evaluation

Diagnostic test assessment is a key component of modern healthcare because clinical decision-making as well as patient outcomes directly depend on it. By ensuring that diagnostic tests are fully validated in terms of their reliability and validity, healthcare workers are able to make informed decisions from accurate information. Reliability addresses the consistency of test results, whereas validity addresses the ability of a test to measure what it is supposed to measure. An assessment that includes these dimensions develops trust both between clinicians and patients, ultimately leading to an enhanced diagnostic process. Furthermore, as evident through recent breakthroughs in rapid diagnostic devices, the incorporation of new technologies can vastly improve test accuracy and turnaround time, which is critical to successful disease management and treatment initiation (Ince et al., 2009). Hence, rigorous evaluation is not just beneficial but essential to optimize diagnostic utility in the clinical environment. Also, the cost burden imposed by the assessment of diagnostic tests is significant and requires thoughtful consideration. The cost dynamics of healthcare are characterized by accelerating costs, with laboratory testing accounting for approximately 3% of the total clinical spending. Ineffective testing can potentially generate unwanted costs and lower aggregate budgetary efficiency (Velazquez et al., 2018). By performing strenuous evaluations, stakeholders can identify instances of overuse and underuse of diagnostic tests and use this information to inform resource allocation that balances patient care without overspending. For instance, employing focused testing methods in diagnostic management teams allows healthcare professionals to select only the most essential tests. This approach not only enhances clinical workflow but also helps healthcare sustainability efforts, offering a solution to reduce waste while ensuring that patients are offered timely and effective diagnostic assessment. Altogether, the importance of evaluating diagnostic tests transcends clinical precision and encompasses deeper implications for both the healthcare system and patients. Rigorous appraisal procedures ensure that diagnostic tests yield correct conclusions, reducing the risk of diagnostic errors leading to uninformed treatment courses. In addition, the financial efficiency achieved through efficient testing protocols holds much promise in addressing increasing healthcare spending pressures. Keeping paramount a strict appraisal framework not only enhances patient care but also fosters an accountability culture within healthcare. With research being more sophisticated, the emphasis on maximizing the development of classical practices and merging new technologies will position diagnostic test evaluation as a cornerstone for effective healthcare interventions, needed to manage both health and economic determinants (Velazquez et al., 2018).

4.1. Types of Diagnostic Tests

The diagnostic testing scene is broad and diverse, encompassing a variety of methodologies directed toward identifying health states, monitoring disease progression, and assessing the efficacy of treatments. At the forefront are laboratory tests that range from simple blood tests to intricate genetic tests. They provide critical quantitative and qualitative data about a patient's health state. For example, blood tests usually provide information about metabolic functions like glucose levels, which are important in controlling ailments like diabetes. However, genetic tests can provide deep insights into inherited risks of certain diseases, thus guiding preventive measures. Diagnostic test development continues to enhance healthcare outcomes and requires an evaluation of its reliability, validity, and overall impact on clinical decision-making and patient treatment (Freeman et al., 2005). Imaging techniques are another essential group of diagnostic tests, providing visual data about the internal body functions. Modalities such as X-rays, CT scans, and MRI allow clinicians to visualize structures and diagnose disease non-invasively. Imaging modalities are able to detect abnormalities such as tumors, fractures, or lesions, and thus allow early intervention. In addition, new imaging modalities, such as 3D imaging and functional imaging, have allowed clinicians to develop a better understanding of pathologies and improve diagnostic accuracy. The importance of imaging tests is also highlighted by their inclusion in multidisciplinary therapy planning, with visual evidence informing therapy plans. Thus, clinicians are required to continually examine the strengths and weaknesses of all imaging modalities to support diagnosis accuracy and overall patient care (Busse et al., 2002). Molecular and point-of-care testing are also essential elements of diagnostic practices. Molecular diagnosis through techniques such as polymerase chain reaction (PCR) and next-generation sequencing allows precise identification of pathogens and genetic abnormalities. They find extensive application in infectious disease management and individualized medicine, delivering treatment regimens according to an individual's genetic makeup or pathogen status. Point-of-care testing, however, allows for the taking of rapid decisions since it can be done away from standard clinical laboratories and can provide real-time results. They are particularly useful in emergency situations or where there is minimal resource availability. The ongoing development of these types of diagnostic tests demands intense scrutiny to establish their conformity with clinical needs, thereby indirectly enhancing patient outcomes (Freeman et al., 2005) (Figure 4.3).

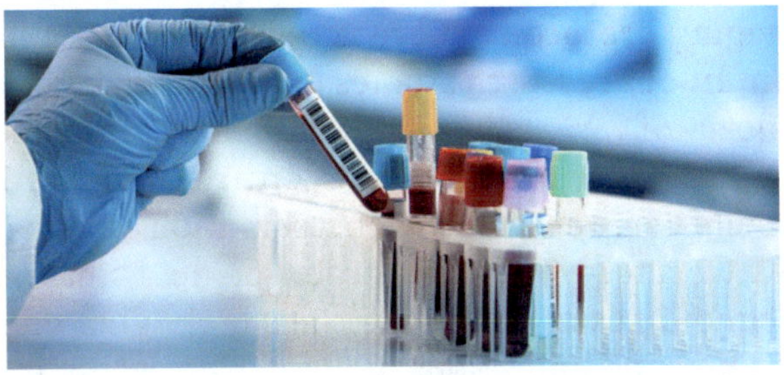

Figure 4.3. Diagnostic tests.

Source: https://images.apollo247.in/pd-cms/cms/2023-10/Shutterstock_1114244621.jpg.

4.1.1. Laboratory Tests

The laboratory test field is a cornerstone in the general architecture of diagnostic test evaluation, where effectiveness and accuracy come first. Laboratory tests are reliable techniques for detecting, diagnosing, and monitoring different health conditions through the examination of several biological samples such as blood, urine, and tissues. The importance of timely and accurate laboratory testing cannot be overstated; it enables informed clinical decision-making and is of crucial importance to patient outcomes. In this regard, quality control and standardization gain paramount importance since variation in laboratory practice can lead to variation in the results of tests, affecting patient care unfavorably. With continuing advances in technology, laboratory testing's accuracy will translate to increased diagnostic certainty and better rates at which conditions can be diagnosed, and thus plays a valuable role in effective healthcare provision. In the realm of laboratory testing, the improvement of diagnostic technologies is perhaps most evident when looking at specific diseases. For instance, the need for improved serological tests to be used in Chagas disease diagnosis also supports the current issues in laboratory diagnosis. The majority of infected persons with *Trypanosoma cruzi* are asymptomatic during the first stages, so it is hard to diagnose and treat in time. The laboratory tests currently in use may lack the sensitivity or specificity to appropriately detect infections, thus leading to untreated cases that become advanced chronic diseases. As put forth in new perspectives from the latest discussions by experts who convened to examine diagnostic issues in Chagas disease, there is a pressing need for new diagnostic solutions. The innovations should focus on rapid tests that address not only the demands for detection of active infection but also for monitoring the efficacy of therapy, enhancing patient management overall (Campaign for Access to Essential Medicines, 2008).

At the same time, incorporation of non-invasive prenatal diagnosis (NIPD) testing represents an excellent example of laboratory testing evolution in maternal-fetal medicine. Such evolution is especially relevant in RhD-negative women, where risk for sensitization has severe implications for the health of both mother and infant. The advent of NIPD has altered the potential for the early detection of fetal RhD status during pregnancy, allowing therapeutic interventions that are able to avert hemolytic disease of the newborn (HDN). Being performed on maternal blood, these tests do not pose risks associated with invasive procedures like amniocentesis and thus are safer in pregnant women. Adequate application of such laboratory tests in clinical settings not only demands improved prenatal care but also points towards a need to integrate new diagnostic methods into the overall healthcare systems to ensure access and improved outcomes for vulnerable populations (Clay et al., 2007) (Figure 4.4).

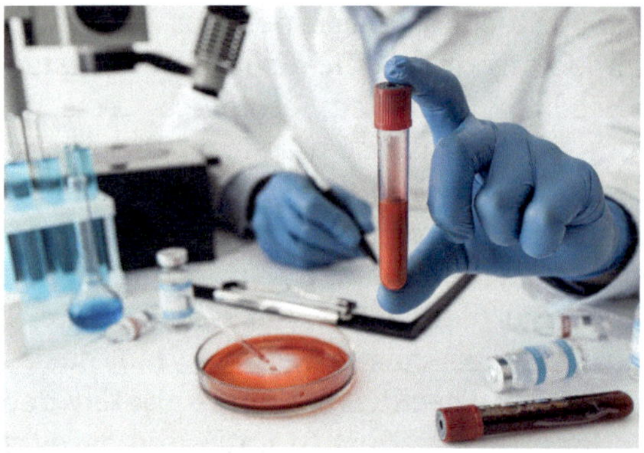

Figure 4.4. Blood tests.

Source: https://cdn-jchih.nitrocdn.com/ytdfWkhjbUydjqTtHRyFWyUdfjAkmQbT/assets/images/optimized/rev-eed486f/abiscans.com/wp-content/uploads/2023/09/coronavirus-vaccine-composition-lab-1-scaled.jpg.

4.1.2. Imaging Tests

Imaging tests have been integrated into the regular evaluation of health and disease of numerous medical conditions, particularly diagnostic and therapeutic decision-making. Such newer modalities, including magnetic resonance imaging (MRI) and computed tomography (CT), can potentially provide valuable information about the anatomical and physiological lesions in patients. Their application is especially relevant in presurgical assessment of conditions such as epilepsy, where identification of the epileptogenic zone will be a defining factor in surgical planning. However, despite the increase in imaging modalities on offer, the cost-effectiveness and unequivocal utility of some of these tests remain questionable, and their use within clinical practice must be closely observed (Chang et al., 2020). With the increasing rise in healthcare costs, the need for judicious utilization of imaging tests that improve patient outcomes at a reduced unnecessary cost is paramount. Critical evaluation of imaging tests is essential, particularly among pediatric patients with UTIs. Data show that routine imaging doesn't provide a substantial benefit in outcomes like recurrent infection or renal scarring. For instance, according to some research, less invasive imaging modalities may not be appropriate alternatives to conventional diagnostic methods, with a negative impact on clinical decision-making (Biggi et al., 2005). Secondly, the challenge lies in creating a balance between investigation comprehensiveness and radiation exposure hazards under conventional imaging protocols. There is a pressing need for continuous research studies to further clarify the efficacy of various imaging modalities, ultimately towards streamlining the entire diagnostic system while ensuring the preservation of patient health safety. The integration of new imaging technologies in clinical settings highlights their benefits and limitations in diagnostic evaluation. Since the medical world is striving towards the design of more efficient diagnostic criteria, there is an increasing need to foster evidence-based practices allowing personalized imaging regimens.

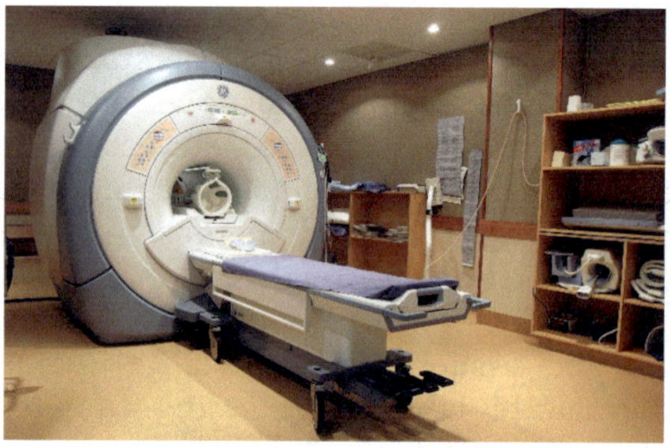

Figure 4.5. Magnetic resonance imaging (MRI).

Source: https://www.datocms-assets.com/117510/1722376162-mri-scanner20160520-5417-10ci1vq.jpg.

For instance, studies that demonstrate the incremental value of imaging in a particular case of individuals support the necessity for a hypothesis-led approach where clinical context in each patient dictates the choice of imaging modality (Chang et al., 2020). Robust evidence is required to identify which imaging tests are of greatest clinical value and weigh their cost and accessibility against one another. As the practice evolves, the generation of quantitative models evaluating the cost-effectiveness of diagnostic tests is sure to play a central role in maximizing patient care in the modern healthcare environment (Figure 4.5).

4.1.3. Clinical Assessments

In the clinical assessment context, the application of brief cognition tools has emerged as a critical element in the early identification of disorders like delirium. The assessments serve as initial screening tests that present healthcare professionals with a rich tool for the assessment of cognitive function in vulnerable groups. It has been established in research that screening older adults, particularly those who are admitted for unplanned hospitalizations, is capable of making a significant contribution to patient outcomes through the facilitation of early intervention. The utilization of various tools like the abbreviated mental test (AMT-4) and the 4 As Test (4AT) has been shown to provide great insights, identifying cognitive impairment that would otherwise escape detection with regular assessment. This first step in the diagnostic process identifies the need for using structured cognitive testing in clinical practice and consequently facilitates better patient care (Burns et al., 2016). The sensitivity and specificity of these clinical assessments are of prime concern, particularly in delirium/dementia differentiation in the presence of common co-morbidity among elderly patients. A comparison between assessment measures reflects a gradient of sensitivity and specificity. The AMT-4, for instance, was found to be sensitive to a level of 92.7% in determining definite delirium with a specificity of only 53.7%. On the other hand, the short Confusion Assessment Method (CAM) provided a more balanced profile with 70.3% sensitivity and greater specificity of 91.4% (Burns et al., 2016). This difference is to say that while certain instruments are excellent at identifying delirium, they may lack the ability to differentiate it from other cognitive impairments. Practically, the selection of the best instrument can thus influence accuracy in diagnosis, ultimately deciding future treatment for patients. Lastly, the role of clinical assessments extends beyond a single diagnosis; they aid in a more nuanced comprehension of the cognitive and functional status of the patient. The addition of tools such as the 4AT and the AMT-10 not only aids in the detection of delirium but also aids in the informing of overall patient management strategies. Data accrued through these assessments aids the clinician in the process of individualizing interventions aimed at addressing both medical and psychosocial dimensions of care. In addition, knowledge gained through routine tests promotes proactive behavior in health care facilities so that critical cognitive dysfunctions get priority during patient screening. As such, incorporating these brief cognitive screens into routine processes emphasizes their function as early detection and long-term care for delirium and other such conditions (Figure 4.6).

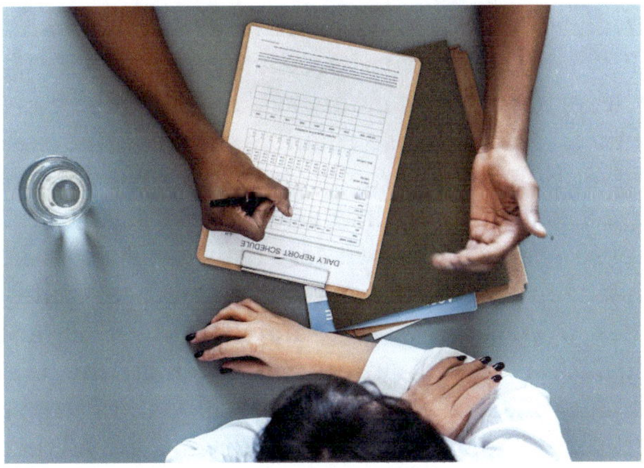

Figure 4.6. Clinical assessments.

Source: https://img.freepik.com/free-photo/aerial-view-doctor-writing-patient-daily-report-checklist_53876-14932.jpg?semt=ais_hybrid&w=740.

4.2. Criteria for Evaluating Diagnostic Tests

Assessment of diagnostic tests is a complex process involving careful consideration of an array of factors in order to determine their overall efficacy and usability in clinical practice. Some of those factors are sensitivity and specificity, such that sensitivity is the test's capacity to correctly identify those with a condition and consequently prevent false negatives, and specificity quantifies the test's capacity to identify those without the condition and therefore prevent false positives. The interrelationship between such parameters is paramount; very sensitive testing may compromise specificity and vice versa. Clinicians thus need to balance these parameters at the same time to realize optimal diagnostic efficiency. In health technology assessment (HTA), the approaches employed to evaluate such tests similarly emphasize analyzing systematically and reporting transparently to facilitate wise clinical decision-making (Busse et al., 2002). Another important criterion for the evaluation of diagnostic tests is positive predictive value (PPV) and negative predictive value (NPV). These are useful measures of the likelihood that a positive test result or a negative test result reflects the true health status of a person. Specifically, PPV estimates the probability that a person with a positive test truly possesses the disorder, while NPV estimates the probability that a person with a negative test is not diseased. The environment in which the test is administered can dramatically alter these predictive values; variation of disease prevalence influences PPV and NPV. Therefore, healthcare providers must cross-translate these values within the epidemiological environment in order to have the outcome of the test converted into meaningful clinical information. Furthermore, development of robust guidelines for reporting and interpreting these criteria, as proposed under HTA protocols, is essential in streamlining the diagnostic process (Freeman et al., 2005). Additionally, the acceptability and feasibility of the diagnostic tests must be added as their criteria for evaluation. This encompasses not only the feasibility of implementing the test in various healthcare settings but also acceptance on the part of providers and patients. Cost, convenience, and time to obtain test results are considerations that can influence the use of diagnostic technologies on a regular basis. Second, the ethical implications of test ordering need to be considered, as uncritical adherence to methodological assessment without regard for social or legal thought has the potential to debase the integrity and deployment of health technologies. As highlighted by HTA debates, an open and consistent approach to evaluating these dimensions serves to promote the credibility and utility of diagnostic tests for clinical application, finally for the good of patient care and healthcare systems (Busse et al., 2002) (Figure 4.7).

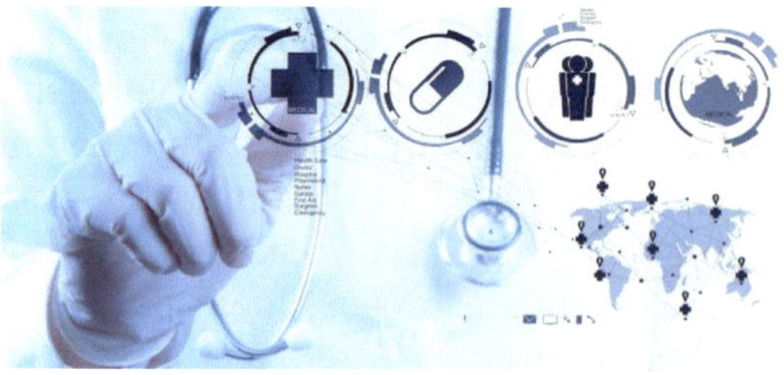

Figure 4.7. Health technology assessment (HTA).

Source: https://www.pgeu.eu/wp-content/uploads/2019/03/17-HTA-1024x607.jpg.

4.2.1. Sensitivity and Specificity

In diagnostic test evaluation, sensitivity and specificity are fundamental measures for determining the validity of a test in detecting the presence or absence of disease. Sensitivity, or the ability of a test to correctly detect individuals with a disease, is crucial in avoiding missing true positive cases. A highly sensitive test is particularly vital in situations where early detection is needed; for example, the diagnosis of life-threatening diseases such as neonatal sepsis. The effectiveness of tests such as interleukin-6 (IL-6) in predicting neonatal sepsis highlights this factor, since it has been established from research work that pooled sensitivity for IL-6 is approximately 0.79 (Ahani et al., 2011). A highly sensitive test thus plays a crucial role in improving outcomes in patients through early interventions and appropriate treatment protocols. Specificity, on the contrary, quantifies the capacity of this test to identify the absence of the disease correctly and, therefore, minimize false positives. Such a property becomes invaluable in scenarios where wrong diagnoses would lead to inappropriate treatments or further invasive interventions. For instance, when testing diagnostic procedures for *Helicobacter pylori*, the ratio of sensitivity to specificity is particularly important because tests with varying levels of these measures could lead to extensive disparity in management plans for patients presenting with dyspeptic symptoms (Ahani et al., 2011). The ideal diagnostic test would possess high sensitivity to identify cases, as well as high specificity to exclude false positives. This delicate balance is important for the formation of effective and appropriate healthcare strategies grounded in evidence-based practice. Finally, incorporating sensitivity and specificity in the evaluation of diagnostic tests is imperative in informing clinical decision-making. Balancing acts between both measures can influence resource allocation, patient care, and the overall efficiency of health care systems. Practically, a highly sensitive test would be desirable in circumstances where failure to make a diagnosis would be catastrophic. For instance, in the diagnosis of infections with H. pylori, a less sensitive rapid test can be employed due to its speed and affordability, thereby underscoring contextual influences on diagnostic tests (Fauli et al., 2025). Hence, understanding and use of sensitivity and specificity are of overriding significance for enhancing the precision of diagnosis and, by extension, patient care in numerous different clinical contexts (Figure 4.8).

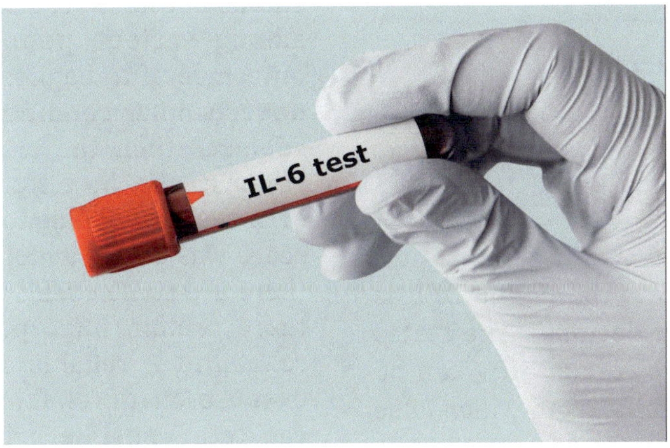

Figure 4.8. Interleukin-6 (IL-6) test.

Source: https://eshop.gentrend.cz/data/produkty/35-40-interleukin-6-il-6-5.jpg.

4.2.2. Positive and Negative Predictive Values

In evaluating diagnostic tests, PPV and NPV are crucial in quantifying the effect of a specific test in a clinical environment. PPV is the chance that patients who test positive have the disease, while NPV is the chance that patients who test negative do not have the disease. These estimates are highly influenced by the prevalence rate of the condition under test, so that with higher prevalence, PPV rises and NPV falls. Estimation of both estimates is helpful to healthcare workers in the making of decisions regarding further diagnostic testing or treatment and thus reveals vital information regarding the utility of tests in everyday situations. Studies confirm the significant role PPV and NPV play in establishing the overall efficiency of diagnostic strategies. For instance, in a study of children with blunt abdominal trauma, a study of abdominal ultrasonography and urinalysis reflected a stunning negative predictive value of 97.5%, evidencing its effectiveness in ruling out injuries, while the positive predictive value was calculated at 63.2% (Zamani, 2019).

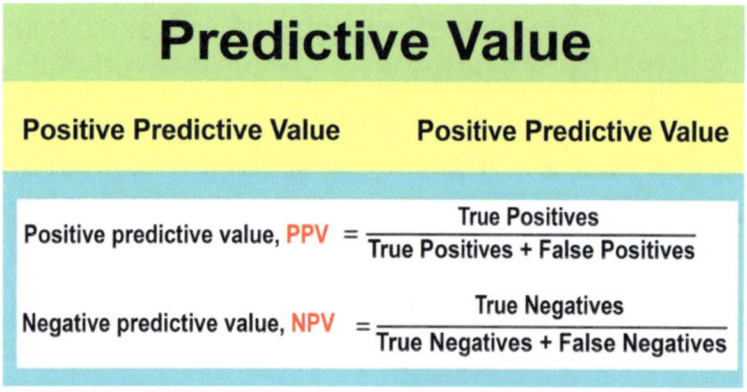

Figure 4.9. Predictive value.

Source: https://microbenotes.com/wp-content/uploads/2021/12/Positive-and-Negative-Predictive-Value-Definition-and-Significance.webp.

These findings indicate that while DPV is particularly important in deciding true states of disease within positive results, NPV can be even more important in contexts in which false negatives can lead to severe underdiagnosis and ultimately jeopardize patient safety. Appropriate assessment of the values is important for establishing effective guidelines in clinical settings. Similarly, the predictive values demonstrate how diagnostic tests must adapt to evolving populations and conditions. For example, in the case of gestational diabetes, one research study highlighted glycosuria's performance indicators as a screening tool, and the positive predictive value only came out to be 23.64% under the International Association of Diabetes Pregnancy Study Groups (IADPSG) criteria (Maranga et al., 2019). Despite the fairly high negative predictive value of 91.04%, which shows low rates of false negatives, the overall failure of PPV to show a good screening test implies that glycosuria is not an effective screening test. Thus, testing for GDM must see that good diagnostic tests like oral glucose tolerance test (OGTT) are used in the right patient assessment, thereby highlighting proper knowledge of both PPV and NPV in making a diagnostic choice (Figure 4.9).

4.2.3. Reliability and Validity

The reliability and validity notions are cornerstones in the evaluation of diagnostic tests and serve as the foundation for their capacity to provide precise identification of individuals' capacities or needs. Reliability entails the test result stability over time and among various populations. Whenever the outcomes of a diagnostic test are inconsistent under similar conditions or among equivalent subjects, then the test reliability is affected. For instance, in a study assessing the quality of a four-level diagnostic test, the reliability score was 0.475, which indicated that although there are some consistent elements of the test, there remain huge problems with the test's reliability. A reliable enough device is crucial because an unreliable diagnostic instrument can cause misinterpretations and inadequate interventions that further worsen problems they were intended to address (Jauhariyah et al., 2024). Validity, on the other hand, assesses whether a test performs what it purports to do. A valid diagnostic instrument ought to accurately reflect the constructs that it intends to measure. The aforementioned study provided a remarkable theoretical validity of 89.29%, which reflects the tests' congruence with the intended learning objectives and measures. Additionally, empirical content validity tests resulted in low false positive and negative rates, namely 6.93% and 6.53%, respectively, bringing credibility to this test as a valid diagnostic tool. To have this twin issue of theoretical and empirical validity is what ensures that the instrument is able to reliably and accurately measure key student misconceptions in Physics, validating the importance of rigorous validation in teaching tests (Jauhariyah et al., 2024). In the area of health assessment, diagnostic testing is further specialized to specific domains, such that focused validity measures are prioritized. As an example, when testing voice and speech function according to the International Classification of Functioning, Disability and Health for Children and Youth (ICF-CY), diagnostic test validity must control for diversities such as fluency and articulation. These factors, including production quality and speech rhythm, need a comprehensive assessment system in order to guarantee clinical applicability and measurement accuracy. By making sure diagnostic tools both possess reliability and validity, practitioners can provide more precise interventions tailored to the individual's requirements, and thus have improved outcomes (Figure 4.10).

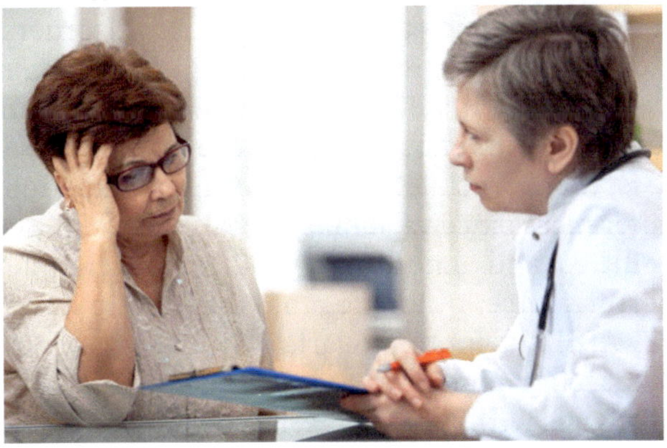

Figure 4.10. Validity and reliability.

Source: https://thinkib.net/media/ib/psychology/images/diagnostic-screening.jpg.

4.3. Challenges in Diagnostic Test Evaluation

The evaluation of diagnostic testing is confronted with a range of issues that impact clinical decisions and patient care. One of these issues is the overuse of testing as a way of excluding severe conditions rather than clarifying the probable diagnosis. Emergency physicians, for example, tend to prefer diagnostic testing to eliminate potentially serious illnesses, but this strategy has been found to not only be more expensive in healthcare terms but also to have the unintended negative effects of creating incidental findings that lead to additional invasive procedures or interventions. Such issues underscore the need for a more sophisticated body of knowledge about when and how to use diagnostic tests appropriately. Also, in the absence of proper shared decision-making models, testing will be hard for clinicians to organize with single-patient conditions, thus impairing patient safety and quality of care within practice environments, particularly in emergency departments, as illustrated in previous work (Arterburn et al., 2016). Although in the background of mounting concerns regarding healthcare delivery, challenges of evaluating diagnostic tests also extend beyond individual patient interactions to involve system-level challenges. In outpatient environments, an area traditionally underrepresented compared to inpatient facilities, there remains a compelling reason to address diagnostic errors and bolster patient safety measures. Since most of the medical practice occurs outside of hospitals, strengthening the diagnostic test requirements within those places could contribute to observable improvements in overall healthcare standards. Nevertheless, isolating the specific variables inherent in successful diagnostics is a formidable task. The complexity of the health environment necessitates multidimensional strategies to augment safety and performance in diagnosis, making it imperative to search for and implement best practices tailored for ambulatory care (Mehdi et al., 2016). Moreover, including shared decision-making (SDM) as part of the evaluation of diagnostic tests brings challenges and opportunities. SDM emphasizes collaboration between clinicians and patients to facilitate the delivery of a more tailored pattern of use of diagnostic tests based on patient risk factors and specific patient requirements. Successful application of SDM in clinical practice is, however, riddled with barriers, from a lack of time for the process to variation in health literacy among patients and clinician familiarity with the process. Overcoming such barriers requires systematic training of healthcare professionals and accessible facilities for patients. The potential advantages of engaging patients in decision-making for their care can result in more judicious use of diagnostic testing and improved health outcomes. Ultimately, the integration of SDM is capable of enabling more nuanced discussion of costs versus benefits of testing, resulting in a patient-centered healthcare system (Arterburn et al., 2016).

4.3.1. Variability in Test Performance

The problem of test performance variability is of utmost concern in the assessment of diagnostic tests, particularly when disorders such as attention-deficit/hyperactivity disorder (ADHD) are involved. This variability typically occurs due to a mixture of variables, including test development, cognitive differences between individuals, and impacts of comorbid conditions. As highlighted by more recent studies, diagnostic accuracy can be significantly enhanced through detailed assessment methods that consider the complexity of disorders. For example, research indicates that alone, individual test scores may not be capable of identifying ADHD in adults. However, when various clinical ratings—e.g., self and informant ratings of symptoms—are integrated, diagnostic accuracy can be as high as 87% (Hoelzle et al., 2019). This renders it very important to measure variability across various measurement procedures so that tests of diagnosis are not merely reliable but valid for application in the clinic. Aside from ADHD, test variability is likewise observed in the diagnosis of medical conditions such as chronic open-angle glaucoma (COAG). The Accelerator 4-Alternative Forced-Choice Flicker Test (A4FTp) demonstrates how test variability influences diagnosis outcomes. Initial tests of this measure showed stable flicker thresholds when tested repeatedly, demonstrating its potential for reliability in detecting glaucomatous changes. With psychometric properties tested, the mean area under the receiver operator characteristic curve (AUROC) of the A4FTp was statistically equivalent to gold-standard diagnostic instruments like the Frequency Doubling Technology (FDT) and Optical Coherence Tomography (OCT) (Ctori et al., 2018). This finding emphasizes the value of measuring variability not only between performances within individual tests, but also between other diagnostic tests and providing information on the best way to test to enhance diagnostic potential. Test performance variability also needs to address implications from the test environment and participants. Anxiety disorders, mood disorders, and the testing environment itself can radically influence outcomes, thus rendering diagnosis even more complicated. It is then crucial to measure inter-individual differences since variability in baseline cognitive abilities and emotional profiles may impact performance outcomes on diagnostic tests. For ADHD, symptom overlap with other mental illnesses provides the potential for incorrect diagnosis without considering variability in test performance (Hoelzle et al., 2019). Furthermore, statistical estimates are invaluable in measuring such variability so that practitioners can distinguish true clinical symptoms from test performance artifacts. All these dimensions demonstrate inherent complexities in diagnostic assessment and the necessity of balanced approaches crafted to be effective to combat variability (Figure 4.11).

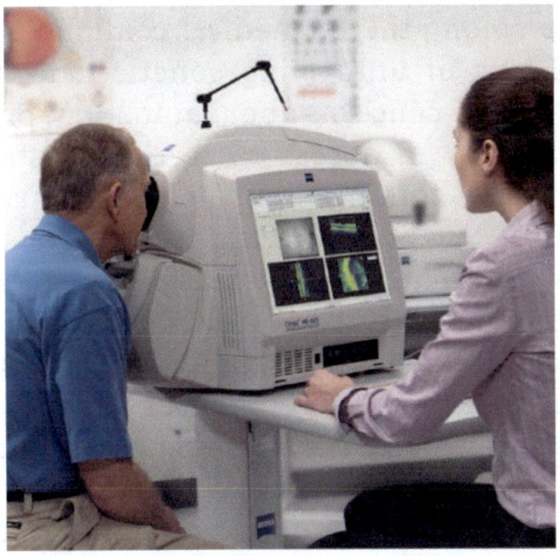

Figure 4.11. Optical coherence tomography.

Source: https://europeaneyecenter.com/wp-content/uploads/2022/12/OCT-Machine_2019-1024x1024-2.jpg.

4.3.2. Cost-Effectiveness Considerations

Cost-effectiveness in diagnostic test assessment features in determining the most beneficial testing approaches. Utilization of models to assess the economic impacts of diagnostic tests allows health professionals to make decisions on cost as well as health outcomes. For instance, the expense of laboratory tests can be represented as a large percentage of the overall healthcare expenditure and is hence paramount in deciding the trade-off between precision, waiting times, and additional healthcare expenditure. The evaluation of tests such as *Helicobacter pylori* tests illustrates how less sensitive but faster tests are cost-effective, where they permit early clinical decision-making, ultimately improving patient care at minimal cost (Fauli et al., 2025). In addition, a systematic review of interventions in different diagnostic settings highlights one of the major determinants of cost-effectiveness: model complexity and how this relates to real-world practice. As seen in colorectal cancer (CRC) screening tests, the procedure applied has a tendency to minimize the complexity of continuing medical practice and potential outcomes. The outcome reminds one of the necessity for ongoing replenishment of evidence on diagnostic performance and consequent treatment. By employing deterministic and probabilistic sensitivity analyses, researchers can better acknowledge uncertainties inherent to test evaluations. However, the need for systemic quality-of-life indicators and management plans for known conditions is a current shortfall to be addressed to enhance the interpretability and usability of cost-effectiveness research (Cairns et al., 2013). The cost-effectiveness analysis of diagnostic testing is not so much a matter of determining the dollar value of tests but of comprehension of the more expansive consequences to patient care and to health systems.

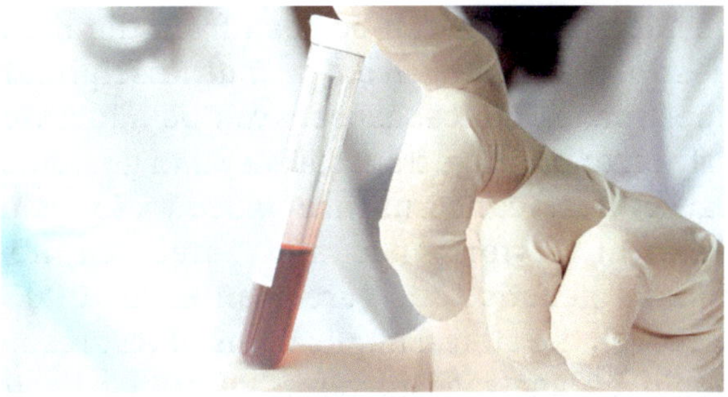

Figure 4.12. Tests for *H. pylori*.

Source: https://www.ucsfhealth.org/-/media/project/ucsf/ucsf-health/medical-tests/hero/tests-for-h-pylori-2x.jpg?rev=e08b2980165b4b73b017c0bbd0489150.

For example, determining the least expensive method of addressing diagnosed adenomas following CRC screenings would greatly affect healthcare provision. With the emergence of new technologies, their cost-effectiveness must be redefined periodically in comparison to current practices in order to achieve optimal usage of healthcare resources. Such situational awareness encourages evidence-based decision-making such that stakeholders can navigate the complexity of diagnostic tests and adopt strategies that optimize health outcomes within an affordable fiscal context (Cairns et al., 2013) (Figure 4.12).

4.3.3. Ethical Implications

The ethical issue of test evaluation for diagnostic tests has significant significance, particularly in the instance of prenatal genetic screening. Increasing application of such testing makes informed consent a critical component of ethical practice. Individuals taking tests should be fully knowledgeable about potential risks and rewards, including impacts on family planning and the psychological influence of results. The Delphi technique used to determine priority questions for health technology assessment (HTA) illustrates how it is possible to use stakeholder involvement to clarify such ethical considerations. As can be seen from the list of questions resulting from a multidisciplinary expert panel, ethical aspects can be addressed early on to promote transparency and guarantee that ethical concerns are placed alongside technical performance and safety in new prenatal genetic tests (Freeman et al., 2005). Moreover, the ethical implications of test results should be analyzed in terms of public health and norms. The distinction between obligatory questions and those deemed desirable in HTA highlights the value judgments involved in diagnostic assessment. This indicates how values can affect the way ahead in health technology assessments. HTA not only assesses technical effectiveness but also addresses legal, social, and ethical considerations that are inherent in the development of new testing technology. Such a holistic approach is required since various purposes among HTA agencies, from consideration for licensure to market to information dissemination to the public, illustrate varying ethics paradigms on which these testing protocols operate (Busse et al., 2002). Finally, the consequences of the evolution of diagnosis technology challenge the rationale of ethics frameworks, with stringent debate among the biomedical community. The complexity of unraveling genetic data raises fundamental concerns about autonomy, privacy, and fairness in access to testing. Testing of the ethical conduct regularly is a priority, particularly when evolving technologies may disproportionately affect marginalized groups and populations. With the development of standard frameworks for HTA, as discussed in efforts to advance best practices in conducting and reporting HTA, the community will be better equipped to manage these complexities. The existence of sound methodologies will not only improve the quality of testing appraisals but also ensure that ethical concerns are suitably integrated along the way, resulting in equitable and just healthcare solutions (Busse et al., 2002).

4.4. Future Directions in Diagnostic Testing

The landscape of diagnostic testing is being revolutionized, particularly with the advent of clinical metagenomic next-generation sequencing (mNGS). This new technique renders a comprehensive characterization of microbial and host nucleic acids, enabling more efficient diagnosis and control of infectious diseases. The potential uses of mNGS are diverse and span from antimicrobial resistance detection to exploring the human microbiome. Through the integration of data collected from mNGS, healthcare professionals are able to create more targeted therapeutic regimens, thus providing improved results for patients. Irrespective, the practice of research transition comes with numerous challenges, such as standardization and integrating advanced data into routine diagnostic procedures. Conquering such hurdles is critical in order to realize the full potential of mNGS, and it is therefore the foundation of next-generation diagnostic technologies that may potentially revolutionize public health programs (Chiu et al., 2019). Aside from mNGS, the intersection of cutting-edge AI and 5G wireless connectivity technology also holds vast promise for the future of diagnostics. As documented by the United Nations Sustainable Development Goals, the provision of equal access to quality healthcare is a global priority. With the integration of 5G technology, high-throughput and low-latency data transmission is made possible, effectively enhancing diagnostic test speed and precision. Paired with AI's ability to analyze data, healthcare providers are able to interpret diagnostic tests more effectively, resulting in faster decision-making and more tailored patient care. But this potential can be attained only by addressing system-wide concerns such as data privacy, interoperability of health information systems, and the need for special training. This coming together of technology presents an unparalleled chance for healthcare transformation, advocating for more efficient and equitable access to diagnostic testing (Farooq et al., 2017). Further, the trends in future diagnostic testing will undoubtedly be propelled by the ongoing need to innovate and adapt to meet global health challenges. The COVID-19 pandemic, for example, has accelerated the use of rapid testing technology and highlighted the importance of flexible diagnostic platforms. Advances in point-of-care and portable testing will likely expand access and convenience, allowing for timely interventions, especially for remote or underserved populations. Integration of learning derived from actual use will be important in the development of these diagnostic tools. Further, encouraging collaboration between academia, industry, and healthcare professionals can offer ways to new mechanisms, allowing diagnostic testing to keep pace with evolving demands of public health. Finally, embracing an innovative, forward-looking stance to diagnostic testing will be required in dealing with the complexity of future healthcare settings (Figure 4.13).

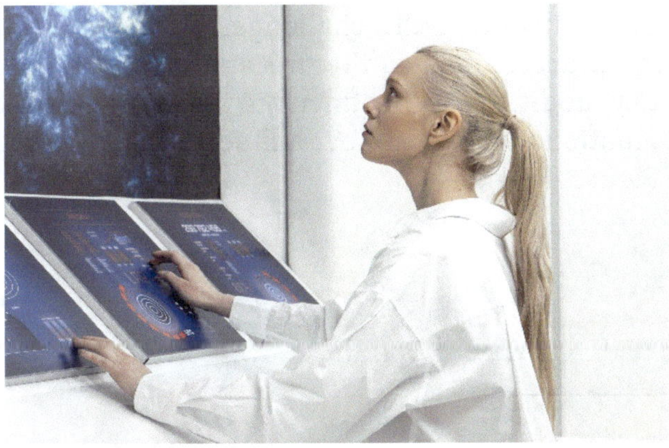

Figure 4.13. The future of diagnostic testing.

Source: https://starmedicallab.com/wp-content/uploads/2024/11/The-Future-of-Diagnostic-Testing-Trends-to-Watch-img-scaled.jpg.

4.4.1. Advances in Technology

Improved technology has profoundly influenced the field of diagnostic test evaluation, particularly concerning infectious diseases like tuberculosis (TB). The demand for rapid and accurate diagnosis is higher than ever, considering the high stakes of public health risks at risk of delayed detection and treatment. Fast-forward to the present, and gold-standard TB tests that are largely laboratory-based are inclined to take extended amounts of time to diagnose. This delay has critical ramifications, as it allows for continued transmission of Mycobacterium tuberculosis among communities, blocking epidemic control. Recent technological advances have facilitated the introduction of new diagnostic technology that not only aims at detecting active TB disease but also aids in screening for latent infection and the detection of drug resistance. However, despite these breakthroughs, a robust, user-friendly point-of-care test remains elusive, emphasizing the ongoing need for innovation in TB diagnostic technology as referenced in Harari et al. (2012). The field of TB diagnostics is also complicated by the development of drug-resistant strains, necessitating re-evaluation of current testing techniques. Drug-resistant tuberculosis, which is increasingly posing challenges globally, emphasizes the importance of appropriate diagnostics as an integral part of clinical management and infection control practices. Advances in diagnostic technology have attempted to enhance the sensitivity and speed of test results. The WHO has embraced automated liquid culture systems and molecular line probe assays as gold standards for contemporary drug susceptibility testing, a sign of heightened dependence on more reliable testing systems. Despite such developments, second-line drug susceptibility testing complexity and cost remain formidable barriers. It would be crucial that future developments address such matters with consideration of the issues of accessibility and rapid diagnostics for effective response measures against tuberculosis, as proposed in Affolabi et al. (2011). New technologies must also consider the varying economic conditions and health system capacities among various countries, especially those that are most affected by TB. The quest for a holy grail test that has all the specifications necessary to be implemented at the point of care is ongoing. The test should carry the attributes of speed, accuracy, cost-effectiveness, and adaptability to different healthcare settings. The integration of new biomarkers and digital health technologies offers potential paths towards fulfilling these needs, potentially transforming the entire TB diagnostic process. Confronting the challenges of providing comprehensive diagnostic solutions is essential for equal access to health care and efficient TB and drug-resistant strain control worldwide. Ultimately, additional investment in technological advancement is needed to improve diagnostic test evaluations within the overall scope of public health programs designed to eliminate tuberculosis (Figure 4.14).

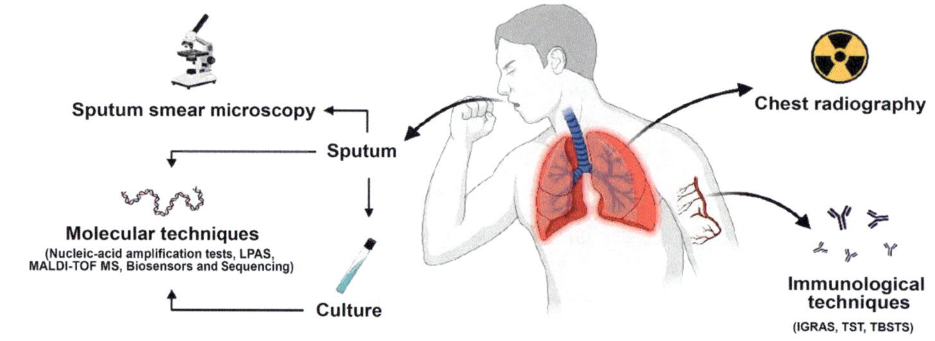

Figure 4.14. This figure illustrates relevant diagnostic techniques employed for pulmonary tuberculosis diagnosis.

Source: https://www.mdpi.com/diseases/diseases-12-00202/article_deploy/html/images/diseases-12-00202-g001.png.

4.4.2. Personalized Medicine Approaches

In the past decade, personalized medicine has emerged as a revolution in healthcare that leverages genetic and molecular information to tailor treatment plans to a given patient. The progress is underpinned by the advancement of high-throughput genetic diagnostics, whereby it is feasible to deeply interrogate the patient's genome. Such technologies allow for the identification of genetic differences that can influence drug action and hence guide therapy. For instance, pharmacogenomic testing becomes more relevant ever with the ability to detect an extremely diverse range of genetic markers, far outpacing our capacity to understand their significance in a clinical practice setting. This mismatch calls for careful scrutiny of how such new diagnostic tests are integrated into patient management algorithms. As we worked through personalized medicine approaches, we found the future of diagnostics not in detection technology, but in the interpretation and application of that genetic information in the clinic (Schrijver et al., 2011). Beyond genetics is proteomics, a component of personalized medicine as well, amplifying the paradigm by which patient care plans are created. By focusing on dynamic molecular characteristics found in proteins, this technique emphasizes real-time differences in patients' biological state. Proteomics has applications for disease prevention, monitoring of disease state, and identification of drug targets. A case in point is in oncology, with conditions such as bladder cancer, where the heterogeneity of the tumor requires precision targeting. Research has referred to the stratification of patients based on protein biomarkers to lead to more effective therapeutic treatment and better outcomes. However, the effectiveness in the use of proteomics-based methods relies on some challenges that must be overcome, including standardization of the test protocols and making clinically significant the discovered biomarkers (Frantzi et al., 2017). The integration of personalized medicine strategies into clinical practice can potentially revolutionize diagnosis processes and enhance patient outcomes. By focusing on the unique proteomic and genetic attributes of patients, healthcare professionals are able to proceed toward a more precise method in selecting treatments. But they come with big challenges as diverse as the need for an integrated protocol in genetic and proteomic analysis to the ongoing demand for interpretative aids that are capable of sensibly adjudicating on the clinical relevance of the data. The success in adopting personalized medicine hinges on a collaborative effort between clinicians, geneticists, and researchers to bridge the gaps, with new diagnostic tests not only having strong data but also being coherent with the overall aim of better patient management. With continuous innovation combined with rigorous testing, personalized medicine can yield revolutionary results in diagnosis as well as treatment (Schrijver et al., 2011; Frantzi et al., 2017) (Figure 4.15).

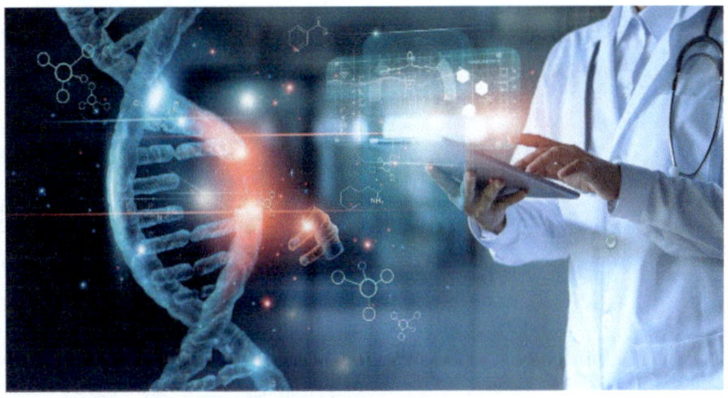

Figure 4.15. Personalized medicine.

Source: https://objective.health/wp-content/uploads/2022/01/objective-health-precision-medicine-future-of-healthcare-personalized-healthcare-scaled.jpeg.

4.4.3. Potential for Artificial Intelligence

The potential for artificial intelligence (AI) to revolutionize diagnostic test evaluation is vast, and it can fundamentally change the manner in which assessments are performed. Traditional assessment practices are rigid and cannot adapt to individual learners' needs, leading to a one-size-fits-all approach that works to disregard the specific learning rates and patterns of unique learners. By applying AI technologies, educators can create dynamic diagnostic environments that not only test students' know-how but also adapt in real-time based on their responses. This strategy facilitates personalized learning experiences, as educators can provide unique support. For instance, student knowledge tracking systems can identify prior knowledge, build individual learner profiles, and offer real-time evaluations, reflecting the customized diagnostic power of AI in education (Fruh et al., 2014). Innovations in cognitive simulation also reflect the potential of AI in the assessment of diagnostic tests. Procedures utilized by tools such as the automated cognitive modeler (ACM) allow a thorough examination of problem-solving strategies among students. This technology deploys the automation of problem space identification and solution paths, thus shedding light on the processes of thinking that students employ when working on intricate tasks. Through the use of machine learning algorithms, AI has the ability to identify patterns in students' approach to problems, separating systematic mistakes from conceptual confusions. The insights gained by cognitive diagnosis are vital for instructors as they inform teaching practices and curriculum design in such a way that teaching methods are better synchronized with learners' needs (Langley et al., 1989). Moreover, the application of AI to diagnostic exams extends beyond the field of personalized learning to enhanced overall assessment accuracy. Standard testing procedures, at times, cannot capture students' subtle understanding and tend to make flawed assessments of their abilities. AI systems can develop sophisticated tests that adapt based on individual performances, revealing more realistic students' learning trajectories. Furthermore, by refining misconception and procedure error assessment, AI enhances the quality of feedback provided to learners. This loop of activity not only enhances a better understanding of the subject matter but also makes the students more interactive towards learning. Thus, the use of AI for diagnostic test evaluation is a significant step towards more reflective and interactive pedagogy (Figure 4.16).

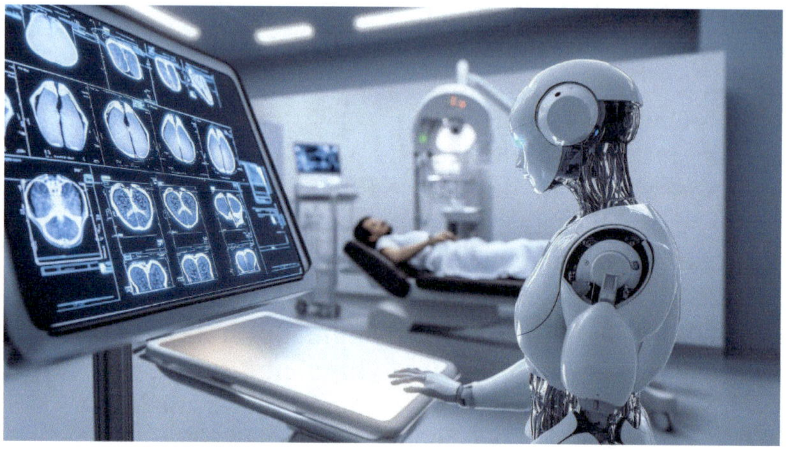

Figure 4.16. The state of AI in medical diagnostics.

Source: https://media.licdn.com/dms/image/v2/D4E12AQHTFHXEe3ffjA/article-cover_image-shrink_720_1280/article-cover_image-shrink_720_1280/0/1725296210279?e=2147483647&v=beta&t=vJuoE7zYATsz0yPgcK5h2DIr8IVBw6BaR7Z8UrMhsiw.

Summary

In encapsulating the evaluation of diagnostic tests, it is important to record the pluralistic nature of health technology assessments (HTAs). These evaluations are pivotal in building an all-encompassing understanding of the technical performance, safety, efficacy, and cost-effectiveness of diagnostic technologies. As the field of medicine becomes increasingly complex, the role of HTA agencies comes into full effect in that not only must they ensure these technologies are performing the functions intended, but also on ethical and economic solid foundations. The ongoing development of HTA methodologies serves to reemphasize the importance of constant upgrading in evaluation practice. As outlined in recent best practice reports, open reporting is vital to the dissemination of HTA results, ultimately for their utility in supporting healthcare decision-making (Busse et al., 2002). Additionally, the integration of expert opinion by way of systematic processes, i.e., Delphi, lends authenticity to HTAs in acknowledging outstanding questions that must be answered during the assessment of new diagnostic technologies. The Delphi exercise facilitates a consensus-based methodology where the importance of different factors concerning diagnostic tools is assessed by the experts to allow questions of priority, necessary for efficient appraisal and implementation. Through the use of a multidisciplinary group of experts, the HTA process not only captures multiple viewpoints but also ensures that the assessments carried out mirror the clinical utility and public health realities. This rigorous method is imperative in the evolving practice of HTA and offers the guideline for quality appraisals that are intended to guide subsequent healthcare interventions (Freeman et al., 2005). Overall, diagnostic test evaluation must align with evolving healthcare, underlining the need for methodological rigor and expert consensus in HTA exercises. By integrating technical performance with clinical, economic, and ethical considerations, decision-makers are able to make choices that enhance the care of the patient. As technology development picks up pace, updates of the HTA frameworks have to be ongoing to stay relevant and helpful. Lastly, a commitment to quality reporting and evidence-based practice in HTA will ensure that diagnostic tests not only be groundbreaking but also beneficial towards the larger goals of enhancing health outcomes and maximizing resource application in healthcare systems. Both systematic review of existing technologies and strategic development of new ones will ensure the strengthening of this essential aspect of current medical practice (Busse et al., 2002).

Evaluation of diagnostic tests is a key means of advancing healthcare results and improving patient safety. A foundational idea behind the evaluation is becoming familiar with the models that guide the interpretation of diagnostic evidence. The PARiHS framework (Promoting Action on Research Implementation in Health Services) is an applicable tool in this area by providing a systematic approach to assessing how different factors, such as evidence and context, influence implementation practices. Although the model is viewed as useful, theoretical contributions to it are poorly quantified, providing scope for further inquiry (Grandos et al., 2008). This suggests the necessity of ongoing dialogue on its application, as implementation science increasingly attempts to bridge practice and theory. Therefore, the creation of the PARiHS framework foretells the shift to more evaluative measures that can be flexible within different healthcare settings. Implementing a two-stage process in diagnostic and assessment measures can also increase the assessment of diagnostic tests further. This process involves a preliminary examination of the factors enclosing evidence and contextual elements prior to an examination of the best facilitation techniques. Through the use of this method, stakeholders are able to customize interventions to the specific conditions of their particular environments, thereby maximizing the applicability and utility of the testing measures. Additionally, this customized method places emphasis on interacting with actors involved in the studies to ensure that the interventions are based on their observations and experiences. Thus, the creation of this two-step process not only stabilizes the framework itself but also strengthens additional cooperative effort among health professionals in the long term, and this, in turn, will result in enhanced diagnostic outcomes (Grandos et al., 2008). Finally, the recurring difficulties in creating efficient diagnostic tests require an approach that is multi-faceted in nature and that employs various methodologies and theoretical perspectives. For addressing such issues, regional and international collaboration becomes essential, particularly in terms of exchanging skills and improving surveillance systems. As an example, initiatives of the FAO during the H5N1 avian flu pandemic emphasize cooperative efforts to laboratory diagnosis as well as epidemiological surveillance. Through the provision of training and support for cooperation among different stakeholders, these kinds of initiatives can enhance public health response capacity overall. This synergy not only goes deeper into the evaluation of diagnostic tests but also paves the way for out-of-the-box thinking in reacting to the evolving paradigm of healthcare problems. This type of collaboration is thus crucial in strengthening both diagnostic evaluation and the field of implementation science as a whole.

CLOSER LOOK

POINT-OF-CARE TESTING

Point-of-care testing (POC testing or POCT) is medical testing conducted with the patient, outside a laboratory. POC testing may also be described as bedside testing, near-patient testing, remote testing, mobile testing, and rapid diagnostics. Generally, the broad term can be used for any patient medical test that is provided ad hoc and provides results instantly. The majority of equipment utilized for POC testing consists of handheld electronics or molecular collection devices. Examples of POC tests that are used frequently include blood glucose meters, thermometers, home pregnancy testing, and rapid strep testing.

For the satisfaction of urgent health requirements, POC testing can be conducted in various locations by first responders, radiologists, nurses, and other paramedics at pharmacies, clinics, ambulances, accident scenes, care facilities, and homes. Remote use devices of POC tests enable doctors to observe, in near real time, important information about their patients, known as remote patient monitoring. It can be combined with telehealth services for the provision of at-home care.

The application of POC testing holds in value-based care where there is heightened demand for timely diagnosis, accurate monitoring, timely detection, and the prevention and care of chronic diseases. For example, rapid strep tests will allow a patient to receive treatment earlier and avoid further risk from misdiagnosis.

The requirement of POC testing was proved during the COVID-19 pandemic. PCR testing in a lab was highly accurate, but the cost and the fact that it was taking several days to get results made it inappropriate. Rapid tests that were performed as POC tests or home tests were more common.

Point-of-care testing is testing at or near the point of patient care, i.e., at the doctor's office or even at home. Patient care is being transformed by the convenience of having instant results for such conditions as diabetes, high cholesterol, and infectious diseases (Figure 4.17).

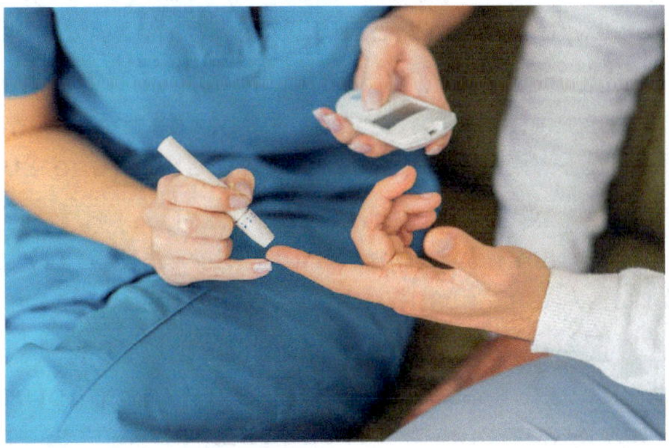

Figure 4.17. A healthcare professional performing a blood glucose test using a finger-prick method.

Source: https://d1ngglk168riv7.cloudfront.net/n/wp-content/uploads/2021/08/31132120/GettyImages-1286543359-scaled.jpg.

References

1. Aceti, F., Bernardini, L., Di Palma, F., Fioriello, A., et al. (2023). Array-comparative genomic hybridization analysis in a cohort of 130 children with autism spectrum disorders: A single center Italian study. https://core.ac.uk/download/614029544.pdf (accessed on 25th June 2025).

2. Adinolfi, A., Bertoldi, I., Cimmino, M. A., Delle Sedie, A., et al. (2016). Ultrasound in the diagnosis of calcium pyrophosphate dihydrate deposition disease: A systematic literature review and a meta-analysis. https://core.ac.uk/download/74318650.pdf (accessed on 25th June 2025).

3. Affolabi, A., Banerjee, R., Blakemore, R., Boehme, C., Brossier, F., Bwanga, F., et al. (2011). New and improved diagnostics for detection of drug-resistant pulmonary tuberculosis. https://core.ac.uk/download/9839057.pdf (accessed on 25th June 2025).

4. Ahani, A., Keshtkar, A., Mirfazeli, A., Roshandel, G., et al. (2011). The role of IL-6 for predicting neonatal sepsis: A systematic review and meta-analysis. https://core.ac.uk/download/52204821.pdf (accessed on 25th June 2025).

5. AIOM-AIRTUM Working Group, AIRTUM Working Group, Alexander, A., Ali, S., Altman, D. G., Attia, J., et al. (2017). Comparative analysis of diagnostic performance, feasibility and cost of different test-methods for thyroid nodules with indeterminate cytology. https://core.ac.uk/download/188830446.pdf (accessed on 25th June 2025).

6. Alicandro, S. (2016). *What is the True Cost to Stay in The Hospital?* https://core.ac.uk/download/56740651.pdf (accessed on 25th June 2025).

7. Arterburn, D., Barton, J., Berkman, N. D., Charles, D., Edmonds, S., Elwyn, G., et al. (2016). The 2016 Academic Emergency Medicine Consensus Conference, Shared Decision Making in the Emergency Department: Development of a policy-relevant patient-centered research agenda–Diagnostic testing breakout session report. https://core.ac.uk/download/155271748.pdf (accessed on 25th June 2025).

8. Berankova, T., Bosse, I., Brotankova, Z., Colaiuda, C., et al. (2016). Case studies of personalized learning. https://core.ac.uk/download/225020853.pdf (accessed on 25th June 2025).

9. Velazquez Berumen, A., Laposata, M., & Verna, R. (2018). Diagnostic error reduction in the United States and Italy through the intervention of diagnostic management teams. https://core.ac.uk/download/160649042.pdf (accessed on 25th June 2025).

10. Biggi, A., Fretzayas, A., Gervaix, A., Haberlik, A., Hitzel, A., Hitzel, A., Piepsz, A., et al. (2005). Further investigation of confirmed urinary tract infection (UTI) in children under five years: A systematic review. https://core.ac.uk/download/57941.pdf (accessed on 25th June 2025).

11. Blondeel, K., Cordero, J., Kiarie, J., Murtagh, M., et al. (2017). Advancing prevention of sexually transmitted infections through point-of-care testing: Target product profiles and landscape analysis. https://core.ac.uk/download/147056121.pdf (accessed on 25th June 2025).

12. Burns, J., Cunnington, A., Evans, J., Hendry, K., et al. (2016). Evaluation of delirium screening tools in geriatric medical inpatients: A diagnostic test accuracy study. https://core.ac.uk/download/46558678.pdf (accessed on 25th June 2025).

13. Busse, R., Drummond, M., Gurtner, F., Jorgensen, T., et al. (2002). Best practice in undertaking

and reporting health technology assessments: Working Group 4 report. https://core.ac.uk/download/58882.pdf (accessed on 25th June 2025).

14. Cairns, J. A., & Jeong, K. E. (2013). Review of economic evidence in the prevention and early detection of colorectal cancer. https://core.ac.uk/download/13111502.pdf (accessed on 25th June 2025).

15. Campaign for Access to Essential Medicines. (2008). *International Meeting: New Diagnostic Tests are Urgently Needed to Treat Patients with Chagas Disease.* https://core.ac.uk/download/pdf/9416984.pdf (accessed on 25th June 2025).

16. Chang, E. F., Jetté, N., & Kwon, C. S. (2020). Cost-effectiveness of advanced imaging technologies in the presurgical workup of epilepsy. https://core.ac.uk/download/323063036.pdf (accessed on 25th June 2025).

17. Chiu, C. Y., & Miller, S. A. (2019). Clinical metagenomics. https://core.ac.uk/download/323062552.pdf (accessed on 25th June 2025).

18. Clay, D., Freeman, K., Hyde, J., et al. (2007). A review of evidence on non-invasive prenatal diagnosis (NIPD): Tests for fetal RHD genotype. https://core.ac.uk/download/49338.pdf (accessed on 25th June 2025).

19. Ctori, I., Fidalgo, B., Jindal, A., Lawrenson, J., et al. (2018). Development and validation of a new glaucoma screening test using temporally modulated flicker. https://core.ac.uk/download/163076801.pdf (accessed on 25th June 2025).

20. Desvaux, S., Goutard, F., & Roger, F. (2005). Workshop to deliver epidemiology and laboratory training for HPAI diagnostic network. http://agritrop.cirad.fr/529308/1/ID529308.pdf (accessed on 25th June 2025).

21. Eggen, T. J. H. M., & Veldkamp, B. P. (2012). Psychometrics in practice at RCEC. https://core.ac.uk/download/pdf/11483225.pdf (accessed on 25th June 2025).

22. Elliott, E., Langhorne, P., & Quinn, T. J. (2018). Cognitive and mood assessment tools for use in stroke. https://core.ac.uk/download/132212026.pdf (accessed on 25th June 2025).

23. Farooq, S., Imran, M. A., Latif, S., Qadir, J., et al. (2017). How 5G wireless (and concomitant technologies) will revolutionize healthcare. https://core.ac.uk/download/143476480.pdf (accessed on 25th June 2025).

24. Fauli, S., & Thue, G. (2025). Economic consequences of near-patient test results–The case of tests for the *Helicobacter pylori* bacterium in dyspepsia. https://core.ac.uk/download/pdf/7107392.pdf (accessed on 25th June 2025).

25. Frantzi, M., Latosinska, A., Merseburger, A. S., Mischak, H., et al. (2017). Clinical proteomics for precision medicine: The bladder cancer case. https://core.ac.uk/download/111557480.pdf (accessed on 25th June 2025).

26. Freeman, K., Hyde, J., Osipenko, L., et al. (2005). Emerging prenatal genetic tests: Developing a health technology assessment (HTA) framework for informed decision-making. https://core.ac.uk/download/105293.pdf (accessed on 25th June 2025).

27. Fruh, W. G., Fylladitakis, E., Hatziapostolou, A., Papadakis, N., et al. (2014). An open learning environment for the diagnosis, assistance and evaluation of students based on artificial intelligence. https://core.ac.uk/download/29092204.pdf (accessed on 25th June 2025).

28. Grandos, A., Kitson, A., Loftus-Hills, A., Oxman, A., Titchen, A., Titchen, A., Van de Ven, A. H., et al. (2008). Evaluating the successful implementation of evidence into practice using the PARiHS framework: Theoretical and practical challenges. https://core.ac.uk/download/48947.pdf (accessed on 25th June 2025).

29. Harari, A., Zumla, A., Armand, M., Axelsson-Robertson, P., Banada, P., Marais, B., Betsou, F., et al. (2012). Tuberculosis diagnostics and biomarkers: Needs, challenges, recent advances, and opportunities. https://core.ac.uk/download/9839032.pdf (accessed on 25th June 2025).

30. Hoelzle, J. B., Marshall, P. S., & Nikolas, M. A. (2019). The role of neurocognitive tests in the assessment of adult attention-deficit/hyperactivity disorder. https://core.ac.uk/download/228028395.pdf (accessed on 25th June 2025).

31. Ince, J., & McNally, A. (2009). Development of rapid, automated diagnostics for infectious disease: Advances and challenges. https://core.ac.uk/download/30633630.pdf (accessed on 25th June 2025).

32. Jauhariyah, M. N. R., & Paramita, U. V. (2024). Identifying student misconceptions on momentum and impulse using four-tier diagnostic test instrument with CRI. https://core.ac.uk/download/599214395.pdf (accessed on 25th June 2025).

33. Kenney, G. M., & Pelletier, J. E. (2010). *Improving the Lives of Young Children: The Role of Developmental Screenings in Medicaid and CHIP*. https://core.ac.uk/download/71347983.pdf (accessed on 25th June 2025).

34. Langley, P., Ohlsson, S., & Wogulis, J. (1989). Rules and principles in cognitive diagnoses. https://core.ac.uk/download/287623394.pdf (accessed on 25th June 2025).

35. Maranga, J. (2019). The predictive value of urine dipstick glucose test in the screening for gestational diabetes mellitus in a tertiary private hospital in Kenya. https://core.ac.uk/download/597995970.pdf (accessed on 25th June 2025).

36. McCartney, E. (2012). *Voice and Speech Functions (B310–B340)*. https://core.ac.uk/download/9040603.pdf (accessed on 25th June 2025).

37. Mehdi, H., Montano, M. F., & Nash, D. B. (2016). Annotated bibliography: Understanding ambulatory care practices in the context of patient safety and quality improvement. https://core.ac.uk/download/83049375.pdf (accessed on 25th June 2025).

38. Read, T. L. (2016). *Emerging Needs in Behavioral Health and The Integrated Care Model* [Master's thesis, Boston University]. https://open.bu.edu/bitstream/2144/17694/1/Read_bu_0017N_11995.pdf (accessed on 25th June 2025).

39. Rowe, A. K., Nkrumah, B., Uzochukwu, B. S. C., Uzochukwu, B. S. C., Sismanidis, C., Chandler, C. I. R., et al. (2012). A cost-effectiveness analysis of provider and community interventions to improve the treatment of uncomplicated malaria in Nigeria: Study protocol for a randomized controlled trial. https://core.ac.uk/download/13546092.pdf (accessed on 25th June 2025).

40. Schrijver, I., & Wiita, A. P. (2011). Clinical application of high throughput molecular screening techniques for pharmacogenomics. https://core.ac.uk/download/323063319.pdf (accessed on 25th June 2025).

41. Zamani, M. (2019). FAST and abnormal urinalysis: The effective screening tools in pediatric abdominal trauma. https://core.ac.uk/download/187725196.pdf (accessed on 25th June 2025).

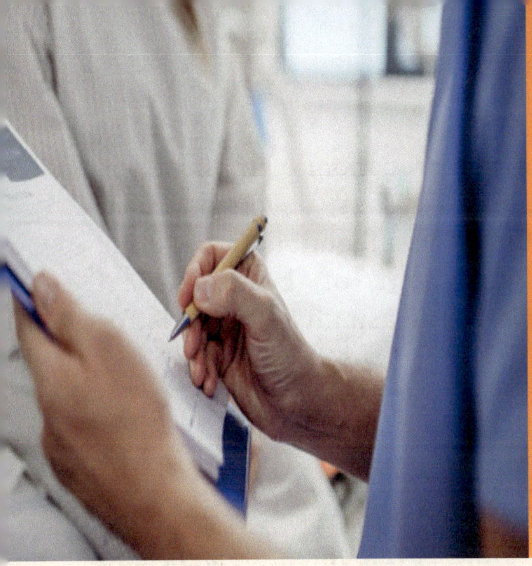

Chapter 5

SCREENING IN EPIDEMIOLOGY

Contents

Introduction

The application of epidemiology largely relies on screening processes as a basic premise of disease control and prevention. Screening enables the identification ahead of time of individuals who may be at risk or already infected with specific health conditions, thus enabling interventions in a timely manner. Early detection is highly necessary for reducing the impacts of diseases since it allows healthcare professionals to initiate interventions or preventive procedures before the manifestation of more severe symptoms. Thus, success for screening procedures can have implications not only on patient health outcomes but on public health as a whole. Through the coordinated application of screening strategies, epidemiologists can enhance the control of disease, make healthcare resources more efficient, and, in turn, reduce morbidity and mortality from the dissemination of different health conditions. For infectious diseases, successful screening and surveillance are also critical in preventing transmission and stopping the outbreak. For instance, the work on hospital-acquired methicillin-resistant *Staphylococcus aureus* (MRSA) focuses on the interaction between these two variables. Surveillance is said to have a very important role in the detection of infected patients, which is most crucial in preventing further transmission in healthcare settings. Besides, different methods of screening are said to play a significant role in the transmission dynamics of both hospital and community settings. Specifically, random screening has been more effective in the control of nosocomial infections and the prevention of epidemic conduct, thereby advocating for robust screening methods in the management of public health emergencies (Jenkins et al., 2006).

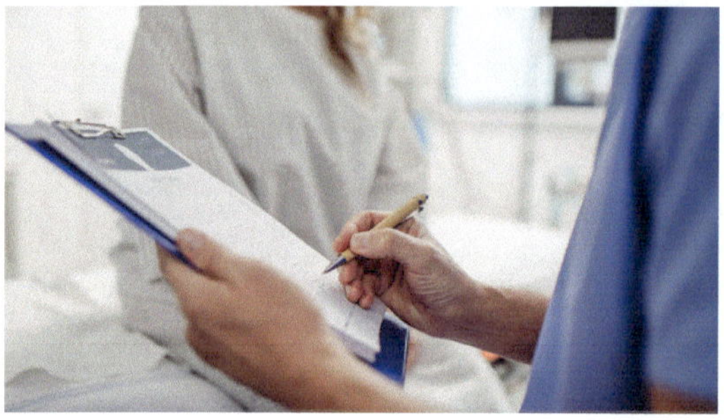

Figure 5.1. Screening tests for common diseases.

Source: https://www.hopkinsmedicine.org/-/media/images/health/2_-treatment/screening-and-diagnostics/provider-going-over-test-results-with-a-patient-teaser.jpg.

Besides, the use of economic appraisals in screening methods is an evolving discipline in epidemiological research, particularly in assessing the effectiveness of varied health interventions. Calibration of decision models, as illustrated in recent studies, can lead to improved predictions of results for public health and resource planning. Through testing input parameters through probabilistic examination, analysts are capable of minimizing uncertainty while maximizing model accuracy, resulting in improved healthcare decisions. This approach not only enhances the validity of epidemiologic models but also identifies the necessity of adapting screening strategies with a broader examination of their economic implications (Karnon et al., 2011). Thus, development in screening practice in epidemiology requires continuing assessment of both clinical effectiveness and cost feasibility (Figure 5.1).

Importance of Screening in Public Health

Public health screening is a primary intervention for the detection of those at risk of contracting diseases prior to the development of signs and symptoms. Screening enables early detection, which is critical in conditions wherein early treatment can significantly improve health outcomes. Public health agencies often effectively reduce morbidity and mortality from prevalent diseases such as cancer, diabetes, and cardiovascular disease through the use of screening programs. The early identification of vulnerable groups in deprived settings enables the effective allocation of resources to guarantee interventions are delivered to those most in need. This not only contributes to individual health but also to the general well-being of populations, as identified through literature on health equity, stressing the interconnectedness of public and individual health results (Akl et al., 2017). Moreover, screening has implications that extend beyond patient-level advantage; it aids in the direction of public health policy and resource allocation. Figures gathered from screening programs enable epidemiologists and public health experts to track disease prevalence and conduct interventions that are evidence-based in reacting to need. Policymakers utilize such data to develop effective programs meant to meet the specific needs of the populations, thereby enhancing health equity. Inclusion of screening in public health systems is also required to address the unique issues of marginalized populations, where health inequities are more extreme. By placing considerable importance on equity-related considerations in screening, public health interventions can advance considerably in improving everyone's health outcomes, particularly those from low-income communities (Akl et al., 2017). In the context of modern epidemiology, screening is as much a healthcare intervention as it is an intrinsic part of healthcare systems that tries to find a balance between equity and efficiency. Clinical epidemiology has also pointed to the mandates of meticulous screening practices in public health programs, enabling an increased understanding of health outcomes. As the field grows, it is important to integrate evidence-based practice to make certain that screening recommendations remain up-to-date and effective. By addressing determinants of health inequities, such as socioeconomic status and care access, public health professionals are able to provide policy recommendations that will protect vulnerable populations. This multidimensional approach not only fosters a healthier society but also embodies the ethical imperative of fairness required in contemporary public health discourse (Figure 5.2).

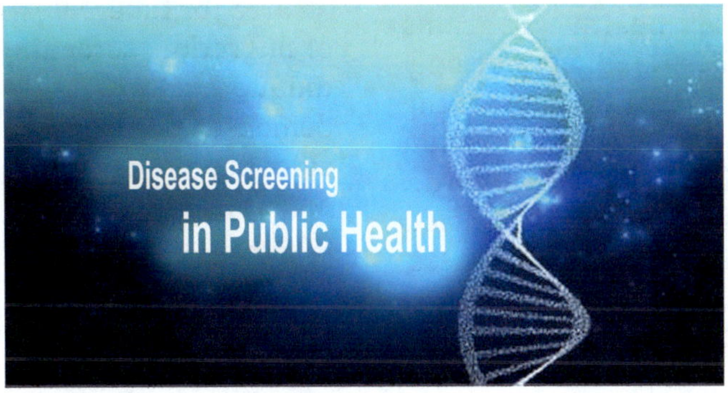

Figure 5.2. Disease screening in public health.

Source: https://i.ytimg.com/vi/9r-4_hGlSfw/hqdefault.jpg.

5.1. Historical Context of Screening

The etiologic context of screening in epidemiology is rooted within the broader conversation about public health trends throughout the 20th century. Early screening was an attempt to respond to the demand for the detection of disease at asymptomatic stages so that intervention could be earlier, and results may improve. The establishment of mass screening for tuberculosis throughout the mid-1900s is a historic realignment of public health policy, advocating for an active approach to disease control. As screening practice evolved, its focus broadened to include a spectrum of long-term illnesses and conditions, emphasizing self-protection by way of preventive healthcare interventions. A review of the evolution of screening methods reveals the progressive move from opportunistic to more systematic screening, commensurate with advances in medical technology and epidemiological research. As insight into the benefits of screening grew, so too did awareness of inequalities in public health programs. Historical evidence illustrates that screening is a powerful disease prevention measure, but that disparities in access and implementation serve to extend health inequities between populations. This was only highlighted by research on various models of screening, for instance, those highlighted in Public Health Gateshead's commissioned research seeking to bring together evidence for organizational structures for Schools of Public Health (Goodall et al., 2011). The findings reflect a longstanding dilemma within epidemiology: ensuring equal access to screening programs alongside addressing the underlying social determinants of health that may preclude successful results. Moreover, the evolution of screening practice has been significantly influenced by technological innovation and shifting public health ideology. Adoption of evidence-based screening guidelines has resulted in a more accurate description of the cost-effectiveness and efficacy of a number of screening programs. As an example, studies have demonstrated excellent interexaminer consistency between dental therapists and gold-standard dentists, which suggests that well-trained non-physician clinicians are able to perform screenings effectively within dental health programs (Curnow et al., 2016). These findings not only contribute to enhanced access for screening but also highlight the importance of calibration and training in maintaining quality standards. This background reveals a consistent tension between policy-making, regulatory effectiveness, and ethical considerations surrounding the equitable application of screening programs (Figure 5.3).

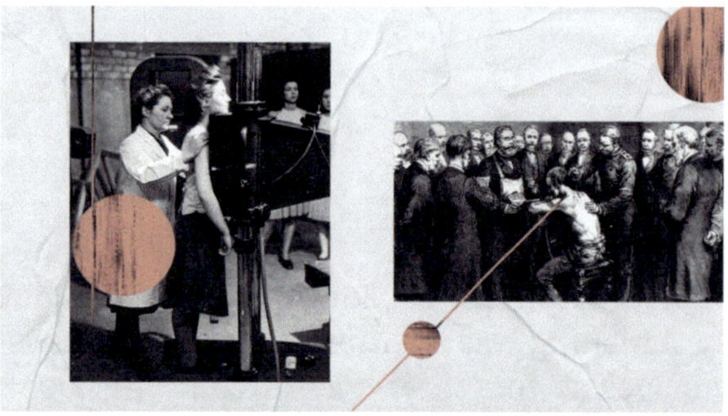

Figure 5.3. Left: 12th February 1944: London factory workers being X-rayed using a mobile radiography unit travelling from borough to borough, during a mass radiography program set up to detect the early stages of tuberculosis. Right: Dr. Koch's Treatment for consumption at the Royal Hospital, Berlin. Dr. Pfuhl is inoculating a patient with the lymph. Undated engraving.

Source: https://post.medicalnewstoday.com/wp-content/uploads/sites/3/2023/10/tuberculosis-history-collage-1296x728-header-1024x575.jpg.

5.1.1. Evolution of Screening Practices

The epidemiological history of screening also reflects a complicated interaction among evolving public health problems over time. Screening itself was at one point nearly solely directed toward established infectious illnesses, whereby initial diagnosis and treatment served to repress outbreaks. An example of required public health control in much of the world is the added screening of migrants recently arriving in an area for tuberculosis. With changing patterns of migration, screening has adapted to address unique health profiles among various groups, demonstrating a trend towards more targeted and evidence-driven practice. Growing recognition of the importance of guidelines is exemplified in the Black Sea and Mediterranean regions, where even the majority of experts advocate for systematic screening guidelines that not only benefit individual health but also minimize potential public health dangers (Napoli et al., 2015). This evolution mirrors an expanding understanding of health determinants, with the implication that screening practice is in a state of continuous improvement to be more effective and reach more people. Furthermore, the science and technology that underpin screening practice have evolved significantly over the decades, leading to improved surveillance and detection techniques. One example is the intense screening of cattle for bovine spongiform encephalopathy (BSE) in Europe, a demonstration of how systematic surveillance is creating further epidemiological insight. By testing nearly 50 million cattle, researchers were actually able to identify significant risk factors and augment passive surveillance programs, revealing the failings of clinical detection methods at the time. Such advances not only facilitate early case identification but also demonstrate the dynamics of disease spread between animal populations, which can be utilized for planning human health policy (Arnold et al., 2008). Thus, the evolution of screening practices is a shift from a reactive response to a proactive response that entails the application of scientific investigation and data analysis to drive public health results. Last but not least, the integration of screening practices into general public health systems is a paradigm shift in addressing and managing health risks within societies. With increasing public health agencies embracing an integrated perspective of disease prevention, screening is increasingly being perceived as part of integrated health approaches and not as an isolated behavior. This change identifies the importance of interprofessional interventions with social, environmental, and biological determinants of health outcomes. The consensus among health professionals that screening for infectious conditions in migrant groups is beneficial points to the necessity of evidence-based interventions to adapt to evolving populations.

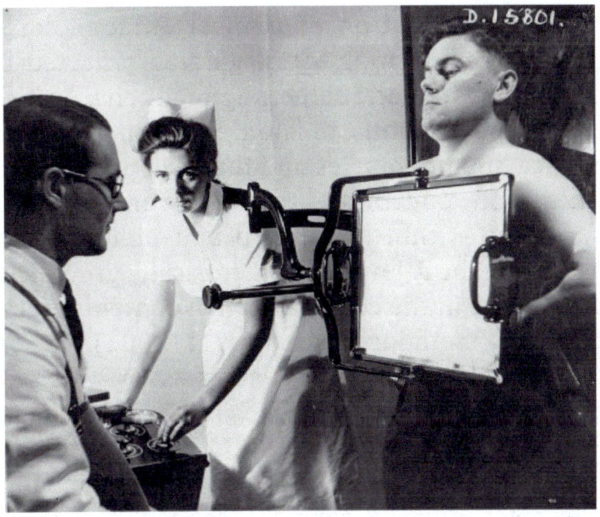

Figure 5.4. Tuberculosis screening.

Source: https://upload.wikimedia.org/wikipedia/commons/c/c7/Treating_Tuberculosis-_Screening_and_Treatment_at_Harefield_Hospital%2C_Hertfordshire%2C_England%2C_UK%2C_1943_D15801.jpg.

The evolution of standardized procedures and enhancing screening programs optimizes individual and population gains, ultimately leading to improved epidemiological solutions and enhanced preparedness for evolving upcoming public health challenges (Napoli et al., 2015) (Figure 5.4).

5.1.2. Key Milestones in Epidemiological Screening

The evolutionary path of epidemiological screening has been characterized by pivotal milestones that have transformed public health interventions among different populations. A basic breakthrough happened in the mid-20th century, mainly through the introduction of screening programs for infectious diseases, including tuberculosis and syphilis. Not only did these programs raise the level of disease detection, but they also highlighted the importance of early intervention in preventing infectious epidemics. The establishment of the Framingham Heart Study in 1948 also contributed to this paradigm shift by publishing on risk factors for cardiovascular disease and emphasizing the population-based data's ability to drive screening protocols. The study prefigured subsequent cardiovascular screening efforts aimed at reducing morbidity and mortality. By demonstrating the benefits of early detection and therapy, these achievements encouraged wider acceptance of mass screening programs within epidemiology. At the same time, advances in technology have made major contributions to the planning of screening programs. The introduction of Pap smears in the 1920s revolutionized screening for cervical cancer by enormously decreasing mortality from cervical cancer through early diagnosis and treatment. As knowledge about different diseases grew, epidemiological screening began to use more advanced technologies, such as imaging methods and genetic testing, to detect previously undiagnosable conditions. The development of mammography in the late 20th century was a prime example of this kind of improvement, as routine screenings dramatically reduced breast cancer fatalities among women. This kind of technology underscores the relationship between scientific advancement and the formulation of effective screening campaigns. Collectively, these important milestones reveal how improvements in screening technologies not only expanded the diversity of conditions treated but also enhanced the impact of public health interventions. The discovery of health inequalities across various populations has also been another important milestone towards the creation of epidemiological screening. Efforts for Indigenous people and disadvantaged groups have revealed significant gaps in health outcomes, especially for long-term conditions such as diabetes and ear disease.

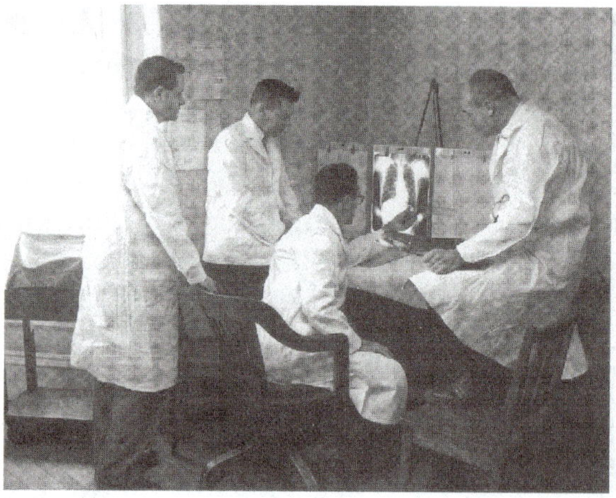

Figure 5.5. Framingham Heart Study physicians.

Source: https://upload.wikimedia.org/wikipedia/commons/1/1c/Framingham_Heart_Study_physicians_%2826548315418%29.jpg.

For instance, in not dealing with environmental, social, and biological conditions driving the disparities, the potency of screening strategies can be undermined. Projects such as the Stronger Futures in the Northern Territory have been initiated, effectively reducing hearing loss and otitis media rates among Indigenous children (N/A, 2025). This emphasis on equity in access to health is also a growing concern for guaranteeing that screening programs are made available, culturally sensitive, and tailored to meet the needs of diverse populations. Ultimately, identification and remediation of such disparities become critical to optimizing overall health outcomes and facilitating the role of epidemiological screening in public health infrastructure (Figure 5.5).

5.1.3. Impact of Historical Events on Current Screening Methods

The advancement of screening methods in epidemiology has been heavily determined by historical events, especially the developments in clinical practice and the impact of various health crises. The reduction of the reliance on traditional observation-driven medicine towards the development of more evidence-based practice was heavily done throughout the 20th century. This was influenced by empiricist and rationalist traditions since Hippocrates' time. The evolution of clinical epidemiology through research-oriented studies reflected a need for systematic screening regimens. As has been reported, this tension between evolving medical methodologies and the need for empiric validation continues to pose fundamental questions within healthcare and policy today regarding the relevance of historically grounded knowledge in the construction of contemporary screening methods (Newton et al., 2001). One of the pivotal events in screening history was the development of the Pap smear by Dr. Georges Papanicolaou during the 1940s. Initially greeted with skepticism, the Pap smear established the discipline of cervical cancer detection and represented a shift toward prevention in women's medicine. By the late 1980s, the official establishment of national screening programs in various countries further solidified the effectiveness of such measures, dramatically reducing the incidence and mortality from cervical cancer. Furthermore, this period of revolution opened up the complexities of medical history, particularly in how evolving attitudes towards women's health in society influenced the sanction and use of such screening techniques.

The discovery of the viral etiology of cervical cancer, namely human papillomavirus (HPV), also spurred decisive advances in screening technology and prevention strategies, marking a significant step in public health campaigns (Reynolds et al., 2009). Moreover, controversy over cervical cancer screening reflects broader social forces on health, gender, and medical innovation. HPV research, as incorporated in the paradigm of screening, illustrates how events have become so intertwined in history that there has been a review and reinforcement of screening techniques. The interaction of virologists, epidemiologists, and health workers in research on HPV in cervical disease set a foundation that not only shattered the common misconception but also stimulated creativity in preventive care. This collaboration is an ongoing process defined by history, indicating that current practice is rooted in past success and failures. The cervical cancer screening history is a key indication of the importance of the past in shaping effective epidemiologic screening modalities to inform future growth (Reynolds et al., 2009).

5.2. Types of Screening

Epidemiological screening is an important intervention for disease detection in its initial forms prior to the onset of symptoms, allowing early intervention and management. Population-based screening is a common type of screening, which entails screening vast segments of the population regardless of symptomatic presentation. It is very effective for conditions like breast cancer, where mammography is provided to women of a certain age. The primary purpose of population-based screening is to reduce morbidity and mortality through early detection. The effective use of this type of screening relies largely on the sensitivity and specificity of the tests to prevent false negatives and false positives, ensuring that healthcare resources are utilized effectively and efficiently in healthcare systems. Opportunistic screening, on the other hand, targets individuals who visit for reasons other than screening, thereby integrating screening into routine healthcare. This method allows medical practitioners to screen symptoms and risk factors at the time of routine consultation. Being less systematic in design than population-based screening, it offers a more personalized approach, allowing for tailored treatment.

Diabetic retinopathy screening through telemedicine is an instance of this. As has been seen in the study of Alavi et al. (2012), teleophthalmology initiatives have been cost-effective through focused screening camps in rural communities, ultimately promoting access and reducing barriers to care among high-risk populations. Opportunistic screening would enhance individual diagnostic yield but is only effective depending upon provider compliance and patient follow-up. The second critical category is that of systematic screening, where rigorous protocols are applied to screen individuals routinely for clearly determined diseases at predetermined intervals. This screening is typically implemented in organized healthcare systems, where policy exists to promote guideline compliance. Systematic cervical cancer screening by Pap or HPV testing, for example, is scheduled to be conducted on given occasions, as recommended by health authorities. The effectiveness of such programs can be enhanced through continued monitoring and evaluation of the implementation process, as has been illustrated in research utilizing calibrated models to evaluate various screening intervals. According to Karnon et al. (2011), the identification of the validity of health economic decision models can help identify the parameters directing these screening processes in a way to achieve the most predictive accuracy and reduce unwarranted variations among patients (Figure 5.6).

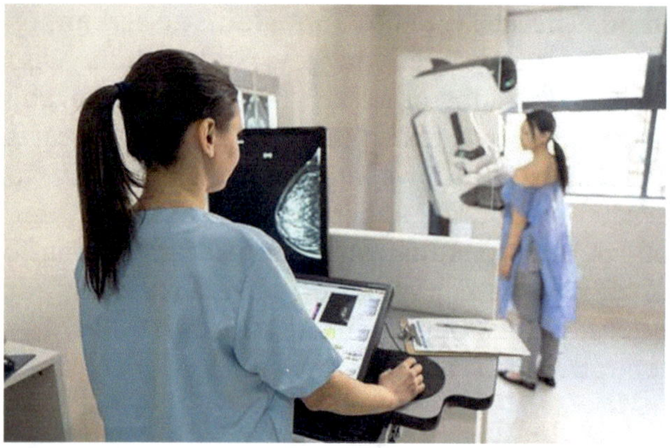

Figure 5.6. Screening mammography has been shown to reduce deaths from breast cancer among women ages 40 to 74, especially those ages 50 to 69.

Source: https://www.cancer.gov/sites/g/files/xnrzdm211/files/styles/cgov_article/public/cgov_image/media_image/100/500/7/files/cancer-screening-test-article.jpg?h=cb2c0a05&itok=uCqnvBQj.

5.2.1. Population-Based Screening

Population screening is a critical element of public health intervention for the avoidance of disease burden by early detection. In addition to making therapy more likely to be effective, the method is also the basis of chronic disease control.

For instance, the application of such screening in renal cell carcinoma (RCC) is promising to prevent mortality through the identification of cases before late-stage presentation. While hope is evident for benefits, opportunities exist for the ideal modalities of screening because the performance of tests can vary greatly in terms of disease stage and population. Evidence shows that while screening technologies, i.e., ultrasound, are very sensitive and specific, high costs of health care and disease prevalence being low pose hurdles to the universal application, suggesting further study and focused screening strategies (Klatte et al., 2018). Furthermore, the economic dimensions of population-based screening must be given significant attention in health policy discourse. The financial expense of delivering screening programs can be reduced by comparing the costs and benefits of alternative methodologies. For instance, from one study using the MISCAN-COLON simulation model, endoscopic colorectal cancer screening can yield net savings for health care systems by preventing costly cancer therapy through early detection.

This also relies on several factors, including screening frequency as well as the natural history of the disease. The review highlights a crucial consideration: the break-even point, where the cost savings from screening equal the initial cost, varies by screening type and duration, posing a dilemma for health policymakers who must ensure efficient resource utilization without compromising patient outcomes (Ballegooijen et al., 2000). Last but not least, risk stratification at the individual level is a rich domain to develop population-based screening approaches. Applying a combination of demographic and clinical risk factors can enhance the precision of screening so that more high-risk groups are identified more accurately.

This personalized method minimizes the harms of overdiagnosis and false positive results, which are key weaknesses of population-based screening methods. As research has demonstrated, understanding and prioritizing individuals based on risk maximizes the use of resources and betterment through facilitating early intervention. This more subtle understanding of population dynamics and the progression of disease sets a path towards more effective screening modalities, ultimately producing stronger public health outcomes among the disparate populations (Klatte et al., 2018) (Figure 5.7).

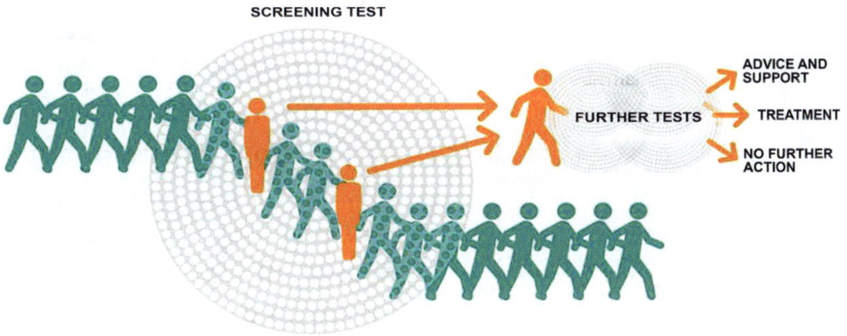

Figure 5.7. Illustration of the screening process.

Source: https://assets.publishing.service.gov.uk/media/63c9560ee90e070718df8a0a/screening_sieve_graphic.svg.

5.2.2. High-Risk Screening

High-risk screening is the focal epidemiological approach, particularly when working with at-risk populations for a specific disease. Screening is the systematic screening process that identifies individuals with a heightened risk for numerous health conditions, creating opportunities to intervene in advance. For example, screening populations using substances may uncover significant health conditions, including viral hepatitis. In one study of American Indian/Alaska Native patients in a chemical dependency treatment center, researchers found that extensive risk factor screening revealed a high prevalence of HCV among study participants, with 28% testing positive for the antibody. This underlines the importance of selective screening guidelines among high-risk populations to better control and limit potential epidemics (Brucker et al., 2012).

Also, the integration of health equity considerations into high-risk screening processes is paramount to improving overall public health outcomes. Owing to the fact that the health status imbalance is usually attributed to poor socioeconomic determinants, the management of these health inequities remains a fundamental part of epidemiological practice as well as research. GRADE framework guidelines encourage recommendations to assess the effects of interventions on health equity to enhance the well-being of marginalized populations. Incorporation of these elements can improve screening by building an entry of services to the neediest, ultimately resulting in more equal distribution of health interventions and resources (Akl et al., 2017). Screening for high-risk is thus not only a diagnostic but an integrated process that involves an understanding of clinical and social determinants of health.

Through reaching more vulnerable populations with certain health issues, researchers and public health officials can deliver targeted interventions that address the precise needs of these groups. The screening activity noted earlier among AI/AN individuals not only cured viral hepatitis but also provided a setting for enhanced health education and prevention, illustrating how focused screening can provide overall health dividends. Ultimately, ongoing innovation in high-risk screening will remain relevant to epidemiology, particularly as we strive for improved health care outcomes in diverse populations (Figure 5.8).

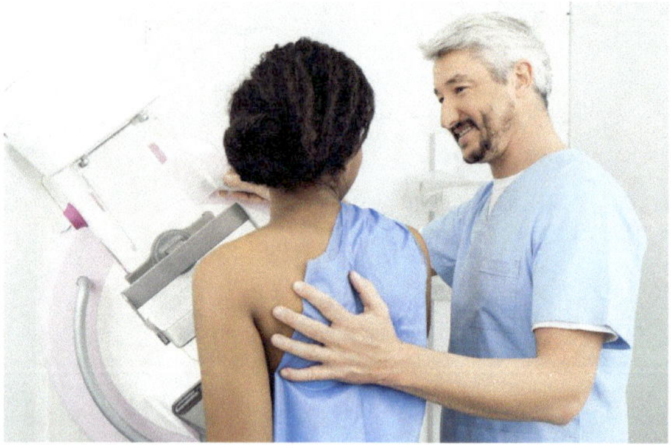

Figure 5.8. Drawing attention to high-risk screening.

Source: https://www.facingourrisk.org/uploads/blog/2013/01/2013-January-Drawing-Attention-1-800x534.jpg.

5.2.3. Diagnostic Screening

Diagnostic screening is a vital element in epidemiology, taking the central role to identify diseases or disease states in asymptomatic individuals. Diagnostic screening is a preventive intervention that can ensure early detection, which can enhance the success of treatments and reduce mortality rates. Diagnostic screening relies on the accuracy of tests employed to identify the presence of indicators of disease among individuals who are asymptomatic.

Moreover, it sets the platform for preventive health planning so that the health professionals can intervene early on before disease development becomes more complicated and advanced diseases. As the etiologies of disease are increasingly understood, diagnostic screening procedures also evolve with more use of evidence-based practice. These innovations reflect the change over the last few decades towards the use of clinical epidemiology to rationalist philosophy, which characterizes modern medicine (Newton et al., 2001). In public health, the use of diagnostic screening goes beyond individual benefits to encompass community health objectives. Successful screening programs can serve as warning systems, making possible the detection of disease outbreaks and enabling preventive interventions to be implemented rapidly. The association between exposure and chronic disease, for example, illustrates the requirement for screening efforts to be comprehensive and to account for multiple avenues of exposure. As highlighted by ongoing endeavors, the Centers for Disease Control and Prevention are trying to create an environmental public health tracking network that integrates disease and environmental information to enhance screening efficacy (Balmes et al., 2004). This approach not only aids in the diagnosis of current health issues but also aids in the general understanding of how environmental exposures are associated with disease patterns and, hence, aids in the development of targeted public health policy.

Additionally, the sustainability and effectiveness of diagnostic screening programs must also continuously be evaluated and innovated to progress as per the shifting paradigm of public health. With the improvement in medical technology, diagnostic devices with increased innovation are able to increase the specificity and sensitivity of screening tests so that improved discrimination between true positives and false alarms is provided. Continuous education campaigns are also essential to inform populations of the necessity for screening and the implications of early disease detection. Health policymakers will be increasingly faced with balancing the benefits with the costs of diagnostic screening. Lastly, harmonizing screening practice with a changing understanding of epidemiological data will allow practitioners to tackle health inequities more effectively and make screening activity worthwhile in bringing about significant health effects for diverse populations (Balmes et al., 2004) (Figure 5.9).

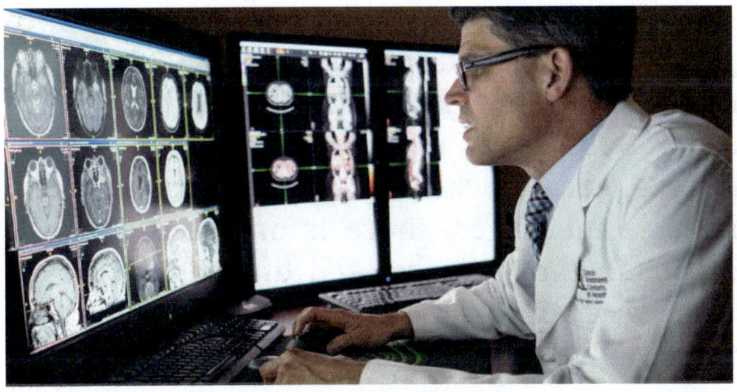

Figure 5.9. During the COVID-19 outbreak, doctors and patients may be faced with the difficult decision of whether to reschedule cancer screening or diagnostic procedures.

Source: https://cdn.cancercenter.com/-/media/ctca/images/others/blogs/2020/04-april/blog-covid-diagnostics-screening-l.jpg.

5.3. Criteria for Effective Screening

Effective screening in epidemiology hinges on some extremely crucial criteria that not only render the screening process valuable, but also address its moral issues. One such fundamental criterion is the accuracy of the screening test, encompassing sensitivity and specificity. The screen test must be able to detect those who have the disease (high sensitivity) with a lower false positive rate (high specificity).

This double requirement safeguards individuals against unwarranted fear and exploitative treatments that may result from incorrect findings. Further, the screening test must be reliable in varying populations to ensure that its universality is not lost and it remains effective. Being inclusive in age, gender, and socio-economic status is crucial to get representative data, ultimately helping lead to more informed public health decisions and interventions that can impact overall disease control and prevention strategies. The other important aspect of good screening is that it is feasible, and this speaks to the realities of implementation. In other words, it involves a cost and accessibility assessment, as well as time for screening and follow-up. If screening and subsequent follow-up are too expensive or take too much time, then a likely event is its limited implementation, thus limiting its potential gain. Second, there is no hierarchy of screening; all screening must be made available to the most-at-risk group due to socio-economic barriers. Proper training of the health workforce is another requirement for a sustainable screening program to ensure proper administration and interpretation of results. When screening programs are constructed with care for these utilitarian aspects, they promote increased participation and collaboration from the population, yielding greater health benefits and improved disease control plans in the long term. Finally, the ethical dimensions of screening cannot be overstated, particularly in the domains of informed consent and the potential psychological impact of screening results. Individuals should be well informed about the risks, benefits, and potential results of opting for a screening scheme. This transparency not only inspires confidence but also enables individuals to make proper decisions about their health. Further, there must be provisions for the follow-up of individuals who receive positive reports, as the psychological burden of such a discovery can be astronomical. Through integrating these ethical considerations with the practical and technical specifications, screening programs can optimize their effectiveness without compromising the dignity and autonomy of the individuals involved. By focusing on the context of dog health surveillance, effective systems are those that achieve a proper balance between data integrity and ethical responsibility, addressing the subtleties of bias and representation towards the goal of effective health interventions (Abo-Shehada et al., 2007; Brodbelt et al., 2014).

5.3.1. Validity and Reliability of Screening Tests

The validity and reliability of screening tests are core concepts in epidemiology, which translate into how effectively they operate in identifying diseases at early stages. Validity refers to how well a test measures what it is supposed to measure. For instance, when screening for ovarian and cervical cancer, the test must effectively identify those who are at risk according to predetermined symptoms and risk factors. It has been established that the development of such measures as the Ovarian and Cervical Cancer Awareness Measures can enhance validity by ensuring that tests are anchored on suitable clinical and epidemiological knowledge (Corker et al., 2011). Reliability, on the other hand, is defined as stability in results yielded by the test over time or between groups. Achieving high reliability entails that a test can be trusted to provide consistent results irrespective of changing circumstances, justifying its application in public health interventions. In order to comprehensively grasp the intricacies of validity and reliability, one must consider the methodologies employed during test development and validation of screening tests. For instance, all screening instruments undergo rigorous psychometric evaluations, which establish various properties such as content validity, internal consistency, and construct validity. One such good example is in Oxford Cognitive Screen-Putonghua, where specialist judgment and empirical testing were employed to ascertain the test's validity in poststroke patients (Chan et al., 2018). With validation against prior-established measures, e.g., valid measures like the Montreal Cognitive Assessment, researchers measure the item difficulty and the correlations. Such stringent tests not only establish the test's reliability in different populations but also ensure that screening measures are robust enough to provide sound clinical decision-making. The importance of validating and establishing the reliability of the screening tests cannot be exaggerated. In the absence of valid and reliable measures, there is an increased risk of misdiagnosis or missed diagnosis, leading to catastrophic public health consequences. Screening tests must yield results that are useful for informing healthcare policy and personal decisions effectively; this requires that tests demonstrate both high sensitivity (to correctly identify persons with the disease) and high specificity (to correctly identify persons without the disease). Ongoing reviews and revisions, as in the case of assessing the Oxford Cognitive Screen, are essential in adjusting instruments to the evolving demographic or clinical settings in order to ultimately maximize their application in epidemiological activities. By placing utmost importance on rigorous validation and reliability, professionals in epidemiology can play an important role in ensuring the accuracy and efficacy of public health screening (Figure 5.10).

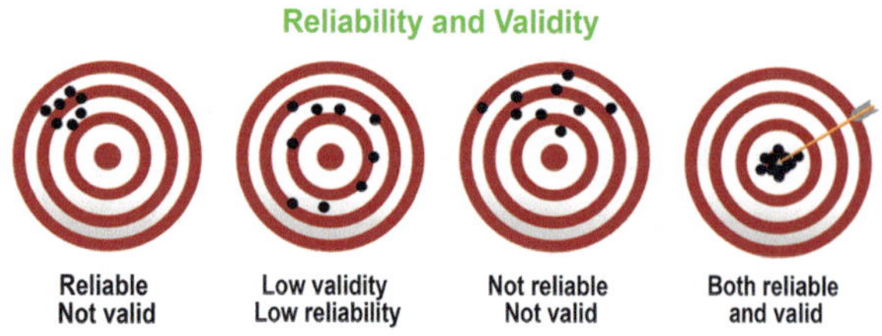

Figure 5.10. Reliability and validity.

Source: https://www.makemyassignments.com/blog/wp-content/uploads/2022/02/Reliability-and-Validity-1200x467.png.

5.3.2. Cost-Effectiveness and Feasibility

The cost-effectiveness principle is central in the context of epidemiological screening because it is only through it that one can determine the economic viability of such interventions. By examining costs incurred in screening programs and what these yield, the policymaker in the health field can utilize limited resources better. The importance of this assessment is highlighted in the GRADE evidence-to-decision framework, where health equity concerns should be included in the balancing of screening programs' effectiveness. Precisely, an awareness of how screening would prove useful for marginalized groups would optimize the overall effect of the public health initiative without amplifying present health disparities (Akl et al., 2017). Thus, cost-effectiveness analysis, which is done appropriately, not only forms a rationale for the implementation of screening programs but also aids in equitable resource allocation to improve health outcomes in varying populations. Feasibility assessment, in terms of operational, technical, and economic factors, is an essential driver of the success of screening interventions. An effective screening program should be practical and sustainable in the provided contexts and thus should be convertible into tangible health improvements. The Malaria Elimination Group prospectus highlights the requirement for countries to conduct comprehensive feasibility studies, particularly with a transition from control interventions to elimination efforts (Feachem et al., 2009).

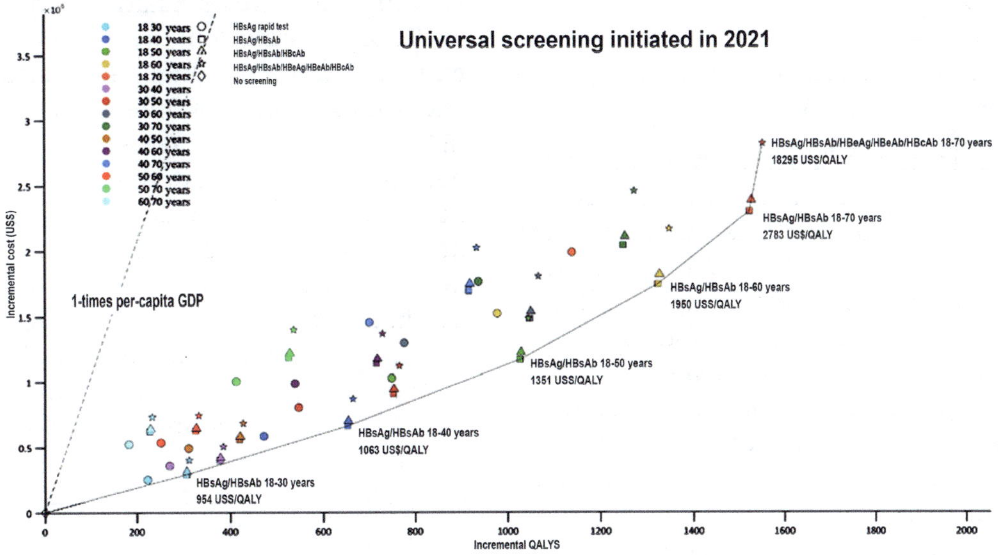

Figure 5.11. Cost-effectiveness plane demonstrating the cost-effectiveness for all screening strategies, subcategorized by the initiation year (2021, 2026, or 2031) of the HBV universal screening program.

Source: https://www.researchgate.net/profile/Jason-Ong-5/publication/352161841/figure/fig1/AS:1038545523326997@1624619956297/Cost-effectiveness-plane-demonstrating-the-cost-effectiveness-for-all-screening.ppm.

This guideline highlights that the studies have to be forward-looking and consider local epidemiology dynamics, available technologies, and the economic sustainability of screening processes. Thus, feasibility evaluations not only outline potential hindrances but also frame methods to change interventions in accordance with local needs, in order that a targeted strategy for screening is formulated as a response to national health objectives. Further, awareness of cost-effectiveness and the feasibility of screening programs encourages decision-making on the part of public health experts and stakeholders. An integrated framework allows best practices to be explored, thereby enlightening future implementations and adoptions of screening procedures. This learning process in cycles is highly essential in the dynamic world of epidemiology, where new approaches and tools are made known on a regular basis. Applying the lessons learned through previous attempts at elimination, such as those documented in malaria eradication campaigns, policymakers can refine their strategies to maximize impact while preventing wastage of resources (Feachem et al., 2009). Lastly, cost-effectiveness and feasibility analysis intertwining dictates a robust strategy for determining the value of screening to address issues in public health, promoting judicious scalability and enhanced health gains (Figure 5.11).

5.3.3. Ethical Considerations in Screening

Ethical considerations in screening precede in epidemiology, more specifically in the context of the question of informed consent and patient autonomy. Screening would generally involve the testing of patients who might not be symptomatic for a disease at all, and therefore raises ethical issues in terms of imposing the burden of subjecting asymptomatic individuals to potentially invasive tests or procedures. It is crucial to ensure that people are educated regarding the benefits, drawbacks, and possible outcomes of screening. This informed consent process, in addition to respecting the autonomy of the patient, also enables people to make more informed decisions regarding their healthcare. Furthermore, communication of the outcomes of screening should be effective in order to prevent potential distress or anxiety likely to be caused by false positives or false negatives, and, therefore, points towards the need for ethical requirements in using screening programs as effectively as they can be used. The ethical situation of screening is also problematic due to access concerns and health disparities among vulnerable groups. Health equity is an ongoing challenge in screening practice, and inequality in access to screening can potentially exacerbate existing inequalities in health. Certain population groups, such as racial and ethnic minorities, may face significant challenges in receiving early and adequate screening services. The ethical consideration of justice demands that these inequalities be removed to enable fair access to health interventions. By the identification of the various socio-behavioral factors that contribute to the health disparities, epidemiologists are in a position to advocate for policy and practice that benefits equitable access to screening for all, thereby advancing toward the elimination of health disparities for the vulnerable populations, as seen through the growing literature on health equity (Borysova et al., 2012). In addition, the impacts of screening on public and individual health also need to be taken into account. While screening is helpful in resulting in early detection and improved health outcomes for the individual, it has population-level effects regarding population health management as well. Ethical screening involves balancing the benefits to individuals against potential societal costs, such as the strain on healthcare resources and implications of overdiagnosis. For instance, in oncogeriatric patients, the mandate to perform geriatric assessments prior to operation is evidence of individualization of screening to focus on populations to attain optimal results while minimizing harm (Lampugnani et al., 2017). By being aware of ethical issues during planning and development of screening programs, public health workers can ensure that the screening processes are not just effective, but also ethical and beneficial both to individuals and to society as a whole.

5.4. Benefits of Screening

Screening in epidemiology is a critical process employed for the early identification of disease, which also enhances the efficacy of treatment and overall health outcomes. Screening programs detect disease at an early stage and hence enhance the likelihood of successful interventions extensively. For example, in cancer of the prostate, screening for prostate-specific antigen (PSA) has uncovered an explosive increase in lifetime risk of diagnosis from 6.1% in 1982 to 19.6% in 2012. The increase demonstrates the power of early screening to detect cancers that otherwise might remain undetected until late in their course and therefore allow individuals to benefit from earlier and often less toxic treatment (Bell et al., 2019). The net impact is the potential for less morbidity and mortality due to disease, highlighting the fundamental role of screening in furthering public health. Further, screening promotes a preventive care culture among the population, likely leading to greater societal investment in health care maintenance. Through routine screening processes, individuals are encouraged to adopt healthier lifestyle choices and obtain routine medical treatment, further heightening the awareness of the public about other health ailments. For instance, malaria-endemic nations that are targeting elimination efforts are targeting surveillance systems that not only identify cases but also enhance community engagement through awareness campaigns of the importance of prevention and treatment (Feachem et al., 2009). These programs foster an educated citizenry more likely to participate in the screening programs, thereby creating a support network and ensuring that more individuals are being provided with essential healthcare services. The subsequent ripple effect of increased health awareness then has the added advantage of reducing the cost of healthcare associated with treating advanced-stage disease. Finally, screening provides a valuable window for monitoring population health trends as well as the evaluation of public health intervention success. Through receipt of information via screening programs, epidemiologists are capable of identifying trends and disparities in disease occurrence, and eventually assist policy-making with scientifically based decisions and focused health programs. With analysis of screening data, public health officials are capable of efficiently allocating resources and responding to specific health concerns within society. Additionally, with advancements in testing protocols, continuous optimization of screening algorithms can result in increased efficiency and accuracy, ultimately maximizing the benefits of such programs (Bell et al., 2019). Thus, the integration of screening into public health interventions not only safeguards the health of a person but also maximizes the capacity of health systems to counter novel epidemiological challenges in advance (Figure 5.12).

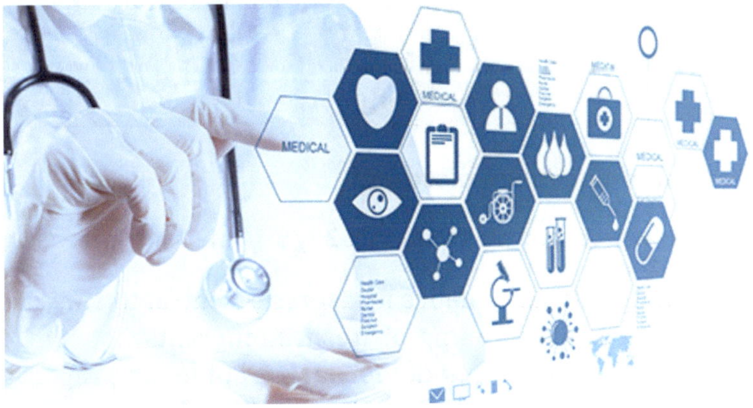

Figure 5.12. Health Screening Benefits.

Source: https://parmanandhospital.com/wp-content/uploads/2023/09/image-1.png.

5.4.1. Early Detection of Diseases

Early diagnosis of illnesses is crucial in enhancing public health outcomes, particularly for infectious diseases. Early detection of pathogens can lead to timely intervention that prevents outbreaks and minimizes their impacts on populations. In recent years, population migration from one country to another has presented new challenges to disease prevention and control. Screening programs are now inevitable, especially among recent migrants, since they facilitate early diagnosis and control, thereby curbing the transmission of infectious diseases. In studies with non-EU countries within the Mediterranean region, the observation was that 61% of the researched nations had implemented screening programs to monitor infectious diseases, thus confirming the important role of screening in population health interventions. This proactive action must be taken in protecting individual and collective health because earlier detection always yields better health and reduced rates of transmission within the population (Napoli et al., 2015). In addition to the surveillance of migrant populations, the emergence of new infectious diseases poses challenges that call for a different approach to surveillance and early detection. Globalization has caused the rapid spread of pathogens, occasionally crossing geographical boundaries and creating new public health issues. The continuous evolution of viruses complicates their early detection, as health authorities need to continuously alter their approach to respond to the shifting threat. This indicates the necessity of advanced technologies in disease surveillance systems, including in silico methods that leverage extensive computational resources. Inter-regional cooperative work has contributed to the creation of global networks for web-based surveillance, especially for illnesses like avian flu. Examination of mutation patterns and comparison of the effectiveness of existing treatments against such mutations, public health agencies can better prepare and respond to outbreaks, ultimately enhancing early detection capacity globally (Breton et al., 2008).

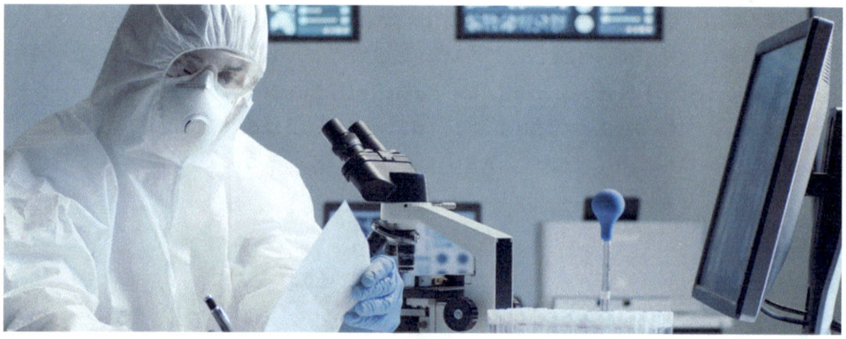

Figure 5.13. Early detection of infectious diseases.

Source: https://mariref.com/wp-content/uploads/2022/10/Infection-disease.webp.

The integration of screening and surveillance measures is central to effective disease prevention and control. As stressed by experts, screening of fresh immigrants not only identifies infectious diseases at the onset but also serves as a model for larger epidemic preparedness interventions. Countries with codified national guidance for screening are well placed to manage public health crises, particularly when the proportion of refugees living in them increases. This connection of screening tactics and health consequences stresses the need for incorporating full-blown public health systems with a bias towards early detection. The implementation of standardized guidelines throughout provinces can make disease diffusion prevention efforts more reasonable and provide individual benefits through timely interventions. By enhancing coordination between screening and information-sharing environments, public health systems can construct robust mechanisms for early detection that lead to healthier communities and fewer outbreaks (Napoli et al., 2015) (Figure 5.13).

5.4.2. Reduction in Morbidity and Mortality

Reduction of morbidity and mortality through targeted screening activities is an important contribution of epidemiology, particularly among high-risk populations. Detection of diseases at the initial stages can play a significant role in the effective control of diseases and consequently the relief of health systems. In rural South Africa, for instance, the prevalence of chronic diseases such as hypertension and diabetes is mind-boggling among the aging population, with self-reported prevalence of hypertension being 31.2% and musculoskeletal pain 41.7% (Clark et al., 2013). The special health issues of the demographics necessitate a robust screening mechanism, promoting stringent systematized health surveys to identify individuals at risk and provide interventions accordingly. Effective screening programs not only result in early diagnosis but also evoke a preventive approach to the management of chronic diseases, ultimately causing a reduction in morbidity. Moreover, minimizing health disparities due to screening leads to improved overall community health, thereby halting mortality rates. Socio-economic factors govern access to healthcare, with at-risk groups usually having several vulnerabilities (Hynes et al., 2012). Lack of proper preparedness and exposure to health risks can also exacerbate existing health conditions, leading to a vicious cycle of deteriorating health outcomes. Utilization of community-based screening interventions has the potential to bridge these gaps by facilitating access to care and improving health literacy among vulnerable populations. Identification of the most burdened chronic disease communities can assist in deploying the resources in a more suitable manner and bridging inequities that result in higher morbidity and mortality. Equipping these populations with the infrastructure and resources to enact healthy behaviors is critical to building an environment where such behavior will flourish. In addition, incorporating principles of environmental justice in screening has the potential to mitigate health dangers as well as stimulate resilience within communities. A comprehensive strategy recognizing the intersection of health, social inequities, and the environment is essential to effective public health intervention. By developing a cumulative risk assessment approach, health researchers can identify communities with interlayered vulnerability and steer a responsive public health strategy (Hynes et al., 2012). Not only does this integrated method help in the identification of areas of immediate concern, but it also highlights the importance of engaging with the community in the research process. Finally, by addressing both the underlying chronic diseases and the socio-environmental determinants that result in them, screening programs can be a powerful tool for reducing morbidity and mortality, thereby fostering better health outcomes for different populations.

5.4.3. Improved Health Outcomes and Quality of Life

Screening protocols in epidemiology significantly enhance health status and quality of life by allowing early detection and intervention. Screening allows for timely medical treatment, which can prevent the further exacerbation of cancers as well as infectious diseases by detecting health issues at their initial stages. For instance, in oncogeriatric patients, the application of comprehensive pre-surgical geriatric assessments is necessary. In spite of the obstacle created by the long and tiring process of performing these tests, their ability to detect risk factors—such as frailty and nutritional status—enables healthcare professionals to tailor treatment procedures suitable for the needs of their geriatric patients. This modification eventually results in improved surgical results and increased living standards for this vulnerable population, justifying the key position of individualized screenings in the new practice area of geriatric oncology (Lampugnane et al., 2017). Similarly, screening for blood-borne viruses (BBVs) and sexually transmissible infections (STIs) in antenatal care is another example where screening programs are capable of yielding improved health outcomes. The Royal Australian & New Zealand College of Obstetricians & Gynecologists' shift in recommendations to also include full STI testing—chlamydia coverage—just demonstrates one aspect of proactive maternal health. In a study, it was demonstrated that prior to revising recommendations, there was a substantial delay in chlamydia screening among pregnant women, with only 18% of pregnant women being subjected to the same. The adoption of new policies aims to close these gaps, ensuring the early detection and treatment of STIs, hence reducing pregnancy complications and generally improving maternal and child health (Combs et al., 2008). Efficient screening procedures, therefore, not only guide clinical practice but also construct healthier communities through the elimination of risks associated with untreated infections. In addition to the above benefits, improved health outcomes arising from screening activities are integrally linked to improved quality of life. Incorporation of effective screening programs ensures individuals have access to care, leading to better management of chronic diseases and increased lifespan. For geriatric patients undergoing surgery, as indicated in the literature, customized tests that consider underlying geriatric conditions allow for individualized treatment regimens that ultimately lead to better recovery and long-term overall health (Lampugnane et al., 2017). Additionally, the focus on maternal and fetal health through comprehensive STI testing underscores the societal emphasis on prevention. By making screening a priority among different populations, public health programs can have several objectives: improvement of the health status of the individuals and improvement of the general level of life in the populations by producing healthier generations to come. This approach requires screening in initiating public health advancement (Figure 5.14).

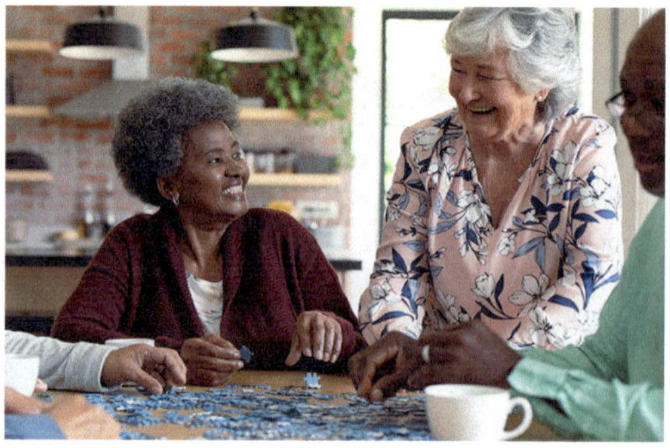

Figure 5.14. Quality of life factors that impact health outcomes.

Source: https://healthdimensionsgroup.com/wp-content/uploads/2022/03/quality-of-life.jpeg.

5.5. Challenges in Screening

The epidemiological screening environment presents several important challenges, with the complexity of identifying and addressing health inequities being the most prominent. Despite technological and methodological advancements in screening, unequal access to health does persist, particularly among ethnic minorities and young adults. For instance, research indicates that sexually active men who have sex with men, as well as black ethnic populations, experience elevated risks for sexually transmitted infections (STIs), with continued access and utilization barriers remaining in screening services. These health inequities usually owe their causation to socioeconomic status, stigma in culture, and poor education, which all lead to preventing early detection and effective intervention (Field et al., 2015). As epidemiologists work to improve screening regimens, a nuanced understanding of the social determinants is at the heart of designing interventions that address the specific needs of diverse communities. In addition, the effectiveness of screening regimens is also complexified by the dynamic nature of disease epidemiology. Since zoonotic diseases and environmental factors keep changing, the suitability of current screening protocols has to be continuously reassessed and updated. The changing epidemiologic landscape demands an active and reactive approach to screening, thereby demanding that stakeholders engage in collective efforts, including researchers, healthcare practitioners, and community-based activists.

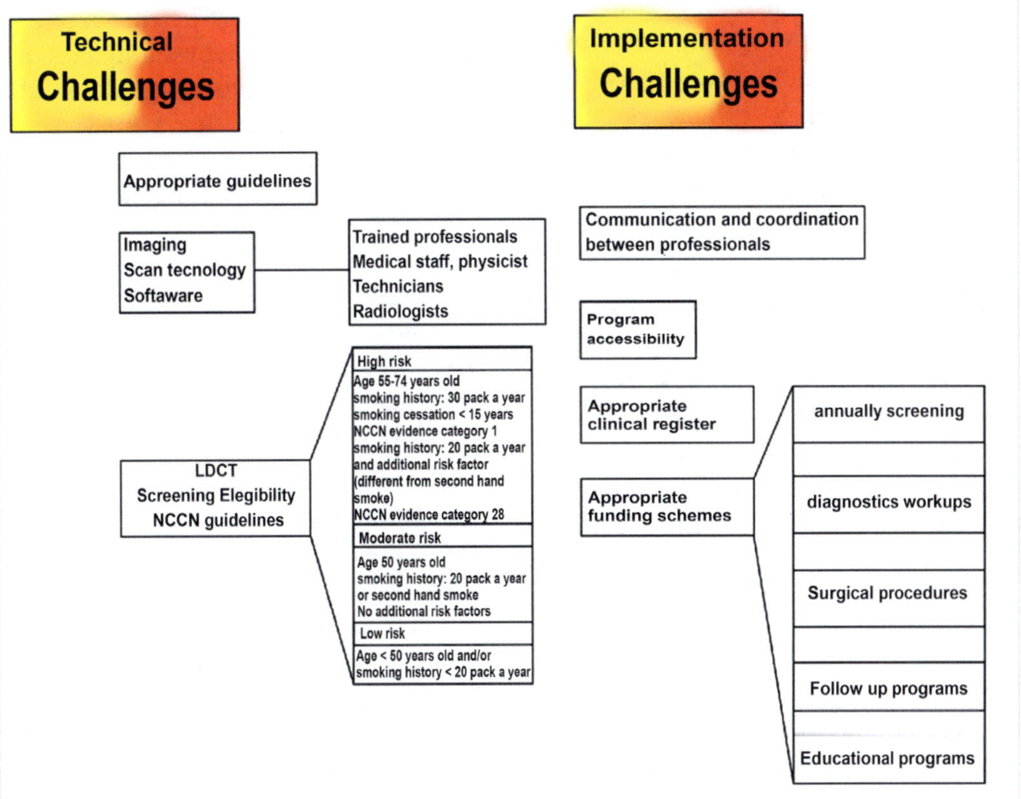

Figure 5.15. Challenges for lung cancer screening implementation. The success of a lung cancer screening program needs several issues to be considered. In order to achieve an adequate flow of the subjects, the coordination of technical, human, and management resources is fundamental.

Source: https://www.researchgate.net/profile/Eva-Bustamante/publication/323265919/figure/fig1/AS:595778389176329@1519056045804/Challenges-for-lung-cancer-screening-implementation-The-success-of-a-lung-cancer.png.

The International Partnership for Dogs, for example, illustrates how various organizations can collaborate to tackle breed-related health issues in dogs, illustrating the importance of collaboration in tackling health issues between species (Bartels et al., 2017). This mirrors a parallel with human epidemiology in which developing partnerships can be succeeded by developing more effective screening strategies that are more responsive to evolving public health problems. In addition to the social and epidemiologic difficulties, logistical considerations are also key to the success of screening programs. Resource allocation, staff training, and limitations of infrastructure are factors that can greatly impact coverage and quality of screening programs. The majority of the screening activities depend heavily on finance, and fluctuations in financial support can lead to services being provided unevenly. Secondly, the use of technology in screening services requires a continuous training system for healthcare personnel to effectively deal with emerging modes of operation. This means that the investments must not only support technological advancement but also work to develop the employees in the public health units. Prioritizing all these logistical issues is the key to supporting an environment where screening programs will be able to flourish and become effective in addressing health problems in communities (Field et al., 2015). With thorough planning and management of resources, the ability to address these challenges in screening can be greatly enhanced (Figure 5.15).

5.5.1. False Positives and False Negatives

For epidemiology, false positives and false negatives are the key to determining the effectiveness of screening programs. When a test detects an individual as developing a particular disease, but they do not, it is referred to as a false positive. Not only does it cause patients unnecessary concern, but it can also lead to additional, often invasive, tests and treatments, which carry their own risk. The effects of false positives also have repercussions for healthcare costs, adding to the burden of overcrowded health systems. For instance, a study had the performance of radiographers interpreting mammograms tested and found that even though their sensitivity levels were comparable to those with experience in radiology, their false positive rates were significantly higher, highlighting a need for diligent training in interpreting screening test results (Mohar et al., 2015). Thus, an understanding of sensitivity and specificity is essential to enhance the validity of screening tests. False negatives are a more malevolent issue in screening. They occur when a test fails to detect a disease that is present, offering a false hope to the doctor as well as the patient. False negatives also lead to delayed treatment, potentially allowing the disease to progress to its later stages and worsening patient outcomes. In tuberculosis screening, scientists have also recognized a need for sensitive and specific tests because cases that are overlooked can be disastrous for public health (Cattamanchi et al., 2011).

To this end, it is also critical to apply effective diagnostic practices together with firm screening tools in order to eliminate the occurrence of false negatives. The implications of these errors reinforce the need for continuous scrutiny and refinement of diagnostic procedures in epidemiology, such that the benefits of screening overcome harm. The impact of false positives and false negatives resonates beyond the level of individual cases, with implications for planning at the population level. Too many false positives result in loss of confidence in screening programs and can lead to discouragement in preventive health screening. False negatives increase the possibility of disease transmission, but more importantly, undermine public health efforts in disease control or eradication. Hence, the design and implementation of screening protocols should aim at reducing both types of errors. This involves integrating advanced technologies, formulating training for staff involved in screening work, and using mathematical models in simulating the effects and costs of various scenarios in screening work (Mohar et al., 2015). By building a culture of ongoing research and development, the profession of epidemiology can enhance the efficacy of public health interventions, thereby leading to better health outcomes in populations.

5.5.2. Access and Equity Issues

Availability of screening in epidemiology remains a significant issue, particularly when examining health disparities between various population segments. All agree that there are institutional impediments based on race, ethnicity, and socioeconomic status that significantly influence the capacity of an individual to gain access to screening programs. For example, breast cancer screening, which is critical for treatment and detection at an early stage, witnesses a discouraging trend of declining rates of participation by racialized and immigrant women. Statistics show that more than half of recent immigrants who were eligible for the screening did not take advantage of the available programs, while 26% of Canadian-born women did so (Mahamoud, 2014). Such disparities underscore the need for interlinked interventions that not only promote awareness regarding screening benefits but also dismantle system barriers that hamper equitable access to health care services. The impacts of unequal access to screening are also compounded by geographical and socioeconomic factors, particularly in health care provision systems. Individuals from rural or underserved cities are inclined to suffer from transportation challenges, limited access to special care, and a lack of insurance, all of which disqualify them from the ability to be part of screening programs. According to the most recent studies, these disparities have a more significant impact on minority patients and lower-income patients than others, leading to preventable disease and even death in serious health disorders such as lung and skin cancer (Carlson et al., 2016). In order to better address these inequities, recognition of the ways that patient activation, bias on the part of providers, and community strengths play a role in shaping health outcomes must occur. Building inclusive cultures within healthcare systems has the potential to profoundly enhance the rates of screening as well as the overall population health. Mitigation of access and equity issues related to screening in epidemiology needs to be multifaceted and evidence-based. Encouraging policies that provide full insurance coverage, expand access to specialty care, and encourage culturally appropriate practices are essential in aiming to make progress. Additionally, research conducted at a community level focusing on the lived experiences of the underserved can be used to inform targeted interventions and policy changes. Attention needs to be directed towards raising awareness regarding screening programs and community partnerships that generate access to care. Moreover, intentional effort to address implicit biases among healthcare providers and integration of quality improvement approaches into the provision of care has been found to significantly reduce disparities in the utilization of screening (Carlson et al., 2016). Since these access and equity concerns remain issues, institutional commitment to reform is needed to ensure everyone has equal opportunity for early disease detection and improved health outcomes (Figure 5.16).

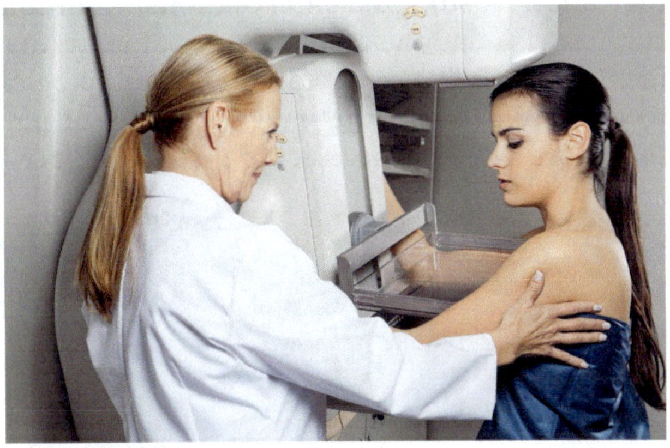

Figure 5.16. Access to breast cancer screening.

Source: https://invisiblepeople.tv/wp-content/uploads/2023/10/Breast-Cancer-Screening.jpg.

5.5.3. Psychological Impact on Individuals

The psychological impact of screening in epidemiology extends beyond mere medical assessment, influencing people's emotional and mental well-being. Once confronted with the risk of disease, particularly life-threatening diseases like cancer, individuals become more anxious, fearful, and stressed. This is most precisely noted in those populations under regular screening, where anticipation of outcome can cause extreme emotional upset. Studies have confirmed that the psychological stress of waiting to learn one's diagnosis leads to negative health outcomes, including increased morbidity and risk of mortality. Moreover, when test outcomes indicate greater levels of risk, the subjects may face hopelessness or feelings of inadequacy, which further destabilize their mental states. Hence, awareness of such psychological impacts is also important for healthcare professionals in order to develop conducive environments for screening sessions. The complexity of psychological responses to screening is further highlighted by the interaction between social factors, such as gender and socio-economic status. For instance, one study established that experiences of gender discrimination significantly detract from women's adherence to mammography screening guidelines, illustrating how negative life stressors might interfere with health-seeking behavior. In studies that followed individuals for several months, women who were subjected to gender discrimination were less apt to adhere to the screening guidelines recommended, particularly in the more affluent groups. This implies consideration of the multifaceted nature of psychological responses, as deeply rooted issues may deter individuals from engaging in essential preventive medical measures. Hence, interventions lowering such barriers may be the secret to improved health outcomes among vulnerable populations, since psychological well-being directly impacts the effectiveness of screening for health. In addition, carrying out geriatric assessments in depth indicates a welcome move toward meeting older persons' psychological needs as they are being screened. As the aging population grows with more health concerns, an understanding of the unique psychological aspects of such a population is paramount. Successful screening, however, requires that the physical well-being of geriatric patients be taken into account alongside their mental and emotional well-being. By carrying out intensive pre-surgical evaluation that incorporates elements like the Geriatric Depression Screening, medical professionals can early detect mental health issues that allow customized interventions. Additionally, such screenings can aid in the prediction of surgical risk and the tailoring of treatment, thereby improving outcomes overall. Thus, it is vital to include psychological factors in epidemiological screening protocols, bringing a holistic approach to treating not only the physical health of patients but also their emotional health, thus leading to a more effective healthcare system (Figure 5.17).

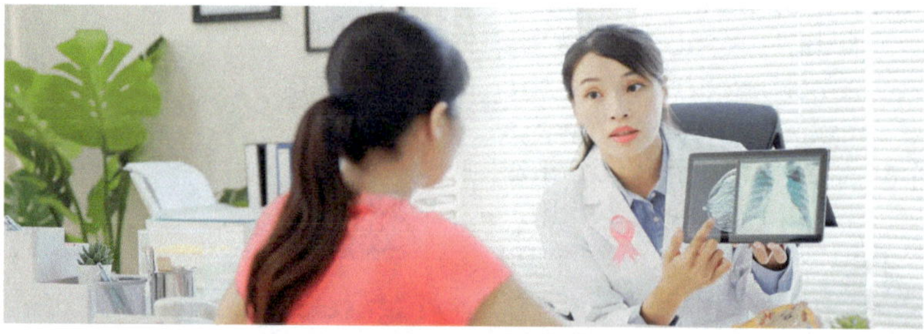

Figure 5.17. Psychological impact of cancer screening.

Source: https://gleneagles.com.my/images/gleneagleshospitalmalaysialibraries/health-digest/why-early-detection-matters-breast-cancer-screening.webp?sfvrsn=797cee92_7.

Summary

To put it briefly, screening in epidemiology is an important strategy for the early identification and prevention of disease. As public health interventions improve, the success of various screening modalities continues to be a focus of research and practice. For instance, newer research highlights the influence of response rates within health surveys, showing that even slight changes, such as questionnaire length or incentives, can lead to a dramatic increase in participation. One such result indicated that the presence of a minimal monetary incentive of £2.50 considerably boosted response rates, underlining the importance of productive participant engagement when designing screening programs (Gatting et al., 2017). These programs can assist in the promotion of demographic and health data collected as representative of the true range of the population, thereby making it possible to produce evidence-based public health policy. Also, the development of predictive measures from genetic risk factors is a promising new frontier in screening practice, particularly in the case of prostate cancer. The inclusion of polygenic risk scores has been shown to accurately predict onset age for severe disease phenotypes, guiding clinical decisions around screening timing (N/A, 2018). This is a massive leap for personalized medicine from the one-size-fits-all approach to a more tailored recommendation based on individual risk profiles. The integration of genetic data into screening programs enables efficient challenges , so that precise targeting is also optimized, while enhancing the potential for successful intervention at an early stage. Finally, the complexities of achieving representative sample populations only underpin the ongoing need for creativity in screening programs. Through the divergence in survey response to different survey methods, screening program design and delivery have to be adaptive enough to address issues of accessibility and participation among the public, so that they can address those concerns. This extends beyond crude rates of participation to encompass more universal questions of equity in health impacts. Through the innovative integration of strategies for maximizing response rates and utilizing leading-edge predictive modeling, epidemiologists can optimize the validity and impact of screening programs. Ultimately, careful evaluation of these measures will enable more effective disease prevention and control, further solidifying the pivotal role of epidemiology in public health.

Screening in epidemiology is a key intervention in the detection of diseases earlier, which finally translates into better patient outcomes and survival. Screening for diseases like breast cancer and healthcare-associated infections is a quintessential example of the importance of detection at an earlier stage. Despite diversity in populations, there still remain inequalities in the access and use of screening, with socioeconomic factors, geographical location, and structural disparities being given. For instance, racialization has deeply impacted women's take-up of Canadian breast cancer screening programs, with significantly varying diagnosis and survival rates. Addressing these disparities calls for an intimate understanding of the obstacles to marginalized groups, as this is the only way measures can be developed that are apt to improve take-up of screening services and general health outcomes (Mahamoud, 2014). Besides, one should admire the various ways through which screening behavior can vary when the disease to be screened for is different. For example, a hand hygiene compliance review cites multimodal interventions as a method to reduce healthcare-associated infection. Practices such as increased availability of hand sanitizers, employee education, and feedback on performance were found to enhance compliance by a narrow margin. Nonetheless, the variation in results from the studies highlights the necessity for solutions that are adapted to the local conditions of healthcare environments. This means that even as general guidelines for screening have been developed, their application needs to be accommodative to suit differences in local and demographic influences affecting health care provision (Chudleigh et al., 2017). Lastly, program effectiveness relies not only on understanding the populations to be served but on implementing follow-through action to involve these populations in prevention efforts. The persistence of inequities in screening utilization emphasizes the need for ongoing study and intervention design. Community-based programs can contribute to an understanding of the daily lives of diverse populations and, in turn, impact the design of more comprehensive screening programs. By resolving these underlying causes, screening has the potential to be the public health imperative it should be, diminishing disparities and enhancing the general well-being of high-risk groups (Mahamoud, 2014).

CLOSER LOOK

FUTURE DIRECTIONS IN SCREENING RESEARCH

With the expanding area of epidemiology, the future of screening studies is destined to witness colossal developments. Scientists are now more interested in creating new methods that utilize technology to enhance screening. New technologies such as artificial intelligence and machine learning have huge potential to scan gigantic databases to identify risk factors more accurately. Such technologies also have the potential to optimize the efficiency of screening programs by detecting populations that are more susceptible to certain illnesses. Through the use of advanced algorithms that can process multifactorial variables, researchers aim to refine screening standards and, in the long term, eradicate false negatives and positives.

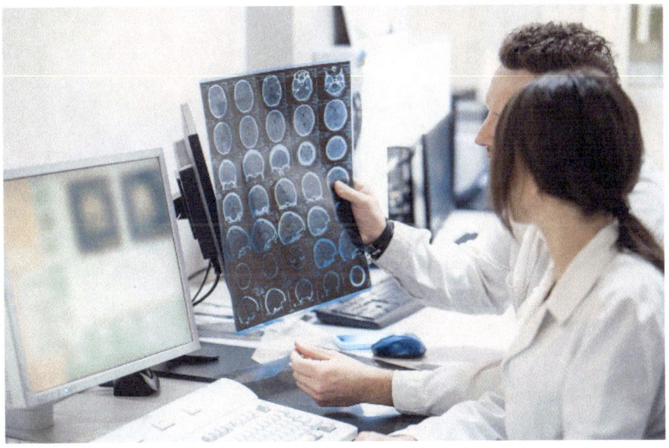

Figure 5.18. Medical researchers are analyzing brain scan images during a clinical screening trial.

Source: https://altusresearch.com/wp-content/uploads/2024/11/altus-research-screening-trials-1-1-scaled.jpg.

The more specific the screening is, the more potential there is to positively impact public health measures, further justifying the pursuit of research in this area of epidemiology. Another promising direction of inquiry in screening research is a greater emphasis on the social determinants of health influencing screening use and outcomes. Socioeconomic status, level of education, and access to healthcare facilities are some of the determinants influencing the compliance and effectiveness of screening. Future studies can benefit from examining the convergence of these social determinants with biological and behavioral risks to provide a comprehensive understanding of screening disparities. For instance, researchers are able to examine the interaction between IQ in childhood and subsequent health outcomes, learning about the effects of cognitive ability on health behavior and exposure to preventive interventions. By shedding light on such complex relations, future screening research can be used to provide more efficient program design, so that intervention is equitable and reaches those in most need of screening (Deary et al., 2005). Furthermore, expanding our knowledge about risk-factor assessment is important for enhancing screening procedures. Conferences such as the ACL Research Retreat have highlighted the importance of ascertaining specific risk factors linked with preventing injuries, demonstrating how concentrated intervention can yield better health consequences. A similar epidemiological strategy can direct disease screening methods based on creating personalized screening processes from person-specific risk profiles. Follow-up research can then concentrate on identifying and verifying new biomarkers and behavior measures that serve as key instruments for health risk prediction. The dual focus on novel risk-factor measurement and individualized screening protocols has the potential for transforming the manner in which we intervene in disease prevention and, in turn, improve public health interventions (NC DOCKS at The University of North Carolina at Greensboro et al., 2010) (Figure 5.18).

References

1. Abo-Shehada, M. N., Guitian, J., Hegazy, Y. M., Holt, H. R., et al. (2007). Systematic review of brucellosis in the Middle East: Disease frequency in ruminants and humans and risk factors for human infection. https://core.ac.uk/download/pdf/36779249.pdf (accessed on 25th June 2025).
2. Akl, E. A., Alonso-Coello, P., Briel, M., Eslava-Schmalbach, J., et al. (2017). GRADE equity guidelines 4: Guidance on how to assess and address health equity within the evidence to decision process. https://core.ac.uk/download/96882593.pdf (accessed on 25th June 2025).
3. Alavi, Y., Kuper, H., Legood, R., Lindfield, R., et al. (2012). The cost-utility of telemedicine to screen for diabetic retinopathy in India.
4. Albert, U., Apergis-Schoute, A., Brakoulias, V., Carmi, L., et al. (2019). Early intervention for obsessive compulsive disorder: An expert consensus statement. https://core.ac.uk/download/287581694.pdf (accessed on 25th June 2025).
5. Arnold, M., Calavas, D., Ducrot, C., Heim, D., et al. (2008). Review on the epidemiology and dynamics of BSE epidemics. https://core.ac.uk/download/pdf/29258720.pdf (accessed on 25th June 2025).
6. Ballegooijen, M. van, Boer, R., Brown, M. L., Habbema, J. D. F., et al. (2000). Endoscopic colorectal cancer screening: A cost-saving analysis. https://core.ac.uk/download/18523767.pdf (accessed on 25th June 2025).
7. Balmes, J., Ritz, B., & Tager, I. (2004). Can lessons from public health disease surveillance be applied to environmental public health tracking? https://core.ac.uk/download/pdf/3775836.pdf (accessed on 25th June 2025).
8. Bartels, A., AIDAP, Clarke, A. J., APGAW, Greko, C., et al. (2017). Moving from information and collaboration to action: Report from the 3rd International Dog Health Workshop, Paris in April 2017. https://core.ac.uk/download/141439096.pdf (accessed on 25th June 2025).
9. Bell, K., Doust, J., Glasziou, P., Hayen, A., et al. (2019). Lifetime risk of prostate cancer overdiagnosis in Australia: Quantifying the risk of overdiagnosis associated with prostate cancer screening in Australia using a novel lifetime risk approach. https://core.ac.uk/download/211066192.pdf (accessed on 25th June 2025).
10. Borysova, M. E., Mitchell, O., Sultan, D. H., Williams, A., et al. (2012). Racial and ethnic health disparities in incarcerated populations. https://digitalscholarship.unlv.edu/cgi/viewcontent.cgi?article=1141&context=jhdrp (accessed on 25th June 2025).
11. Breton, V. V., Da Costa, A. L., De Vlieger, P., Hai, R., et al. (2008). Innovative *in silico* approaches to address avian flu using grid technology. https://core.ac.uk/download/49299291.pdf (accessed on 25th June 2025).
12. Brodbelt, D. C., Church, D. B., McGreevy, P. D., O'Neill, D. G., et al. (2014). Approaches to canine health surveillance. https://core.ac.uk/download/36777547.pdf (accessed on 25th June 2025).
13. Brucker, R., Buffington, J., Castor, M. L., Forquera, R., et al. (2012). Integrating viral hepatitis screening and prevention services into an urban chemical dependency treatment facility for American Indians and Alaska Natives. https://digitalscholarship.unlv.edu/cgi/viewcontent.cgi?article=1013&context=jhdrp (accessed on 25th June 2025).

14. Carlson, C., Sholk, J., Nanni, J., Peterson, K., Smith, L. A., & Bhavaraju, N. (2016). *Breaking the Barriers to Specialty Care: Practical Ideas to Improve Health Equity and Reduce Cost–Ensuring High-Quality Specialty Care*. https://core.ac.uk/download/75785771.pdf (accessed on 25th June 2025).
15. Cattamanchi, A., Dowdy, D. W., Pai, M., Steingart, K. R., et al. (2011). Is scale-up worth it? Challenges in economic analysis of diagnostic tests for tuberculosis. https://core.ac.uk/download/323075169.pdf (accessed on 25th June 2025).
16. Chan, C. C. H., Chen, L., Chien, C., Demeyere, N., et al. (2018). Psychometric properties of the Chinese (Putonghua) version of the Oxford Cognitive Screen (OCS-P) in subacute poststroke patients without neglect. https://core.ac.uk/download/212868643.pdf (accessed on 25th June 2025).
17. Chudleigh, J. H., Drey, N., Gould, D. J., Moralejo, D., et al. (2017). Interventions to improve hand hygiene compliance in patient care. https://core.ac.uk/download/160607161.pdf (accessed on 25th June 2025).
18. Clark, B., Gómez-Olivé, F. X., Kahn, K., Thorogood, M., et al. (2013). Self-reported health and health care use in an ageing population in the Agincourt sub-district of rural South Africa. https://core.ac.uk/download/13117710.pdf (accessed on 25th June 2025).
19. Combs, B. G., Giele, C. M., Kwan, K. S. H., Mak, D. B., et al. (2008). Audit of antenatal testing of sexually transmissible infections and blood borne viruses at Western Australian hospitals. https://core.ac.uk/download/61303469.pdf (accessed on 25th June 2025).
20. Corker, E., Grimmett, C., Matheson, L., Menon, U., et al. (2011). Ovarian and cervical cancer awareness: Development of two validated measurement tools. https://core.ac.uk/download/1669224.pdf (accessed on 25th June 2025).
21. Curnow, M. M., Jones, C. M., Macpherson, L. D., McMahon, A. D., et al. (2016). Evaluation of dental therapists undertaking dental examinations in a school setting in Scotland. https://core.ac.uk/download/46164933.pdf (accessed on 25th June 2025).
22. Dailey, A. B., Holford, T. R., Jones, B. A., Kasl, S. V., et al. (2010). Neighborhood and individual level socioeconomic variation in perceptions of racial discrimination. https://cupola.gettysburg.edu/cgi/viewcontent.cgi?article=1002&context=healthfac (accessed on 25th June 2025).
23. Dailey, A. B., Jones, B. A., Calvocoressi, L., Centers for Disease Control and Prevention (CDC), Department of Health and Human Services, Consedine, N. S., & Kasl, S. V. (2008). Does gender discrimination impact regular mammography screening? Findings from the Race Differences in Screening Mammography Study. https://cupola.gettysburg.edu/cgi/viewcontent.cgi?article=1020&context=healthfac (accessed on 25th June 2025).
24. Deary, I. J., Hart, C. L., Hole, D., Smith, G. D., et al. (2005). Childhood IQ and social factors on smoking behavior, lung function and smoking-related outcomes in adulthood: Linking the Scottish Mental Survey 1932 and the Midspan studies. https://core.ac.uk/download/1393705.pdf (accessed on 25th June 2025).
25. Desvaux, S., Goutard, F., & Roger, F. (2005). Workshop to deliver epidemiology and laboratory training for HPAI diagnostic network. http://agritrop.cirad.fr/529308/1/ID529308.pdf (accessed on 25th June 2025).
26. Feachem, R. G. A., Phillips, A. A., & Targett, G. A. (2009). *Shrinking the Malaria Map: A*

Prospectus on Malaria Elimination. https://core.ac.uk/download/pdf/11307280.pdf (accessed on 25th June 2025).

27. Field, N. M., & Hughes, G. (2015). The epidemiology of sexually transmitted infections in the United Kingdom: Impact of behavior, services and interventions. https://core.ac.uk/download/29410608.pdf (accessed on 25th June 2025).
28. Gatting, L., Robb, K. A., & Wardle, J. (2017). What impact do questionnaire length and monetary incentives have on mailed health psychology survey response? https://core.ac.uk/download/80697202.pdf (accessed on 25th June 2025).
29. Goodall, D., Lombardo, C., & Steven, A. (2011). Models for schools of public health: A scoping review and synthesis of existing evidence. https://core.ac.uk/download/5900218.pdf (accessed on 25th June 2025).
30. Hynes, H. P., & Lopez, R. (2012). Cumulative risk and a call for action in environmental justice communities. https://digitalscholarship.unlv.edu/cgi/viewcontent.cgi?article=1111&context=jhdrp (accessed on 25th June 2025).
31. Jenkins, D. R., Medley, G., & Robotham, J. (2006). Screening strategies in surveillance and control of methicillin-resistant *Staphylococcus aureus* (MRSA). https://core.ac.uk/download/48834.pdf (accessed on 25th June 2025).
32. Karnon, J., & Vanni, T. (2011). Calibrating models in economic evaluation: A comparison of alternative measures of goodness of fit, parameter search strategies and convergence criteria.
33. Klatte, T., Rossi, S. H., Stewart, G. D., Usher-Smith, J. A., et al. (2018). Epidemiology and screening for renal cancer. https://core.ac.uk/download/162912487.pdf (accessed on 25th June 2025).
34. Lampugnale, C. A. (2017). Surgical assessment of the geriatric oncology patient. https://open.bu.edu/bitstream/2144/26707/5/Lampugnale_bu_0017N_13146.pdf (accessed on 25th June 2025).
35. Mahamoud, A. (2014). *Breast Cancer Screening in Racialized Women: Implications for Health Equity*. https://core.ac.uk/download/71365142.pdf (accessed on 25th June 2025).
36. Mohar, A., Chapman, A. H., Dowdy, A. H., Bogart, A., Angeles-Llerenas, A., Mucci, B., Hillman, B. J., et al. (2015). Radiographers supporting radiologists in the interpretation of screening mammography: A viable strategy to meet the shortage in the number of radiologists. https://core.ac.uk/download/323073234.pdf (accessed on 25th June 2025).
37. N/A. (2018). Polygenic hazard score to guide screening for aggressive prostate cancer: Development and validation in large scale cohorts. https://core.ac.uk/download/151178451.pdf (accessed on 25th June 2025).
38. N/A. (2025). *Ear disease in Aboriginal and Torres Strait Islander children*. https://core.ac.uk/download/pdf/30673322.pdf (accessed on 25th June 2025).
39. Napoli, C., Riccardo, F., Dente, M., Rossi, P., Declich, S., & Kärki, T. (2015). Screening for infectious diseases among newly arrived migrants: Experiences and practices in non-EU countries of the Mediterranean basin and Black Sea. https://core.ac.uk/download/54525874.pdf (accessed on 25th June 2025).
40. NC DOCKS at The University of North Carolina at Greensboro, Schmitz, R. J., & Shultz, S. J. (2010). ACL Research Retreat V: An update on ACL injury risk and prevention, March 25–27,

2010, Greensboro, NC. https://core.ac.uk/download/345082581.pdf (accessed on 25th June 2025).

41. Newton, W. (2001). Rationalism and empiricism in modern medicine. https://core.ac.uk/download/62568601.pdf (accessed on 25th June 2025).

42. Reynolds, L. A., & Tansey, E. M. (2009). *History of Cervical Cancer and The Role of The Human Papillomavirus, 1960–2000*. https://core.ac.uk/download/30696170.pdf (accessed on 25th June 2025).

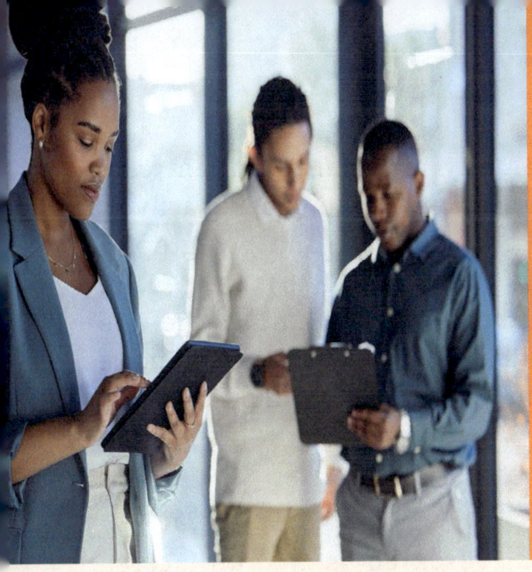

Chapter 6

BIAS IN CLINICAL STUDIES

Contents

Introduction

The starting platform for considering bias in clinical trials is the setting for an intense examination of how such biases can influence treatment outcomes and patient treatment. In clinical research, the integrity of findings matters most because findings have a tendency to drive clinical practice decisions and policy directions. However, biases can take many forms, and by doing so can distort outcomes and challenge the integrity of a study's findings. To illustrate, where outcomes are influenced by misleadingly optimistic reporting on the part of clinicians, reported effect quality can make it difficult to interpret true patient experience. This dualism brings into focus the necessity for bias deeply rooted in clinical research to be countered, and hence the necessity for methodological stringency that buffers against such dangers and aids constructivist evidence in the medical arena (Howick et al., 2017). With the focus of study lying in the impact of positive messaging in clinical environments, the necessity for extensive meta-analysis becomes evident. The effectiveness of such approaches is typically negated by variability in study design and inherent biases of heterogeneous trials. Systematic assessment of the literature is imperative, with sound methods being employed to synthesize evidence effectively. Systematic reviews and meta-analyses not only assign importance to findings but also carry with them transparency and objectivity in the evaluation of clinical interventions. In evaluating the potential benefits of positive messaging, it is essential to think about the heterogeneity of reported outcomes because differing methods can obscure the true effectiveness of treatments for pain relief. These rigorous methods inform clinical practice critically and determine directions of research in the future (Lunet, 2025).

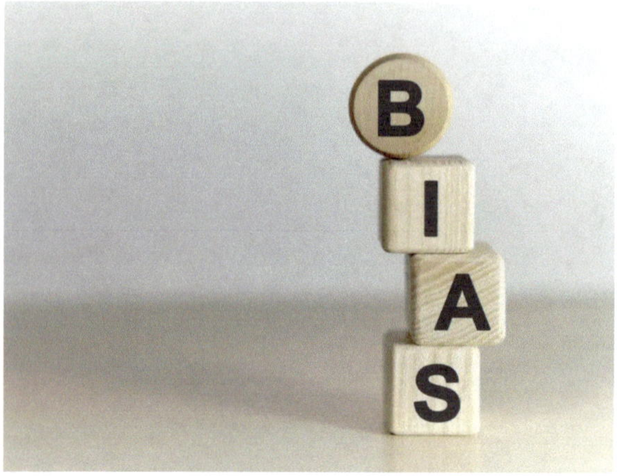

Figure 6.1. Bias in clinical research studies.

Source: https://417studies.com/wp-content/uploads/2022/05/Wood-blocks-spelling-BIAS-stacked-up.jpg.webp.

Lastly, the alignment of evidence with respect to bias underscores the need to adopt complex practices in clinical research. Researchers have the responsibility to be vigilant for and remove biases that could compromise the reliability of their findings. There is a need for better-quality research; increased methodological rigor can go towards validating or invalidating existing hypotheses regarding intervention effectiveness. Putting precedence on creating standards that reduce bias allows the clinical research community to advance patient care and the field as a whole. Through being actively checked on recent literature and being open, researchers can contribute to a more precise and informative base of clinical knowledge, and thereby an evidence-based practice-conducive climate (Howick et al., 2017; Lunet, 2025) (Figure 6.1).

Definition of Bias in Clinical Studies

Bias in clinical research is a multifaceted one and often the determining factor in the validity of the results of studies. Bias can be defined as a systematic departure from reality in findings or conclusions drawn from a study, to the extent of providing biased conclusions. Such differences can be attributed to multiple sources, including selection bias, performance bias, detection bias, and attrition bias, all of which can threaten the data quality obtained. For instance, selection bias occurs when participants who are chosen for the study do not represent the intended population. The inability to represent true to form distorts outcomes and limits the generalizability of findings, ultimately threatening their applicability in real-world settings. Awareness of such biases and their implications is important for study designers so that the frequency of these biases is reduced to make the clinical evidence stronger. In observational studies, the identification of bias is quite challenging, as investigators need to deal with confounding variables that may influence outcomes with care. This complexity warrants the application of strong methodological approaches to minimize bias. Researchers may be able to use statistical techniques to hold confounding variables constant, but controls can only partly remove bias due to unmeasured variables. One example comes from sibling studies of the causal effect of schooling on wages, where unmeasured heterogeneous ability can create significant bias to make causal estimates invalid. These issues highlight the need for continuing research in research methods to develop new ways of detecting and preventing bias so that results from clinical studies become more accurate (Hasegawa et al., 2019). Bias is also measured in randomized controlled trials (RCTs), which are regarded as the standard against which all other study designs should be measured. Although RCTs aim to eliminate most forms of biases through randomization, they are not immune to biases that may occur during the process of design and implementation. For example, poor case definition in studies may result in ambiguities influencing the assessment of treatment efficacy. Systematic review of randomized controlled trials of probiotics in the management of diarrheal in children illustrates how differences in definitions and reporting of outcomes can lead to statistically significant heterogeneity, ultimately to evidence of low certainty (Alam et al., 2024). Hence, this illustration points out the need for designing arduous protocols and employing extensive assessment tools so that both the risk of bias and the quality of evidence in clinical trials may be evaluated so that the conclusion reached forms a realistic representation of reality (Figure 6.2).

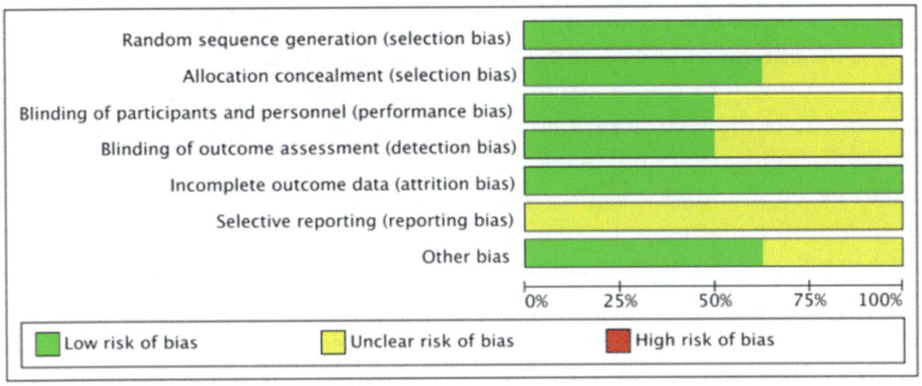

Figure 6.2. Risk of bias graph including selection bias, performance bias, detection bias, attrition bias, and reporting bias.

Source: https://www.researchgate.net/publication/340672314/figure/fig3/AS:960114626412568@1605920573924/Risk-of-bias-graph-including-selection-bias-performance-bias-detection-bias-attrition.png.

Importance of Addressing Bias

Battling bias in clinical studies is of paramount concern with profound implications for medical outcomes and patient care. Bias can take many different forms, including selection bias, publication bias, and outcome assessment bias, all of which potentially compromise the integrity of research results. Misleading clinical practice and compromising patient safety could be the consequences of these biases, particularly when treatment guidelines are developed on the basis of biased evidence. The literature closely illustrates that biases often remain unaddressed, raising concerns about the applicability of results to diverse populations. Ensuring biases are identified and mitigated, therefore, allows for wider representation of clinical safety and efficacy, ultimately enhancing patient care and medicine development. In clinical research, applying systematic approaches to reading literature plays a critical role. Traditional literature searches can fail or inadequately assess the effect of biases, leading to inconclusive or misleading findings in research. As proposed by new evidence, the use of systematic reviews can significantly enhance research reproducibility and transparency. Through the use of rigorous methodologies in literature searches, researchers can minimize the influence of biases, particularly when determining the effects of interventions in vulnerable populations. This shift in methodology not only underpins research designs but also ensures that clinical advice considers the diverse experience and needs of all patients, thus providing fairer healthcare delivery. The reliance on systematic reviews provides a helpful platform for gaining insight into cumulative evidence, which is crucial for evidence-based clinical decision-making. Moreover, addressing bias in clinical studies is an inseparable adjunct to researchers' and practitioners' ethical obligation. Encouraging unprejudiced research methods is not only a scientific cause; it is an ethical one that impacts patient trust and the honesty of the healthcare system. The creation of transparent reporting guidelines and open dialogue regarding possible bias not only makes research more credible but also supports accountability among researchers. Finally, fostering a sensitivity to bias in clinical trials encourages a culture of ethical research that places importance on patient welfare and informed consent. With greater demand for solid, unbiased studies, it is increasingly clear that working against bias must happen in order to advance evidence-based medicine as well as the overall progress of healthcare outcomes for patients from all walks of life.

6.1. Types of Bias

The presence of bias in clinical studies can be perceived from a variety of perspectives, significantly impacting the validity of research results and the subsequent applicability of outcomes to clinical practice. Selection bias occurs when subjects participating in a study are not representative of the overall population, thereby skewing results and avert generalizability. This issue will occur in studies where recruitment methods predispose groups or clinical characteristics, leading to over- or underrepresentation of specific groups. The bias can occur in outcomes regarding real-world effectiveness, and it is therefore critical to have rigid study designs that yield heterogeneous and representative populations in all phases of clinical trials. Addressing selection bias is the most critical because it directly influences the quality of the evidence produced and its validity to inform healthcare decisions. Performance bias, another important type of bias in clinical trials, relates to variations in the way care is provided across different study groups. This kind of bias may occur when the participants are aware of the intervention that they are receiving, leading to differential treatment conditions due to expectations or participant and researcher biases. For instance, differences in monitoring or other treatments given to one but not another group in trials evaluating the efficacy of new medications can unintentionally influence the outcomes. To eliminate performance bias, the participants and researchers are typically blinded, as a strategy to prevent outside interference with the study findings. Validity of trial outcomes relies on reducing this bias, thereby emphasizing the need to maintain objectivity throughout the research process. Measurement bias, whereby methods of data collection are substandard or unreliable, is another significant problem in clinical research. This prejudice can be due to numerous sources, like abuse of the measurement tools, observer prejudice, or utilization of self-reported information, which are often inaccurate measures of real outcomes. As an example, if a study measuring pain relief employs subjects' personal reports, variation in perception and reporting variation may lead to errors in conclusions. For more valid and reliable findings, standardized measurement procedures and good training of the person conducting the measurement need to be instituted. Measurement bias reduction not only increases the credibility of the outcome of studies but also enhances the overall quality and usefulness of the research conducted, ultimately enhancing evidence-based clinical practice (Figure 6.3).

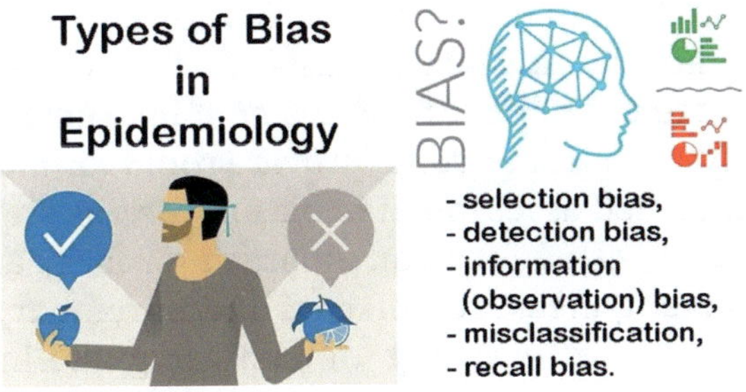

Figure 6.3. Types of bias in epidemiology.

Source: https://microbenotes.com/wp-content/uploads/2021/12/Types-of-Bias-in-Epidemiology.webp.

6.1.1. Selection Bias

Selection bias is a widespread issue in clinical studies since it can lead to misleading conclusions regarding the intervention's efficacy. Selection bias occurs when the participants of the study are not representative of the population to which the results aim to be generalized. For example, if a clinical trial has strict inclusion criteria, it may exclude certain demographic groups or individuals with comorbidities prevalent in the targeted population. Such biases will skew results, and this can result in overestimation or underestimation of the treatment's actual effect. By not controlling for the variation of participant attributes, researchers can unwittingly produce results that are not externally valid, thus reducing the general applicability of the study findings. The effects of selection bias have serious implications for practice and policy formation. When a clinical trial demonstrates the efficacy of a treatment through a non-representative sample, doctors will implement recommendations that fail to yield the same positive outcomes in the broader population. This can aggravate health disparities, particularly if particular groups are systematically underrepresented. For instance, in research on chronic diseases such as chronic obstructive pulmonary disease (COPD), where the focus is primarily on a homogeneous population, the findings may not reflect the opinions of heterogeneous patient populations being exposed to a range of biological or environmental hazards. Hence, accessing ethical and effective healthcare intervention is inextricably linked with fighting and minimizing selection bias by adopting inclusive research designs and rigorous recruitment processes. To assist in managing selection bias, several strategies can be implemented by researchers during study design and conduct. Randomized controlled trials (RCTs) are an effective tool since the randomization process theoretically distributes the participant attributes to intervention groups in equal proportions. This research approach makes it less likely for the effect of systematic bias to affect the outcome measures.

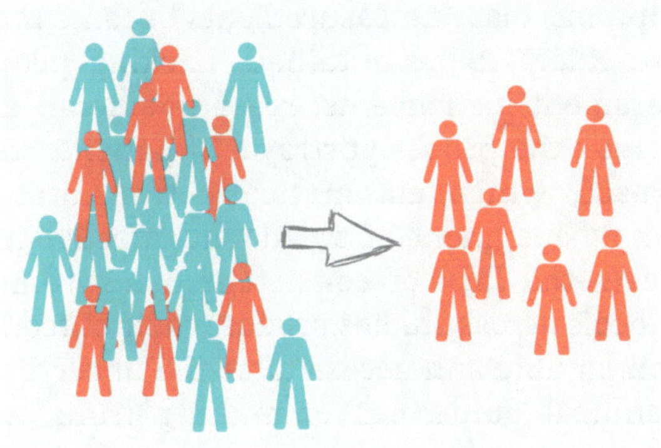

Figure 6.4. Selection bias.

Source: https://databasecamp.de/wp-content/uploads/population-and-sample-1-1024x709.png.

Additionally, researchers can perform sensitivity analyses to ascertain the extent to which various demographic variables can affect findings. For instance, in examining results of thyroidectomy, researchers can distinguish between experiences of different patient subgroups since comparative studies on subtotal and total thyroidectomy results for multinodular non-toxic goitre show (Arezzo et al., 2015). Moreover, comparisons of telecare with traditional care modalities for conditions like COPD can identify the importance of multi-dimensional selection of participants in determining treatment effect among various populations (Car et al., 2011). By prioritizing inclusive approaches, the integrity and validity of clinical research can be best guaranteed (Figure 6.4).

6.1.2. Measurement Bias

Measurement bias is a serious issue in clinical trials because it can systematically distort findings, resulting in erroneous conclusions about efficacy and safety. When data collection techniques subtly favor particular results or groups, the validity of the findings is severely compromised. As an example, if a trial uses unvalidated questionnaires to evaluate patient symptoms, biased measurements become much more likely to be obtained. Lacking proper assessment instruments, researchers can also overlook the proper portrayal of patients' true statuses, which automatically translates to their misjudgment of treatment effectiveness. Indeed, the lack of consistent measurement protocols across studies renders their outcomes incomparable and necessitates the uncertainty of clinical guidelines emanating from such analyses, thereby underscoring methodological prudence in crafting assessment instruments for the fight against measurement bias in clinical research.

A shared framework to evaluate bias that was suggested in the current literature can enhance the understanding of measurement bias in clinical research. The integration of inquiry into measurement bias with other forms of bias—e.g., selection and confounding bias—can help scientists enhance their insight into how systematic errors influence study findings. According to new paradigms, methodological improvements involve the application of causal diagrams in explaining relations among variables and suggesting potential sources of bias. The technique is particularly crucial as it allows scientists to define hypotheses prior to analysis and thereby invalidate biases that may result from the use of poor measurement instruments. Lastly, such frameworks provide room for more harmonized assessment of bias in various study designs, with a focus on embracing robust and consistent measures of data measurement to enhance the integrity of clinical guidelines and treatment protocols (Burger et al., 2020). Emerging evidence within clinical research underscores the necessity of critically appraising measurement bias via systematic reviews and meta-analyses. For instance, a therapeutic interventions meta-analysis in gaming disorder highlights the importance of measuring within-study bias rigorously with well-established tools like RoB2 and ROBINS-I. However, the effects were moderate to large across treatments, publication risk for bias and heterogeneity in study methods nuanced the findings. This example illustrates measurement bias, whereby the lack of stability in outcome measures can distort relative treatment results. This also adds weight to the calls for better methodological conduct and transparent reporting in clinical trials in order to avert the effect of measurement bias effectively. Firm appraisal and sound study design can potentially fortify the foundations of evidence-based medicine, ultimately to produce more precise clinical guidelines (Danielsen et al., 2022) (Figure 6.5).

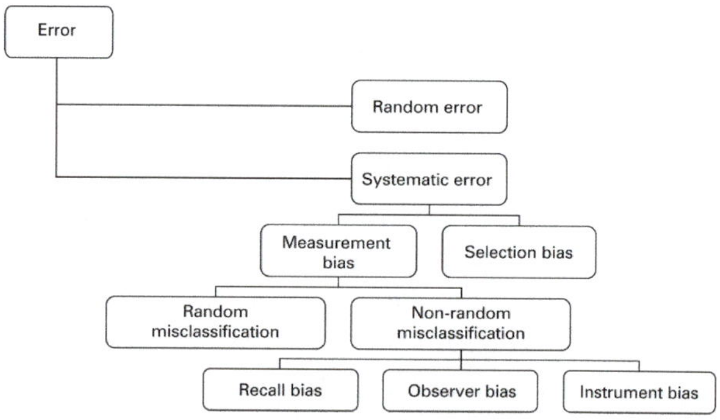

Figure 6.5. A systematic approach to bias.

Source: https://mentalhealth.bmj.com/content/ebmental/11/2/36/F1.large.jpg.

6.1.3. Confounding Bias

Confounding bias is a significant threat to the internal validity of clinical trials that diminishes the reliability of findings on treatment effects. Confounding bias occurs when there is an extraneous variable or confounder that affects the independent and dependent variables in the same direction, thus creating a spurious relationship between them. For instance, when measuring the impact of a new treatment on health status, confounding factors such as age, comorbidities, and socio-economic status may skew the result. By failing to adjust for such factors, researchers can end up assigning effects to the treatment where these effects are the result of the confounding factors. This misrepresentation can mislead clinical decision-making and counsel, thus making it important to have robust methodological designs within clinical studies.

The use of an example case to demonstrate confounding bias is through observational studies aimed at examining treatment efficacy in patients with COVID-19. In one such analysis, researchers had the option to explore the assessment of treatment efficacy without any regard to competing risks and confounding variables, hence making biased estimates of mortality risk between treated and untreated groups. Using unadjusted naive statistical methods that failed to account for these biases produced an overestimation of mortality risk to the point of gross exaggeration, with treated patients possessing a misleadingly unconservative high risk, which was made all the worse by confounding variables. With a trial emulation platform, researchers would be able to more effectively deal with confounding bias, offering a more accurate characterization of treatment effect and moving the interpretative context regarding their findings (Hazard et al., 2024). The relevance of confounding bias is also seen in research examining periodontal intervention effectiveness during pregnancy. In one recent review of clinical trials, low-risk and high-risk trials were both tested for bias, and it was determined that high-risk trials were especially susceptible to confounding bias, with the power to distort outcomes with regard to preterm birth and low birth weight. While some subgroups resulted in potential gains from periodontal treatment, the aggregate evidence was unclear due to the omnipresent risk of confounding. The findings highlight the need for a robust trial design that strictly regulates confounding variables in an effort to produce more accurate, actionable findings. In light of this, confidence and rigorous testing of confounding bias should be on top of both interpretation and result reportage in clinical trials, with a key emphasis on continued research into methodological developments that mitigate this kind of bias (Allareddy et al., 2015) (Figure 6.6).

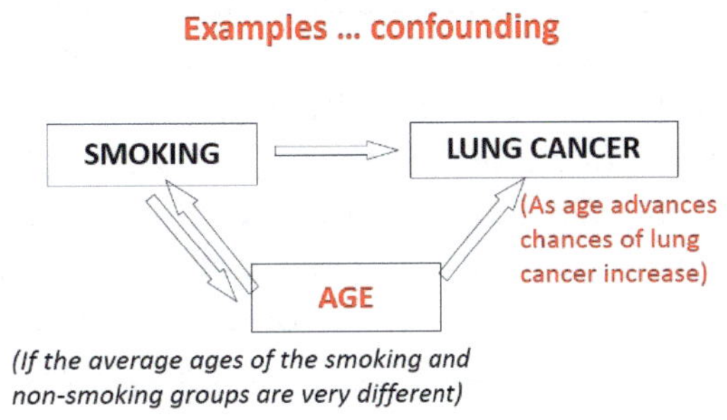

Figure 6.6. Example of confounding bias.

Source: https://howmed.net/wp-content/uploads/2013/07/bias-example.jpg.

6.2. Sources of Bias

Identification of potential sources of bias in clinical research is significant to the interpretation of the quality and credibility of the evidence. Selective publication is one source of bias, where statistically significant trials are published preferentially over those yielding null results. This can result in systematic reviews that do not reflect the true evidence base, skewing the conclusion from the data. As emphasized in the literature, evidence selection bias is more likely to occur in systematic reviews that fail to include unpublished data, and suggests that researchers should actively seek out these unpublished studies from diverse sources like clinical trial registries and regulatory agency databases like the EMA and FDA, as compiled in Abuabara et al. (2016). Eliminating this bias is an attempt to ensure that all information deemed relevant is brought to light and reviewed when synthesizing evidence.

Differences in study design and reporting requirements constitute another principal source of bias in clinical research. For instance, in the case of neuraminidase inhibitors (NIs), oseltamivir and zanamivir, poor reporting protocols led to high selection and performance bias risks as seen from analysis of clinical trial reports. More specifically, the trials did not remain blinded, or placebo interventions were not inert, invalidating results. As noted in Mar et al. (2014), such deficiencies can be biased and lead to incorrect conclusions regarding treatment safety and effectiveness, particularly where sponsors are directing the trials they fund. Therefore, the study design and reporting need to be open to minimize the threats of these biases. Additionally, selective reporting and attrition bias are frequent defects that invalidate the integrity of clinical studies. Attrition bias occurs when there are significant differences between those who take part in a study and those who drop out, affecting the reliability of the results overall. For example, research into NIs revealed that attrition was more prevalent within some of the trials, and thus it was uncertain whether results could be generalized to the population as a whole. Furthermore, selective result reporting, in which some results are presented and others are left out, can also add to the problem. This was seen in the literature of oseltamivir and zanamivir trials, where selective outcome reporting concealed the true effectiveness and safety profile of the interventions, as seen in Mar et al. (2014). Combating such issues involves strict adherence to preregistered plans and reporting all results, regardless of their outcomes, to gain a full perspective of any intervention's impact (Figure 6.7).

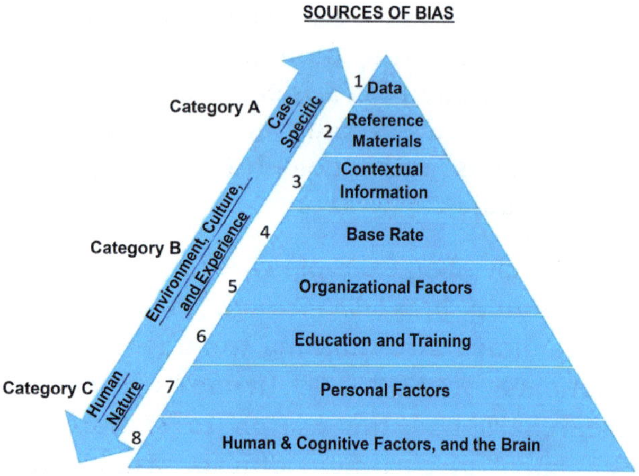

Figure 6.7. Sources of bias.

Source: https://jaapl.org/content/jaapl/early/2025/05/05/JAAPL.250019-25/F1.large.jpg?width=800&height=600&carousel=1.

6.2.1. Research Design Flaws

Clinical research validity relies heavily on research design, as flaws in research design have the potential to introduce powerful biases that make the results invalid. Randomization, allocation concealment, and blinding flaws are particularly destructive because they have the potential to introduce systematic variability among study groups. For instance, poor randomization can result in selection bias, which often favors some results while hiding true therapeutic effects. Studies across various disciplines have explained such issues, indicating that improved methodological quality research provides more reliable outcomes. The assessment of systematic reviews and meta-analyses for acupuncture interventions in stroke demonstrates that the majority of primary studies are beset by such design flaws, particularly those from the Chinese literature, which documented higher discrepancies in the criteria employed to avoid bias and ensure a stringent search strategy (Chen et al., 2017). Another vital element of study design is the operationalization of outcomes, which can add further to the weakening of validity in clinical research. If researchers fail to define outcomes clearly or employ low-quality measuring instruments, the evidence is prone to being skewed or even manipulated and, in practice, introduces bias. Assessor reliability is pertinent in measuring the quality of research to make conclusions drawn from the evidence valid and applicable for use in clinical practice. These developments underscore the necessity of creating quality assessment methods that reflect inter-rater reliability and agreement validity. Hence, assessment tool adaptation is essential in order to enhance international methodological excellence of clinical studies, which indirectly affects opinions and acceptance of medicine interventions (Arora et al., 2012). Furthermore, the implications of study design flaws in clinical research go beyond immediate results, influencing even policy-making and clinical guidelines. Where biases contaminate published studies, they can affect medical guidelines and public health policy based on dodgy evidence. It is increasingly important, therefore, to improve the research quality of clinical trials so that evidence-based practice is based on solid research findings. The ongoing prevalence of study design errors indicates a need for better training of researchers and a collective effort to adopt best practices in trial design. The world of clinical research can only improve by further debate around methodological transparency and publication of studies less susceptible to bias, hence leading to more robust and applicable medical innovations for the patient.

6.2.2. Participant Recruitment Issues

Effective participant recruitment is an important aspect of clinical trial integrity since it will have a direct influence on the validity and generalizability of findings. Bias can easily be introduced through the recruitment process, particularly if convenience samples or geographic locations are utilized. A particular hospital or clinic may be used in a study to recruit participants, resulting in a homogenous patient population. This setting limits the diversity required for treatment effect interpretation by groups. The pilot study of repetitive functional task practice (RFTP) demonstrated these limitations, indicating that 4–6% of screen-in patients were enrolled, ultimately achieving recruitment targets at only two of three study sites (Pollock et al., 2016). These low recruitment rates can skew outcomes, suggesting effectiveness when no such effect might exist in broader populations and thus emphasizing the value of more representative recruitment protocols. Lastly, the rise of virtual clinical trials represents a significant shift in participant recruitment strategies, offering benefits and risk factors. Such trials spur democratization of clinical research, enhancing access for those who live far from research centers (Andrews et al., 2017). Yet, the virtual aspect of recruitment can introduce specific biases, above all regarding demographic representation and socioeconomic status. Participants with restricted access to the internet or technical skills might be systematically excluded, and hence, the sample might be skewed and result in biased findings. Additionally, virtual trials impose strong means of securing informed consent, but participants might not really understand the consequences of taking part, which further complicates the ethical context of recruitment. Therefore, the balance between accessibility and stricter ethical and scientific standards must be achieved in preventing bias. Lastly, participant dropout represents another serious issue throughout clinical trials that also contaminates biases and validity. Systematically elevated dropout rates will interfere with treatment group equilibrium as well as create missing data, again causing bias in study outcomes. For instance, in the RFTP pilot study, although there was limited initial recruitment, follow-up rates showed that outcome assessors were unblinded for a high percentage of participants, potentially compromising the study's validity and integrity (Pollock et al., 2016). Attrition must be addressed with careful planning, including procedures to continue to engage participants and to communicate continuously over the course of the study's duration. Moreover, trials also have to report and track adherence to interventions, as varying degrees of commitment may result in further bias and eventually weaken the validity of the trial conclusion. All these multifaceted problems of participant recruitment should be properly addressed to enable the potency of clinical research and avert bias (Figure 6.8).

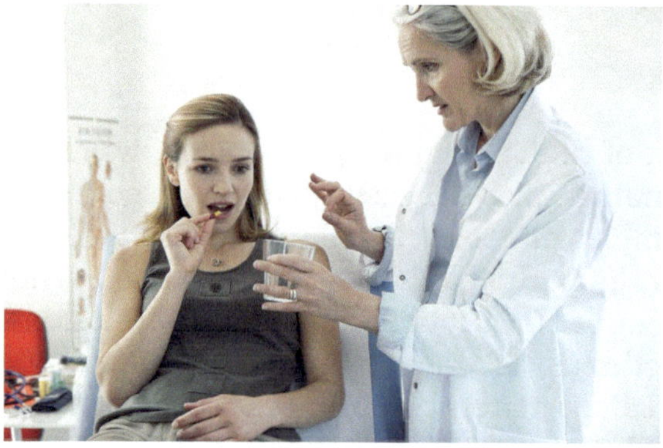

Figure 6.8. Recruitment of study participants is vital to phase 1 and 2 clinical trial success.

Source: https://www.biopharmaservices.com/wp-content/uploads/2022/05/Recruitment-of-Study-Participants-Is-Vital-to-Phase-1-2-Clinical-Trial-Success-blog-image.jpg.

6.2.3. Data Collection Methods

Data collection methods are of utmost concern in establishing the validity and reliability of clinical study findings. The choice of whether or not to utilize a given method has significant impacts on data integrity that can ultimately generate biases that predispose study outcomes. For instance, antiquated oral and written records of dietary history may result in recall bias, where patients may provide inaccurate accounts of what they have been consuming through memory gaps. Alternatively, computer-assisted history taking systems (CAHTS) aim to surmount these barriers by providing a formatted environment that may allow for more accurate self-report data. Even though one study found patients created more accurate food diaries once familiarized with CAHTS, overall risk of bias was moderate, with the note that stronger research is required to validate the usefulness of CAHTS in clinical practice (Alberti et al., 2011). Apart from nutritional measurements, other methods of data collection, like direct observation, have also been criticized for inducing inherent biases. A systematic review highlighted that direct observation of hand hygiene adherence in healthcare environments often faces selection as well as information biases. These biases are produced due to constraints such as weekday observations only and specific specialties, ultimately providing an incomplete status in terms of compliance behavior across various environments. To contribute to the distortion of data, variables such as observer training and measurement criterion variation are significant. These inconsistencies threaten the validity of inferences drawn from clinical practice research, necessitating the establishment of standardized procedures that would enhance the credibility of outcomes in clinical studies (Abela et al., 2018). The impact of biased data collection techniques is immense, particularly in developing effective interventions for managing diseases. When biases come into information, they can deflect clinical decision-making and policy formulation, which ultimately will be reflected in the quality of patient care. For example, based on faulty diet recommendations, tools could result in ineffective diet advice on diabetes management, leading to compromised patient results. It is therefore essential for researchers and practitioners to identify and rectify biases in data collection mechanisms. Future research must focus not only on enhancing data collection techniques but also on performing rigorous validation processes to determine reliability. With this approach, a more practical clinical practice and understanding of patient behavior will translate to interventions that are genuinely reflective of patient needs and settings, paving the way to better healthcare outcomes overall.

6.3. Impact of Bias on Study Results

Bias drastically affects the outcome of clinical trials and has a tendency to negatively affect the validity of results. Various forms of bias, including selection bias, measurement bias, and reporting bias, tend to denigrate the credibility of research results. For instance, when researchers inadvertently select a non-representative sample, the study results' applicability to larger populations becomes questionable. The implications of such biases also appear in the success of clinical interventions; outcomes that appear wonderful in biased research will not necessarily be true in real life, and consequently mislead healthcare professionals and patients alike. Detection and correction of these biases are critical to improve the quality of clinical research and support evidence-based practice in healthcare facilities. Furthermore, the complexity of clinical questions typically enhances the level of bias, particularly in communication among healthcare professionals. For example, one study that aimed to investigate whether email communication was effective among health professionals identified significant biases in blinding and concealment of allocation (Atherton et al., 2012). The study demonstrated that while the application of e-mail enhanced conformity to clinical guidelines, its applicability and validity were limited by an extremely high risk of bias. This highlights the importance of stringent design in clinical studies where biases might distort not only certain study results but even the overall conclusion inferred from a body of literature. If biases permeate many studies, collectively they are forcing a healthcare-knowledge trend that can affect patient care. The consequences of bias extend beyond the research effort to clinical decision-making and to patient outcomes. Interventions to modify cognitive bias, such as cognitive bias modification for interpretation bias (CBM-I), have shown varied efficacy in reducing levels of hostility among clinical populations (Cougle et al., 2021). The evidenced gains, as modest and variable as they are, mirror the richness of psychological and medical interventions in biases. Without strict controls to prevent them, results can pick up bias that distorts perceived benefit or harm, and the decision-making process becomes even more burdensome for clinicians. This emphasizes a need for ongoing vigilance in recognizing and removing bias from clinical trials so results fully reflect the effectiveness of interventions and ultimately enhance patient care.

6.3.1. Alteration of Treatment Efficacy

The variation in the efficacy of treatments in clinical trials is a significant problem that can occur as a result of various sources of bias, hence affecting the validity of the results. A significant determinant of treatment efficacy is the quality of trials conducted. Evidence indicates that low-quality studies are much more likely to generate biased results, which can lead to an exaggeration of the treatment effects as observed in small animal models, as seen in clinical studies within the stroke research field (Bahor et al., 2020). The methodological errors, say, inadequate randomization and lack of blinding, not only influence the noted effectiveness of interventions but also raise questions on the clinical significance of findings drawn from such research. Hence, it is apparent that methodological strictness plays a very important role in ensuring adequate measurement of treatment effects in clinical trials. Compliance with treatment protocols, besides that, is central to establishing the noted effectiveness of interventions. More specifically, the management of long-term conditions, such as spondyloarthritis (SpA), often relies on patients' adherence to exercise interventions as prescribed by professionals. It has been shown in a systematic review how adherence rates may vary significantly, depending on the level of disease severity and the duration of diagnostic delay (Coulter et al., 2019).

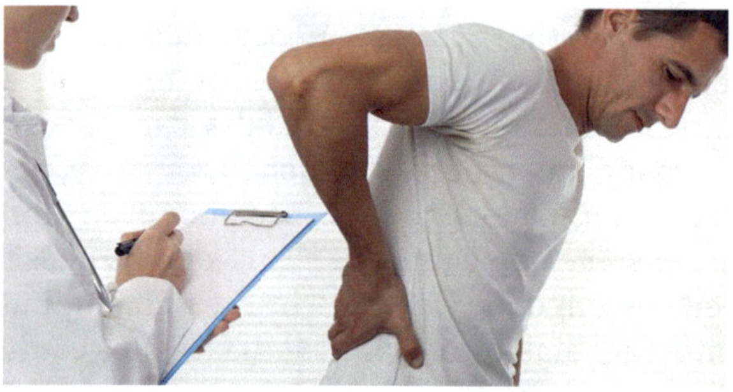

Figure 6.9. The effectiveness of TNF inhibitors for axial SpA can vary significantly between men and women, depending on which disease activity measure is used.

Source: https://www.healio.com/~/media/slack-news/stock-images/rheumatology/b/backpain2.jpg?w=800.

While some studies suggest that education does improve compliance, variation in findings and the numerous intervening factors influencing compliance make it difficult to measure treatment effectiveness. This inconsistency not only distorts data but also taints the essential aim of enhancing patient outcomes with effective interventions and eventually alters what is being perceived as treatment effectiveness. In clinical research, the intersection of study design quality and patient adherence describes the complexity of treatment efficacy. The intersection of these two variables indicates that activity aimed at preventing bias must aim to maximize both the methodological quality of studies and adherence strategies to follow treatment protocols. Because higher-quality studies usually correlate with higher-quality results, methodological improvements in most clinical trials can actually enhance the validity of treatment efficacy claims (Bahor et al., 2020). Likewise, identifying and eliminating obstacles to adherence can result in improved patient outcomes, thereby painting a better picture of how effective interventions are in the long run. Coordination of such efforts is key to building a more robust and consistent evidence base in clinical research (Figure 6.9).

6.3.2. Misleading Conclusions

The presence of fallacious conclusions usually contaminates the reliability of clinical research, particularly when studies are done or analyzed without rigorous methodological oversight. Researchers and practitioners may unintentionally draw false conclusions from data due to prejudice that enters all study design, data gathering, and analysis levels. For instance, the patterns of behavior in subjects with obsessive-compulsive disorder (OCD) indicate how biases of cognitive process interpretation may result in incorrect conclusions. In another experiment on eye movement patterns of subclinical checkers, subclinical checkers possessed atypical fixation behaviors that were wrongly attributed to the realm of memory and not specific attentional bias. These incorrect interpretations not only fail to account for the nuances of initial observations but also have the potential to create erroneous recommendations of treatment modalities, which can become detrimental to patient care in the long term. Moreover, the biasing of results can be further exacerbated by the selective reporting of data, an all-too-familiar scenario in publication bias. This practice enables scientists to selectively choose results that are supportive of their hypotheses and reject negative results, creating the impression of efficacy without the backing of the entire body of evidence. As highlighted by the growing concern about medical ghostwriting and deceptive information it disseminates, distorted publication practices can have quite substantial health policy and clinical guideline implications. These practices not only mislead practitioners but also erode the patient's right to effective and safe treatment. Without strong regulation and ethics within the publication process, the medical literature is tainted, and a vicious cycle of misinformation erodes the foundation of evidence-based medicine and patient care. Finally, to alleviate the issue of misleading conclusions in clinical trials, there needs to be concerted efforts towards greater accountability and transparency among the research community. As demonstrated in discussions on the legal implications of medical ghostwriting, tougher enforcement of more stringent rules for authorship contribution and data submission is called for. Also, stimulating an environmentally friendly approach to the planning of studies, as done by a study of eye movement of high checkers, can function to elucidate the complex interaction between reported outcome and cognitive bias. By creating a culture of integrity and rigor in clinical research, the danger of forming incorrect conclusions can be significantly minimized, developing more dependable interpretations of evidence. Besides, stakeholders like regulatory bodies and learning institutions must prioritize coming up with frameworks for encouraging ethical publishing behavior to safeguard public health and trust in medical research (Harkin et al., 2012; Minasi et al., 2017).

6.3.3. Implications for Patient Care

The impact of bias in clinical research transcends the clinical context and has tragic consequences for patient care and outcomes. Identification of ethical issues posed by biased clinical research conduct is necessary to advance best practices for patient care. Vulnerable populations, such as children or individuals unable to make decisions regarding their own health, demonstrate the urgent need for an ethical paradigm for clinical research. By prioritizing patient interests and keeping personal, cultural, and religious biases aside, health professionals can practice more objective care. It is imperative to develop a standardized code of practice in ethical decision-making when the health resources utilized need to be stretched parsimoniously to meet the individual's and community's needs. This delicate equilibrium ensures that treatment of patients is still effective, as well as addressing the systemic effects of bias in clinical research (Montalto et al., 2014). Furthermore, health disparities initiated by biases in clinical research can generate significant disparities in patient treatment. For instance, minority communities and socio-economically disadvantaged groups tend to face challenges in accessing proper healthcare services. These disparities are fueled by a vast array of reasons, like geographical limitations, inadequate insurance coverage, and biased providers, all of which work synergistically to promote undesirable health outcomes. Such patients suffering from critical diseases are subjected to heightened risks related to these disparities, eventually leading to deteriorated general health and an upsurge in healthcare costs. Redress of these disparities is crucial since, in addition to causing unnecessary morbidity and mortality, they also place excessive costs on the healthcare system. The solutions that address these disparities will improve the quality and availability of patient care for marginalized groups as a testament to the need for systemic reform of medical practice (Carlson et al., 2016). To address the impact of bias in clinical research and the implications of patient care, healthcare providers and policymakers are required to work proactively toward equity-enhancing activities. Activities involved in widening specialty care access, ensuring quality treatment, and patient engagement are relevant in such cases. In addition, by removing implicit bias among providers and promoting culturally competent care, health systems are able to begin dismantling systemic barriers that disadvantage groups. Not only do these interventions improve patient outcomes, but they also increase the overall quality of healthcare, ultimately reducing unnecessary costs associated with healthcare disparities. When stakeholders of the health care system identify the importance of integrating equity into practices of care, they will be in a better place to accommodate the varied needs of all patients and neutralize the consequences of bias inherent in clinical research (Carlson et al., 2016) (Figure 6.10).

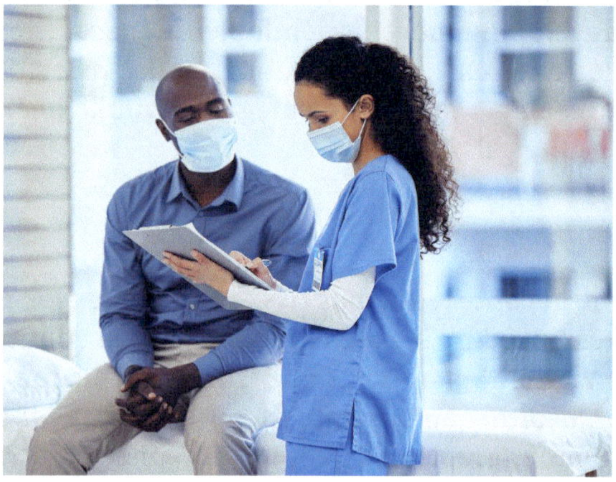

Figure 6.10. Implications for patient care.

Source: https://www.intelycare.com/wp-content/uploads/2024/02/what-is-a-nursing-implication.jpg.

6.4. Strategies to Minimize Bias

Eliminating bias in clinical trials is required to offer confidence in the validity and reliability of findings. One of the efficient ways is employing distributed networks that conduct analyses across various sites while ensuring that data is kept confidential. These networks, according to Brown et al. (2020), enhance research quality by using common protocols and analysis plans, therefore providing consistency in methodology. By combining large and diverse populations to study, such networks can substantially reduce sample selection biases. Not only is this method conducive to transparency, but it also facilitates auditing and replication of studies, which is a prerequisite for building findings. As more researchers employ distributed approaches, the likelihood of site-specific processes culminating in biases is reduced, giving way to more credible evidence to inform clinical and regulatory decisions. Another extremely important way of reducing bias in clinical studies is implementing rigorous conflict of interest and blinding policies. Blinding treatment assignments to researchers, participants, and evaluators reduces the influence of preconceived notions and individual biases on the outcome of studies to a great extent. As noted by Brown et al. (2020), adherence to blinding protocols is particularly crucial in clinical trials where subjective assessment of outcomes might lead to varying interpretations depending on the observer. Additionally, transparent conflict of interest policies help avoid outside pressures distorting the research findings. These all coalesce into an even more objective research environment, one that ultimately enhances the validity of research results and encourages public trust in clinical research. Rigorously standardized methods are a second essential method for mitigating bias in clinical trials. Randomized controlled trials (RCTs), for instance, are the best standard for determining cause-and-effect relationships using random assignment of patients to treatment and control groups. As discussed, employing RCTs, particularly where interventions like community paramedic interventions for chronic disease management, help illuminate the actual effects of a treatment by controlling confounding variables. Further, employing strong statistical analysis like Poisson regression and negative binomial regression allows the researcher to analyze outcomes effectively and to eliminate bias further in inferential statistics. By methodically adopting these methodological protections, researchers will be able to more closely position their studies to reflect high levels of scientific rigor, thus promoting the credibility and usefulness of their results in actual clinical practice (Figure 6.11).

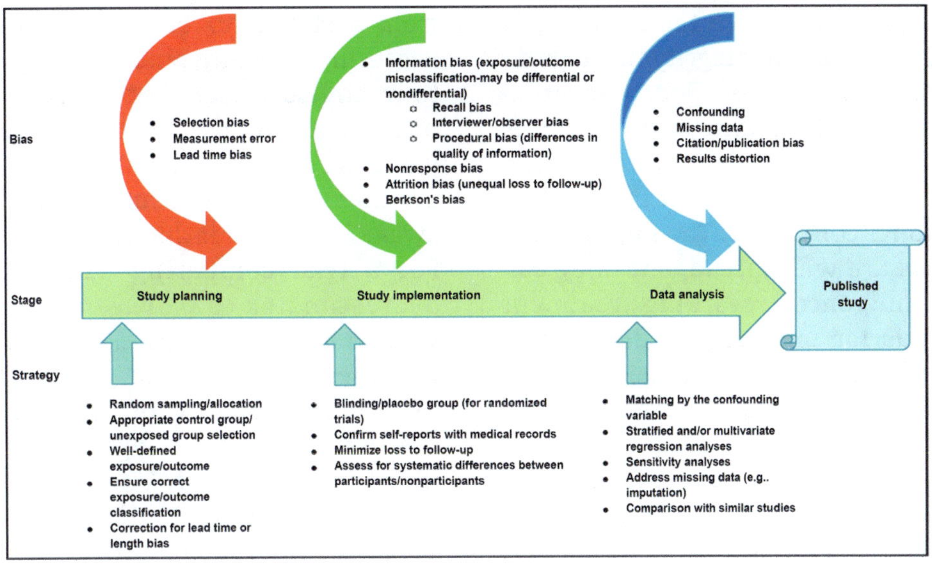

Figure 6.11. Strategies to minimize biases common to observational research. Methods for addressing various biases in epidemiologic research are shown, although this list is not exhaustive.

Source: https://www.researchgate.net/profile/Milad-Asgari-3/publication/331448148/figure/fig1/AS:870868532076550@1584642646650/Strategies-to-minimize-biases-common-to-observational-research-Methods-for-addressing.png.

6.4.1. Randomization Techniques

Randomization techniques are important in clinical trials by minimizing bias and increasing the validity of findings from research. Random allocation to treatment groups ensures that attributes are spread evenly, minimizing systematic differences that could result in biased outcomes. The strict method works to ensure internal validity by preventing selective participation based on confounding variables. Randomization procedures may be in various forms, e.g., simple randomization, block randomization, and stratified randomization. All have some merits and demerits that decide the overall study result. As Bahor et al. (2020) stress, inappropriate randomization can lead to biased results, particularly in extensive animal models, where random assignment may be overlooked in favor of convenience, highlighting the extreme significance of observing methodological rigor in any research. Also, the handling of covariates by the randomization process has become a hot topic of discussion for statisticians. Supporters of stratification argue that balancing known covariates can enhance the precision of treatment comparison. There are counterarguments regarding the efficiency of such procedures, as balance alone is insufficient to guarantee optimal outcomes or increased treatment assignment probability. Whereas traditional randomization concentrates on non-biased assignment, newer approaches like covariate-adaptive randomization make things more complicated by attempting to balance and account for treatment effect simultaneously. The need for familiarity with these procedures, however, is clear, as in Rosenberger et al. (2011), where tension between ethical and statistical efficiency interests is addressed. Lastly, the choice of a randomization scheme must align with the study-specific goals of the clinical study in order to yield valid and sound results. Aside from the varying methodologies, the challenge of maintaining randomization integrity throughout a study cannot be overstated. Poor allocation concealment or lack of blinding of participants and researchers are some of the factors that can cause bias, which is precisely what the process of randomization is combating. The implications of these failures are widespread, and they can result in false inferences regarding treatment efficacy. Methods for ensuring randomization integrity involve the use of independent central randomization services and automated methods of allocation that reduce the need for human involvement. In addition, the establishment of a methodological culture among researchers, as proposed by the examination of large animal stroke studies in Bahor et al. (2020), can greatly enhance study quality. Lastly, the efficient application of the randomization techniques is not only crucial in minimizing bias but also enhancing the credibility and validity of clinical research results (Figure 6.12).

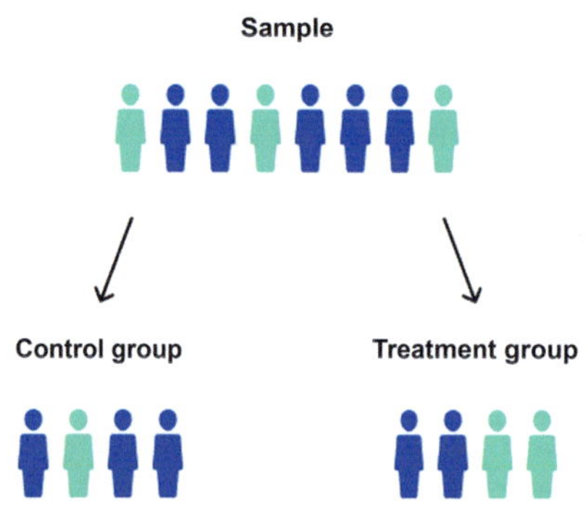

Figure 6.12. Simple randomization uses arbitrary random methods to assign participants to either a control or a treatment group.

Source: https://blog.greenlight.guru/hubfs/randomization%20blog%20img%201.png.

6.4.2. Blinding Methods

Effective blinding procedures are critical in clinical trials in order to minimize bias and ensure the validity of results. Blinding involves concealing the treatment assignment from participants, caregivers, and researchers assessing the outcomes. This practice works to minimize biases that result from treatment effect expectations, commonly referred to as the placebo effect. In poorly blinded trials, subjects are able to report results influenced by being aware of their treatment and introducing bias. For a trial comparing nasal decongestants, overestimates of drug effect may occur when patients, aware they receive an active treatment, report relief from symptoms due to their expectation of response rather than the actual pharmacologic effect of the drug (Sutter et al., 2016). Therefore, incorporation of sound blinding methods not only enhances the validity of study findings but also improves replication and clinical research acceptability in general. Second, the success of blinding can vary depending on the intervention type as well as the participants. Occasionally, blinding caregivers and assessors could yield more objective outcomes compared to subjective ratings. Still, in intervention trials such as cryotherapy or keratinocyte growth factor for cancer patients, blinding may be tougher due to the physical nature of the interventions and their impact. If the subjects can identify whether they receive treatment or a placebo, the risk of report bias is present, which eventually affects the study's conclusion regarding the intervention's effectiveness (Abramoff et al., 2010). Thus, researchers have to plan studies with appropriate blinding methods in consideration that deal with these unique challenges, to raise reliability and produce valid data accurately reflecting actual treatment effects. As much as blinding is included in bias reduction, so also is it important to recognize circumstances under which blinding cannot be applied. For certain research, e.g., those assessing cognitive or behavioral treatments in relation to effectiveness, blinding is simply not feasible since participants know they are part of an active process of intervention. For such studies, a mix of other measures, e.g., the objective and subjective outcomes, may be used to minimize bias. Researchers may also use strict statistical methods to account for confounding that arises from poor blinding. By appreciating the subtleties of blinding and adapting methodologies suitably, researchers can maximize the evidence base for clinical interventions and publish more accurate results to inform future practice in healthcare (Figure 6.13).

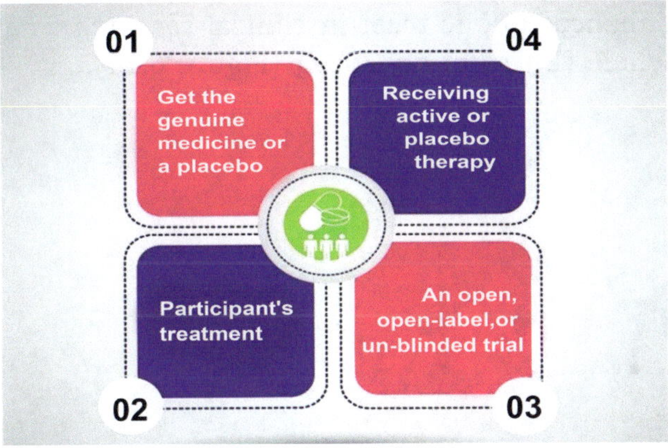

Figure 6.13. Blinding in clinical trials.

Source: https://pubrica.com/academy/wp-content/uploads/2021/11/aca5-1-768x576.jpg.

6.4.3. Standardization of Protocols

The standardization principle of clinical trial protocols is highly essential in preventing bias and enhancing the validity of results. Standard protocols create a framework for the form of the design and conduct of studies, therefore ensuring minimal variability and maximum consistency across diverse sites of study. When procedures are consistently applied, this ensures that methods of data collection, participant inclusion criteria, and outcome measures are identical, a prerequisite in drawing accurate conclusions. An example of how stringent methods in a study, such as one evaluating genetic markers for renal cell carcinoma, illustrates how standardization can bridge gaps in translational utility in the end and increase the potential for clinically relevant results (Cunningham et al., 2014). The scrupulous use of standardized protocols not only enables comparability between studies but also reduces the risk of systematic errors that arise from differences in methodology. In addition, the use of standardized protocols enables researchers to pool data from heterogeneous populations, thus enhancing the statistical power of clinical studies. In the context of umbilical artery Doppler indices, for instance, the INTERGROWTH-21st Project illustrated how a rigorous standard methodology in different geographical locations gave us robust normative information that minimized site-specific biases (Barros et al., 2020). Pooled data is particularly important when examining subtle clinical outcomes where sample sizes are small. When standardized, demographic and clinical characteristics can be adequately controlled, allowing for improved understanding of variation and outcome. In this way, adherence to standardized procedures can improve the overall validity of research findings to yield more generalizable results that can more effectively inform clinical practice and policy. Beyond improving validity and comparability, standardization of procedures is also essential to address ethical problems in clinical research. It assists in providing a baseline for informed consent such that participants' rights and comprehension of study procedures are addressed uniformly for all study sites. By minimizing variation in the ways trials get conducted, bias through differential participant recruitment and treatment processes is reduced to a large degree. Alignment of methodologies, as in the studies herein, can enhance trust within the scientific community and with participants and may facilitate improved recruitment and retention (Cunningham et al., 2014; Barros et al., 2020). Common protocol development not only increases the quality of clinical science but also enhances the ethical responsibility of protecting participants and research integrity.

6.5. Ethical Considerations

The moral consequences of bias in clinical trials are multifaceted and crucial in ensuring the validity of study findings. Researchers should demand strict compliance with ethical norms requiring openness, complete disclosure, and equitable treatment of subjects. Above all, biases are conceivable if subjects included in a study are not representative of the entire population. This is capable of producing biased outcomes, which puts into question the effectiveness of the tested intervention and eventually influences clinical guidelines. Ethical evaluation thus requires that all populations, including vulnerable groups, should be represented so that they do not continue contributing to disparities in health. In addition, scientists must embrace best practices in health technology assessment (HTA) to handle the complexities of these ethical demands while producing credible and applicable results in clinical trials (Busse et al., 2002). In addition to participant representation, public and patient involvement in the design of studies is equally an important ethical requirement. Public input in clinical trials enhances the applicability of research results by aligning studies with patient priorities. Although this inclusion is difficult, e.g., role confusion of lay-volunteers and doubt about the real added value of their work, evidence pointed out that public involvement could improve the research design process and the quality of outcome, but only if researchers clearly establish roles and expectations to overcome tokenism and representation bias (Albarqouni et al., 2017). Therefore, ethical issues transcend compliance; they require robust systems of conducting public involvement optimally and ethically in clinical research contexts. Finally, conflict of interest remains a vital component in maintaining ethical integrity in clinical investigations. Researchers must be acutely sensitive to the influence of sponsorship and funding sources because these can be causes of bias in the research endeavor. Financial pressure can inadvertently lead to the manipulation of study design, data analysis, or interpretation of findings, undermining the validity of the results. It is the moral obligation of researchers to disclose any potential conflicts, and to pursue transparency in their approaches. Creation of oversight mechanisms, e.g., independent ethical review boards, can also guarantee studies' adherence to ethical principles while avoiding bias. Thus, maintaining ethical standards in managing conflicts of interest not only insulates the integrity of research findings but also enhances public trust in clinical research as a whole (Busse et al., 2002) (Figure 6.14).

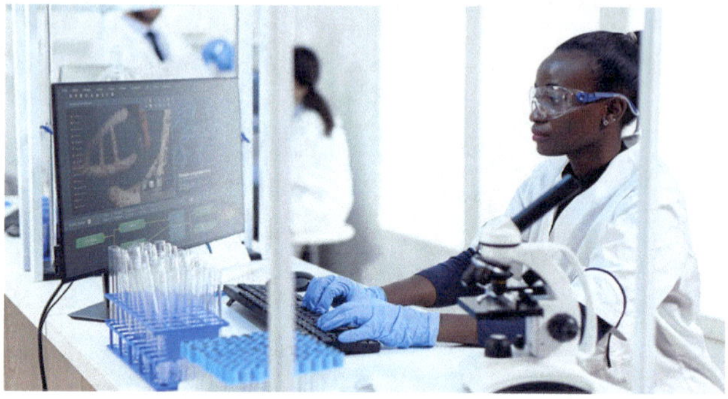

Figure 6.14. The importance of ethical considerations in research and clinical trials.

Source: https://lpsonline.sas.upenn.edu/sites/default/files/2024-07/lpso-ethical-clinical-trials.jpg.

6.5.1. Responsibility of Researchers

The role of researchers is not only to gather data but also to assume the ethical duty to make sure that their research is done with the highest integrity and respect for plural populations. In clinical research, researchers have to be highly sensitive to how their design, sampling, and interpretation of data might innocently introduce bias. Such bias may invalidate research outcomes, ultimately affecting patient treatment plans and healthcare policy. According to the literature, nursing educators have to develop an environment in which competence in being knowledgeable about patient safety is the top priority, beginning with alertness to possible biases in clinical research settings (Bagnasco et al., 2016). Such a mandate obliges researchers to embrace practices of openness and inclusiveness in research. The other ethics concern that cannot be overlooked in clinical research is bias. Researchers have a crucial obligation to think about how their work affects various communities, particularly marginalized communities that may be underrepresented in clinical trials. As researchers fail to consider ethnic diversity and other demographic factors, they end up actually guaranteeing that health inequalities are replicated, rather than decreased. The literature is in favor of using evidence-based studies that reflect the population's diversity (Allmark et al., 2009). In doing so with due consideration, researchers guarantee more equitable health outcomes and gain trust among the populations that they serve. Such a preemptive approach not only enhances the quality of clinical research but also aligns with the overall healthcare goals of efficacy and safety for all. In addition, the consequences of the duties of researchers extend to reporting. The manner in which clinical study findings are relayed is a critical determinant of public comprehension and healthcare policy direction. Researchers must ensure that conclusions are drawn from accurate data and be careful not to claim more for their results than is warranted, especially in instances of bias. This is something that demands critically scrutinizing their work against an ethical and just mindset. Doing so enables researchers to facilitate informed dialogue between scholars and policymakers, ensuring that decisions are made based on careful and objective evidence. The need for rigorous methodological requirements and ethical research guidelines is most essential in facilitating the validity and generalizability of clinical studies in alleviating biases that have significant implications for patient care and health in general (Figure 6.15).

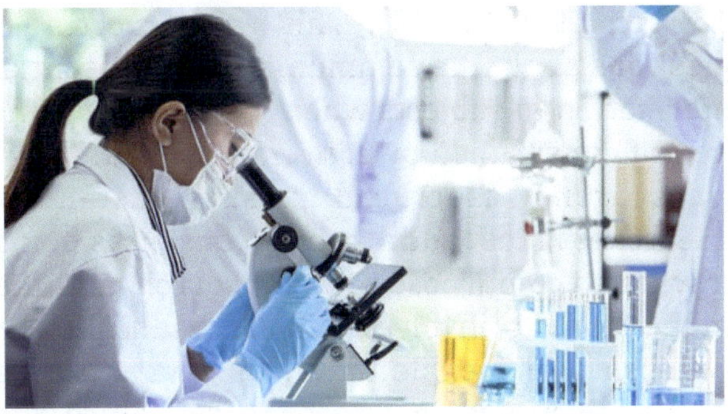

Figure 6.15. Obligations and responsibilities of the clinical researchers.

Source: https://joethomas.in/wp-content/uploads/2008/05/Clinical-trial.jpg.

6.5.2. Informed Consent and Transparency

Informed consent and transparency are inherent parts of ethical clinical research practice, especially in avoiding bias. The informed consent process is not an empty ritual; it is a valuable exchange between researchers and participants that builds trust and clarity. Participants have a better opportunity to make fully informed decisions if they understand the risks, benefits, and what the study is about. However, modern practices such as virtual clinical trials, where recruitment and consent are electronic, complicate this interaction. As discussed, where these can extend access to most individuals who might otherwise not participate, they raise issues of transparency and understanding, particularly with regard to participants' rights as well as potential risks from the study design (Andrews et al., 2017). Hence, a well-informed balance in informed consent must then be crafted to guarantee that participants are actually informed. The complexity of informed consent is then compounded again with implementation research, where the traditional ethical codes may not necessarily apply directly. In cluster randomized trials, for instance, the problem of individual consent may be addressed by broader concerns of justice and fairness

(Iversen et al., 2008). This raises pertinent questions about the communication of essential information to subjects when recruitment plans are not constrained by conventional standards. Transparency is crucial in such instances; researchers must address how consent is being provided, the purpose of the research, and the implications to involved subjects. Additionally, ownership and exploitation of data must be openly discussed in efforts to safeguard the interests of participants as well as remain within ethical research standards. As the clinical research environment evolves, so too must the ethical framework underlying informed consent.

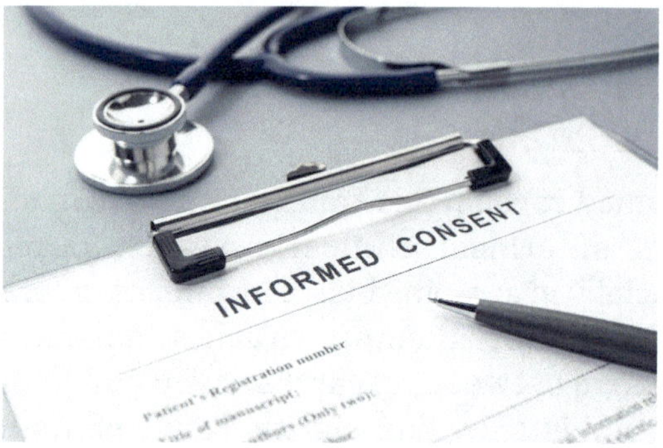

Figure 6.16. Informed consent form.

Source: https://www.consent-vault.com/wp-content/uploads/2024/01/informed-consent-form-on-desk-2023-11-27-05-26-18-utc.jpg.

Ultimately, it is the double value of transparency and informed consent that is necessary to minimize bias in clinical research. Strong informed consent allows participants to be stakeholders within the research process, as well as promoting ethical practice. Transparency, however, allows for scrutiny of the research design and execution, which are able to expose and offset any outside biases that might skew study findings. This crossroads is particularly important in a day when the incorporation of technology into clinical trials continues to increase. By ensuring that subjects not only understand what is happening but are also an integral part of an open-ended process, researchers can create a trusted environment. Such an environment is crucial to the promotion of the validity of results and the creation of a more equitable clinical research playing field. In this new environment, the intersection of informed consent, disclosure, and bias must remain a high-priority subject to discuss and improve upon (Figure 6.16).

6.5.3. Regulatory Oversight and Guidelines

Effective regulation plays a crucial role in minimizing bias in clinical trials so that research findings become valid as well as applicable across various populations. Regulator bodies such as the Food and Drug Administration (FDA) and European Medicines Agency (EMA) have established guidelines for ensuring the integrity of clinical research. These regulations include ethical treatment of subjects, open reporting, and rigorous review of study design. They also mandate diversity in populations for clinical trials, which helps detect potential biases caused by demographic variables. Regulation of this kind is important for building confidence in the biomedical research enterprise and safeguarding public health outcomes because it tackles systemic biases that can compromise research findings. Thus, these regulatory frameworks are patient-centered in facilitating fair health interventions and guaranteeing that clinical trials represent the populations upon whom they are performed. Additionally, the evolving clinical research environment, particularly with the integration of artificial intelligence (AI), presents new regulatory challenges. The use of AI allows one to examine vast quantities of data, which might lead to a greater identification of bias that would not be identified by traditional methods. However, as the RUSI study carried out on behalf of GCHQ demonstrates, the use of AI within medical contexts raises significant ethical questions. The application of machine systems can have the unintended result of introducing bias if the data used is based on past injustices or if the algorithms used are biased. Therefore, regulatory bodies must ensure that guidelines catch up with technological advancements, with consideration of both efficacy and ethical implications. Regulation must include regular monitoring of AI techniques to actively detect and counter biases most likely to arise from their use in medical research, thereby guaranteeing healthcare responsible innovation. In addition to regulatory frameworks, standards for data transparency play a critical role in warding off bias in clinical trials. Requiring researchers to disclose their practices, data sources, and potential conflicts of interest raises the overall responsibility of the research community collectively. Transparency benefits not only peer review, but also independent examination, where biases that were overlooked in the course of the original study, or perhaps even were there but unrealized, can be uncovered. Furthermore, adherence to rigorous reporting standards, such as those defined by the Consolidated Standards of Reporting Trials (CONSORT), guarantees that all clinical trials are reported adequately and accurately. The interplay between rigorous regulatory measures and rigorous openness policies provides a setting conducive to the recognition and elimination of bias, which enhances the validity of clinical research findings in the long run. This holistic approach is paramount in taking equitable healthcare practice forward; thus, stakeholders must place such key areas at the forefront of clinical study design and implementation.

Summary

In defining an examination of bias in clinical research, it is essential that the intricate nature of this issue and its implications for clinical practice and research validity be acknowledged. Bias can take a number of forms, including selection bias, performance bias, and reporting bias, ultimately distorting the findings and hindering the ability of researchers and clinicians to make soundly informed judgments. For instance, the inconsistency in study design and protocols in the prevention of hamstring injury review illustrates how methodological variation can produce ambiguous findings and compromise the' reliability of conclusions (Arnason et al., 2012). Such variations affect not just the validity of individual studies but also complicate the total synthesis of studies, with practitioners finding it challenging to adhere to inconsistent advice based on biased information. Furthermore, stringent methodological standards are also highlighted in positive messaging findings for pain control because bias was a major determinant of reported results. Although there were a few studies that indicated a positive effect of messages delivered by clinicians to alleviate pain, overall results were inconsistent, and caution was applied more generally due to inherent biases. The identification of high-risk studies within the meta-analysis is evidence that calls for a close examination of research designs and reporting protocols since such biases have the potential to mislead therapeutic benefits and patient outcomes (Howick et al., 2017). Ultimately, inclusion of so many biased studies may lead to ineffective or harmful clinical recommendations, further spreading evidence-based practice issues. With such important problems, it is vital that future clinical studies put the highest priority on employing appropriate methodologies and clear reporting to ensure that bias does not dominate. The implementation of randomized controlled trials (RCTs), as suggested in the review of hamstring injury prevention, is imperative in ascertaining more credible and generalized outcomes. This approach not only enhances the quality of one's research but also creates credibility among clinicians and patients (Arnason et al., 2012). With evolving times in research, a focus on improving study designs and utilising strict methods to counterbalance biases should always be the fundamental mantra of clinical research. By seeking excellence in research integrity, healthcare professionals can bridge the gap between evidence and practice, leading to improved patient outcomes and care.

In understanding the ramifications of clinical research bias, it is evident that the measurement instruments used greatly determine the findings of research. This is particularly important in the instance of cancer patient mental health screenings in oncology. For instance, a meta-review on mixed depression assessments in cancer patients determined that one of the most frequently tested, but with shortcomings related to variable cut points in studies, was the Hospital Anxiety Depression Scale (HADS). The review also determined that the Beck Depression Inventory and the Center for Epidemiologic Studies Depression Scale were more generalized in applicability and responsiveness. Such variations demonstrate how bias might not only emerge from study design but also from selecting and validating measuring instruments, potentially skewing results and conclusions drawn during clinical research (Andersen et al., 2015). Recognizing these biases is key to allowing findings to be generalizable and applicable in clinical practice. Furthermore, bias generally occurs in the methodology employed in clinical trials, and this has been noted within studies evaluating acupuncture in pain control.

A combination of some promising results suggested that acupuncture had an effect in relieving pain, but the inherent problems with the quality of methodological issues allowed doubts to be raised as to whether these findings were valid. Issues such as small sample sizes, inadequate reporting, and unblinding of certain groups can lead to large-scale bias, making it difficult to conclude on the effectiveness of the intervention (Akhileswaran et al., 2011). Such outcomes emphasize the need for strong study designs that minimize bias adequately and thus enhance the data validity acquired. In addition, such methodological flaws highlight the importance of design choices in the apparent efficacy of treatments, ultimately influencing clinical guidelines and patient care. Finally, the potential biases' impact extends to clinical practice, both affecting treatment protocols and health disparities. Since clinical research produces clinical guidelines, research results biases can reinforce inequalities, particularly among populations already susceptible to disenfranchisement from good-quality healthcare. For instance, a lack of adequate evaluation of the outcomes of mental health or the efficacy of acupuncture can rule out some of the treatment modalities that are likely beneficial to specific patients (Andersen et al., 2015; Akhileswaran et al., 2011). Hence, researchers and clinicians must be aware of the potential biases in the design, conduct, and interpretation of trials. By creating a culture that emphasizes research as being of top quality, the medical community will be able to more effectively protect clinical findings' integrity and ultimately improve patient outcomes in heterogeneous populations.

CLOSER LOOK

THE EFFECTS OF BIAS AND CHANCE ARE CUMULATIVE

The two sources of error, i.e., bias and chance, are not distinct. In most instances, they occur together. The way the two interact is depicted by the figure below. Consider the measurement of diastolic blood pressure in one patient as an example. Each dot is an observation for that patient. True blood pressure, in this patient, 80 mm Hg, can be measured with an intra-arterial cannula, but not for routine measurement. Blood pressure is measured indirectly, by a sphygmomanometer (blood pressure cuff). As shown in a previous example, the simpler device is inaccurate or deviates from the true value. On the graph, error is indicated by all of the sphygmomanometer measurements dropping below the actual value. Deviation of sphygmomanometer readings to higher values (bias) may have a multitude of explanations (e.g., improper cuff size, patient anxiety, or "white coat hypertension"). Individual measurements of blood pressure are also subject to error with random variation in measurement, as evidenced by the spread of the readings from the sphygmomanometer around the mean (90 mm Hg) (Figure 6.17).

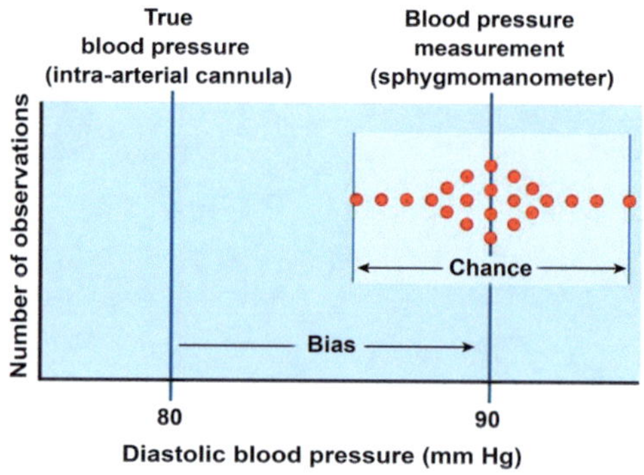

Figure 6.17. Bias and chance. True blood pressure by intra-arterial cannula and clinical measurement by sphygmomanometer.

Source: https://alraziuni.edu.ye/uploads/pdf/book1/%D8%B5%D8%AD%D8%A9-%D8%B9%D8%A7%D9%85%D8%A9/Robert-H.-Fletcher-MD-MSc-Suzanne-W.-Fletcher-MD-MSc-Grant-S.-Fletcher-MD-MPH-Clinical-Epidemiology_-The-Essentials-LWW-2012.pdf.

The main reason for distinguishing between bias and chance is that they are handled differently. In theory, bias may be eliminated by conducting clinical trials carefully or repaired after data analysis. If not eradicated, bias generally can be uncovered to the keen observer. Most of this book addresses how one may detect, avoid, or restrict bias. Chance cannot be eliminated, but its impact can be minimized through good design of research, and what is left can be approximated with statistics. There is no statistical adjustment for unexpected data biases. Some statisticians would actually advise against applying statistics to data that are subject to bias in the design of the study, or risk conferring spurious respectability on, in effect, fraudulent work.

References

1. Abela, S., Aboumatar, H., Al-Wazzan, A., Albert, H., Allegranzi, B., et al. (2018). Validity of hand hygiene compliance measurement by observation: A systematic review. https://core.ac.uk/download/161771316.pdf (accessed on 25th June 2025).
2. Abramoff, M., Adamietz, I., Ahmed, S., Ahn, J., Aisa, N., et al. (2010). Interventions for preventing oral mucositis for patients with cancer receiving treatment. https://core.ac.uk/download/20451371.pdf (accessed on 25th June 2025).
3. Abuabara, K., Drucker, A. M., Doney, E., Hart, J., Hartung, D. M., Williams, H. C., Ioannidis, J. P. A., et al. (2016). Research techniques made simple: Workflow for searching databases to reduce evidence selection bias in systematic reviews. https://core.ac.uk/download/76975094.pdf (accessed on 25th June 2025).
4. Abuja, B., Akdemir, M., Anthony, H., et al. (2018). The physiological mechanisms of effect of vitamins and amino acids on tendon and muscle healing: A systematic review. https://core.ac.uk/download/287581405.pdf (accessed on 25th June 2025).
5. Akhileswaran, A., Alimi, D., Aung, S., Bardia, A., Beuken-van Everdingen, M. H., et al. (2011). Acupuncture for cancer pain in adults. https://core.ac.uk/download/29018651.pdf (accessed on 25th June 2025).
6. Alam, R., Ariff, S., Das, J. K., Ishaq, M., et al. (2024). Efficacy of probiotics for treatment of acute or persistent diarrhea in children from birth till 10 years: Systematic review and meta-analysis. https://core.ac.uk/download/631324741.pdf (accessed on 25th June 2025).
7. Albarqouni, L., Burls, A., Clarke, M., Kirkpatrick, J., et al. (2017). Patient and public involvement in the design of clinical trials: An overview of systematic reviews. https://core.ac.uk/download/196605461.pdf (accessed on 25th June 2025).
8. Alberti, K. G. M. M., American Diabetes Association, Auerbach, A. D., Bachman, D. L., Bakker, A. J., Beasley, J. M., Benaroia, M., et al. (2011). Computer-assisted versus oral-and-written dietary history taking for diabetes mellitus. https://core.ac.uk/download/130975129.pdf (accessed on 25th June 2025).
9. Allareddy, V., Gluud, C., Karimbux, N., Schwendicke, F., et al. (2015). A meta- and trial sequential analysis. https://core.ac.uk/download/199411796.pdf (accessed on 25th June 2025).
10. Allmark, P. J., Barley, R., Ellison, G., Gerrish, K., et al. (2009). Social research for a multiethnic population: Do the research ethics and standards guidelines of UK learned societies address this challenge? https://core.ac.uk/download/100463.pdf (accessed on 25th June 2025).
11. Andersen, B. L., Becker, M. H., Carey, T. S., Carlson, R. W., Cella, D. F., et al. (2015). Patient-reported depression measures in cancer: A meta-review. https://core.ac.uk/download/42138163.pdf (accessed on 25th June 2025).
12. Andrews, L., Franco, A., Kostelecky, K., Spritz, R., et al. (2017). Virtual clinical trials: One step forward, two steps back. https://core.ac.uk/download/128127841.pdf (accessed on 25th June 2025).
13. Arezzo, A., Avenia, N., Barczyñski, M., Cirocchi, R., et al. (2015). Total or near-total thyroidectomy versus subtotal thyroidectomy for multinodular non-toxic goiter in adults. https://core.ac.uk/download/54521026.pdf (accessed on 25th June 2025).

14. Arnason, A., Askling, C., Bandy, W. D., Beaulieu, J., Bennell, K., Bixler, B., Brooks, J. H., et al. (2012). Static stretching of the hamstring muscle for injury prevention in football codes: A systematic review. https://core.ac.uk/download/14529557.pdf (accessed on 25th June 2025).
15. Arora, R., Barkhordarian, A., Chiappelli, F., Giroux, M., et al. (2012). Reliability of quality assessments in research synthesis: Securing the highest quality bioinformation for HIT. https://core.ac.uk/download/323077996.pdf (accessed on 25th June 2025).
16. Arunogiri, S., Baldacchino, A., Bates, M. E., Bowden-Jones, H., et al. (2019). A roadmap for integrating neuroscience into addiction treatment: A consensus of the Neuroscience Interest Group of the International Society of Addiction Medicine. https://core.ac.uk/download/286356092.pdf (accessed on 25th June 2025).
17. Atherton, H., Car, J., Majeed, A., Sawmynaden, R., et al. (2012). Email for clinical communication between healthcare professionals. https://core.ac.uk/download/30317357.pdf (accessed on 25th June 2025).
18. Montalto Attard , S. (2014). Ethical principles in pediatric practice. https://core.ac.uk/download/46603075.pdf (accessed on 25th June 2025).
19. Atzema, C. L., Barrette, N., Dainty, K. N., Drennan, I. R., et al. (2014). Expanding Paramedicine in the Community (EPIC): Study protocol for a randomized controlled trial. https://core.ac.uk/download/323071062.pdf (accessed on 25th June 2025).
20. Babuta, A., Janjeva, A., & Oswald, M. (2020). Artificial intelligence and UK national security: Policy considerations. https://core.ac.uk/download/305121521.pdf (accessed on 25th June 2025).
21. Bagnasco, A., Bianchi, M., Bressan, V., Cadorin, L., et al. (2016). Patient safety competencies in undergraduate nursing students: A rapid evidence assessment. https://core.ac.uk/download/151161157.pdf (accessed on 25th June 2025).
22. Bahor, Z., Boltze, J., Herrmann, A. M., Kringe, L., et al. (2020). Quality and validity of large animal experiments in stroke: A systematic review. https://core.ac.uk/download/323058004.pdf (accessed on 25th June 2025).
23. Barros, F. C., Berkley, J. A., Carvalho, M., Drukker, L., et al. (2020). International gestational age-specific centiles for umbilical artery Doppler indices: A longitudinal prospective cohort study of the *INTERGROWTH-21st Project*. https://core.ac.uk/download/294756260.pdf (accessed on 25th June 2025).
24. Boly, M., & Seth, A. K. (2012). Modes and models in disorders of consciousness science. https://core.ac.uk/download/30613167.pdf (accessed on 25th June 2025).
25. Britton, W. B., Brown, A. C., Chou, J. C., Deluca, M., et al. (2013). Contemplative science: An insider's prospectus. https://core.ac.uk/download/185244991.pdf (accessed on 25th June 2025).
26. Brown, J. S., Henry, D. A., Klungel, O. H., Platt, R., et al. (2020). How pharmacoepidemiology networks can manage distributed analyses to improve replicability and transparency and minimize bias. https://core.ac.uk/download/196607041.pdf (accessed on 25th June 2025).
27. Burger, H., Koolman, X., Luijendijk, H. J., Page, M., et al. (2020). Assessing risk of bias: A proposal for a unified framework for observational studies and randomized trials. https://core.ac.uk/download/519035518.pdf (accessed on 25th June 2025).

28. Burns, D. S., Docherty, S. L., Haase, J. E., Robb, S. L., et al. (2010). Ensuring treatment fidelity in a multi-site behavioral intervention study: Implementing NIH Behavior Change Consortium recommendations in the SMART Trial. https://core.ac.uk/download/46962319.pdf (accessed on 25th June 2025).

29. Busse, R., Drummond, M., Gurtner, F., Jorgensen, M., et al. (2002). Best practice in undertaking and reporting health technology assessments: Working Group 4 report. https://core.ac.uk/download/58882.pdf (accessed on 25th June 2025).

30. Car, J., Liu, J. L. Y., McLean, S., Nurmatov, U., et al. (2011). Telehealth care for chronic obstructive pulmonary disease. https://core.ac.uk/download/20453590.pdf (accessed on 25th June 2025).

31. Carlson, C., Sholk, J., Nanni, J., Peterson, K., Smith, L. A., & Bhavaraju, N. (2016). *Breaking the Barriers to Specialty Care: Practical Ideas to Improve Health Equity and Reduce Cost–Ensuring High-Quality Specialty Care.* https://core.ac.uk/download/75785771.pdf (accessed on 25th June 2025).

32. Chen, X. L., Gao, R. Y., Hu, Y., Li, M., et al. (2017). Methodological quality of systematic reviews and meta-analyses on acupuncture for stroke: A review of reviews. https://core.ac.uk/download/96884712.pdf (accessed on 25th June 2025).

33. Cougle, J. R., Lobbestael, J., Peeters, F., van Teffelen, A., et al. (2021). Interpretation bias modification for hostility: A randomized clinical trial. https://core.ac.uk/download/479287089.pdf (accessed on 25th June 2025).

34. Coulter, E. H., McDonald, D. A., McDonald, M. T., Paul, L., et al. (2019). Level of adherence to prescribed exercise in spondylarthritis and factors affecting this adherence: A systematic review. https://core.ac.uk/download/293886085.pdf (accessed on 25th June 2025).

35. Cunningham, J., El-Mokadem, I., Fitzpatrick, J., Fleming, S., et al. (2014). Significance of chromosome 9p status in renal cell carcinoma: A systematic review and quality of the reported studies. https://core.ac.uk/download/30661759.pdf (accessed on 25th June 2025).

36. Danielsen, P. A. (2022). Treatment effects of therapeutic interventions for gaming disorder: A systematic review and meta-analysis. https://core.ac.uk/download/573317810.pdf (accessed on 25th June 2025).

37. Sutter De , A., Deckx, L., Guo, L., Mir, N., et al. (2016). Nasal decongestants in monotherapy for the common cold. https://core.ac.uk/download/55850304.pdf (accessed on 25th June 2025).

38. Mar Del , C. B., Doshi, P., Hama, R., Heneghan, C. J., et al. (2014). Neuraminidase inhibitors for preventing and treating influenza in healthy adults and children. https://core.ac.uk/download/196601387.pdf (accessed on 25th June 2025).

39. Harkin, B., Soriano-Mas, C., Kessler, K., & Miellet, S. (2012). What checkers actually check: An eye tracking study of inhibitory control and working memory. https://core.ac.uk/download/9650770.pdf (accessed on 25th June 2025).

40. Hazard, D., Mansourian, M., Marateb, H. R., Martinuka, P., et al. (2024). Methodological biases in observational hospital studies of COVID-19 treatment effectiveness: Pitfalls and potential. https://core.ac.uk/download/613974426.pdf (accessed on 25th June 2025).

41. Howick, J., & Mebius, A. (2017). Positive messages may reduce patient pain: A meta-analysis. https://core.ac.uk/download/200759475.pdf (accessed on 25th June 2025).

42. Iversen, A., Vahratian, A., American Statistical Association, Briesacher, B., Woodward, B.,

Junghans, C., Verity, C., et al. (2008). Ethical issues in implementation research: A discussion of the problems in achieving informed consent. https://core.ac.uk/download/48972.pdf (accessed on 25th June 2025).

43. Koppl, R. (2012). Leveraging bias in forensic science. https://core.ac.uk/download/144228363.pdf (accessed on 25th June 2025).
44. Lunet, N. (2025). Teaching meta-analysis using Stata. https://core.ac.uk/download/pdf/6314113.pdf (accessed on 25th June 2025).
45. Minasi, D. (2017). Confronting the ghost: Legal strategies to oust medical ghostwriters. https://core.ac.uk/download/144232628.pdf (accessed on 25th June 2025).
46. Pollock, A., Pollock, A., Turton, A., French, B., Langhammer, B., Bradley, C., et al. (2016). Repetitive arm functional tasks after stroke (RAFTAS): A pilot randomized controlled trial. https://core.ac.uk/download/42138432.pdf (accessed on 25th June 2025).
47. Polonioli, A. (2019). A plea for minimally biased naturalistic philosophy. https://core.ac.uk/download/146502275.pdf (accessed on 25th June 2025).
48. Rosenberger, W. F., & Sverdlov, O. (2011). Handling covariates in the design of clinical trials. https://arxiv.org/abs/1102.3773 (accessed on 25th June 2025).
49. Smith, E. (2020). Traditional Chinese medicine and its role in women's health. https://core.ac.uk/download/322850890.pdf (accessed on 25th June 2025).
50. Stafford, G. L. (2014). Review found little difference between sandblasted and acid-etched (SLA) dental implants and modified surface (SLActive) implants. https://core.ac.uk/download/213055765.pdf (accessed on 25th June 2025).

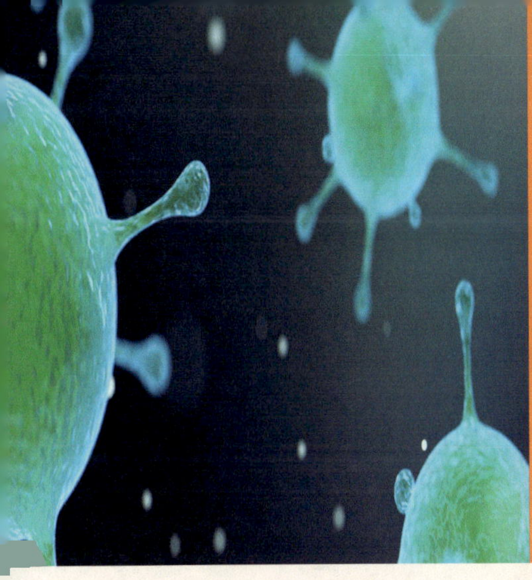

Chapter 7

CAUSATION IN EPIDEMIOLOGY

Contents

Introduction

Causation in epidemiology is a vital topic that creates much interest because it forms the basis of public health interventions and policies. Defining the association between exposures and health outcomes enables investigators and practitioners to distinguish risk factors, guide health behaviors, and utilize resources more efficiently. Causation also presents particular challenges because of the complexity of biological systems and the occurrence of confounding variables. To be able to make substantive progress in this field, it needs to be accurately established that a specific exposure does result in the subsequent health outcome. This preliminary examination will explore some of the varying frameworks and methodologies applied in epidemiological research, with the foundation for subsequent examination of how causality is established and interpreted in health research. Models such as Bradford Hills have enabled researchers to cut through the complicated process of establishing cause-and-effect relationships in the past. In 1965, Bradford Hill set down nine points of causation as a general guideline for assessing epidemiological proof and making causal assumptions. These points have become widely utilized but are open to refined interpretation of their epistemological grounding. With the application of modern methods to the Hills framework, researchers can address the difficulties inherent in epidemiological evidence, such as those encountered in Zika virus research and its association with birth defects, or the frequent observation of the relationship between lung cancer and smoking (Dammann et al., 2019).

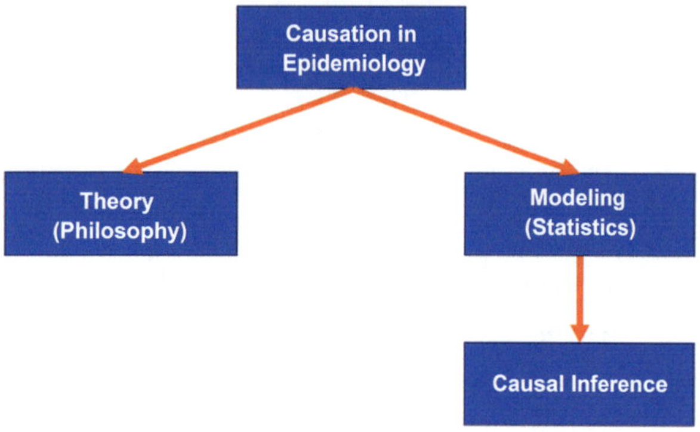

Figure 7.1. Causation in epidemiology.

Source: https://www.goldsteinepi.com/blog/notes-on-causal-inference-in-observational-epidemiology/hierarchy.png.

These applications illustrate the necessity of enhancing causal inference models to meet the demands of current epidemiological problems. In addition, considering causation in a legal environment adds another layer of complexity to the landscape. Causation has to be proven scientifically but balanced within legal frameworks that necessitate specificity and clarity. Legal situations differentiate between types of causation, including negligence with exposure, risks at the population level, and individual plaintiff cases. Through the application of adaptations of the Bradford Hill criteria, as proposed, researchers can formulate systematic approaches to evaluating causality in epidemiological evidence in order to facilitate informed connections between statistical findings and legal judgments (Mengersen et al., 2007). These observations underscore the importance of an integrated causation approach that strikes a balance between scientific rigor and utilization in both public health and legal contexts, referencing the multidimensional character of this important topic (Figure 7.1).

Definition of Epidemiology

The word epidemiology entails extensive inquiry into the determinants and distribution of health-related events or states among defined populations. The discipline is extremely relevant to public health, as it helps in understanding the interaction of various factors, including environmental, biological, and social determinants of health outcomes. Epidemiology not only facilitates the quantification of disease prevalence but also explores underlying causes, thereby facilitating the planning of targeted interventions. As a foundational science, it employs multiple methodologies, from observational and experimental research studies, in the course of discovering patterns of disease and health, ultimately informing public health policy and practice aimed at improving population well-being. The epidemiologic theory of causation is multifaceted, dependent upon the ability to ascertain an association between exposures and effects on health. A number of frameworks are used to estimate causation, such as the Bradford Hill criteria, which necessitate examination of such things as strength, consistency, and specificity of association by researchers. Determination of causation demands an advanced level of understanding of both group-level and individual effects. Specifically, epidemiologists seek to identify not only whether or not there is a correlation, but how that correlation translates into causal relationships. As discussed in the literature, varying definitions of cause are present, especially when examining legal cases where exact probabilistic judgments are needed. Thus, epidemiology is a core discipline that sheds light on pathways of causation in disease and health, and broader horizons for research conduct and application in other fields like law and public health (Mengersen et al., 2007). In addition, causation in epidemiology involves grappling with probabilistic measures that define risk and outcome relationships. For example, medical scientific evidence relies upon the application of two probabilities: the probability of injury due to exposure and the potential to create spurious associations due to confounding variables. The two-probability model assists in the causation of the preponderance of the evidence needed for causal claims. Such sophistication is a main rationale for why cautious statistical methods are an absolute necessity in epidemiological studies. The complexity of cause factors is additionally augmented when these intersect with legal notions of causation because these paradigms must grapple with entrenched scientific methods while adhering to legal standards. It is therefore paramount to gain a fuller comprehension of how causation is framed and applied in epidemiology for investigators as well as practitioners working with public health, policy-making, and legal settings (Barnes et al., 2001) (Figure 7.2).

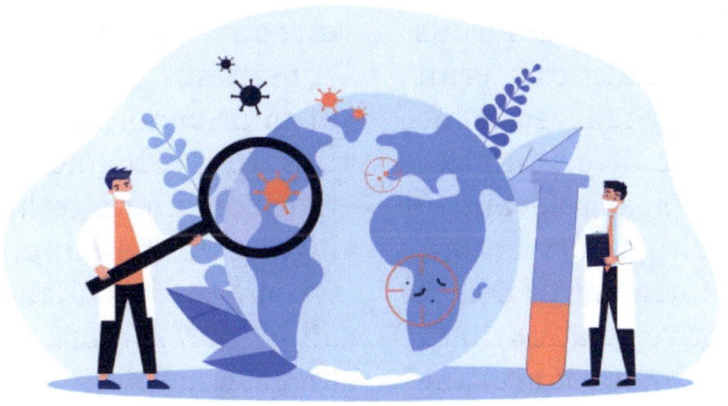

Figure 7.2. Epidemiology.

Source: https://assets.everspringpartners.com/dims4/default/72e4ed3/2147483647/strip/true/crop/954x501+337+0/resize/1200x630!/quality/90/?url=http%3A%2F%2Feverspring-brightspot.s3.us-east-1.amazonaws.com%2F33%2Fa5%2F7c66b322456da074d93dfe7de0af%2Fadobestock-348362021-1600x500.jpg.

Importance of Causation in Public Health

Causation is critical in public health because it helps practitioners identify the underlying causes resulting in health outcomes. The information is not only crucial in the design of interventions but also in the application of disease prevention policies. Epidemiological techniques provide one with the tools necessary to establish associations between exposures and health outcomes. The evidence-based medicine paradigm stresses causation because, in the medical profession, experts require solid data to make scientific judgments regarding treatment modalities and public health interventions. The longtime empiricist-rationalist association, from the Hippocratic tradition, has been instrumental in shaping today's medical practices. Clinical epidemiology has sped up this progress by illuminating causal associations behind health burden and disparities, making healthcare systems aware of how to react to priority health issues (Newton et al., 2001). Secondly, recognition of causation aids in prioritizing public health issues if several potential risk factors are present. Epidemiologists commonly need to find associations among heterogeneous exposures that are potentially causing chronic diseases, which also typically feature multiple causes. Because most chronic diseases result from interactions between genetic, environmental, and lifestyle exposures, such causation knowledge enhances the potential for developing holistic public health interventions. Environmental epidemiology, as a specialty, focuses on the importance of assessing external factors, such as water and air quality, that impact health outcomes. This is important, especially where populations are exposed to more than one environmental risk factor, possibly making it hard to determine causation (Amiri et al., 2016). By focusing on the interaction of numerous influences, public health officials can craft interventions that are specifically tailored to the needs of communities that have diverse health issues. Secondly, causation is also relevant in the evaluation of public health interventions as well as the continuous refinement of health policy. By establishing causative relationships, public health authorities can measure the effectiveness of health campaigns and legislation interventions. For instance, causal explanations of why smoking causes lung cancer have promoted mass public health campaigns to quit smoking. The evaluation of the impact of interventions relies heavily on causal models, which provide specificity to what interventions produce desirable health outcomes. Moreover, the dynamic nature of global health calls for epidemiologists to be adaptable at all times, integrating new evidence into public health practice. As exemplified by developments in environmental epidemiology, the integration of population health with molecular biology perspectives deepens the understanding of causation, and thereby informs broad health public policies that address short-term as well as long-term health implications (Amiri et al., 2016).

7.1. Historical Perspectives on Causation

Causation in epidemiology has varied greatly through the ages, as a testament to the altered paradigms of scientific thought and societal issues. In the past, the concept of causation tended to be simplistic, often simplified to a linear system in which a sole factor or event was the direct cause of an outcome. For example, in the initial research of infectious disease, the germ theory of the 19th century dictated the causative understanding, linking disease directly to pathogens. But this perspective sometimes underestimated the complexities of multifactorial diseases, and offered a trend toward a recognition of cumulative risk factors that contribute to health conditions. This shift highlights the importance of placing causation within the broader historical contexts, which allow for a more nuanced understanding of disease etiology in modern epidemiological studies. This causal complexity of health outcomes is also exacerbated by social values and norms, which historically have guided scientific inquiry. For instance, the need to control some of the health-related variables tends to predispose researchers toward particular causes over others. This concept is supported in the discussion of Collingwood's control principle, which holds that the selection of causes is not fully objective but largely defined by social interest and priority. This insight is realized in the discursive history of causation, which reflects the convergence of scientific objectives and normative settings that together frame epidemiological events. Therefore, a history of causation in epidemiology must consider how these social forces have influenced the research field. Further, placing such history within contemporary epidemiological practice improves our understanding of causation. One exemplary example is research on perfluoroalkyl substances (PFAS) like perfluorooctanoic acid (PFOA) and their link to kidney function. Subsequent studies have shown more recently that correlations between measured concentrations of PFOA and decreased kidney function may be caused by reverse causation, implying fundamental questions about interpreting such causal relationships. That difficulty strengthens the need to use advanced methods, adjusting for exposure levels in the past, without allowing such cross-sectional analysis biases. Through a critical examination of historical points of view, more powerful models of causation can be developed by epidemiologists, eventually promoting stronger public health interventions and policies that dynamically react to changing scientific and social environments (Figure 7.3).

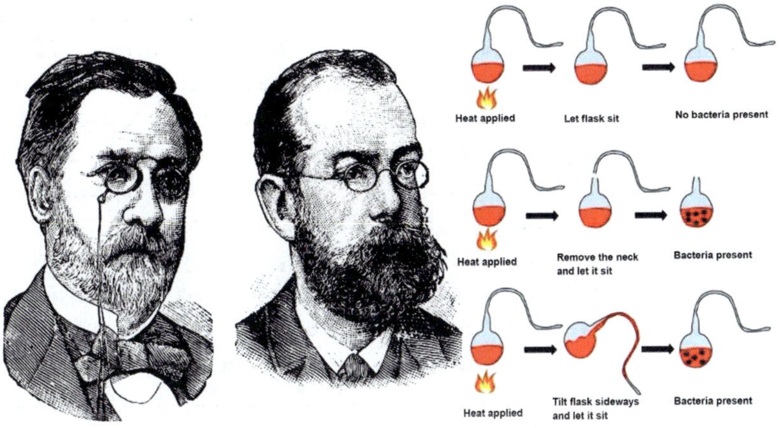

Figure 7.3. The germ theory of disease replaced the concept of spontaneous generation.

Source: https://biologynotesonline.com/wp-content/uploads/2023/07/Germ-Theory-of-Disease-Spontaneous-Generation.jpg.

7.1.1. Early Theories of Disease Causation

Historical disease causation has evolved significantly from ancient hypotheses to modern-day epidemiological paradigms. Early explanations were in terms of religious and humoral theories, where disease was believed to be a punishment from God or the result of out-of-balance body fluids, called humors. The Hippocratic school was a major landmark in this way of thinking by encouraging rational examination of signs and influences of the environment, paving the way for physicians to practice clinical epidemiology. The emphasis on reason and observation at this point was crucial because it laid the groundwork for later strides in disease research and treatment. In addition, the rationalist thinking ensured that clinical practice began to rely on empirical fact rather than mystical reasoning, offering a valuable foundation that would influence healthcare practice for centuries to come (Newton et al., 2001). With the development of medicine, the mechanical disease causation models emerged in the Enlightenment era and became very much in command with the introduction of microbiological research findings in the 19th century. This period was characterized by the move away from mystical causes and towards a focus on concrete biological agents as direct causes of disease. The germ theory developed by scientists such as Louis Pasteur and Robert Koch firmly established that microbes caused the development of some diseases, thus revolutionizing public health practices. But rigid reliance on mechanistic models sometimes led to the overlook of disease etiology's complex causation, not just biological but also environmental and social. The mechanistic dogma, while pioneering, has produced concerns regarding the need for the application of the understanding of health to cover variables such as lifestyle and socio-economic status that are commensurate with advances in mechanistic explanation (Ehsani et al., 2018). In a recognition of the limitations of early and mechanistic models, contemporary epidemiology has adopted more integrated approaches to the causation of disease. The interplay between biological, environmental, and social factors is now addressed in order to better explain the emergence and progression of disease. Mechanism-plus-X conceptualization promotes expanding mechanistic models with qualitative factors as well as quantitative biological explanations. This perspective acknowledges that while microbial agents contribute largely, they are not independent forces and exist within a broad array of other inputs with causative capacities to generate health outcomes. By marrying multiple dimensions of causation, scientists aim to better explain channels of disease development and prevention, emphasizing contextuality in health. This method not only elucidates the conceptualization of disease dynamics but also informs successful public health interventions and policy (Ehsani et al., 2018).

7.1.2. The Role of Koch's Postulates

The enduring significance of Koch's postulates in epidemiology lies in their foundational role in establishing a causal relationship between pathogens and diseases. Formulated in the late 19th century, these postulates delineate a systematic approach to demonstrate that a specific microorganism is the causative agent of a particular disease. All postulates represent integral factors in the testing of a microorganism's pathogenic potential, fostering an atmosphere of scientific precision. For instance, through careful observation and experimentation, scientists can ascertain that a microorganism can be found in infected subjects but not in their uninfected counterparts, thereby hypothesizing a potential cause-and-effect relationship. This systematic methodology not only enlarges our understanding of disease cause but also forms the basis of formulating targeted public health interventions, enhancing the overall impact of epidemiological investigation. Even though historically important, the application of Koch's postulates has been altered in consideration of the latest developments in genetics and metagenomics. Modern epidemiology takes advantage of genetic information to demystify the complexities of disease that may not necessarily adhere to Koch's original postulates. For example, genetic mutations can significantly influence an individual's susceptibility to infectious diseases, which signifies a broadening definition of causation to extend beyond the absolute presence or absence of the causative agent. As Parkinson et al. (2022) have it, genetic factors could play a substantial role in determining immune responses, thus emphasizing the interface of infectious agents and genetics. Consequently, while Koch's postulates remain at the forefront of early causal association identification, they must be placed against the backdrop of modern times that incorporate an understanding of the contribution of genetics to disease, further elevating epidemiological discourse. Moreover, the introduction of metagenomics represents a major departure from disease causation science, introducing new tools into the researcher's toolkit. Through analysis of complex microbial communities in human tissues, metagenomics facilitates a more advanced investigation of the roles that different organisms play in expressing disease. As it is pointed out in Morfopoulou et al. (2015), the potential to profile complex samples and identify low levels of pathogens is a paradigm shift for epidemiologic studies. The new strength abrogates ancient power enshrined in Koch's postulates with an appeal for an integrated view of causation encompassing both microbial agents and host interactions. This transition draws attention to the fact that epidemiological frameworks must transform and adapt, adopting multi-dimensional viewpoints that guide our knowledge concerning health and disease among populations (Figure 7.4).

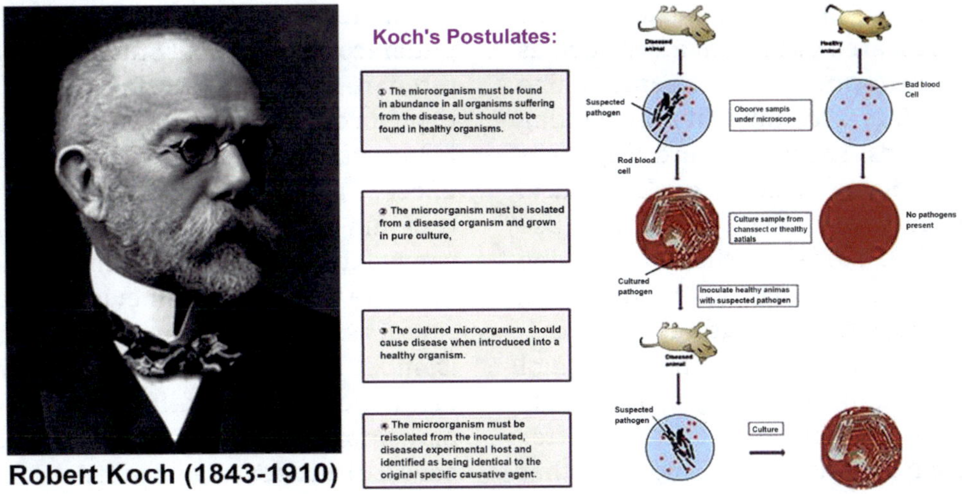

Figure 7.4. Robert Hermann Koch was a German physician who developed Koch's postulates.

Source: https://microbenotes.com/wp-content/uploads/2019/01/Robert-Koch-and-Koch%E2%80%99s-Postulates.jpg.

7.1.3. Evolution of Causal Inference in Epidemiology

The advancement of causal inference in epidemiology is a testament to the discipline's ongoing endeavor to understand and make clear the complex relationships between exposures and health outcomes. Early endeavors in the field, very clearly explicated in the early classics of Greenwood and Hill in the first generation of epidemiologic textbooks, were directed towards the building of foundational ideas such as bias and confounding. These early definitions lay the groundwork for increasingly nuanced descriptions of causality, laying the groundwork for classical epidemiology. Morris, MacMahon, and Pugh, Susser, and Lilienfeld, several of the most prominent members of this second generation, contributed to the discussion by elucidating designs like cohort and case-control studies, enabling scientists to investigate causal relationships systematically as they pertain to disease. This advancement indicates how earlier frameworks set by early epidemiologists created a crucial platform for a more diverse concept of causation in subsequent scholarly discussions (Baldi et al., 2018). With the growth of the discipline, so too did its methodological refinement in drawing causal conclusions. The third generation of epidemiologic textbooks, represented by Miettinen and Rothman, was a major step forward in the integration of study designs and outcome measures. This modern approach emphasizes the requirement to formalize concepts of confounding and interaction, realizing that the determinants of health are such multifaceted things that they cannot possibly be addressed with simplistic models. As statistical techniques improved and the use of more sophisticated methodologies became widespread, the researchers began to adopt a multi-dimensional perspective for causal inference, encompassing the interaction among various biological, environmental, and social factors. This shift not only represents a more advanced sophistication in epidemiologic inquiry but also an acknowledgment that causal relationships are often context-dependent and nonlinear, with sophisticated analysis tools needed for accurate interpretation (Baldi et al., 2018). The contemporary causal inference debate is also guided by the research of investigators such as Bradford Hill, who formulated an arsenal of nine criteria to take into account when evaluating causal relationships. These standards highlight the multiform nature of evidence to place causal claims in epidemiology on firm foundations. Use of Thagard's ECHO model provides a unifying interpretation to jumps over such standards, facilitating a systematic exploration of claims—such as those between Zika virus and congenital defects, and smoking and lung cancer. This synoptic model is used by researchers to better traverse the complex evidentiary landscape that characterizes epidemiological inference. With advances in the field of epidemiology, causation is increasingly realized to require an integrated strategy that permits complexity, thereby enhancing public health policy and intervention aimed at disease prevention.

7.2. Types of Causation

In epidemiology, understanding the causation types is needed to correctly determine the relationships between exposures and health outcomes. Usually, causation can be classified into several categories: necessary causes, sufficient causes, and probabilistic causes. A necessary cause needs to occur for a specific outcome to manifest; i.e., if this cause fails to occur, the outcome fails to happen. On the contrary, a sufficient cause is a cause capable of producing the outcome independently, even if other causes lead to the same outcome. This distinction is important in epidemiology studies since it governs the interpretation of findings and assists in planning interventions to prevent or reduce risk factors towards the occurrence of most diseases. Moreover, probabilistic causation is also gaining more prominence in recent years, particularly in the domains of public health and legal discussion. Probabilistic causation recognizes that disease tends to be multi-causation and implies that it is insufficient to define causation as a dualism. As underscored by recent studies, results in groups often result from a combination of multiple exposures occurring at the same time, and hence, the process of determining cause-and-effect relationships can be especially difficult. By providing the odds of an effect being caused by some determinants, epidemiologists are able to evaluate the strength of evidence for particular causal associations. This nuanced understanding is most relevant in law cases, whereby the distinction between different types of causation may impact expert testimony admissibility and have a direct bearing on judicial rulings (Henifin et al., 1998).

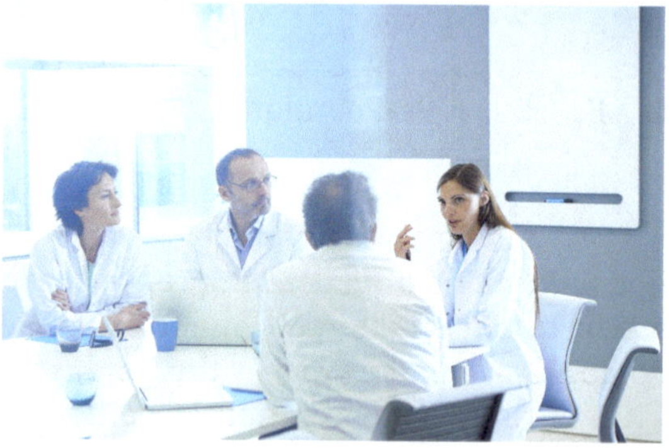

Figure 7.5. Necessary and sufficient causes in science and medicine.

Source: https://www.verywellhealth.com/thmb/H9Fnhg7lu-9PhLwfBfTEZp4hnac=/1500x0/filters:no_upscale():max_bytes(150000):strip_icc()/GettyImages-512136801-59cf48aa22fa3a001182a19d.jpg.

Secondly, the union of epidemiologic methodology and law principles reveals to us another facet of causation—individual versus population effects. In legal cases, causation can be considered to fall under three categories: exposure-related negligence, statistical associations that are potential indicators of increased risk, and plaintiff-specific claims. Each of these categories of causation has particular implications for the imposition of legal liability on individuals. Recognizing the role that epidemiological data can play in assisting legal criteria for causation allows the integration of the adjudication of health-related claims cases. The systematic examination of causative associations, as envisioned under the Bradford Hill approach, integrates scientific rigor and openness in the differentiation between collective proof and single relevance and the application of sound epidemiological evidence in judicial decision-making (Mengersen et al., 2007) (Figure 7.5).

7.2.1. Direct vs. Indirect Causation

The study of causation in epidemiology is more about the distinction between direct and indirect causation and its far-reaching significance for understanding the etiology of disease. Direct causation is where an exposure causes an outcome directly without mediation, and indirect causation is through intermediary variables that create a pathway between the exposure and the outcome. For example, in the analysis of how socioeconomic status affects health, one must differentiate between whether or not poverty directly leads to health inequality or if this correlation is mediated by intervening variables such as education and access to healthcare. Such pathways, when identified, not only help delineate disease mechanisms but also facilitate targeted intervention strategies that help mitigate risk factors for unhealthy outcomes. The relationship between direct and indirect causation can be explained in relation to socioeconomic status and mental health.

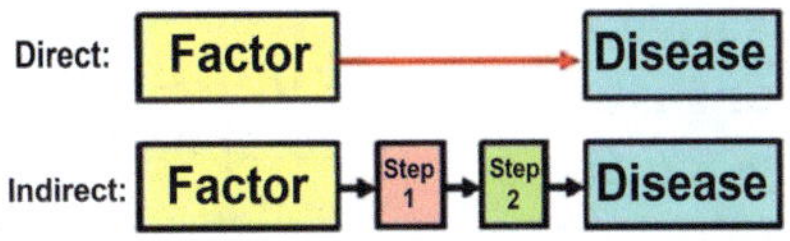

Figure 7.6. Direct vs. indirect causation.

Source: https://q2a.s3.us-west-1.amazonaws.com/keepnotes/doc-page-preview/45098-1page_11.webp.

A sample study that investigates the question of whether or not socioeconomic status influences depression is helpful when it comes to these concepts. Specifically, it proposes two competing hypotheses: social causation, in which economic disadvantage leads to negative mental health directly, and social drift, which proposes that individuals with mental illness may drift into lower socioeconomic groups. The research findings confirm that the two processes are concurrent and that individuals can find themselves in a cycle of deprivation where economic disadvantage feeds mental illness, and mental illness perpetuates economic disadvantage (Bachmann et al., 2019). When this duality is realized, then there can be a synoptic examination of the public health responses that will address both economic disparities and mental illness. In addition, the nuances of direct and indirect causation can also be observed in how asthma is influenced by wealth. Studies on this relationship indicate that wealth can both be a direct protective factor against severe asthma and an indirect one through easier access to health services and environmental quality. The research indicates that poorer asthma is related to lower wealth, confirming the idea that wealth has a direct impact on health (Smith et al., 2016). Alternatively, changes in wealth following diagnosis do not alter the likelihood of the person having asthma, meaning that while wealth can act as a buffer for the disease, asthma does not negatively affect wealth growth. They highlight the complexity of causal associations in epidemiology, calling for a conservative analytical approach to disentangle the multi-dimensional effects of direct and indirect causation (Figure 7.6).

7.2.2. Necessary and Sufficient Causes

It is important to know the distinction between necessary and sufficient causes in epidemiologic studies, because it plays a vital role in comprehending causal associations in public health. A necessary cause is a condition that must be present for an outcome to occur, while a sufficient cause can independently bring about the described outcome. This fine distinction in epidemiology assists the researchers in identifying risk factors and the causative roles that they play in disease etiology. For instance, certain pathogens may be necessary causes of some diseases, while certain lifestyle factors may be sufficient causes of chronic diseases like heart disease. This distinction shifts the focus beyond mere association to more substantial determinations of causation, often employing instruments such as the Bradford Hill criteria in investigating such relations to a greater extent and accuracy, ultimately informing effective public health intervention. The application of the necessary and sufficient cause model also interfaces with legal concepts of causation in epidemiology. By strict analysis according to statistical paradigms, scientists can account for how exposure to particular risk factors may be assigned causality to health effects in populations. Notably, the model distinguishes between negligence as a cause at law, scientifically established risk factors, and an individual's perception of these risks. As suggested, the population-based approach to causation allows for epidemiologists to establish arguments of causation statistically, hence bridging the scientific knowledge and legal accountability gaps. Under such circumstances, it is indispensable to use systematic model testing in conformity with scientific investigation as well as legal requirements to make causative claims based on sound statistical principles while addressing community health concerns in an integrated way (Mengersen et al., 2007). Furthermore, the complexity of causal inference necessitates the belief in consistent models in order to combine multi-faceted sources of data and apply them in actual contexts.

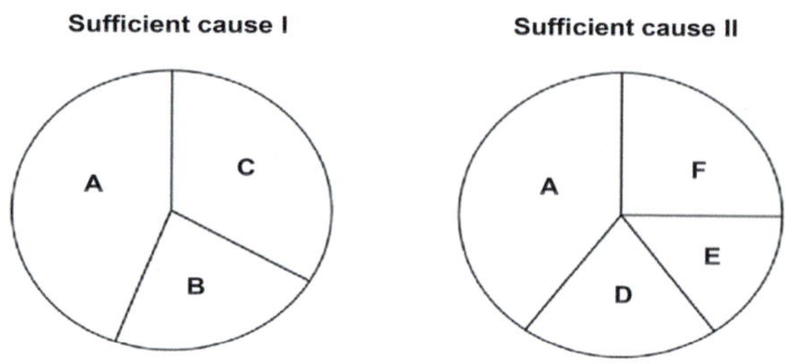

Figure 7.7. Causal pies. A-F represent component causes, of which A is a necessary cause. Sufficient causes can be composed of various causes.

Source: https://www.researchgate.net/profile/Bianca_Arrhenius/publication/363212779/figure/fig2/AS:11431281082683267@1662107261872/Causal-pies-A-F-represent-component-causes-of-which-A-is-a-necessary-cause-Sufficient.png.

The ECHO model, as proposed by Thagard, is a model for understanding how various causes come into action in delivering causation in epidemiology. By applying this model to understand prominent case histories, such as the link between the Zika virus and birth abnormalities or the historical inference between cancer and smoking, researchers are able to penetrate the intricate network of evidence supporting assertions of causation. This model describes the disease processes as multidimensional, supplementing standard models to include the dynamic interaction among risk factors and disease outcomes. Moreover, the inclusion of necessary and sufficient causes in this rich epistemological heritage speaks to the contemporary demands of scientific discipline and policy for public health (Dammann et al., 2019) (Figure 7.7).

7.2.3. The Role of Confounding Factors

Confounding factors are a key issue in causation analysis in epidemiology. They are variables extraneous to an experiment that obscure the true relationship between the outcome and exposure of concern, thereby creating biased effects. For instance, when researchers are examining the relationship between respiratory infections and vitamin D levels, confounding factors such as healthcare access, geographic location, or socioeconomic status can mislead the causality. When confounders are not adequately controlled, the observed relationship could be spurious, and thus suggest a relationship that does not exist in reality. Therefore, identification and management of confounding factors become important in making valid causal inferences in epidemiology to ensure proper public health interventions based on accurate information. Numerous methodological approaches towards controlling confounding variables exist in epidemiologic research, each contributing to the causal validity of the inferences. Researchers may employ techniques such as randomization, stratification, and multivariable regression analysis to mitigate the effects of confounders. Randomization, which is frequently applied in clinical trials, minimizes the confounding effect by allocating confounding variables equitably across study treatment groups. Alternatively, employing stratification, where groups are analyzed individually, allows for confounding factors within a specific setting to be viewed. In addition, multivariable regression models allow statistical adjustment for multiple confounders simultaneously. Nevertheless, difficulties persist, particularly with latent confounders—unmeasured variables with an impact on exposure and outcome, precluding the process of causal inference. Coping with these subtleties is essential to the validity of epidemiologic study (Wunsch, 2025). Even the legal implications of confounding variables address their significance in epidemiologic analysis. Epidemiologic evidence of causation in a courtroom involves a complete understanding of the role of confounding in outcomes.

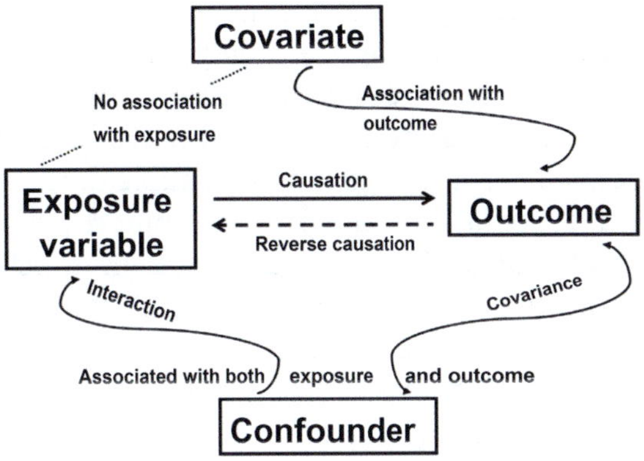

Figure 7.8. Possible relationships of a covariate and a confounder to an exposure variable and an outcome.

Source: https://www.researchgate.net/profile/Ian-Wilson-30/publication/299415540/figure/fig1/AS:349820582678528@1460415134350/Possible-relationships-of-a-covariate-and-a-confounder-to-an-exposure-variable-and-an.png.

Legal systems will rely on probabilistic assertions subject to statistical estimates, which could be confounded by confounders (Mengersen et al., 2007). Unscrambling the interaction between exposure, outcome, and confounders is essential in legal cases with the burden of proof on the demonstrated causal association. The sensitive estimation of confounders not only enhances the quality of the scientific evidence of assertions but also the credibility of expert testimony. It is thus critical to determine the impact of confounding variables, not only in epidemiology but also at the points where it meets law and public policy, in order to reach conclusions on the basis of good evidence and clear thinking (Figure 7.8).

7.3. Causal Models in Epidemiology

Causal models of epidemiology serve as the central guiding frameworks that enlighten researchers regarding the complex interaction between exposures and health outcomes. By limiting channels along which exposures influence health, causal models enable detecting causal associations despite the messiness of the real world. A widely accepted method in epidemiology is the Bradford Hill criteria, a formalized process of deciding causation for observational studies. This model encourages consideration of multiple factors, such as strength, consistency, and specificity of associations, and comprehension of the potential for confounding variables to obfuscate actual causal relationships. With these models, epidemiologists are better able to walk the often-muddy terrain of observational data, telling more straightforward stories of the determinants of health outcomes and laying the groundwork for evidence-based public health policy. Besides, the concept of causation must also be understood within the social contexts, as social epidemiology emphasizes the impact of societal determinants on health outcomes. Social epidemiology is interested in how social and economic characteristics—i.e., discrimination and income inequality—affect population health. By incorporating theories of social sciences, social epidemiologists advocate for a multi-dimensional investigation of determinants of health as opposed to the purely biological approach. This is particularly valuable when working with health inequities caused by structural inequalities, which are most often neglected in traditional causal models. Thus, by including social determinants within causal models, one is able to appreciate more fully how individual and collective exposures converge to create health outcomes, which is important for effective epidemiological practice and intervention design. Finally, the legal implications of epidemiological evidence need a robust causal modeling framework. Causation in court cases is typically based on probabilistic conclusions drawn from epidemiological data. The distinction between competing interpretations of causation—e.g., negligence due to exposure, population causation, and individual claims—highlights the complexity of legal cases based on epidemiological evidence. As proposed in dominant legal thought, the challenge is between statistical quantifications of causation and legal standards that may not align. This takes a nuanced system of analysis that can explain under what conditions exposures result in health outcomes, as outlined in the alternative Bradford Hill criteria approach proposed for forensic use. This convergence of epidemiology and law is crucial to recognize in order to ensure the scientific evidence is used properly within court systems, particularly when addressing public health issues.

7.3.1. The Bradford Hill Criteria

The Bradford Hill criteria are a cornerstone of epidemiology that provides a methodology for determining causation between exposure and an outcome in health. The criteria were established by Sir Austin Bradford Hill in 1965 and comprise a series of dimensions that researchers may examine to ascertain whether or not a causal association is present beyond correlation. The dimensions are strength, consistency, specificity, temporality, biological gradient, plausibility, coherence, experiment, and analogy. All these parts are essential in constructing a robust foundation for the evaluation of potential causal associations, yielding clarity amidst epidemiologic analytic ambiguity. While the criteria are internationally standardized and used, they also stimulate persistent debate regarding interpretation and use across settings, underscoring dynamic growth in causal inference within public health research. The most striking aspect of the Bradford Hill criteria is how it focuses on temporality, such that for the purposes of attributing causation from an exposure, the exposure should precede the development of the disease. This becomes especially important in the context of long-latency diseases, where the time lag between the exposure and the effect could be several years and could be hard to directly establish. Besides, consistency and strength of association are most significant, as greater correlations in several studies raise the prospects of a causal relationship. Still, even though these criteria provide a systematic approach, one must have some flexibility in their application, especially in areas of developing health problems, where new pathogens or risk factors might be ill-fitting to traditional paradigms of causation, as demonstrated by recent research employing these criteria to examine complex cases like the Zika virus and resulting birth malformations (Dammann et al., 2019). Apart from their practical application to epidemiology, the Bradford Hill criteria extend to legal domains, where the determination of causation matters. Causality may be considered in the legal arena through three different lenses: negligence, scientific proof of risk, and individual responsibility. The application of a Bradford Hill-based structure in court cases may help courts determine causal claims, in particular, by reviewing statistical evidence from epidemiological studies. The structures help balance probabilistic findings with legal standards and eventually aid practitioners in grasping the subtleties of causation in litigation. There is a need to identify and negotiate the intersecting, but distinct, senses of causation in science and law, demonstrating the scope of use the Bradford Hill criteria continue to have (Mengersen et al., 2007) (Figure 7.9).

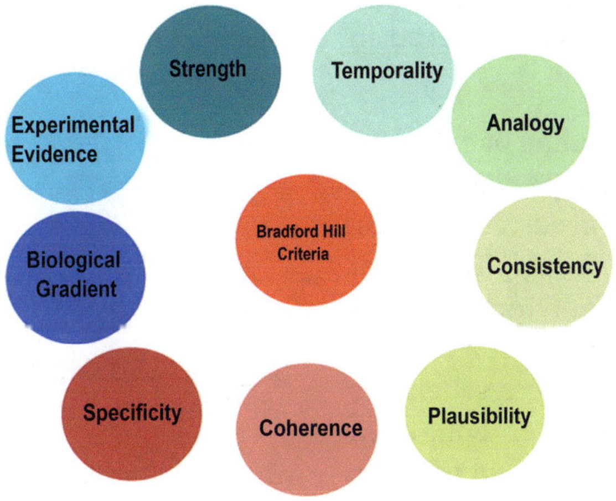

Figure 7.9. The Bradford Hill criteria.

Source: https://res.cloudinary.com/less-likely/image/upload/f_auto,q_auto/v1554700109/Site/BradfordHillCriteria.png.

7.3.2. The Causal Pie Model

In epidemiology, the causal pie model is a simple model to explain the multifactorial causation of disease. Proposed by Kenneth Rothman, the model explains causation in terms of a pie consisting of independent slices, each for different contributory factors in the etiology of a disease. In this analogy, any one slice can signify one of a variety of things, such as environmental agents, host factors, and endogenous biological processes. By depicting these factors in combined states, the model enables researchers to depict the synergy of a 1000 causes behind complex diseases caused by an enormous number of factors working synergistically together, rather than causation by one single agent. This dimensional depiction conforms to contemporary thought behind exposure-disease relations, whereby there are possibilities of making fine judgments of cases of multiple influence occurring jointly, ultimately adding more sophistication to epidemiologic accounts of causation. The use of the causal pie model in epidemiology allows for a transition from one-dimensional causal models to an integrative approach to understanding health outcomes. It is possible to classify and quantify causal factors—biological, social, or environmental—and results accordingly match results found with biomarkers and sociomarkers covered in the literature.

For instance, the understanding of oxidative stress under the scenarios of type one to type four biomarkers, as illustrated in current studies, is significant in pointing out the application of models in illustrating how individual factors might cumulatively be responsible for disease development. This understanding is crucial as it not only contributes to further enhanced risk factor identification but also guides specific prevention and health promotion interventions. The causal pie model thus encourages epidemiologists to think through the interplay of various factors and their relative importance, which is essential for effective public health intervention. In addition, the causal pie model enables us to address the complexity of causation systematically. It stresses the potential for partial explanations in epidemiologic research, in line with the notion that causes can explain part but not all of an effect, as stressed in modern contrastive theories of causation. This perspective allows more examination of how varying degrees of causation interact with some exposures, which is at the center of epidemiology's goal to reveal associations between risk factors and disease outcomes. Comprehending these subtleties can contribute to the improvement of risk estimates and the formation of precision public health strategies. Therefore, the model is an invaluable asset for maneuvering the complex aspects of causation, promoting theoretical advancement and practical implementation in epidemiology (Figure 7.10).

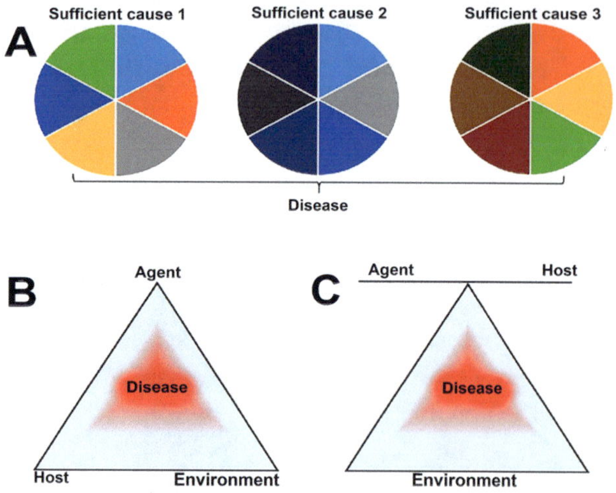

Figure 7.10. Models of disease causation. A The Rothman pie. B, C The epidemiological triad.

Source: https://www.researchgate.net/publication/338939405/figure/fig1/AS:864853870796802@1583208639351/Models-of-disease-causation-A-The-Rothman-pie-1-B-C-The-epidemiological-triad-From.png.

7.3.3. The Role of Directed Acyclic Graphs (DAGs)

The application of DAGs in epidemiology

represents a significant step in the understanding of causal relationships among various outcomes of health. By providing a clear graphical representation of the postulated causal pathways, DAGs allow the identification of confounders, mediators, and colliders in a given data set. This graphical approach enables researchers to systematically analyze the impact of various variables without the ambiguity of traditional statistical analysis, which tends to veil underlying causal mechanisms. Furthermore, the potential for modeling these causal relationships along a directed acyclic graph enhances the rigor of epidemiologic analysis, enabling the formulation of more accurate hypotheses and more targeted interventions. The use of DAGs is also helpful in navigating complex epidemiological data, where causal inference is typically masked by confounding factors. Central to creating informative DAGs is the convergence of empirical evidence and causal inference principles, as highlighted in innovative methods such as the Evidence Synthesis for Constructing Directed Acyclic Graphs (ESC-DAGs) protocol. This process focuses on the organized process of converting study results into DAG form, thus making causal relations more ethical and accountable. With three major phases—mapping literature results, assessing causal structures, and incorporating synthesized DAGs—scholars are in a position to enhance the depth and accuracy of their analytical models. This procedure not only allows DAGs to be developed but also gives researchers a robust foundation for strengthening epidemiological evidence.

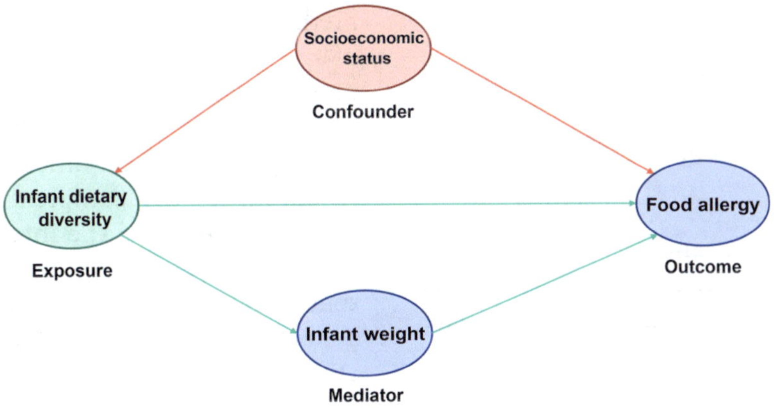

Figure 7.11. Simplified directed acyclic graph depicting the conception of confounder and mediator. Confounder (socioeconomic status): The shared causes of both exposure (infant dietary diversity) and outcome (food allergy). Counfounders should be adjusted in the analysis. Bias pathway (red line): The "exposure←confounder→outcome" pathway. Mediator (infant weight): The results of the exposure (infant dietary diversity) and the cause of the outcome (food allergy). Mediators should not be adjusted in the analysis. Direct causal pathway (mid green line): The "exposure→outcome" pathway. Indirect causal pathway (bottom green line): The "exposure→mediator→outcome" pathway.

Source: https://onlinelibrary.wiley.com/cms/asset/5ee7946f-799e-4c91-9532-a116801d31e5/all16025-fig-0003-m.jpg.

The use of this protocol in real-world settings further highlights the importance of evidence synthesis in refining causal assertions in public health research (Ferguson et al., 2020). In the case of complex diseases, increasing identification of DAGs is joined by advances in causal discovery methods, more importantly, as they relate to microbiome research. The ability to make use of flexible causal architectures allows richer representation of the intricate interaction among genetic, environmental, and microbial determinants leading to disease outcomes. Coupled with the integration of sophisticated causal inference mechanisms, scientists are capable of overcoming the issues of observability that are common in microbiome studies. Here, DAGs not only serve as a foundation for hypothesis formation but also reinforce methodological innovation to enhance causal thinking in large-scale biological systems. Such advancements validate that through appropriate utilization, DAGs are crucial in identifying causal mechanisms, thereby enhancing our approach towards disease prevention and cure (Corander et al., 2022) (Figure 7.11).

7.4. Statistical Methods for Causal Inference

Statistical methods for causal inference are central to understanding relationships in epidemiology, for which causation has implications for public health and policy. The Bradford Hill criteria, for instance, provide a set of considerations to frame causality by assessing factors such as strength, consistency, and specificity of association. The criteria help researchers establish whether observed correlations are indicative of a causal association. However, application of such criteria tends to require a delicate understanding of the underlying data and potential confounders that may generate biased results. Furthermore, the inherent nature of human health data requires robust statistical analysis capable of separating true causal effects from association, the reason why careful methodological care is paramount in epidemiological research (Mengersen et al., 2007). Researchers in public health regularly utilize different statistical designs to determine causal relations, among which nonrandomized study designs are common. Such designs largely come under two categories: confounder-control strategies and instrumental variable methods. Confounder-control methods, such as regression adjustment and propensity score matching, are intended to match groups on the basis of observed covariates, thereby reducing bias. In contrast, instrumental variables and these designs leverage external variables that influence treatment assignment but not outcome, a seemingly durable method for causality inference without manipulating variables. The comparative advantage of the methods points to statistical power, internal validity, and generalizability trade-offs. A consideration of the differences invites interdisciplinary communication required for the advancement of epidemiological research methodology (Adler et al., 2020). The integration of statistical approaches to causal inference not only enhances the strength of epidemiological investigation but also bridges disconnects among diverse disciplines within public health research. As the complexity of health-related data increases and the interdisciplinary nature of health issues, adopting a pluralistic position that allows for diversity in methodologies is a necessity. Statistical methods are typically employed in conjunction with thoughtful attention to the substantive setting, ultimately enabling researchers to make more valid inferences regarding causal relations. As epidemiologists seek to refine their methods for causal inference, thoughtful attention to empirical data and methodological decisions remains vital. This dynamic exchange will not only enhance the scientific rigor of public health evidence but also inform decision-making that influences population health outcomes in the real world (Mengersen et al., 2007).

7.4.1. Randomized Controlled Trials (RCTs)

The efficiency of RCTs in epidemiology has been described as the gold standard for determining causal associations. RCTs offer a structured means of isolating the effect of interventions through random allocation to treatment or control groups. Randomization eliminates biases and confounding variables that otherwise define observational studies, hence making the results more valid. For example, to evaluate the impact of new medications or public health measures, RCTs enable more accurate attribution of results to specific treatments. Without this methodological precision, the discovery of the true causal processes is plagued with pitfalls, and erroneous interpretations of public health policies and programs pose a threat. Despite their apparent advantages, RCTs have some limitations when applied to public health research, especially when confronted with complex social interventions. The rigid design of RCTs may overlook the complex context variables shaping health outcomes, particularly in diverse populations. With the complexity of HIV transmission captured by the issues of understanding the nuances of HIV transmission from one area to another, sole reliance on behavioral factors can lead to incomplete or inaccurate conclusions (Sawers et al., 2018). RCTs can also end up excluding the universal social determinants of health that are central to managing health disparities comprehensively. The gap between trial outcomes and the realities of day-to-day situations challenges the generalizability of RCT outcomes to wider public health settings. Furthermore, the emphasis on RCTs as the gold standard in public health evaluation has the potential to stifle innovation in methodology. Critics argue that strict adherence to RCTs restricts the exploration of alternative assessment methods that could better capture the complexities of multi-faceted interventions, such as microcredit schemes (Biosca et al., 2017). The concern relies on the presumption that an exclusive emphasis on randomized trials risks obscuring important elements of health equity and effectiveness. As epidemiology continues to evolve, the use of alternative methodologies alongside RCTs will be instrumental in constructing an integrated understanding of causation and creating more effective public health policies. Emphasizing this multiplexity of methods can ultimately lead to a more satisfying debate in causal inference in public health (Figure 7.12).

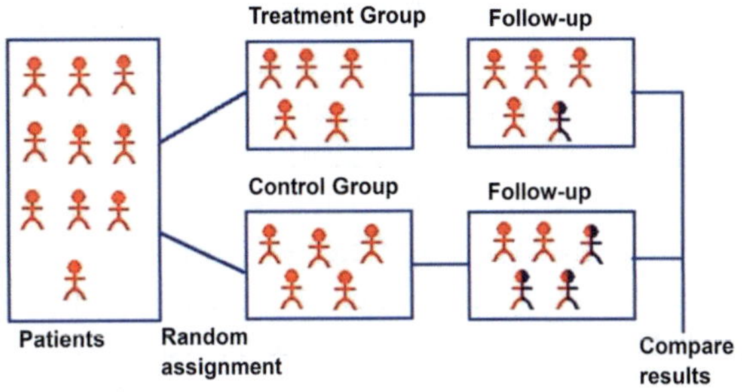

Figure 7.12. Randomized controlled trials.

Source: https://microbenotes.com/wp-content/uploads/2021/12/Randomized-Controlled-Trial-RCTs-Features-Principle-Steps-Bias.webp.

7.4.2. Observational Studies and Their Limitations

Observational studies are the cornerstone of epidemiology, yielding rich evidence of potential causal relationships between exposure and outcome. Through analysis of data collected from populations without altering variables, observational studies can establish correlations that need to be investigated further. However, their design weaknesses make it hard to interpret the findings easily. With confounding variables distorting the observed correlations, it becomes harder to distinguish between correlation and causation. Additionally, selection bias and recall bias may impact the outcomes, potentially misrepresenting the true relationships. Henifin et al. (1998) examine critically how these issues not only impinge on the scientific understanding of causation but also in legal affairs, highlighting that there is a need to be cautious when making judgments based on observational data. Application of observational studies in epidemiology is also plagued by issues of reverse causation and confounding variables. For instance, when one seeks to quantify the effect of lifestyle factors on health outcomes, it becomes impossible to ascertain whether the exposure really precedes the health status or whether the latter influences the former. This lack of clarity may result in misinterpretation of evidence, eventually sabotaging good public health counsel. Apart from that, limitations like small sample sizes or lack of generalizability can affect the generalizability of results. Such limitations must be addressed; researchers seek alternative approaches like Mendelian randomization (MR), which prevents confounding and bias by employing genetic variations as instrumental variables (Bowden et al., 2016). Highlights how MR offers a cheap means of strengthening causal inference, but advises that it is still subject to some assumptions that, if violated, can lead to misinterpretation. Apart from research design and data interpretation issues, observational studies are also at risk for ethical problems, particularly where intervention based on outcomes is contemplated.

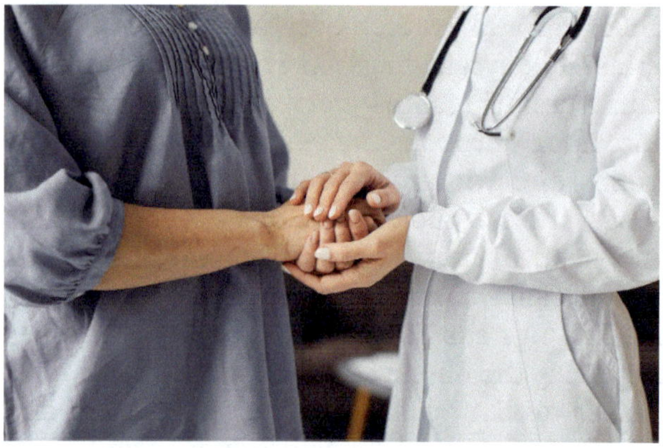

Figure 7.13. The role of observational studies in modern epidemiology.

Source: https://propharmaresearch.com/sites/default/files/no-responsivas/2148847832.jpg.

For instance, while observation data can indicate that a specific treatment is beneficial, the lack of controlled environments raises ethical concerns when such data is applied to practice. This is further compounded by potential political or economic interests that can influence the manner in which public health interventions are prioritized. As Henifin et al. (1998) observe, history in theories of disease causation within public health mirrors the complexity involved in distinguishing expert opinion from empirical evidence. Thus, as important as observational studies are to epidemiology, their limitations require delicate handling. Researchers need to balance carefully alternative approaches and ethics to ensure rigorous validity and reliability of outcomes (Figure 7.13).

7.4.3. Techniques for Controlling Confounding

The presence of confounding variables can potentially strongly distort the causal relationship of exposure and outcome in epidemiology. For this reason, confounding needs to be controlled through some techniques if proper causal inference is to be made. One of the common practices is stratification, where data are separated into independent subgroups based on the confounding variable. Through this, researchers can consider the effect of the exposure in each stratum and eliminate or control confounding effects. Above all, stratification facilitates visualization of the relationship of different strata of the confounder with the exposure, making it possible to untangle patterns otherwise obscured in aggregated data. Stratification introduces sample size and complexity issues, especially where there are many confounders, and this leads towards auxiliary control methods that will bypass these issues in different settings (Wunsch, 2025). One of the strong ways of managing confounding in epidemiologic analysis is the application of multivariable regression models. The models allow the researchers to manage many confounders simultaneously, providing an estimate of the effect of exposure and adjusting for the effect of other variables. Regression adjustment may involve various types of factors, such as demographic and socioeconomic factors, which may influence the outcome of interest. An advantage of the method is that it can easily consider vast amounts of data, gaining insights that one may miss with stratification. It should be noted here that regression analysis heavily depends on correctly specified models. Missing key confounders or misspecification of functional forms may lead to biased estimates, accentuating the importance of rigorous model specification and selection in causal inference methods (Adler et al., 2020). Instrumental variable analysis is an advanced method to manage confounding through variables that correlate with exposure but are not directly influenced by the outcome. This technique is one method of controlling for unmeasured confounding through the use of natural experiments or external data to provide a better causal relationship estimate. Instrumental variables may prove useful when randomization is unavailable or where control methods can be ineffective in addressing confounding.

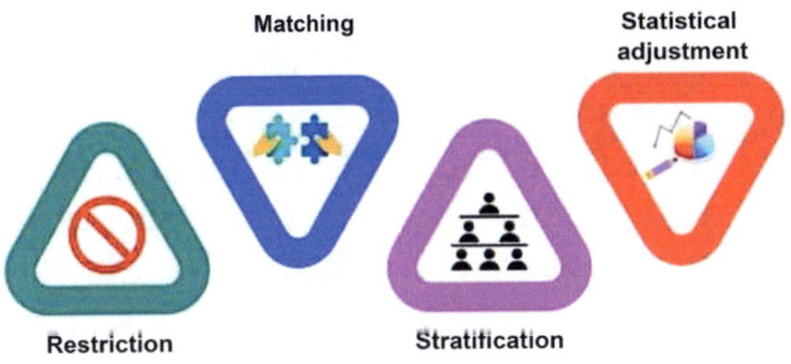

Figure 7.14. Controlling for confounding.

Source: https://b1879915.smushcdn.com/1879915/wp-content/uploads/2015/03/Controlling-for-Confounding.jpg?lossy=2&strip=1&webp=1.

Nevertheless, the effectiveness of this approach hinges on the selection of an adequate instrument—one that influences the exposure but not the effect in any other way. Comprehension of trade-offs among confounder control methods, including instrumental variables, is critical in facilitating researchers to make informed decisions in comprehending causal associations in epidemiology (Adler et al., 2020) (Figure 7.14).

7.5. Challenges in Establishing Causation

The causal structure of epidemiology is full of confounding intricacies that confound researchers in their quest for truth. One of the major obstacles is the issue of confounding variables, which can mask the actual relationship between exposure and effect. Confounders may be correlated with both the exposure and the effect, and thereby confounders make causal conclusions wrong. For instance, one study may determine that increased exercise is linked with lower heart disease rates. However, if socioeconomic status, a confounding variable, isn't controlled for, researchers may mistakenly attribute causality to exercise as the sole causal factor. This shows that a proper study design to hold potential confounders constant is necessary in order to make proper causal inferences. The second significant challenge of establishing causation is the observational nature of most epidemiological studies. Observational studies contrast with randomized controlled trials (RCTs) since they are susceptible to biases such as selection bias and information bias. These biases can significantly contort the observed association between variables. For example, a cohort study examining the link between smoking and lung cancer could be underreported in smoking behavior among participants due to stigma. Such misreporting could weaken the seemingly present association and lead to an overestimation of the risk. Without the tight controls provided by RCTs, observational studies must be approached with skepticism, and this limitation necessitates the development of advanced statistical techniques to adjust for biases and infer causation accurately. The synergy of interdisciplinary approaches holds the promise of being a good path to surmounting some of these hindrances to causation definition in epidemiology. Interdisciplinary work with natural scientists can bring methodological strength, providing evidence that might reveal hidden biological processes or causal pathways that traditional epidemiological techniques do not pick up. For instance, researchers working together with biologists may carefully evaluate the philosophy of science within causation, taking on board such prominent issues as the problem of agency and the individualistic fallacy. In addition, the convergence of person-centered healthcare (PCH) and evidence-based medicine (EBM) places the foregrounding of contrasting ontological frameworks that shape causal understanding. While EBM moves in a positivist epistemology, PCH may advance perspectives in line with more reticent causal dispositions, thereby pushing forward causal inference discussion in epidemiology (Grant et al., 2010; Anjum et al., 2016) (Figure 7.15).

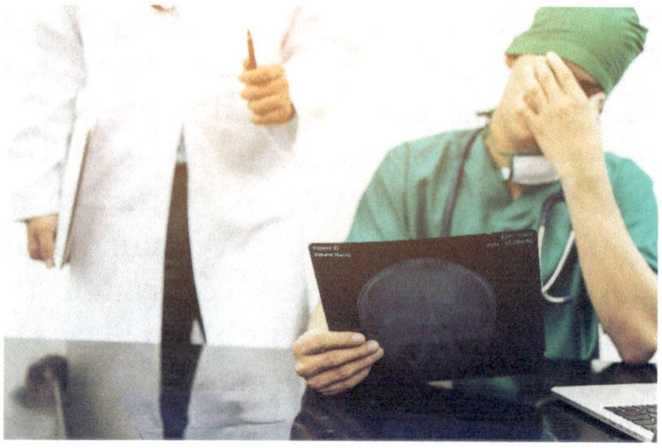

Figure 7.15. The challenges in establishing causation in TBI claims.

Source: https://emirabellalaw.com/wp-content/uploads/2024/07/bigstock-Doctor-Covering-His-Face-With-196811011.jpg.

7.5.1. Complexity of Biological Systems

The complexity of biological systems presents epidemiology with very challenging problems, particularly the identification of causal relationships. Biological systems themselves are complex with interacting nonlinearities among numerous variables such as genetic determinants, the environment, and lifestyles. The complexity necessitates sophisticated models to understand and infer potential causal pathways. As Bradford Hills' nine points indicate, the intricate nature of the relations mentioned hinders causation determination in epidemiological research. Researchers are not only required to identify correlations but also to contend with confounding variables and events' temporal order. The explanatory coherence model of ECHO presents itself in this instance as a valuable tool, providing a formal means of breaking through the multifaceted weave of connections that define biological events, finally to aid in the assessment of causality in various health outcomes (Dammann et al., 2019). Lastly, the philosophical underpinnings of contemporary paradigms in medicine also impact how causality is framed within epidemiology. Evidence-based medicine (EBM) has had a long hold on this ground, emphasizing positivist approaches founded on statistical analysis of data and clinical trials. However, as the limitations of EBM become apparent when they are confronted with the complexity of individual patient experiences, approaches such as person-centered healthcare (PCH) can be accessed as alternatives. PCH also enjoys a more nuanced understanding of health that takes into account the interplay of biology, psychology, and sociality. Such a movement towards a holistic vision triggers a reconsideration of causative models in epidemiology, opening to scrutiny of ontological visions that emphasize the complexity of disease and health (Anjum et al., 2016). The contemporary contest between EBM and PCH thus portrays an increased realization of the complexity of biological systems. Finally, understanding the complexity of biological systems requires interdisciplinary collaboration, essential to the conduct of epidemiological research. Fields such as systems biology, computational modeling, and bioinformatics give tremendous insights into the effects of multifactorial interactions on health outcomes. Converging knowledge and methodologies from different scientific disciplines enable scientists to better model biological interactions and uncover subtle patterns suppressed by homogenized methods. Converging not only enhances the robustness of epidemiological research but also illuminates new avenues for interventions and public health policies. As the field moves forward, embracing this complexity and promoting interdisciplinary discussion will be crucial in crafting and refining our definition of causation, leading to improved health outcomes for populations with complex diseases (Dammann et al., 2019).

7.5.2. Issues with Data Quality and Availability

In epidemiology, issues associated with the availability and quality of data greatly hinder establishing causative associations between disease determinants and environmental factors. One major challenge arises from inconsistency in data collection processes in different regions that may lead to variability in the datasets. For instance, epidemiological studies rely on self-reported data, which may possess biases that affect the accuracy of outcomes. The impact of these biases is particularly significant when assessing chronic diseases that call for accurate and multidimensional data. The validity of dietary reference intakes (DRIs) and other model approaches can thus be questioned, as argued in the dialogue in setting up DRI values for chronic disease endpoints. The dialogue attaches importance to solid data (Ard et al., 2016). Also, health and environmental data integration remains a prime but difficult task in epidemiological research. Efforts, such as the creation of the national environmental public health tracking (EPHT) network, try to bridge the gap between chronic disease surveillance and the collection of environmental data. But uniting these disparate sources of data is a single issue of methodological consistency and technological complexity required to properly bring them together. Chronic diseases, for their part, are often multifactorial in etiology in their environmental and lifestyle antecedents, and do not easily conform to the strictures of conventional data analysis. Therefore, as the EPHT initiative suggests, a dynamic process facilitating ongoing updating and sharing of integrated data is essential to improve population-level exposure estimations and assist in risk community identification (Balmes et al., 2004). Aside from data integration deficits, the sustainability of chronic disease surveillance systems remains under constant scrutiny. Epidemiological work is generally reliant on established paradigms that may fail to capture new health threats linked to environmental aetiologies. Toaddress this, surveillance activities need to prioritize not only the accuracy of their data collection, but also the ability to respond to evolving public health crises and technological development. In the wake of the crucial role of data in guiding public health interventions, it is important to maintain emphasis on ongoing evaluation and investment in such systems. The ultimate goal is to keep enhancing our understanding and prevention of chronic diseases, with the confidence that data quality and availability are at the forefront of epidemiologic research efforts (Ard et al., 2016; Balmes et al., 2004).

7.5.3. Ethical Considerations in Causal Research

Causal epidemiological research is mostly concerned with uncovering the relationship between variables, but it is also important to deal with the ethical consequences that accompany such studies. When researchers try to establish causality, they must operate in an environment that is neither too relaxed in scientific procedure nor too yielding to moral demands. Ethical concerns are implicated when participants' welfare is at stake, particularly in nonrandomized observational studies. Risk of harm must be properly assessed because all confounding factors influencing health cannot be controlled through experimentation by researchers. A balance is to be ensured between scientific progress and safeguards for participants, for which ethical guidelines and regulation schemes are all the more important to ensure that studies are not only scientifically acceptable but also clearly ensure human rights and dignity, serving as the basis for responsible epidemiological practice in determining causative agents and associated health hazards (Canela et al., 2017). The complexities of causal inference in turn also demand strict ethical scrutiny, especially while using a variety of methodological methods. In epidemiology, various study designs such as confounder-control and instrument-based approaches each have their respective merits and demerits (Adler et al., 2020). The ethical consequences of such a decision are significant, in that researchers have an obligation to make such choices as will affect both the validity of their results and the integrity of their work. For instance, the application of observational studies is challenging when it comes to representing those vulnerable groups , where certain groups may either be overrepresented or underrepresented and therefore taint the results. Ethical investigation demands openness and thorough reporting, allowing for critical scrutiny of the methods employed and their potential implications for the varied populations being examined. Further, the ethical principle of beneficence, which entails minimizing harm and maximizing benefit, is the underpinning of all causal research in epidemiology. Researchers have to consider societal implications of the findings, particularly where causality is related to public health interventions. Misuses or misinterpretations of causal associations have the potential to lead to harmful or even deleterious health policy. For this reason, maintaining an ethical approach remains pertinent not only to the integrity of the research process itself but also to the population health impacts such research may have. It is the duty of epidemiologists to convey their findings meaningfully such that the evidence so created is utilized in advancing health equity while managing the moral complexities involved in causal research designs (Canela et al., 2017).

7.6. Case Studies in Causation

When one explores Case Studies in Causation, it is important to realize how the studies illuminate the multiple facets of causation in epidemiology. Epidemiological investigation often encounters the complicated causation of disease, where factors may be dependent on each other and not isolated. Case studies are helpful since they provide real-world practical insights into the application of the sufficient-component cause model, a conceptual model that expounds the set of necessary and sufficient causes of disease. By studying specific instances of illness, scientists are better able to visualize how individual components are pieced together to form health. In addition, these case studies emphasize the value of sophisticated approaches that consider contemporary challenges, including biases and misinterpretations that occur in classical research strategies. Indeed, as observed in recent arguments, new epidemiological methods are the pillar to further enhance our capability in assessing disease causation and prevention strategies (Alrawahi et al., 2020). The application of statistical evidence in constructing causation is particularly relevant in legal contexts, as has been argued in the argument on the application of epidemiological contributions to legal proceedings. Here, causation divides into various meanings: negligence in terms of exposure, scientifically supported elevated risk in populations, and implications for plaintiffs as individuals. The subtle distinctions in establishing causality can get in the way of legal determinations, especially as these apply to epidemiological evidence. Through the use of case studies to illustrate these varied definitions of causality, one gains a perspective on how legal boundaries cross into epidemiological examination. These case studies provide critical context for how observation data might be employed to shape legal standards and highlight the importance of statistical discipline. A full understanding of causation is thus obtained that accounts for both population-level observations and also for implications at the individual case level, thereby adding strength to the nuance involved in translating epidemiological results into legal conclusions (Mengersen et al., 2007). Secondly, causation case studies allow for the application of varied analytic techniques, providing richer insights into the risk determinants of specific health events. Specifically, the creation of novel study designs, i.e., the exposed case-control design, captures the changing nature of epidemiological techniques. The new approach is intended to analyze the interaction of future component causes and their role in disease occurrence, refining models of risk prediction. Causation models within epidemiology need to be fine-tuned to address the evolving health challenges. As seen in current literature, the requirement for systematic reviews and meta-analyses focusing specifically on causation studies is crucial. Through the employment of case studies with fine-tuned approaches, researchers can contribute more significantly to the understanding of disease mechanisms, hence guiding public health activities towards more efficient preventive interventions. Therefore, case studies not only summarize existing knowledge but also contribute to the advancement of the science of epidemiology (Alrawahi et al., 2020).

7.6.1. Tobacco Use and Lung Cancer

The link between tobacco smoking and lung cancer is the classic one of causation in epidemiology. The link has been a subject of widespread research, and robust evidence supports the argument that smoking significantly increases the risk of lung cancer. Epidemiological studies consistently indicate a dose-response relationship; that is, more consumption of tobacco is found to have increased rates of lung cancer. The theories constructed by influential thinkers, such as Bradford Hill, provide valuable tools for understanding the nuances of causation. The criteria established by Hill identify such factors as strength, consistency, and biological plausibility, and collectively these point to the causal link between smoking and lung cancer. By applying these requirements to epidemiological evidence, researchers can build strong cases that not only outline the risks of tobacco consumption but also identify it as a primary causative factor in lung cancer incidence (Dammann et al., 2019). In legal and scientific discussions about causation and tobacco consumption, different senses of cause need to be distinguished from one another. From a public health point of view, tobacco is a major cause of lung cancer because it has clearly established risk factors. That is well captured in population studies documenting the increase in lung cancer in smokers compared with non-smokers. When, however, individual cases are examined, the legal system often has difficulty in establishing legal causation. This is about linking negligence in exposure to tobacco and relating it to the results in individual plaintiffs. The causation terminology in court environments replicates scientific practice, where stringent statistical tests are utilized in support of claims. Through incorporating these perspectives, the public health community is in a better position to advance policy initiatives reducing tobacco use and hence lung cancer incidence (Mengersen et al., 2007). Despite the established association between smoking and lung cancer, many still hinder smoking reduction in public health efforts. Tobacco consumption is greatly determined by many sociocultural influences that impact smoking, including peer pressure, advertising, and finances. Antitobacco interventions should thus be holistic, not only going after the biological consequences of smoking but also targeting factors within society that facilitate smoking. Public health campaigns, legislation, and education initiatives all have crucial roles to play in this process by enhancing awareness and access to quitting. As the evidence base in epidemiology is still evolving, it is increasingly clear that an effective strategy will have to tackle these complexities. Merging epidemiologic understanding with effective public health action can largely curb the burden of lung cancer caused by tobacco use, ultimately bringing about health outcomes on a higher scale (Dammann et al., 2019) (Figure 7.16).

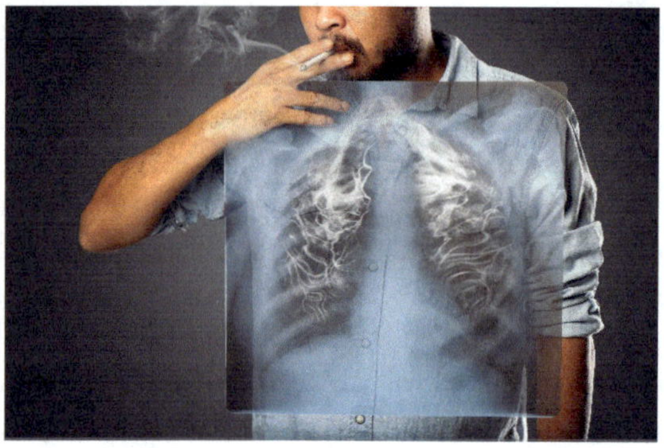

Figure 7.16. Smoking and lung cancer.

Source: https://www.compassoncology.com/hubfs/AdobeStock_122035640-1.jpeg.

7.6.2. Obesity and Diabetes

The link between obesity and diabetes has been the focus of important exploration in epidemiological research, which has identified a complex interaction between obesity and diabetes as twin public health challenges. Obesity has been shown to be a relevant risk factor for type 2 diabetes based predominantly on the mechanisms by which additional fat tissue influences insulin sensitivity. Obese persons usually have a condition of chronic low-grade inflammation, and this may impair insulin action, further worsening glucose tolerance. Further, since the rate of obesity has increased at an alarming rate worldwide, so too has the problem of diabetes, necessitating strong public health measures. However, care has to be taken in navigating this relationship on the tightrope because confounding factors, such as environment and genes, obscure the direct causative relationship between obesity and diabetes (Linden et al., 2017). Recent research has identified sociodemographic factors and food choice as significantly affecting the obesity-diabetes profile. Urbanization and changes in eating habits, especially the adoption of Western diets high in sugars and unhealthy fats, have been cited as key drivers of the rise in obesity and diabetes. Food market size analysis showed that increased income often leads to greater consumption of calorie-dense foods, and this can divert consumption towards products that are not so healthy. Notably, the rising consumption of sugars, particularly from imported foods, has been quantitatively linked to rising diabetes incidence, so while lifestyle factors are important, it would appear that the economic and sociopolitical context also has to be considered (Basu et al., 2012). These results add to the complexity of solving these health conditions in an environment with multiple factors. Other than individual lifestyle variables, public health programs thus have to take an integrated approach that explicitly deals with the more overarching societal determinants of diabetes and obesity. Prevention strategies involving nutrition and exercise may be too limited and overlook certain important areas, such as the food environment and socioeconomic status, which exert significant influences on food intake and physical activity levels. Furthermore, epidemiologic evidence of associations between obesity and diabetes must be framed in some depth so that it is possible to control for potential confounding variables, including age, cultural factors, and existing health disparities. Additional research has to be conducted in order to define causal pathways from obesity to diabetes and suitable policies aimed at these interlinked diseases. It is only by such concerted efforts that we can possibly improve public health outcomes and minimize the impact of these two diseases (Linden et al., 2017) (Figure 7.17).

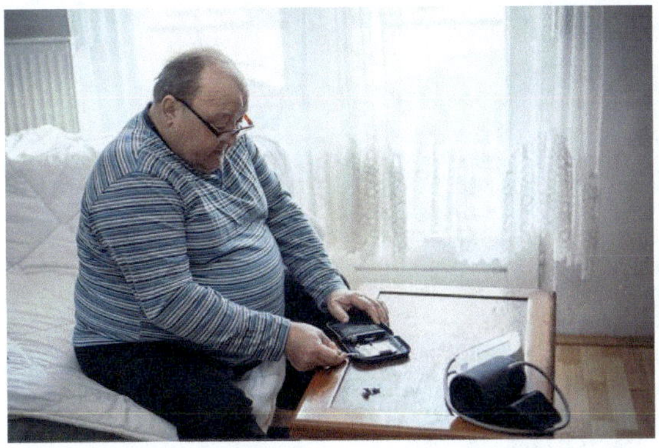

Figure 7.17. Obesity and diabetes.

Source: https://www.templehealth.org/sites/default/files/styles/without_crop/public/older-man-checking-blood-sugar-levels_0.jpg?itok=3jZNU2cj.

7.6.3. Environmental Factors and Respiratory Diseases

Environmental factors are held accountable for the causation and exacerbation of respiratory disorders, impacting public health levels to a considerable extent. Of central importance among them are air pollutants, which generally follow directly from industrial activities, vehicular emissions, and domestic heating systems. These are particulate matter, nitrogen dioxide, sulfur dioxide, and ozone, each carrying a different respiratory disorder like asthma, chronic obstructive pulmonary disease (COPD), and lung cancer. Epidemiologic studies have consistently shown that populations with high levels of exposure to air pollution have higher morbidity and mortality rates associated with respiratory disease. For instance, chronic exposure to fine particulate matter has been associated with the development of asthma in children and symptom worsening in adults with pre-existing conditions. Hence, understanding the causal mechanisms of environmental toxins can lead to the development of efficient public health strategies. Indoor air quality has also been in the spotlight as an important environmental determinant responsible for causing respiratory illnesses, especially in developing countries. Biomass and coal are used by numerous households as primary sources of energy, leading to foul indoor air pollution. Exposure to smoke from these processes has been linked to severe health risks, particularly for women and children who remain indoors a majority of the time while cooking and performing domestic cleaning. Research indicates that improving indoor air quality through interventions has a notable effect on diminishing respiratory symptoms and overall disease burden. Of those interventions, cleaner cooking stoves as well as ventilation systems have been found to be effective (Ezzati et al., 2025). This raises the call for an integrated strategy that fuses technological, behavioral, and environmental assessment to mitigate indoor air pollution's health impacts holistically. In addition to the overt pollutants, the socioeconomic determinants of health and environmental determinants of health in community design also affect respiratory health outcomes. Urbanization increases traffic density, which in turn results in increased exposure to outdoor air pollution. Low-income communities tend to bear a disproportionate burden of environmental hazards on the basis of housing quality and proximity to industrial operations. Consequently, individuals living in such communities are exposed to a higher risk of respiratory disease. Interventions at the community level that aim at both the environmental and social factors of health, such as housing quality improvement and enhanced green space, can minimize the exposure to toxic substances as well as enhance lung function. It is essential to synthesize data from multidisciplinary fields, including epidemiology, urban planning, and public health, in order to formulate effective strategies that address the complex relationships between environmental determinants and respiratory diseases (Al Kandari et al., 2014). This multidisciplinary approach is core to advancing public health interventions that reduce the burden of these diseases (Figure 7.18).

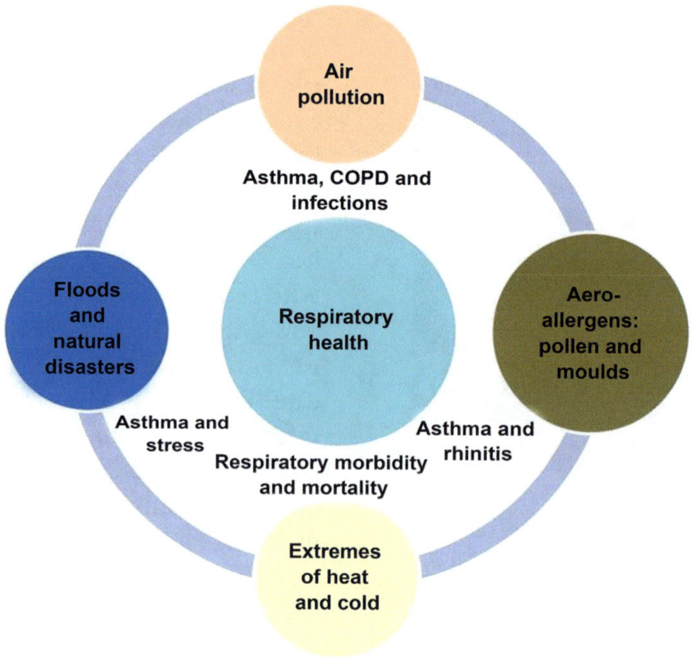

Figure 7.18. Potential respiratory health effects of climate change.

Source: https://publications.ersnet.org/content/errev/23/132/161/F1.large.jpg.

Summary

In finalizing the quest for causation in epidemiology, it is essential to note the intricacy of establishing causal relations in this field of science. Epidemiological studies are tasked with establishing associations between exposures and effects, but attributing causation is complex. The necessity of rigorous statistical techniques to establish a causal association is even greater when outcomes can have implications for public health policy or the law. Different conceptions of cause within context—ranging from negligence to science-informed risk—highlight the variety of demands for evidence across the fields. Nonetheless, adopting a formal approach, such as the Bradford Hill criteria, will assist in applying causation to systematic examination and enhancing the intelligibility of results within epidemiology, especially where informed evidence is required for public health and legal judgment (Mengersen et al., 2007). Moreover, the integration of biopsychosocial models into epidemiological screening improves causation knowledge by perceiving biological, psychological, and social factors as interacting determinants of health outcomes. Not only does this model elaborate on causality examination, but it also facilitates multidimensional treatment planning, particularly for complex health conditions. For instance, for upper limb disorders, a biomedical management alone may not be sufficient without psychosocial factors that play a critical role in influencing the outcome for the patient. Synthesis of evidence from systematic reviews points out that biopsychosocial management plans are more likely to have better occupational outcomes and quality of life for individuals with these disorders. Thus, identification of psychosocial determinants in epidemiology becomes crucial to informing effective interventions and closing the research discovery to useful applications that meet the needs of vulnerable populations (Burton et al., 2008). Last but not least, the implication of the conclusion that can be drawn from the discussion of causation in epidemiology is that there is a need for constant adjustment in study designs that acknowledge the complexity of health determinants. Successful communication between researchers, policymakers, and the public regarding the findings of epidemiological studies is essential to inform health interventions as well as legislative responses. Moreover, the need for an aggregate technique—securing the involvement of various stakeholders like healthcare workers, researchers, and affected groups—is essential to make the control of disease scientifically valid but also applicable to the situation. Emphasis on working together and considering causation holistically can lead to enhanced health outcomes and equity in health policy. As the field develops, a continued requirement for refinement in statistical techniques as well as integration of multiple factors that influence health to inform effective public health interventions and strategies (Mengersen et al., 2007; Burton et al., 2008).

To understand causation in epidemiology means having a keen examination of the diverse determinants of health outcomes. To the forefront of these are risk and exposure, factors that combine to explain why particular variables cause illness in populations. An integral aspect of such investigation is the recognition of the multifactorial nature of health conditions like upper limb disorders (ULDs) and breast cancer. For ULDs, the evidence suggests that neither biomedical treatments nor ergonomic treatment alone is effective; instead, it is a biopsychosocial model that is advisable for effective management (Burton et al., 2008). Breast cancer, on the other hand, captures the complexity of causation, where incidence depends on a range of factors, including genetic, hormonal, and environmental factors. Hence, both conditions underscore the importance of employing an integrated approach to unveil the intricate web of causative factors. The causation analysis also elucidates the necessity for context-specific determinants of health outcomes. For instance, in the management of upper limb disorders, there is a strong interaction between psychosocial determinants and biological determinants. The emerging evidence corroborates the assumption that effective management of ULDs requires a concerted effort by surgeons, physiotherapists, employers, and patients to work together on treatment goals (Burton et al., 2008). An integrated effort emphasizes the point that disease management transcends isolated intervention and depends instead upon a systemic understanding of how the various components interact. Similarly, the causation image of breast cancer illustrates historically the move towards the embracement of man-made chemicals as significant risk factors in environmental exposures. The embracement that such chemicals can alter hormonal levels not only redefines risk assessment procedures but also calls for ongoing research on the causation determinants of disease incidence. Ultimately, incorporating such knowledge into causation establishes the role for dynamic paradigms to encompass multiple forces of influence. The traditional mechanisms of health are prone to overlooking the complex interplay among the various factors, such as social behaviors, environmental exposures, and biological vulnerabilities, shown along the course of diseases like breast cancer. Shifting the direction of attention toward a conceptual framework that consolidates such factors can enhance prevention strategies better adapted to modern epidemiological requirements. In summary, knowledge of the multifaceted nature of causation bestows strength to public health efforts and policy-making, as evidenced by the demand for new insights towards disease mechanism explanation, hence strengthening the field of epidemiology and application to real-world issues of health.

CLOSER LOOK

IMPLICATIONS FOR PUBLIC HEALTH POLICY

The intricate dance of causality in public health policy and epidemiology reiterates the importance of evidence-based paradigms. With progress in medicine in the recent past, particularly the last three decades, the scientific grounding of clinical epidemiology has solidified the necessity for health policies to be evidence-based. This has made possible the elucidation of causal associations that can guide interventions and prevention. For instance, understanding the causal pathways to chronic illness can lead to specific health promotion interventions for the target populations at risk. These evidence-informed interventions can maximize the use of resources and improve health outcomes within populations and ultimately illustrate the triumph of rationalist thought that underlies much contemporary public health endeavor (Newton et al., 2001).

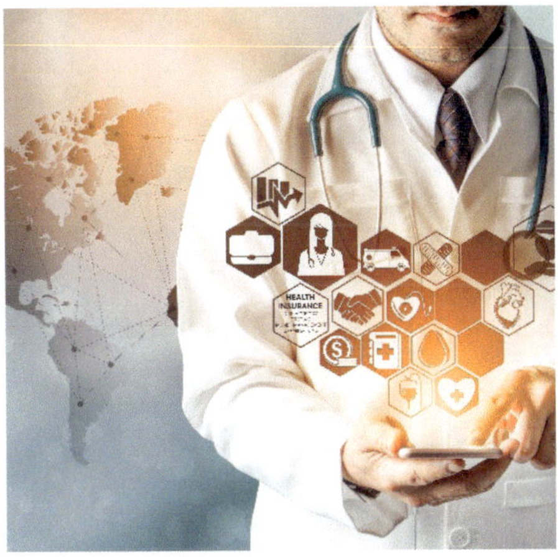

Figure 7.19. Physician using digital health technologies to access and manage global healthcare data.

Source: https://www.climateone.org/files/images/media/Pod-Implications%20for%20Public%20Health.jpg.

In addition, the complexity of health issues creates an urgent necessity for a more nuanced understanding of the interdetermination among various health determinants, as well as among the social, economic, and environmental determinants of these. Hence, public health policy must take an interdisciplinary input that is attuned to these intricate interdeterminations. The integration of socio-economic considerations in epidemiological studies allows policymakers to formulate interventions that address the roots of health disparities instead of merely addressing the symptoms. This approach can lead to more cohesive health policies with enhanced abilities for promoting health equity. While the public health environment is being molded, the need for policies that not only react to health information but also address socioeconomic and environmental conditions increases more and more (Beth et al., 2013). Public health policy implications extend beyond immediate health interventions and necessitate that the legislative framework that supports health be assessed. Policy-makers are under pressure to prioritize the creation of guidelines that not only respond to current epidemiological trends but also those that foresee and prevent impending future health risks from future infectious and chronic diseases. This preemptive measure is urgent in a globalized world where health issues refuse to respect national borders. A clear understanding of causative determinants, underpinned by strong epidemiologic evidence, can allow health agencies to develop policies that strengthen healthcare systems. Health systems need to be strong enough to survive and change with the modification in health trends while effectively solving social determinants. Last but not least, causation and epidemiologic information are a powerful force that serves as a basis of necessary stimulus toward broad public health action for population health (Newton et al., 2001) (Figure 7.19).

References

1. Adler, N. E., Glymour, M. M., Gottlieb, L. M., Hagan, H., et al. (2020). Alternative causal inference methods in population health research: Evaluating tradeoffs and triangulating evidence. https://core.ac.uk/download/323062870.pdf (accessed on 25th June 2025).
2. AlKandari, F., Ayres, J. G., Cowie, H., Dick, F., et al. (2014). A systematic review of associations between environmental exposures and development of asthma in children aged up to 9 years. https://core.ac.uk/download/29465901.pdf (accessed on 25th June 2025).
3. Alrawahi, A. H. (2020). New approaches to disease causation research based on the sufficient-component cause model. https://core.ac.uk/download/352125479.pdf (accessed on 25th June 2025).
4. Amiri, M., & Arbabi, M. (2016). *Environmental Epidemiology: An Introduction*. https://core.ac.uk/download/143844367.pdf (accessed on 25th June 2025).
5. Anjum, R. L. (2016). Evidence based or person centered? An ontological debate. https://core.ac.uk/download/131207993.pdf (accessed on 25th June 2025).
6. Ard, J., Atkinson, S., Bier, D., Carriquiry, A., et al. (2016). Options for basing Dietary Reference Intakes (DRIs) on chronic disease endpoints: Report from a joint US-/Canadian-sponsored working group. https://core.ac.uk/download/323080977.pdf (accessed on 25th June 2025).
7. Bachmann, M. O., Clark, A., Elwell-Sutton, T., Fairall, L., et al. (2019). Socioeconomic position and depression in South African adults with long term health conditions: A longitudinal study of causal pathways. https://core.ac.uk/download/131078994.pdf (accessed on 25th June 2025).
8. Baldi, G., Chatterjee, A., Diaz, A., Dounel, A., et al. (2018). Evolution of epidemiologic methods and concepts in selected textbooks of the 20th century. https://core.ac.uk/download/159156667.pdf (accessed on 25th June 2025).
9. Balmes, J., Ritz, B., & Tager, I. (2004). Can lessons from public health disease surveillance be applied to environmental public health tracking? https://core.ac.uk/download/pdf/3775836.pdf (accessed on 25th June 2025).
10. Barnes, D. W. (2001). Too many probabilities: Statistical evidence of tort causation. https://core.ac.uk/download/62568618.pdf (accessed on 25th June 2025).
11. Bartell, S. M., Elston, B., Fletcher, T., Josson, J., et al. (2013). Exposure to perfluoroalkyl acids and markers of kidney function among children and adolescents living near a chemical plant. https://core.ac.uk/download/13109873.pdf (accessed on 25th June 2025).
12. Basu, S., Galea, G., McKee, M., Stuckler, D., et al. (2012). Nutritional determinants of worldwide diabetes: An econometric study of food markets and diabetes prevalence in 173 countries. https://core.ac.uk/download/13114335.pdf (accessed on 25th June 2025).
13. Beth, A., Dandouras, I., Garnier, P., Mazelle, C., et al. (2013). "Whose data is it anyway?" The implications of putting small area-level health and social data online. https://core.ac.uk/download/pdf/29026859.pdf (accessed on 25th June 2025).
14. Biosca, O., Donaldson, C., & McHugh, N. (2017). From wealth to health: Evaluating microfinance as a complex intervention. https://core.ac.uk/download/293860192.pdf (accessed on 25th June 2025).

15. Bowden, J., Burgess, S., Davey Smith, G., Haycock, P., et al. (2016). Best (but oft-forgotten) practices: The design, analysis, and interpretation of Mendelian randomization studies. https://core.ac.uk/download/33131892.pdf (accessed on 25th June 2025).

16. Burton, A. K., Abasolo, I., Alizadehkhaiyat, O., Pearce, B. G., Baldwin, A., Beaton, D., Bonde, J. P., et al. (2008). Management of work-relevant upper limb disorders: A review. https://core.ac.uk/download/1649687.pdf (accessed on 25th June 2025).

17. Canela i Soler, J., & Monleón Getino, T. (2017). Causality in medicine and its relationship with the role of statistics. https://core.ac.uk/download/83829966.pdf (accessed on 25th June 2025).

18. Corander, J., Hanage, W. P., & Pensar, J. (2022). Causal discovery for the microbiome. https://core.ac.uk/download/565397940.pdf (accessed on 25th June 2025).

19. Dammann, O., Poston, T., & Thagard, P. (2019). How do medical researchers make causal inferences? https://core.ac.uk/download/186330941.pdf (accessed on 25th June 2025).

20. Ehsani, S. (2018). The challenges of purely mechanistic models in biology and the minimum need for a 'mechanism-plus-X' framework. https://core.ac.uk/download/237182316.pdf (accessed on 25th June 2025).

21. Ezzati, M., & Kammen, D. (2025). The health impacts of exposure to indoor air pollution from solid fuels in developing countries: Knowledge, gaps, and data needs. https://core.ac.uk/download/pdf/9308128.pdf (accessed on 25th June 2025).

22. Ferguson, K. D., Green, M. J., Katikireddi, S. V., Lewsey, J., et al. (2020). Evidence synthesis for constructing directed acyclic graphs (ESC-DAGs): A novel and systematic method for building directed acyclic graphs. https://core.ac.uk/download/222882203.pdf (accessed on 25th June 2025).

23. Garfinkel, A., Shipley, B., Van Fraassen, B., Hitchcock, C., Hitchcock, C., Sober, E., Dretske, F., et al. (2012). Degree of explanation. https://core.ac.uk/download/9346831.pdf (accessed on 25th June 2025).

24. Ghezzi, P. (2020). Environmental risk factors and their footprints *in vivo*–A proposal for the classification of oxidative stress biomarkers. https://core.ac.uk/download/287600956.pdf (accessed on 25th June 2025).

25. Grant, W., & Greaves, J. (2010). *Crossing the Interdisciplinary Divide: Political Science and Biological Science*. https://core.ac.uk/download/46694.pdf (accessed on 25th June 2025).

26. Henifin, M. S., & Lynch, R. M. (1998). Causation in occupational disease: Balancing epidemiology, law and manufacturer conduct. https://core.ac.uk/download/72056434.pdf (accessed on 25th June 2025).

27. Karlsson, M., Mayhew, L., & Rickayzen, B. D. (2007). In sickness and in health? Dynamics of health and cohabitation in the United Kingdom. https://core.ac.uk/download/9983072.pdf (accessed on 25th June 2025).

28. Kronfeldner, M. (2014). How norms make causes. https://core.ac.uk/download/146502161.pdf (accessed on 25th June 2025).

29. Linden, G., & Winning, L. (2017). Periodontitis and systemic disease: Association or causality? https://core.ac.uk/download/77603157.pdf (accessed on 25th June 2025).

30. Link, B., Morroni, C., Myer, L., Susser, E., et al. (2008). *Social Epidemiology*. https://core.ac.uk/download/1670083.pdf (accessed on 25th June 2025).

31. Mengersen, K., Moynihan, S. A., & Tweedie, R. L. (2007). Causality and association: The statistical and legal approaches. https://core.ac.uk/download/10883828.pdf (accessed on 25th June 2025).

32. Morfopoulou, S. (2015). *Bayesian Mixture Models for Metagenomic Community Profiling*. https://core.ac.uk/download/79497914.pdf (accessed on 25th June 2025).

33. Newton, W. (2001). *Rationalism and Empiricism in Modern Medicine*. https://core.ac.uk/download/62568601.pdf (accessed on 25th June 2025).

34. Parkinson, N. J. (2022). *Functional Genomics in The Regulation of The Immune Response*. https://core.ac.uk/download/533445451.pdf (accessed on 25th June 2025).

35. Plant, J., Stanley, E., & Voulvoulis, N. (2016). Environmental chemical exposures and breast cancer. https://core.ac.uk/download/77011572.pdf (accessed on 25th June 2025).

36. Sawers, L., & Stillwaggon, E. (2018). Understanding HIV/AIDS in the African context. https://cupola.gettysburg.edu/cgi/viewcontent.cgi?article=1030&context=econfac (accessed on 25th June 2025).

37. Smith, P. K., & Zagorsky, J. L. (2016). Does asthma impair wealth accumulation or does wealth protect against asthma? https://open.bu.edu/bitstream/2144/40247/3/Asthma_Paper_Aug_21_2014.pdf (accessed on 25th June 2025).

38. Wunsch, G. (2025). Confounding and control. https://core.ac.uk/download/pdf/7127328.pdf (accessed on 25th June 2025).

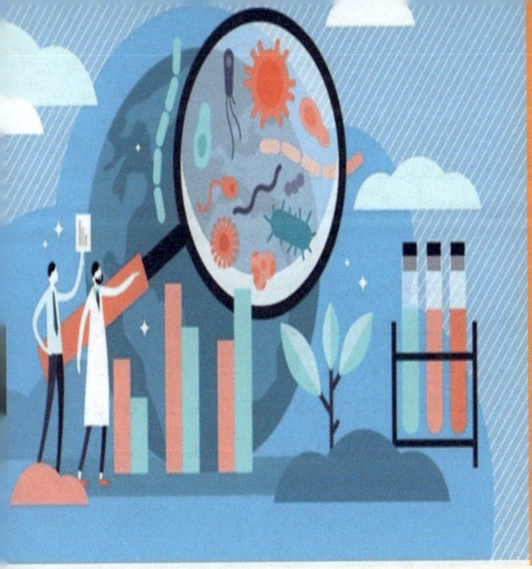

Chapter 8

STATISTICAL METHODS IN EPIDEMIOLOGY

Contents

Introduction

Epidemiology examines a foundational pillar of public health, paying particular attention to examining the determinants and distribution of health-related states or events within specific populations. In the strict emphasis on determinants and incidence of disease, epidemiologists measure health outcomes, track trends, and ultimately aid in informing the overall picture of public health issues. This initial foray into epidemiology emphasizes descriptive and analytical techniques that facilitate the discovery of patterns and associations in public health data. Statistical analysis has a key role in such processes, not only for disease occurrence analysis but also in determining causality. These methods enable epidemiologists to assess various factors impacting health outcomes that, in turn, enable proper interventions and well-informed policy choices that can help increase community health and well-being. A wide variety of statistical methods are used within the epidemiological field to assess data appropriately. Of these, techniques such as propensity score methods have gained popularity due to their usefulness in estimating causal relationships where randomized control trials cannot be conducted due to ethical considerations or logistical constraints. Rosenbaum and Rubin developed propensity score methods, and these help researchers account for confounders so they are able to make more valid inferences from observational data. By balancing covariates within treatment groups, the above methods significantly reduce selection bias, hence enhancing the validity of findings. These sophisticated statistical methods are required in the evaluation of public health intervention effectiveness because they allow epidemiologists to identify the likely impact of multiple determinants on outcomes, thereby guiding possible future study and practice in this area (Rubin et al., 2006).

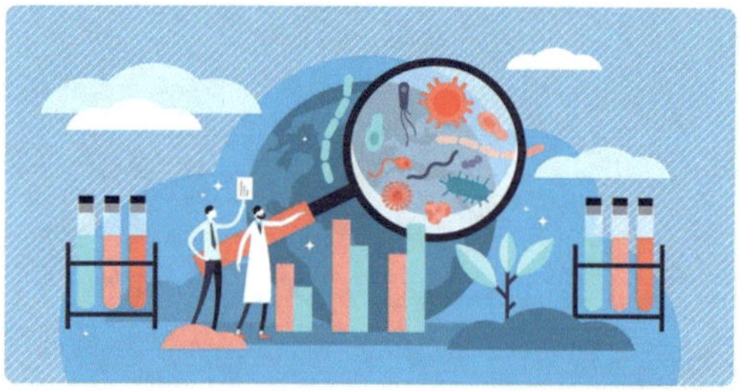

Figure 8.1. Statistics and epidemiology.

Source: https://www.news-medical.net/image-handler/ts/20211007071956/ri/673/picture/2021/10/shutterstock_1398762395.jpg.

The application of statistical techniques in epidemiology is also evident in research into zoonotic pathogens such as Shiga toxin-producing *Escherichia coli* (STEC). Research into STEC prevalence within dairy farming, for example, applies the application of molecular and statistical techniques in making sense of the risk factors of human infections. By the utilization of novel diagnostic tests and stratified cross-sectional analysis, researchers were able to define the prevalence of the Top 7 STEC serogroups and their association with environmental factors. These studies highlight the important contribution of statistical methods in the disentanglement of complex associations among organisms, environments, and human well-being. Lastly, rigorous statistical analysis in epidemiology not only aids in the identification of diseases' causes but also supports interventions that are meant to decrease risks and improve public health outcomes (Browne et al., 2018) (Figure 8.1).

8.1. Types of Epidemiological Studies

Epidemiology is a heterogeneous collection of study designs, all carefully tailored to meet some research question and public health problem. Observational studies are crucial among them, classified broadly into cohort, case-control, and cross-sectional studies. Cohort studies observe groups prospectively to quantify health outcomes, effectively building temporal associations and risk factors. Conversely, case-control studies retrospectively compare individuals with a specific condition to those without, thereby identifying potential exposure determinants. Cross-sectional studies provide a snapshot in time, observing population characteristics and health outcomes simultaneously. This diverse toolkit allows epidemiologists to analyze data flexibly and holistically, ensuring robust insights into disease patterns and determinants that are essential for intervention strategies. Within the last few decades, the emergence of the exposome idea further enriched the field of epidemiologic studies by highlighting the sum total of environmental exposures an individual experiences during a lifetime. This methodology combines different methodological advances, borrowing methods across various fields of the life sciences. More importantly, the exposome defies conventional models by not only taking into account genetic influences but also how many nongenetic environmental factors combine to affect disease onset. By applying statistical methodology to analyze complex exposure data, researchers can identify patterns and associations beyond those of simple association. Gradual as these progressions are, they have the potential to uncover a nuanced understanding of health endpoints and advance understanding of complicated diseases, as elucidated in the commentary by Canali et al. (2020). The application of network theory to epidemiological research has revolutionized the study of disease dynamics. By modeling transmission of infectious disease among connected populations, researchers can develop in-depth insight into disease dynamics and focus interventions effectively. Different network structures like social, geographical, and transport networks provide structure for representing contacts that spread or hinder the spread of disease. The statistical methods used to estimate parameters of epidemiology from the networks have seen phenomenal progress, enabling researchers to model epidemic dynamics realistically. This focus on network epidemiology can potentially guide more effectively informed public health policy, identifying main intervention and control pathways within populations. As noted in recent literature, the marriage of network theory and epidemiological insight holds much promise for future directions (Danon et al., 2010) (Figure 8.2).

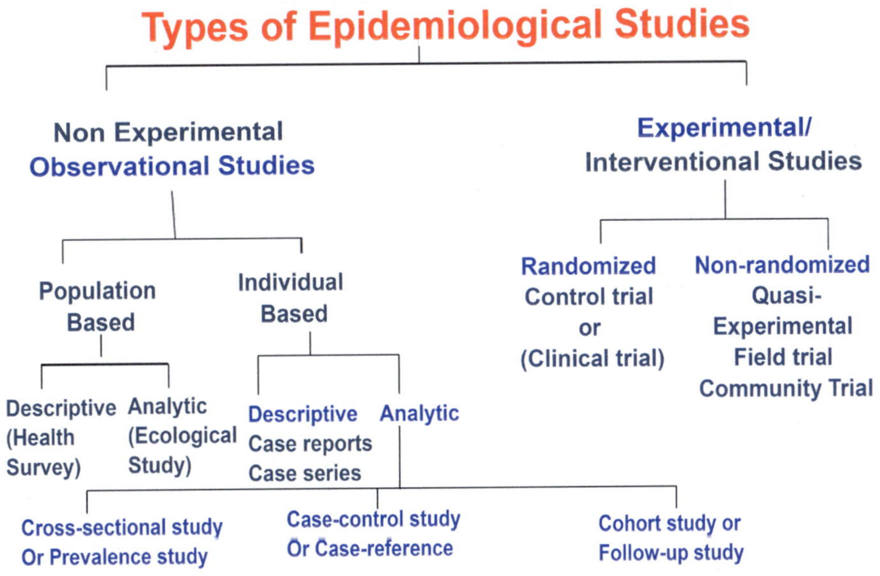

Figure 8.2. Types of epidemiological studies.

Source: https://lo.unisa.edu.au/pluginfile.php/1020294/mod_book/chapter/110421/Epidemiological%20study%20types.jpg.

8.1.1. Descriptive Studies

Descriptive studies play a crucial role in epidemiology because they provide detailed descriptions of health-related events within populations. Descriptive studies are employed to describe disease and health outcome distribution through factors such as age, sex, ethnicity, and place. Descriptive studies enable scientists to identify patterns and trends that serve as building blocks for more complex epidemiological questions. With descriptive statistics, epidemiologists are able to summarize large amounts of data, reporting information regarding the incidence and prevalence of disease. The results of such research are likely to point out prominent public health problems, which necessitate additional studies and intervention strategies. In addition, they form the foundation for hypothesis generation, igniting the research activity needed to establish the etiology of differences in the health of various populations. Even though descriptive studies are informative, they also have limitations. The natural lack of control of variables obstructs the construction of causality between exposures and outcomes. Descriptive studies, on the contrary, are based more on observation than on experiments. For example, in a descriptive study of the frequency of a disease, researchers can uncover patterns indicating potential risk factors, but they cannot conclude that these factors cause the disease. It is important for researchers to deliberately recognize such limitations, leading to misinterpretation of data. As stressed by the STROBE guidelines, reporting transparency is essential in ensuring that the findings of descriptive studies are clearly stated and interpreted so they can be effectively used within public health practice and policy (Cevallos et al., 2016). In epidemiological studies, methodological adequacy in conducting descriptive studies is a prerequisite to the formulation of valid findings. Careful planning needs to be done in formulating clear inclusion and exclusion criteria so that the study population accurately reflects the population from which it is being sampled. Moreover, necessary sampling techniques need to be employed to prevent biases common in observational studies. As stated, certain biases—such as selection bias and information bias—may exert huge influences on the validity of findings. Together with the demand for groundbreaking approaches to research design, researchers need to strive to apply sound methods in order to maximize the value of their descriptive studies. Ultimately, they continue to evolve, high-quality descriptive studies that produce valuable findings will enable us to better understand health phenomena in addition to guiding future research directions (Amanda et al., 2018) (Figure 8.3).

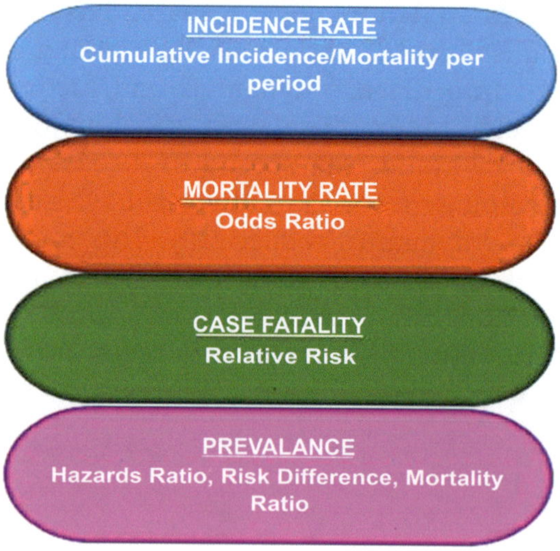

Figure 8.3. Types of quantifying and comparison measures.

Source: https://i0.wp.com/www.projectguru.in/wp-content/uploads/2017/09/1-2.jpg?w=372&ssl=1.

8.1.2. Analytical Studies

Analytical studies are the most important building blocks of epidemiology, paving the way for understanding the intricate relationships between health effects and exposure. Analytical studies make use of a wide range of statistical methods to establish the effect of various factors on health, including demographics and lifestyles. Through the use of sophisticated designs, scientists are able to test hypotheses under controlled settings, thereby distinguishing causation from correlation. For instance, an area effects study of health has increased in vigor, which states that individual factors do not, by themselves, account for health differences. As noted in previous research, a lot of the inter-area variation in health is accounted for by area context and socio-economic determinants outside the individual risk profile, which suggests the use of broad-brush analytical frameworks in epidemiologic studies (Cangelosi et al., 2001). This integrated approach enhances the examination of public health issues and is critical in developing focused interventions. Further, analytical studies commonly emphasize advanced methodologies such as multilevel modeling and logistic regression to analytically cut through complex health data. Such advanced statistical analysis enhances the capacity to control for individual and community-level variances, thus yielding more accurate health inequality insights. A good example is the incorporation of metabolomics and lipidomics into clinical intervention studies to further enhance patient stratification and optimize therapeutic strategy. Via the elucidation of metabolic profiles, scientists are able to predict responses to pharmacotherapies more accurately while unveiling drug action mechanisms or adverse effects. Despite their potential, the majority of existing studies have been criticized for underpowerment and poor study designs, whence strong methods in generalizing evidence to larger populations are a reflection of the significance (Preiss et al., 2016). As such, the implementation of new statistical methods in analysis studies is at the forefront in guiding epidemiological research. Lastly, knowledge derived from analytical studies is central in guiding public health policy as well as clinical practice. As there is an increasing emphasis on population-level interventions, the findings derived from research can inform resource planning as well as health promotion policy. The evidence for area-based effects upon health, as developed through analytical research, also highlights the interplay between health outcomes and social determinants. While public health institutions aim for fair health care provision, the statistical approaches used in such study designs provide a bridge to solving inequalities in health access and outcomes. The investigation of new metrics and sound study designs can provide more precise predictions and, hence, better health interventions. Here the ongoing evolution of analytical research not only ennobles scholarly discourse but also has some extremely profound implications for practical applications in public health (Cangelosi et al., 2001; Preiss et al., 2016) (Figure 8.4).

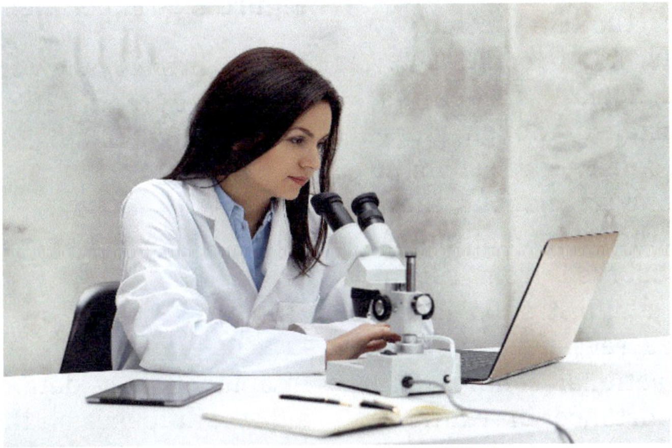

Figure 8.4. Analytical research.

Source: https://blog.researcher.life/wp-content/uploads/2024/12/analytical-research.jpg.

8.1.3. Experimental Studies

Experimental research is a pillar in epidemiology, particularly in establishing causal relationships between exposures and outcomes. Unlike observational studies that only observe and report, experimental studies intervene and manipulate variables to ascertain the impact of an intervention under controlled environments. The defining characteristic of a true experimental design, such as randomized controlled trials (RCTs), is the random allocation of participants into treatment or control groups. This randomization minimizes selection bias and enhances the internal validity of the findings in a way that scientists can make more definitive conclusions about the exposure-outcome relationship. To be sure, the practical and ethical constraints of certain health interventions can make full experimental designs unadvisable, and as such, a mixture of methodologies must draw from both experimental and observational study designs in epidemiology. In the general setting of statistical methods in epidemiology, the finer points of experimental designs allow for important concerns regarding interpretation and data validity. Even within randomized trials, there is a risk of confounding factors, requiring stringent analytical models to demonstrate that the treatment effects separated are indeed an outcome of the intervention at hand. Observational research, though limited by the self-designing biases, has become a key complementary tool, particularly in defining real-life settings. For instance, though meta-analyses of observational studies and systematic reviews can produce strong correlations, these are more likely to reflect the design limitations of these studies. As observed from recent research, corticosteroid administration in the management of influenza revealed increased mortality among observational cohorts and noted the marked importance of cautious interpretation of empirical evidence derived from such studies (Leonardi-Bee et al., 2015). Also, the integration of different study designs within epidemiological studies promotes further insight into public health processes. By employing diverse methodologies, researchers can address questions of substance on causation and effect more comprehensively. As indicated in the literature, employing multiple statistical techniques involving confounder-control or instrumental variables allows for richer analysis and comparison across fields (Adler et al., 2020). This versatility not only enhances causal inference validity but also facilitates interdisciplinary collaboration and cross-pollination, an essential element in the creation of population health studies. Equilibrating the trade-offs between different observational and experimental designs finally helps epidemiologists choose the most suitable designs to resolve specific research questions, thus optimizing the contribution of their findings to public health interventions (Figure 8.5).

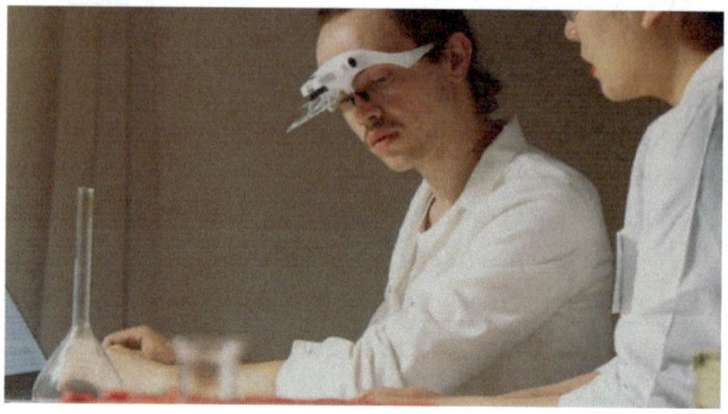

Figure 8.5. Experimental research designs.

Source: https://www.enago.com/academy/wp-content/uploads/2022/11/ResearchDesign_Global-1280x720.jpg.

8.2. Data Collection Methods

In epidemiology, data collection methods have a direct influence on the validity and reliability of study findings. Various methods may be employed, and each has consequences for study findings and interpretations. Surveys, interviews, and direct observation are common methods for obtaining quantitative and qualitative data that allow scientists to quantify health indicators and risk factors in populations. The choice of data collection approach is normally guided by the research question under consideration, the population under consideration, and available resources. For instance, while surveys can facilitate the collection of a substantial amount of data in a short period of time, their value is subject to the accuracy of questions and response rates. Furthermore, the application of technology in data collection, for example, the utilization of mobile health apps, has altered the data collection speed and quality, thus creating stronger statistical analysis in epidemiological studies. Further, nonrandomized study designs provide a less subtle approach to data collection within epidemiology, particularly for studies of causal inference. Techniques such as confounder-control methods, with regression adjustment and propensity score matching, are commonly employed in order to balance potential biases.

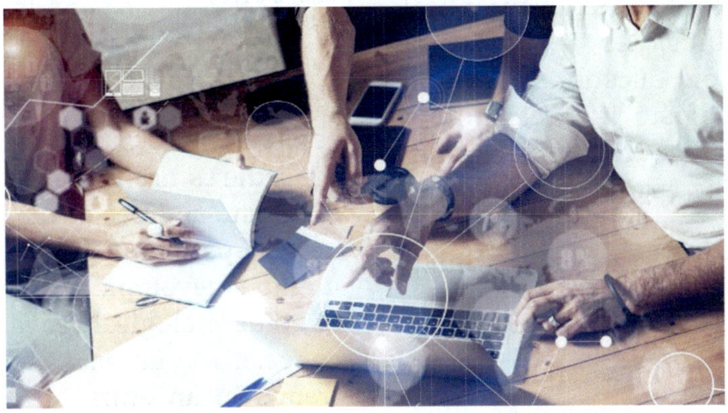

Figure 8.6. Data collection methods.

Source: https://cdn.prod.website-files.com/64022de562115a8189fe542a/6417b34d181646346e0028e6_Data-Collection-Methods-In-Research.jpeg.

Both of these processes involve a rigorous regard for variables potentially influencing outcome, thus enhancing internal validity of findings. There must be an awareness, however, that excessive reliance on a single methodology will be limiting since each method has limitations and biases inherent to it. For example, even though confounder-control offers a good platform to analyze, it cannot fully address unmeasured confounders, and so one is compelled to explore instrument-based methods, such as instrumental variables or regression discontinuity. The diverse methods have to be explored against existing studies so that one has a full picture of causal relationships (Adler et al., 2020). In addition, the role of capacity development in the processes of data collection cannot be overstated in epidemiology. Capacity development for epidemiological data collection and analysis capabilities by public health practitioners is vital through training workshops such as those conducted by bodies like the FAO with international research institutions. Such programs not only promote standardization of the practice but also facilitate practitioners to adopt state-of-the-art methods for data collection and analysis. For instance, the emphasis on modern epidemiological practices equips public health authorities with the tools needed to effectively respond to new emerging health challenges. The ongoing education and teamwork fostered by such workshops bridge gaps across disciplines and facilitate valid application of best practices in data collection. This interdisciplinary approach ultimately enhances the overall quality of epidemiological research and its public health policy and practice implications (Desvaux et al., 2009) (Figure 8.6).

8.2.1. Surveys and Questionnaires

Surveys and questionnaires are the most important tools in epidemiological studies, as they facilitate the collection of quantitative and qualitative information related to health outcomes and health-related behaviors. By facilitating inquiries of specific questions from a specified group, the tools are capable of generating responses that cover a range of variables, including lifestyle, environmental risk, and demographics. As a principal method of data collection, questionnaires and surveys aid epidemiologists in determining correlations and trends that are not clear from clinical observation. The process of creating such instruments, however, must be carefully prioritized in an effort to achieve maximum reliability and validity for the data collected. Carefully constructed questionnaires and surveys eventually contribute significantly towards maximizing our understanding of public health problems, allowing us to implement evidence-based interventions and policies. The ChiBS study highlights the versatile role of questionnaires and surveys in epidemiological research, particularly in examining the interaction between child obesity and chronic psychosocial stress. By utilizing both child- and parent-proxy-reported stress questionnaires and objective biomarkers in this longitudinal study, scientists explored how chronic stress can impact body composition among children. By taking a dual approach, it proves the merit of using diverse methodologies to collect a comprehensive view of health determinants. Notably, the study design allowed for the collection of additional contextual data, such as socio-economic status and dietary intake, through other questionnaires. Consequently, the integration of these various sources of data enhances the quality of findings and allows for specific interventions to prevent obesity in young people while emphasizing the difficulty of achieving honest responses in high-risk groups (Henauw et al., 2012). Moreover, the validity of questionnaires and surveys is based not only on their design but also on the resolution of potential limitations incorporated in data collection instruments. Mathematica Policy Research, Inc.'s project highlights the necessity of assessing current disability data collection procedures in order to enhance the credibility of such surveys. Through analysis of strengths and weaknesses within existing practice, researchers are better positioned to lead the development of innovative data improvement methods that allow for a more informed use of the information already being amassed. Continuous refinement of survey technique ensures that procedures are aligned with best practice and eliminate sources of bias, ultimately producing better epidemiological results. As such, survey method development tracks the development of epidemiological research, reflecting ongoing concern for understanding population health trends in an enlightened and evidence-based manner (Bleeker et al., 2006) (Figure 8.7).

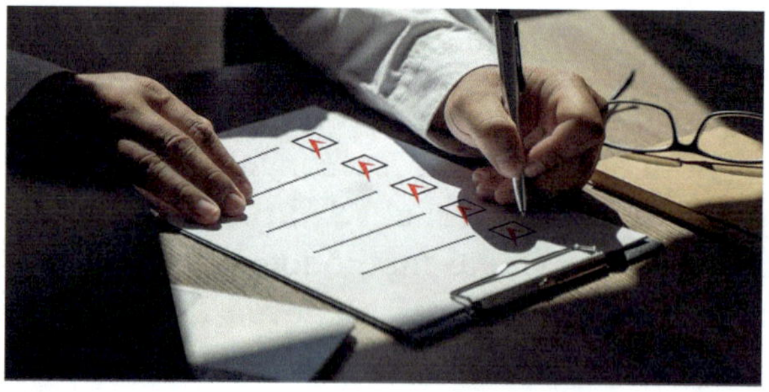

Figure 8.7. Survey and questionnaire.

Source: https://blog.justfeedback.com/wp-content/uploads/2024/01/36207911-1140x570.jpg.

8.2.2. Observational Data

In epidemiology, observational data are a fundamental cornerstone of identifying associations between exposures and health. They are collected in real-world settings free from the intervening manipulations of randomized controlled trials. This difference allows scientists to explore weak, subtle associations in heterogeneous populations. Observational studies commonly comprise a range of study designs, including cohort studies, case-control studies, and cross-sectional surveys, each able to answer unique questions. For instance, they are capable of determining trends in disease occurrence by eating habits or health consequences due to environmental factors. Finally, whether one is able to draw sound conclusions with observational data hinges on adequate design and analysis that enables researchers to identify potential causal relationships without the constraints of experimental research designs. The use of Mendelian randomization is a new tool in applying observational data to measure questions of causality. By leveraging genetic variants as instrumental variables, researchers are capable of excluding confounding biases characteristic of traditional observational studies. Such was aptly shown in studies on dietary elements and multiple sclerosis (MS), where authors utilized summary statistics to assess the possible causal effects of pork intake and fish/liver oil supplements on risk of MS (Ye et al., 2025). With great attention to analytical approaches such as the inverse-variance weighted method and sensitivity analyses, the study underscored the importance of robust statistical methods for ascertaining causal pathways. These applications show the ways in which observational data can be effectively used for deeper insights, moving from associations to useful evidence for public health interventions and preventive practices. Furthermore, internet search patterns provide an empirical basis for research into public knowledge and interest in medical interventions, as seen in studies of treatments for migraine. Based on Google Trends information, scientists pointed to significant fluctuations in public interest, particularly for the drug Nurtec, which reflect coincidence with marketing campaigns and regulatory approvals (Anthony et al., 2024). Nevertheless, search volume for migraine surgery reflected a steadily low level of interest, reflecting possible public education and awareness deficits regarding surgical options. These results illustrate the potential of observational data not only to measure health outcomes but also to comment on the wider implications of health communication measures. By recognizing how data like these provide insight into societal patterns and attitudes, epidemiologists can inform policy and education more effectively in order to contribute to better public health (Figure 8.8).

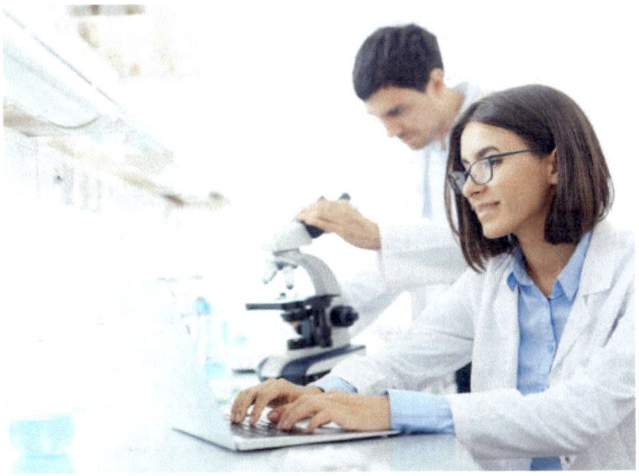

Figure 8.8. Observational study design.

Source: https://scientific-publishing.webshop.elsevier.com/wp-content/uploads/2021/08/22-Clinical-Questions-560x420.jpg.

8.2.3. Secondary Data Sources

Secondary sources of data in epidemiology are also important to boost the power of statistical analysis. Secondary data sources are data collected previously and, hence, available to be used for different purposes. Typically created from various disciplines like insurance records, clinical trials, public health publications, and observational studies, secondary data enable researchers to work with huge datasets without experiencing primary data collection logistical constraints. For example, insurance information can yield information about widespread health issues within various population groups, hence promoting a deeper understanding of disease trends. Nevertheless, researchers should be keenly aware of the intrinsic biases in these datasets, for example, selection bias and misclassification bias, as discussed in research regarding dog health surveillance systems, which emphasize caution regarding close scrutiny of data validity and representativeness (Brodbelt et al., 2014). Further, the cost-effectiveness and efficiency in epidemiological research are emphasized by the use of secondary data. By making use of readily accessible datasets, researchers will be able to reduce resource use and still conduct statistically valid analyses. Secondary sources such as national health surveys and electronic health records provide potential avenues for epidemiological research. These data typically have rich information on developments over time in disease trends. However, findings from secondary data must be interpreted with caution. Researchers are then responsible for working through the possible shortcomings of these data sets, specifically data integrity and the applicability of the demographic contexts in which the data were collected. Hence, adherence to recognized reporting guidelines, like the STROBE guidelines adapted to veterinary studies, is essential for enhancing the transparency and consistency of observational studies based on secondary data (Cevallos et al., 2016). Secondary data sources also enable interdisciplinary research across various fields of epidemiology. Integration of multiple datasets has the potential to offer a better comprehensive image of the health issue by consolidating knowledge across different populations and settings. Scientists may explore health disparities, assess the impact of interventions, or examine relationships between environmental factors and outcomes using sophisticated statistical analysis. However, the accuracy of such analysis rests on the selection of appropriate data consistent with research questions being considered, as judicious as it is supposed to be. As seen in the case of surveillance in canine health, the entire population is well represented in secondary data, so conclusions can be derived reliably. The need for continued improvement of data collection technology and development of stable frameworks for secondary use remains important to ensure that the findings contribute to adding value to the body of epidemiologic knowledge as well as public health interventions (Brodbelt et al., 2014).

8.3. Statistical Techniques in Epidemiology

The application of statistical techniques in epidemiology is central to the understanding of health-related events in populations. With varying study designs, e.g., cross-sectional, cohort, and case-control studies, epidemiologists can obtain and analyze data for recognizing patterns in disease occurrence. Statistical techniques are irreplaceable in ascertaining associations between exposures and outcomes, which allow the identification of disease risk factors. For instance, statistical analysis of prevalence rates can inform public health policy by bringing to the fore risk populations. Through these techniques, epidemiologists also ascertain the effectiveness of interventions employed in reducing disease incidence, thus providing evidence-based recommendations for health behavior. This reliance on sound statistical techniques places significant importance on precise data analysis in reaching meaningful conclusions from epidemiologic investigations. Additionally, the complexity of actual data demands advanced statistical techniques to manage confounding factors, interactions, and non-linear relationships among a range of factors. In the area of epidemiology, one has to apply analytical techniques that address these problems, as neglecting confounding variables may yield inaccurate results. Various statistical software packages enable researchers to convert output into useful conclusions in a proper manner, turning raw data into useful inferences.

A proper grasp of such techniques enables epidemiologists to conduct analyses that capture the heterogeneity of the health process. In addition, the creation of statistical strategies like molecular and genetic epidemiology has even enabled additional probing into disease dynamics at an even more intense level, revealing pathways that otherwise might have remained undetected employing conventional techniques. Integration of advanced statistical paradigms into epidemiology research is instrumental in further enhancing public health science. Recent research, such as research on Shiga toxin-producing *Escherichia coli* (STEC) in New Zealand, demonstrates statistical methods in use. The study used a culture-independent assay combined with statistical and microbiological techniques to analyze the incidence and transmission dynamics of STEC in dairy farms, highlighting the importance of good data analysis to reach public health interventions. The study found certain STEC serogroups to be prevalent in young dairy calves, an example of how statistical analysis can identify associations between animal husbandry and human health risk. The analysis of prevalence data helped scientists establish regional patterns and routes of transmission, which in turn helped design strategies for reducing risks. This is clear evidence of the critical role of statistical application in epidemiology, justifying its significance in guiding effective public health interventions and encouraging safe agricultural applications while protecting human health (Figure 8.9).

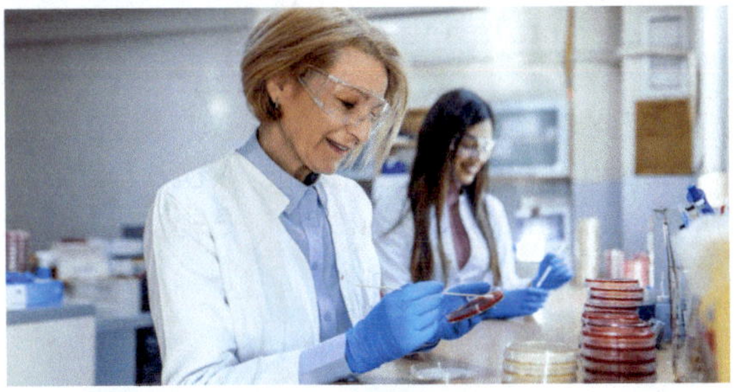

Figure 8.9. Statistical techniques.

Source: https://llri.in/wp-content/uploads/2024/06/BLOG-THUMBNAIL-5-2-1024x536.png.

8.3.1. Descriptive Statistics

Descriptive statistics form the foundation of statistical analysis in epidemiology, which provides important information to researchers. Descriptive statistics condense and present aspects of datasets to clearly outline information regarding disease incidence, prevalence, and outcome. Differences between populations or groups within studies can be addressed using normal measures such as means, medians, and modes. Moreover, measures of dispersion such as standard deviation and interquartile ranges give a sense of data variability, which is critical to accurately interpret epidemiological outcomes. As described in recent studies, descriptive statistics are applied extensively in evaluating clinical data in terms of diseases like community-acquired pneumonia (CAP), providing evidence of the significance of researchers being proficient in these simple methods to be able to make meaningful contributions towards the field of research (Chandler et al., 2017). In epidemiologic investigation, the application of descriptive statistics is not a crude operation; it contributes to the construction of methodologies and conclusions of studies. Descriptive statistics provide the groundwork for inferential analysis, such that trends and patterns can be identified before more complex models are applied. For instance, frequency distribution and percentage determination indicate the prevalence of some of the risk factors and thus guide public health programs. Most of the frequently reported descriptive statistics in clinical studies on CAP, according to the findings, were frequency (100%) and median values (73%) (Chandler et al., 2017).

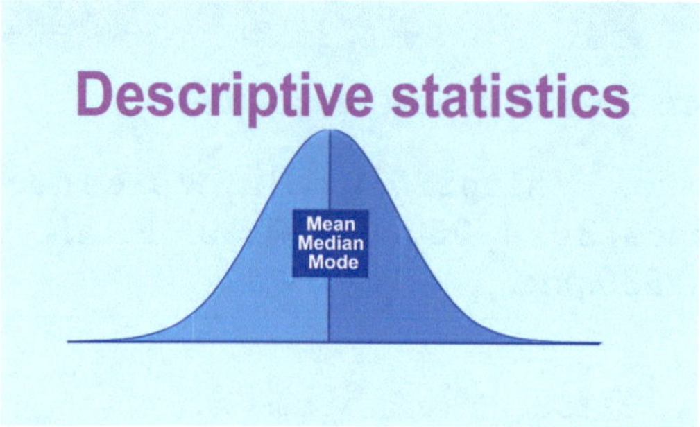

Figure 8.10. Descriptive statistics.

Source: https://miro.medium.com/v2/resize:fit:707/0*y7uQT5sY093YN6N3.png.

This prevalence suggests that a standard method in data analysis ensures findings are clearer and more applicable. Thus, overcoming descriptive statistics may enable new researchers so that they may be able to confidently manage more advanced statistical techniques . Secondly, the reliability of descriptive statistics relies on strict adherence to pre-prescribed reporting requirements, such as the STROBE statement, which demands meticulous data presentation in observational studies. This way ensures that scientists present their methods in an effective way, thus enhancing the reproducibility and accuracy of findings. By using descriptive statistics in conjunction with good reporting procedures, researchers can illuminate meaningful associations and trends in health data and thus contribute to the overall understanding of the disease epidemiology. Combining good statistical practices with good reporting not only enhances the transparency of studies but also facilitates effective decision-making by policymakers and public health practitioners. Overall, descriptive statistics form a crucial instrument within the statistical toolkit utilized in epidemiology and upon which further analyses and interpretations are built (Figure 8.10).

8.3.2. Inferential Statistics

Inferential statistics play a critical role in epidemiology because they allow scientists to make inferences about a population from sample information. Inferential statistics enable epidemiologists to make inferences about health-related status and outcomes based on variability and uncertainty in population behavior. Precisely, inferential techniques enable confidence interval estimation, hypothesis testing, and regression analysis, which are all part of establishing causal associations among risk factors and outcomes. The ability to make inferences from sample data regarding larger populations is invaluable, especially in research where a complete population assessment is unfeasible. Thus, the employment of inferential statistics not only enhances epidemiological findings' strength but also allows for the creation of effective public health interventions and policies to stop disease transmission and improve population health outcomes.

Application of instrumental variables (IV) for the establishment of causality is one of the most important elements of inferential statistics in epidemiology. The IV approach is focal, particularly where randomization in experiments is not feasible or hard to achieve. Literature reports that traditional methods of inference have largely relied on asymptotic approximations, creating structural modeling assumptions. Recent advances have offered randomness inference methods that rely on randomized treatment assignments as a point of analysis. This shift is a recognition of increasing awareness of the pitfalls in traditional statistical significance tests, which have a tendency to mask the nuance of causal inference. Through the integration of these newer methodologies, epidemiological research is in a position to generate outputs not only statistically meaningful but also of substantive value, thus enhancing the capacity of the discipline to address health inequalities (Kang et al., 2018; Abelson et al., 2012). Controversy over statistical significance testing also calls for close scrutiny of inferential statistics in epidemiological research. Critics have argued that such tests promote a mechanistic approach to decision-making without taking the needed step of distinguishing between statistical and substantive significance. Such a shortcoming can lead to misinterpreting the meaning of statistical findings, potentially reducing valuable insight into health concerns in the public. Taking such limitations into consideration, epidemiologists are forced to be more advanced in interpreting statistical results, with standard errors and confidence intervals as tools for inference. This shift towards a broader appreciation of inferential statistics has the potential to foster greater critical thinking and enhance the quality of epidemiological research. The redefinition of statistical practice in the field then has the potential to make research findings more relevant and applicable to real public health issues (Abelson et al., 2012) (Figure 8.11).

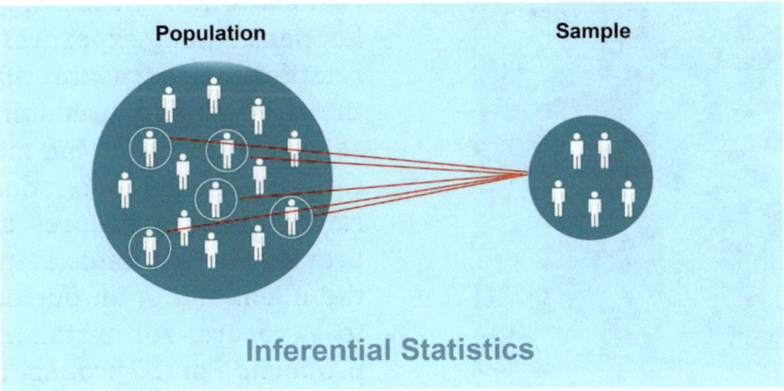

Figure 8.11. Inferential statistics.

Source: https://www.analytixlabs.co.in/wp-content/uploads/2022/08/Inferential-Statistics-analytix-labs.jpeg.

8.3.3. Multivariate Analysis

Multivariate analysis is one of the main statistical instruments in the epidemiological field that enables researchers to investigate complex relationships between many variables simultaneously. It is the main approach, since in every study, there is a multifactor etiology of health outcomes, which is affected by a variety of connected determinants from demographic, environmental, and biological perspectives. With techniques such as multiple regression, factor analysis, and multivariate analysis of variance (MANOVA), epidemiologists are better able to uncover patterns and relationships that would be unattainable if only univariate analyses were employed. The capacity to model such complicated relationships increases the ability to predict more accurately and to make disease etiology a more understandable phenomenon, ultimately leading to improved public health interventions and policy. One of the significant applications of multivariate analysis in epidemiology involves its function in monitoring patterns in health through surveillance data. The effective utilization of statistical techniques enables the detection of aberrations within health outcomes, which is a significant element in identifying outbreaks as well as analyzing patterns of disease over time. A case of application of the Farrington algorithm and Poisson cumulative sum schemes for rabies surveillance of the fox population is presented by Held et al. (2007). Such techniques not only account for seasonal patterns and spatial factors but also enable retrospective examination, which informs health authorities to make informed decisions. Incorporation of multivariate techniques thus enhances the sophistication of epidemiological surveillance and ultimately supports effective public health interventions.

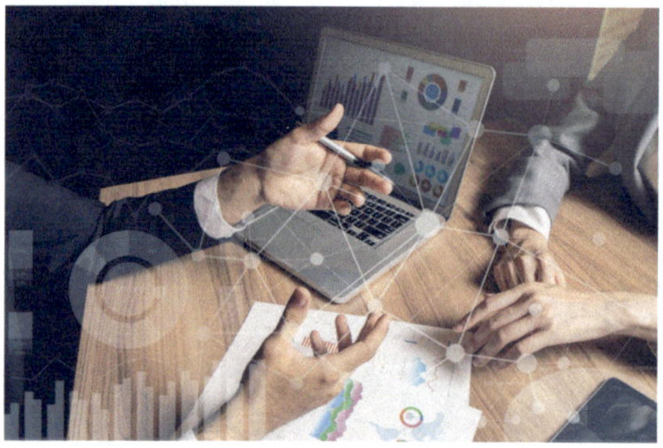

Figure 8.12. Multivariate analysis.

Source: https://www.mygreatlearning.com/blog/wp-content/uploads/2020/07/iStock-861092542.jpg.

The utility of multivariate analysis also extends into diagnostic test evaluation that supports decision-making at the level of healthcare. Especially in situations where there are several tests with different thresholds that have to be contrasted, multivariate approaches offer a stable basis for analysis. As Cooper et al. (2018) suggest, an application of a bivariate network meta-analysis model allows us to make a joint comparison of the efficacy of such tests as the Mini-Mental State Examination (MMSE) and the Montreal Cognitive Assessment (MoCA). By comparing multiple diagnostic criteria simultaneously, scientists are able to establish that certain tests work better under certain conditions, enhancing clinical judgment. Thus, the application of multivariate analysis in this context not only enhances data evaluation but also profoundly influences diagnostic accuracy and patient outcome (Figure 8.12).

8.4. Measures of Association

In the discipline of epidemiology, an understanding of the concept of measure of association is necessary to interpret what happens among exposures and health outcome relationships. Measures of association quantify the strength and direction of such associations so that researchers can make inferences about causality. Risk ratios, odds ratios, and hazard ratios are all measures commonly used that provide varying kinds of information regarding the likelihood of an outcome event in relation to exposure. For instance, a risk ratio is the proportion of the probability of the event in the exposed group compared to the non-exposed group and gives a direct interpretation of risk. With these metrics, scientists are in a better position to assess public health interventions more effectively and progress evidence-based practice, illustrating the pivotal role of good statistical methods in informing health policy and clinical practice. Choice of appropriate measures of association is important in ensuring the validity of epidemiologic research. Various study designs, whether observational or experimental, dictate the type of measure that should be applied in order to accurately quantify the relationship between variables. For instance, risk ratios are the preferred option in cohort studies because of their ease of interpretation and straightforward application in measuring time-to-event outcomes. Alternatively, case-control studies use odds ratios most frequently as a measure of the odds of exposure in cases relative to controls. Accordingly, authors must also consider the resultant biases and confounding variables that can distort their conclusions, thereby necessitating careful methodological preparation. Since different measures can yield different conclusions about the same associations, understanding their details helps to address the misinterpretations that might ultimately impact public health claims. Furthermore, the context in which measures of association are applied remains paramount in the interpretation of epidemiological data. From studies that examine area effects on health, the role of ecological settings is emphasized across a number of health outcomes, with the demand for inclusive designs of analysis. Notably, the inclusion of multilevel modeling techniques allows assessment of the interaction between individual-level contexts and broader socioeconomic environments and provides a more sophisticated investigation of determinants of health. As evidenced by current findings, the spatial scope and measures of exposure significantly influence observed associations. Accordingly, researchers must exercise caution in selecting the appropriate context and method to ensure the complexity of the determinants of health is portrayed accurately, ultimately leading to more effective public health programs and policy-making (Adler et al., 2020; Cangelosi et al., 2001) (Figure 8.13).

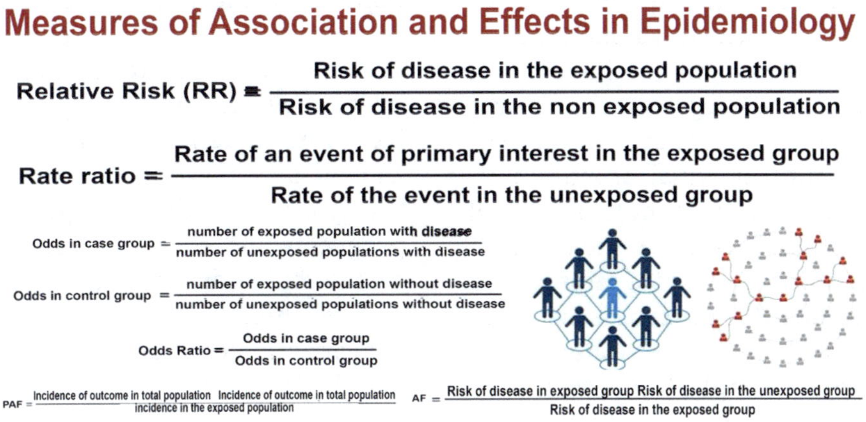

Figure 8.13. Measures of Association and effects in epidemiology.

Source: https://microbenotes.com/wp-content/uploads/2024/10/Measures-of-Association-and-Effects-in-Epidemiology.jpeg.

8.4.1. Risk Ratios

It is essential within epidemiological studies to understand risk ratios since they provide an easy measure of association between exposure and outcome. Risk ratios, which are defined as the probability of an event's occurrence in the exposed relative to the non-exposed group, make relative risk interpretable within various health scenarios. Since scientists can express the magnitude of associations between disease incidence and single risk factors using risk ratios, these are able to convey the strength of associations in a meaningful way. Such an approach has been seen to be particularly valuable in infectious disease epidemiology, where ascertaining the impact of vaccination campaigns, e.g., as observed with the Serengeti Health Initiative, can illustrate marked contrasts in health status among populations found within and outside zones of vaccination. These investigations underscore the importance of understanding and reporting risk ratios clearly to guide public health intervention and action (Younce et al., 2018). Additionally, the application of statistical models in the estimation of risk ratios has evoked controversy on the efficacy and applicability of several measures of association, particularly in cross-sectional studies. In the past, odds ratios have been used, but with more recent practices emphasizing the utilization of prevalence ratios (PR) because they are potentially more intuitive as relative risk in certain populations. This shift from the utilization of odds ratios to PR is not without difficulty, in that issues with model convergence and adequate statistical tools being available typically prevent straightforward methods of calculation. Nonetheless, the estimation of PR directly from logistic regression not only simplifies but also ensures that calculated risks are in closer proximity to actual probabilities, hence increasing the validity of epidemiological findings (Bastos et al., 2014). The inclusion of risk ratios in epidemiology serves to improve the comprehension of health risk processes more effectively, hence enabling more informed public health decisions. For example, the detection of significant differences in awareness of animal cases of rabies among communities bordering vaccination zones illustrates the way risk ratios can direct education campaign efforts. Such differences underscore the importance of using powerful statistical measures, like risk ratios, to estimate the sustainability of health interventions over time. Researchers who take an integrated approach to the analysis of risk ratios stand a better chance of evaluating the effectiveness of public health interventions, and the applied use of their research transcends academia to reach real-life health policy and outcomes. This intersection of statistical metrics and day-to-day use is the soul of the benefit of risk ratios to public health (Younce et al., 2018) (Figure 8.14).

$$\text{Relative Risk (RR)} = \frac{\text{Risk of disease in the exposed population}}{\text{Risk of disease in the non} - \text{exposed population}}$$

Figure 8.14. Relative risk formula.

Source: https://microbenotes.com/wp-content/uploads/2024/10/Relative-Risk-Formula.jpg.

8.4.2. Odds Ratios

Odds ratio (OR) is an important statistical indicator utilized heavily in epidemiology for quantifying the association between exposure and outcome. Through comparison of the probability of an event happening (e.g., disease occurrence) in an exposed vs. an unexposed group, researchers can elucidate potential risk factors. For instance, in a study of toxic air pollutants, the data employed binary logistic regression to test the relationship between maternal exposure to lead and toluene before pregnancy and adverse pregnancy outcomes like preterm delivery and low birth weight. The ORs of associations in such analyses can be highly critical indicators, guiding public health programs and clinical practice. When properly calculated, odds ratios can define the extent of relationships and ultimately contribute to the prioritization of interventions intended to lower health risk, making the value of this method in epidemiologic analysis (Carman et al., 2009). In the evaluation of public health data, odds ratios can also reveal important demographic trends otherwise left unrevealed. For instance, in the study of HIV prevalence in Zambia, application of a generalized geo-additive semi-parametric model yielded results that were better than typical analytical approaches. Spatial auto-correlation was captured, and confounding risk factors such as age, gender, and geographical area were adjusted for by scientists, enabling them to precisely adjust HIV prevalence estimates. This advanced understanding of dynamics in a situation puts odds ratios center stage in the depiction of health outcome complexity across populations. By illuminating the interaction between variables and how they might influence prevalence, odds ratios help us to gain a deeper appreciation of the disease mechanisms, greatly enhancing the quality of epidemiological evidence (Cappuccio et al., 2008). Moreover, the application of odds ratios is extended to public health policy formulation and intervention development. With the determination and quantification of the relationship between risk determinants and health outcomes, ORs provide a concrete basis for the allocation of resources and targeted action. With the hazardous air pollutants study, specific odds ratios can help policymakers establish regulations that aim to reduce exposure to harmful environmental factors. Similarly, in the estimation of HIV prevalence in different geographic environments, the explanation of prevalence variation as it pertains to demographic factors informs strategic health responses. The implications highlight the pivotal role of odds ratios in not just formulating scientific knowledge but also in disseminating research findings into actionable public health interventions so that health priorities remain empirically informed (Carman et al., 2009; Cappuccio et al., 2008) (Figure 8.15).

$$\text{Odds in case group} = \frac{\text{number of exposed population with disease}}{\text{number of unexposed populations with disease}}$$

$$\text{Odds in control group} = \frac{\text{number of exposed population without disease}}{\text{number of unexposed populations without disease}}$$

$$\text{Odds Ratio} = \frac{\text{Odds in case group}}{\text{Odds in control group}}$$

Figure 8.15. Odds ratio formula.

Source: https://microbenotes.com/wp-content/uploads/2024/10/Odds-Ratio-Formula.jpg.

8.4.3. Attributable Risk

Attributable risk (AR) is a critical epidemiological concept referring to that portion of disease occurrence in the exposed group that is due to an individual risk factor. Statistical estimation thereof enables one to estimate the impact on public health of such exposures, and thus it is critical in the formulation of preventive strategies. By quantifying AR, scientists can determine to what extent a specific disease, e.g., cardiovascular disease or infections, is directly caused by modifiable risk factors such as smoking or lack of personal hygiene. Measurement not only clarifies the cause-and-effect relationship between disease and exposure, but it is also necessary for planning resources and decision-making regarding health policy to minimize risk factors in populations. The estimation of AR is largely dependent on incidence data obtained from epidemiological research, where careful methodology must be employed to avoid inaccuracies. Population-based cohort studies or case-control studies are often used to obtain these estimates and highlight the importance of sound data collection procedures. Careful conduct of such studies, as advocated by guidelines like the STROBE statement, increases the validity of findings pertinent to AR. These standards are necessary guidelines to report observational studies in order to achieve completeness and transparency. Following predetermined report protocols is thus crucial to obtaining accurate estimations of attributable risk that can be employed to inform upcoming studies and interventions (Cevallos et al., 2016). The investigation of the relationships between attributable risk and healthcare burdens is highly crucial in the understanding of the healthcare burden exacted by specific diseases. For instance, research into infections like Clostridium difficile illustrates how attributable risks can signify to the stakeholders the significant impact of such infections on healthcare resources. Systematic review of literature showed that the hospital-acquired rate of C. difficile infection not only affects patient outcomes but is also linked with increased hospital duration of stay and increased healthcare costs (Balkenende et al., 2020). This relationship is important in stressing the importance of responsible estimation of attributable risk as it forms the foundation of public health intervention priorities towards the prevention of infection incidence as well as its resultant impacts on healthcare systems. Understanding these dynamics guides the institution of effective prevention policies and resource allocation within the clinical setting.

8.5. Confounding and Bias

In epidemiological research, bias and confounding are issues that will significantly affect the validity of study findings. Confounding occurs when there is an extraneous factor that has an impact on both the independent and dependent variables, creating a spurious relationship that can conceal the true relationship under research. For instance, in researching lung cancer and smoking, such confounding variables as age, socio-economic status, and even genetic predispositions may influence results if not accounted for. This makes it important to employ robust statistical analysis to account for potential confounders, thereby making the study outcomes more solid. The STROBE guidelines highlight standard reporting, which assists researchers in dealing with such issues in observational studies in a systematic manner and increases trust in epidemiological findings through transparency and methodological reliability (Cevallos et al., 2016). Bias, however, refers to systematic deviations from truth in findings or measurements, which can arise from various sources, starting from study design and selection of participants. The most prevalent form of bias is selection bias, in which the sample population is not an accurate reflection of the population under observation. This holds particularly for nonrandomized trials, whereby members will self-select into groups and controls based on specific characteristics. Such biases can mask the true effect of an intervention and can misguide public health policy and practice. As noted in recent literature, proper correction of such biases is crucial to make good causal inferences in epidemiology. By employing good strategies to minimize bias, scientists can provide improved perspectives into health consequences and interventions and, in turn, maximize public health interventions and public funds (Adler et al., 2020). To properly address confounding and bias, scientists must apply both confounder-control and instrument-based study designs, the former and latter of which have their respective strengths and weaknesses. Confounder-control methods such as regression adjustment or propensity score matching allow for the explicit control of confounders in statistical models, effectively keeping the relation of interest constant.

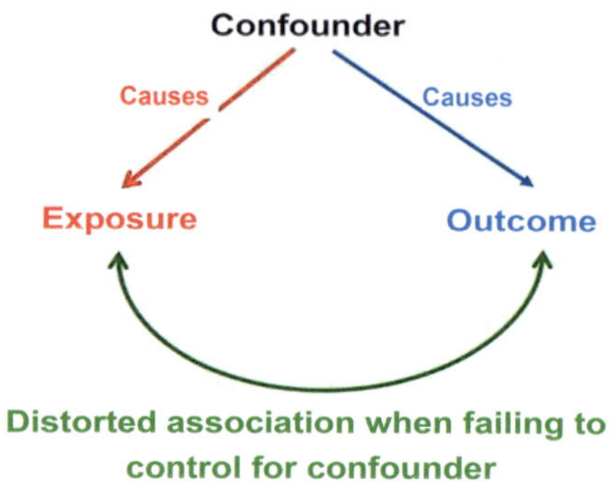

Figure 8.16. The principle of confounding; the confounder makes the exposure more likely and, in some way, independently modifies the outcome, making it appear that there is an association between the exposure and the outcome when there is none, or masking a true association.

Source: https://catalogofbias.org/wp-content/uploads/sites/2/2018/05/Picture2-e1534244135583.jpg.

However, these methods rely strongly on the accurate identification and measurement of confounders, which might be unachievable in practice. On the other hand, instrument-based methods like instrumental variables and regression discontinuity offer alternative avenues for causal inference from natural experiments or exposure differences. Although these methods may be capable of adjusting for unobserved confounders, they have assumptions that can make their validity questionable. Balancing such methodological approaches is key to advancing epidemiological studies and determining that research findings mirror causal relationships in populations (Cevallos et al., 2016; Adler et al., 2020) (Figure 8.16).

8.5.1. Types of Confounding Variables

In the area of epidemiological research, confounding factors play a critical role in establishing the validity of the findings. Confounding exists because the extraneous factor is linked to the exposure and outcome of interest and may lead to a spurious or overestimated association between the two. A variety of types of confounding factors exist, including demographic factors, socioeconomic status, and lifestyle. For instance, age and sex can have a major effect on risk of exposure and susceptibility to disease and are therefore omnipresent confounders of health research. Failing to control for such factors, scientists may draw incorrect conclusions that do not accurately reflect the true causal relation. This serves to emphasize the importance of good study planning and analytical approach to identify and control for hidden confounders in an effort to establish sound epidemiological proof. Among the standard practices of addressing confounding variables in observational studies is the use of confounder-control strategies, which involve statistical strategies such as regression adjustment and propensity score matching. These strategies aim to regulate the impact of the principal exposure variable by systematically adjusting for known confounding variables. Regression methods, for example, allow researchers to identify covariates that may bias the outcomes and therefore provide a better estimate of variable relationships. However, there are limitations to the application of these methods. Statistical controls used may force one to make certain assumptions about the relationships between variables, and these are usually hard to validate. Researchers must identify such trade-offs in internal validity and statistical power and reflect on the setting of their study carefully in order to make appropriate decisions regarding their analytical approach (Adler et al., 2020). Besides confounder-control methods, researchers also use instrument-based methods to minimize confounding impacts. Instrumental variable analysis, regression discontinuity designs, and differences-in-differences methods serve as alternatives that yield causal results even when there are unmeasured confounders.

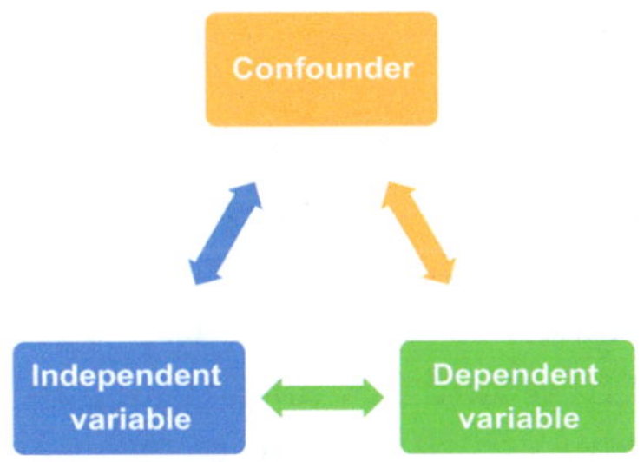

Figure 8.17. Confounding variable.

Source: https://i0.wp.com/statisticsbyjim.com/wp-content/uploads/2018/09/confounding.png?w=837&ssl=1.

These methods rely on certain assumptions, say, the strength of the instrument and its independence from confounding, which must be properly assessed. While instrument-based methods can enhance causal inference in epidemiologic studies, they also carry their own subtleties, involving careful interpretation of results. According to Cevallos et al. (2016), as researchers navigate the intricacies of observational studies, adherence to established reporting guidelines, such as the STROBE statement, can facilitate transparency and rigor in study design, thereby aiding in the identification and discussion of confounding variables. The convergence of various methods and guidelines aims to foster a common understanding of confounding and promote robust epidemiological research (Figure 8.17).

8.5.2. Sources of Bias in Epidemiological Studies

The prevalence of bias in epidemiologic studies will significantly influence the validity of study results, which will lead to faulty conclusions and uninformed public health actions. Selection bias is a frequent reason for bias, as the study population is not representative of the overall population. This could occur as a result of non-random sampling methods such as convenience sampling or self-selection, leading to biased results. For instance, when participants are sampled by researchers from a specific population or social group, outcomes cannot be generalized across groups. Also, selection bias can propagate to downstream analyses, leading to false positives between the outcome and exposure. It would require rigorous sampling practices and stratification for the participants, such that a fair representation of the population is obtained, which is important in making an informed conclusion while carrying out epidemiological studies. Information bias is also a crucial source of bias, and it occurs when there is systematic overestimation or underestimation of exposure or outcome variables.

This could be due to participants' false self-reporting, faulty calibration of measuring instruments, or differential misclassification because participants know their health status. For instance, disease-diagnosed individuals may remember their past exposures more than healthy controls and hence tend to over-report more, which can cause a divergence between reports and reality. Such divergence can bias the perceived associations between risk factors and health outcomes. In order to minimize information bias, researchers are required to employ rigorous data collection instruments, such as validated questionnaires and objective measure scales, to gather accurate and standardized data in groups, and hence enhance the reliability of study outcomes. Moreover, publication bias is another significant source of bias in epidemiological literature since studies with statistically significant results are over-represented compared to studies with null results. This creates an imbalanced representation of the evidence present, and this can lead to intervention overestimation of the effectiveness or association among variables. A study that conducted a review of systematic reviews found that 43% had formally examined publication bias, with numerous reasons for this not being tackled, like low numbers of studies and low awareness of the biases (Ayorinde et al., 2020). Additionally, scientists can consciously or unconsciously assign greater significance to studies supporting their hypotheses and overlook those that contradict them, leading to a biased view of evidence. For the sake of integrity in epidemiological research, it is quite crucial to adopt openness in study reports and strive deliberately to publish negative findings, and this results in a better understanding of public health status (Lewnard et al., 2019) (Figure 8.18).

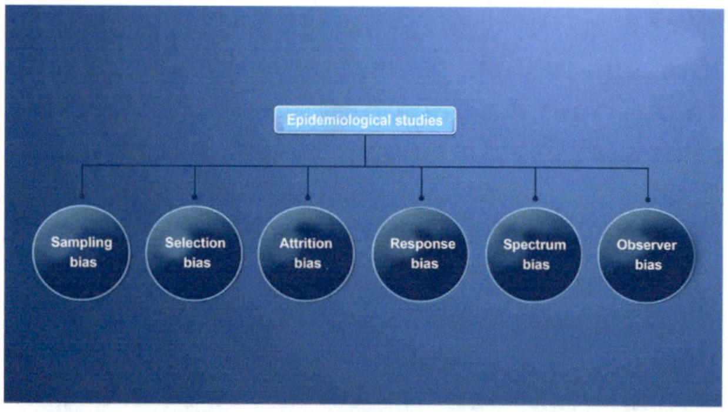

Figure 8.18. Bias in epidemiological studies.

Source: https://www.jove.com/files/media/science-education/science-education-thumbs/17609.jpg.

8.5.3. Methods to Control for Confounding and Bias

Methods to manage confounding and bias in epidemiologic research are required to preserve the validity of findings. Confounding occurs when an external factor has an influence on both the exposure and the outcome and obscures the true relationship between them. For this, researchers employ statistical techniques such as stratification more frequently, by dividing the study population into strata based on possible confounders. For instance, in occupational epidemiological studies, identification of the healthy worker survivor effect (HWSE) is critical. G-methods, or novel statistical strategies, are capable of addressing time-varying confounding and dampening the effect of HWSE, thus providing improved estimations for target parameters in populations with different characteristics (N/A, 2025). Application of these methods indicates the value of researchers providing clear study design descriptions for enhancing the quality of their evidence. The other extremely popular method for the control of confounding and bias is the randomized controlled trial (RCT), which remains the "gold standard" in epidemiological research. The participants in RCTs are assigned to treatment and control groups at random, thereby effectively preventing confounding by the even spread of both known and unknown factors within groups. But when it is not possible to conduct RCTs or is ethically not permissible, observational studies become inevitable. In these cases, the application of strong statistical analysis, including matching techniques and regression analysis, may be employed to balance the effect of confounders. The Strengthening the Reporting of Observational Studies in Epidemiology (STROBE) guideline provides a list of guidelines to enhance transparency and rigor in reporting results of observational studies and ensure that biases have been addressed and reported appropriately (Cevallos et al., 2016). This is of extreme importance for scientific credibility and public trust in epidemiologic findings. Finally, one should also value the worth of sensitivity analyses for ascertaining the stability of study outcomes against bias. Sensitivity analysis involves modifying assumptions or conditions of the statistical model to see how variation over these modifications affects the results. This method is particularly useful in ascertaining whether the conclusions reached are sensitive to confounding variables or biases. By applying this technique, researchers can ascertain how confident they can be of their results. Along with sensitivity analysis, employing methods such as inverse probability weighting can also reverse the effect of confounding and bias, particularly in observational studies when randomization is not possible. An unambiguous understanding and application of these different methodologies are needed in advocating the credibility and application of epidemiological research results to public health policy and clinical practice.

8.6. Interpretation of Epidemiological Data

Epidemiologic data analysis is a critical component of public health trend interpretation and policy-making. Underpinning the interpretation is the application of statistical methods that transform raw facts into meaningful information. Epidemiologists make use of descriptive and inferential statistics to summarize the occurrence of public health events and relate factors of exposure to disease outcomes. Through pattern identification from such analysis, researchers can identify potential risk factors or trends that need to be addressed by public health. However, the validity of such interpretations is heavily contingent upon methodological accuracy and the avoidance of error types such as overgeneralization or misconstruction of correlation with causation. Epidemiologists' critical evaluation of these aspects allows them to make conclusions from evidence that are actionable, ultimately leading to preventive interventions tailored to specific populations. In addition, the' validity and accuracy of epidemiologic inferences are also influenced by intrinsic limitations of the field, in addition to data error and sampling issues of data collection. Variation in sources of data, reporting trends, and populations can conceal the true patterns in disease and health outcomes. Most significantly, the inclusion of more advanced methodologies such as machine learning and multi-omics is proving to be revolutionary in making epidemiologic studies more accurate. For instance, Kang et al. (2020) respond to quality control in metabolomics studies with the assertion that a reliable methodological framework is capable of greatly strengthening interpretation validity. This becomes imperative for epidemiologists to not only select appropriate statistical analysis but also exercise care over potential pitfalls that may compromise their conclusions, thus ensuring their inferences reflect true and authentic health information. In addition, ethics are a core issue in the analysis of epidemiological data, particularly in studies of toxic substances.

As highlighted in Cranor et al. (1990), researchers must be certain to know and discuss normative issues that arise at the time of analysis. They include ethical considerations of risk assessments and the potential impacts on society upon disclosure of results to the public. For instance, neglecting to put epidemiological information about exposure to toxic substances into perspective may result in unnecessary alarm or misappropriation of resources. Therefore, effective communication plans are vital to interpreting complicated statistical results into understandable data for stakeholders such as policymakers and the general public. By integrating moral consideration alongside statistical subtlety, epidemiologists can potentially ensure that their inference meets scientific criteria and resonates with public concerns, ultimately reinforcing the public's faith in epidemiology.

8.6.1. Statistical Significance vs. Clinical Significance

For epidemiology, the distinction between statistical significance and clinical significance ought to be closely noted. Statistical significance is generally used to indicate the likelihood of a finding or association observed in data not occurring by chance and is typically measured through p-values. Though statistical significance is a very important benchmark in hypothesis testing, it does not necessarily tell us about the practical relevance of findings within a clinical context. For instance, a statistically significant result will indicate that there is a difference across treatments, but the difference may be so minimal that it makes no difference in practice. Thus, researchers must think critically about the salience of their findings, beyond statistical significance per se, to what their implications are for patient treatment and care. Clinical significance, in contrast, speaks to the practical importance of an effect of treatment or intervention to clinical practice. While statistical significance can detect associations within data, it is clinical significance that specifies the applicability of such findings to patient populations. For example, in cancer medicine, an intervention may be statistically significant for enhancing survival durations in patients with hepatic cell carcinoma (HCC), but a minimal difference in survival duration does not necessarily equate to a quantifiable benefit to patients and families, leading to concerns about the utility of interventions. This reflection is of specific significance in the case of high-dimensional molecular information and models involving clinical predictors, as the actual added value of such information is more likely to be representative of its clinical relevance rather than its statistical nature (Boulesteix et al., 2010). Apart from distinguishing between these two forms of significance, there is also a need for rigorous evaluations of prognostic models in which both statistical and clinical factors are considered. One such need is illustrated in research comparing the performance of several staging systems for HCC, pointing out that statistical measures themselves may not be sufficient in deciding on treatment (Göke et al., 2012). The ordering of staging systems by their performance as predictors of survival rates, for instance, is illustrated to necessitate a demonstration of how such systems impact clinical outcomes in practice. Correspondingly, a balanced viewpoint that considers both statistical data and clinical implications enables clinicians and researchers to make very informed choices that improve patient care ultimately. Understanding the limits of statistical significance provides the entry point into greater immersion in the realities of clinical significance and emphasizes the worth of thorough evaluation in epidemiological research (Figure 8.19).

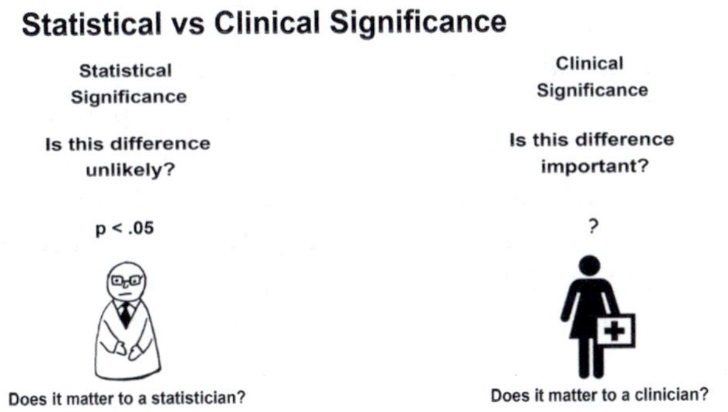

Figure 8.19. Statistical significance vs. clinical significance.

Source: https://i.ytimg.com/vi/E7934CSKkN4/maxresdefault.jpg.

8.6.2. Confidence Intervals

Confidence intervals (CIs) are at the heart of epidemiology since they give a means of estimating population parameter uncertainty. In that they give an interval over which the actual parameter is likely to be located, CIs add to the meaning of statistical findings. For instance, in the analysis of mortality rates using the Standardized Mortality Ratio (SMR), CIs may demonstrate the precision of observed as opposed to expected rates in a standard population. The construction of these intervals, particularly for Poisson-distributed data, is critical as the underlying distributions affect estimation as well as results interpretation. Scientists have been arguing over a number of methods to ascertain such confidence limits so that scientists can clearly inform the reliability of their epidemiological estimates, ultimately resulting in more informed public health decision-making (Wang et al., 2002). In the analysis of epidemiological data, confidence intervals assist in gaining a more precise comprehension of the variability of potential results inherent in statistical estimates. This is especially true when one is dealing with cases where the observed data may differ randomly or due to bias. For example, by calculating confidence intervals with the parameter of the Poisson, researchers are in a position to express not just the magnitude of the effect but also uncertainty over that magnitude, which is necessary when one is calculating risk and making decisions about public health. The application of different techniques, such as conventional normal approximations and chi-square distribution, enables researchers to estimate more precise confidence intervals of the SMR. These intervals, thus, are not statistical artifacts; they are the important bounds within which public health policy and preventive interventions may be formulated (Kang et al., 2018). The utility of confidence intervals is more than mere statistical analysis; it is a means of communication that informs stakeholders about the reliability of epidemiologic findings. By presenting a quantitative measure of uncertainty, CIs enable scientists to communicate the likelihood of their estimates. This is particularly necessary when reporting epidemiologic investigations in which direct causal inference may be obscured by confounding or bias. In such applications as occupational epidemiology, interpretation of SMR based on confidence intervals can have regulatory policy and workplace standards implications. Moreover, developments in statistical approaches and simulation studies have made it possible to calculate more accurate confidence interval estimates. With researchers striving to create more accurate and computationally meaningful methods, the utility of CIs in summarizing uncertainty in epidemiologic data remains a cornerstone of sound public health research (Wang et al., 2002).

8.6.3. Limitations of Statistical Analysis

Statistical analysis is a critical part of epidemiologic studies, but it has limitations intrinsic to it that must be recognized. One of the fundamental limitations might well be excessive reliance on assumptions that underlie numerous statistical methods. For example, when making causal inferences, most strategies are dependent on assumptions that are empirically untestable and therefore prone to biases. Researchers employ nonrandomized study designs, including confounder-control approaches such as regression adjustment or propensity score matching. However, these methods could not adequately deal with hidden bias or confounding variables, further making it challenging to form valid conclusions. The balance between using confounder-control and instrument-based methods, as established in research, identifies the challenge in maintaining both internal validity and the results' generalizability. Therefore, the inherent restriction in statistical analysis has a far-reaching effect on the results of epidemiological studies and the subsequent public health interventions derived from these outcomes. A second limitation arises from the issue of data quality and measurement bias, which can have adverse effects on statistical results. Accurate data collection is paramount to the validity of epidemiology studies, yet various factors, such as misreporting or incomplete data, have the potential to introduce bias. For instance, in veterinary epidemiology, there have to be specific reporting regulations that ensure observational studies clearly report their methods and findings. The adaptation of items in the STROBE statement to enhance how the unique aspects of veterinary research are communicated is a reflection on how statistical regulations can adapt to address challenges pertaining to data integrity and reporting quality (Ersbøll et al., 2016). When there are problems in data quality, the validity and application of the statistical analyses decrease, yielding conclusions that can misrepresent the actual relationships between health outcomes, exposures, or interventions. Additionally, the selection of statistical methodology can also hide the limitations inherent in epidemiological research. Different disciplines can have different priorities of study designs and statistical approaches, creating barriers to interdisciplinary dialogue and collaboration. This is so in causal inference approaches, in which varying methods can cause ambiguity or misinterpretation of findings across researchers from different disciplines. Although openness to selecting statistical approaches is necessary, it may also make comparative studies across research a burden. The literature on causal inference necessitates an in-depth understanding of different statistical approaches and hence supports methodological pluralism and critical evaluation of existing studies. By creating a common understanding of these limitations, researchers can enhance the quality of epidemiologic studies and minimize the chances of forming incorrect conclusions (Adler et al., 2020).

Summary

In summarizing the critical role of statistical methods in epidemiology, it is critical to evaluate the various statistical methods employed in the study of health-related data. Statistical methods not only provide a framework for the comprehension of disease distribution and determinants but also enable researchers to provide meaningful conclusions from their results. For instance, the use of quasi-experimental designs and meta-analysis strategies highlights the challenge introduced by confounding variables and biases in combining findings from studies. By using rigorous design techniques, researchers ensure that the results are both valid and reliable, thereby adding to the body of knowledge in epidemiological research. Therefore, a good understanding of statistical techniques is imperative to epidemiologists who aim to not only detect patterns but also inform public health interventions. Moreover, the influence of demographic variables, such as gender and severity of functional impairment, can influence epidemiological findings in different populations. As cited in other research, such as that focusing on the severity of shoulder pain in adhesive capsulitis, gender may contribute to the role in determining the severity of pain and distribution, as a result of the multifaceted relationship between biological indicators and health outcomes (Candela et al., 2017). This is the significance of obtaining deep demographic considerations that are to be implemented in statistical analysis. It becomes significant that epidemiologists adjust their approaches to enable such complexities to be captured so that the summations that are obtained are sensitive to varying population characteristics. Lastly, the integration of deep demographic data into statistical analysis strengthens the evidence base in favor of epidemiological conclusions and ultimately enables more effective public health intervention. Essentially, the inferences derived from statistical methods in epidemiology determine not only successes but also limitations of health research. The synthesis of results from quasi-experimental studies demonstrates the interactive nuances of bias and confounding issues, which require precise methodological controls in analysis (Aloe et al., 2017). Epidemiologists thus need to update their approaches on a regular basis in order to be able to keep up with evolving research environments and advancing levels of health-related issues. The importance of a meticulous and methodologically stringent method cannot be overstated because such activities contribute to more accurate interpretations and public health policy implications. Therefore, with advancement in the discipline on the move, compliance with stringent statistical analysis will remain at the forefront in building knowledge in epidemiology and improving health outcomes globally.

Statistical methods in epidemiology are also highly critical in identifying health-related data and communicating research findings. At the center of these methods is the application of good statistical principles that assist in uncovering disease patterns, risk factors, and intervention effectiveness among populations. Epidemiologists employ techniques such as regression analysis, stratified sampling, and survival analysis to draw valid inferences from complex data sets. These strategies not only ensure the validity and reliability of findings but also the quality of the study in general. The effectiveness of epidemic surveillance to a large extent relies on such statistical tools, and these are thus critical tools in public health decision-making. Furthermore, reporting guidelines such as the Strengthening the Reporting of Observational Studies in Epidemiology (STROBE) statement cannot be discounted. The STROBE initiative focuses on full reporting of observational studies with emphasis on major issues such as study design, data collection methods, and data analysis. This has particular relevance to veterinary epidemiology owing to the fact that particular problems are posed by animal health studies in terms of the complexity of animal nature and food safety, as well as animal welfare concerns. Increased transparency through maintaining high reporting standards not only adds credibility to the results but also instills confidence within the scientific community and stakeholders in health-oriented research (Cevallos et al., 2016). Furthermore, the extension of the STROBE statement for veterinary research shows elevated sensitivity to the need to modify statistical reporting guidelines per discipline. Consensus opinion resulted in recommendations to modify STROBE items so as to capture the special characteristics of observational studies in veterinary medicine. The modifications ensure that key areas of veterinary research, including health outcomes, production parameters, and animal welfare issues, are sufficiently addressed. Through adopting such tailored reporting guidelines, the field of veterinary epidemiology would be in a better position to improve the quality of observational studies, and ultimately public health and food safety programs (Ersbøll et al., 2016).

CLOSER LOOK

THE ROLE OF STATISTICAL METHODS IN PUBLIC HEALTH DECISION-MAKING

Statistical methods are key to public health decision-making. They provide the quantitative basis for analyzing health data and making practical conclusions. Statistical procedures enable epidemiologists to identify patterns and associations in complex data sets so that it is known how to impact health outcomes through a number of variables. This information is crucial in creating targeted public health interventions. For instance, using statistical models, scientists can quantify the impact of environmental determinants on chronic diseases such as asthma and predict the chances of exacerbation among select groups. Such predictive analysis is invaluable in equipping health officials with the information necessary to develop effective strategies aimed at improving public health interventions.

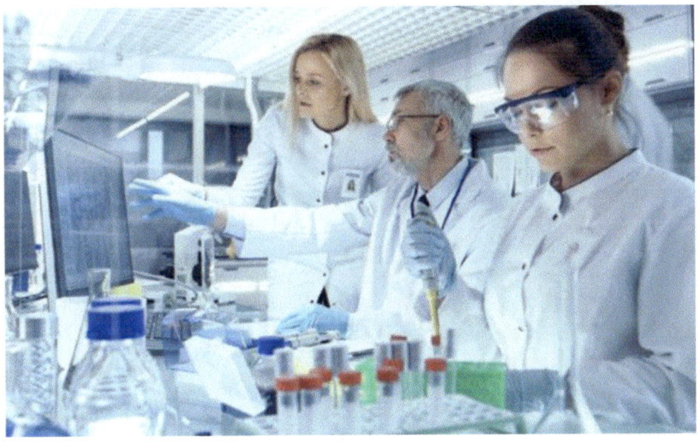

Figure 8.20. A team of scientists collaborating in a modern laboratory to conduct biomedical research.

Source: https://infinity-medical-academy.s3.me-central-1.amazonaws.com/2024/09/ad12964a2c4dd2a1902dbd664777b427_1727638844270.jpg.

In general, statistical methods are the key to closing the gap between the collection of data and evidence-based decision-making for public health. The COVID-19 pandemic highlights the immense importance of statistical methods in guiding public health interventions. With the inclusion of in-silico epidemiological modeling, health policy makers have now shifted the way in which infectious diseases are forecasted. Applying advanced statistical techniques, such as simulation-based inference, scientists have considered the epidemiology of disease spread and potential intervention techniques. Not only do these models provide critical information on how varied containment policies function, but they also enhance the readiness of health systems to face future epidemics. Moreover, software interface development to enable Bayesian inference in epidemiological models is a significant achievement towards closing the gap between statistical methodology and public health decision-making. With the infectious disease environment ever-evolving, utilizing statistical models will continue to be a key tool for developing successful public health measures. Besides, the overlap between epidemiological and statistical methodologies holds a huge potential for advancing health service delivery using evidence-based techniques. For example, understanding temporal asthma occurrence may involve modification by environmental factors is made possible using strong statistical techniques that accommodate historical data as well as current data. The newer idea of semistructured black-box models, as seen in recent literature, identifies the need for adaptive forecasting techniques in the management of chronic conditions. Such models have the capability to help create early warning systems that notify health professionals of impending disease epidemics or worsening health trends. Ultimately, the capacity to combine various statistical techniques into health prediction will not only improve public health decision making but also make a proactive approach to manage and prevent health hazards in populations (Figure 8.20).

References

1. Abelson, R. P., Adler, N. E., American Psychological Association, Anderson, N. B., Armstrong, T., et al. (2012). Caveats for using statistical significance tests in research assessments. http://arxiv.org/abs/1112.2516 (accessed on 25th June 2025).
2. Abu-Rmeileh, N., Islek, D., Kilic, B., Korkmaz, B., et al. (2014). Research capacity and training needs for non-communicable diseases in the public health arena in Turkey. https://core.ac.uk/download/42362877.pdf (accessed on 25th June 2025).
3. Adler, N. E., Glymour, M. M., Gottlieb, L. M., Hagan, H., et al. (2020). Alternative causal inference methods in population health research: Evaluating tradeoffs and triangulating evidence. https://core.ac.uk/download/323062870.pdf (accessed on 25th June 2025).
4. Aloe, A. M., Becker, B. J., Duvendack, M., Fretheim, A., et al. (2017). Quasi-experimental study designs series – Paper 10: Synthesizing evidence for effects collected from quasi-experimental studies presents surmountable challenges. https://core.ac.uk/download/80686520.pdf (accessed on 25th June 2025).
5. Ayorinde, A. A., Chen, Y. F., Lilford, R. J., Mannion, R., et al. (2020). Assessment of publication bias and outcome reporting bias in systematic reviews of health services and delivery research: A meta-epidemiological study. https://core.ac.uk/download/287602325.pdf (accessed on 25th June 2025).
6. Balkenende, E., Blevins, A. E., Chiang, H. Y., Chorazy, M., et al. (2020). Incidence and outcomes associated with *Clostridium difficile* infections: A systematic review and meta-analysis. https://core.ac.uk/download/288845936.pdf (accessed on 25th June 2025).
7. Bastos, L. S., de Oliveira, R. de V. C., & de Velasque, L. S. (2014). Obtaining adjusted prevalence ratios from logistic regression model in cross-sectional studies. http://arxiv.org/abs/1409.6239 (accessed on 25th June 2025).
8. Baydin, A. G., Darzi, A., de Witt, C. S., Dokania, R., et al. (2020). Simulation-based inference for global health decisions. https://core.ac.uk/download/396289157.pdf (accessed on 25th June 2025).
9. Beck, A. P., Gröne, A., Caswell, J. L., Meyerholz, D. K., Dohoo, I. R., LaDouceur, E. E. B., Origgi, F. C., et al. (2018). Observational study design in veterinary pathology, Part 1: Study design. https://core.ac.uk/download/160499856.pdf (accessed on 25th June 2025).
10. Bell, M. L., Dominici, F., & Samet, J. M. (2003). Time-series studies of particulate matter. https://core.ac.uk/download/61318357.pdf (accessed on 25th June 2025).
11. Bishay, A. E., Fijany, A. J., Holan, C., Mubang, R. N., Montorfano, L., Olsson, S., Troia, T., et al. (2024). Analyzing Google search trends for migraine surgery and Nurtec in response to public announcements. *Plastic and Reconstructive Surgery Global Open, 12*. https://www.semanticscholar.org/paper/6e74254f0204934ed81d0ed508d2caa12ab22d3a (accessed on 25th June 2025).
12. Bleeker, M., Cashion, J., & Markesich, J. (2006). *Surveying Persons with Disabilities: A Source Guide (Version 1)*. https://core.ac.uk/download/5118447.pdf (accessed on 25th June 2025).
13. Boulesteix, A. L., & Sauerbrei, W. (2010). Added predictive value of high-throughput molecular data to clinical data, and its validation. https://core.ac.uk/download/12172403.pdf (accessed on 25th June 2025).

14. Brodbelt, D. C., Church, D. B., McGreevy, P. D., O'Neill, D. G., et al. (2014). Approaches to canine health surveillance. https://core.ac.uk/download/36777547.pdf (accessed on 25th June 2025).

15. Browne, A. S. (2018). *A Food Chain Approach to Control of Shiga Toxin-Producing Escherichia coli In New Zealand: A Thesis Presented in Partial Fulfilment of The Requirements for The Degree of Doctor of Philosophy in Veterinary Science at Massey University, Palmerston North, New Zealand.* https://core.ac.uk/download/186668373.pdf (accessed on 25th June 2025).

16. Canali, S. (2020). What is new about the exposome? Exploring scientific change in contemporary epidemiology. https://core.ac.uk/download/323306328.pdf (accessed on 25th June 2025).

17. Candela, V., Giannicola, G., Gumina, S., Passaretti, M., et al. (2017). Adhesive capsulitis of the shoulder: Pain intensity and distribution. https://core.ac.uk/download/188822733.pdf (accessed on 25th June 2025).

18. Cangelosi, A., Plaut, D. C., Floreano, D., Kolen, J. F., Rueckl, J. G., Jacobs, R. A., Van Fraassen, B., et al. (2001). Toward the next generation of research into small area effects on health: A synthesis of multilevel investigations published since July 1998. https://core.ac.uk/download/65683.pdf (accessed on 25th June 2025).

19. Cappuccio, F., Ji, C., Kandala, N. B., Stones, R. W., et al. (2008). The epidemiology of HIV infection in Zambia. https://core.ac.uk/download/49398.pdf (accessed on 25th June 2025).

20. Carman, A. E. (2009). Ambient air toxic releases and adverse pregnancy outcomes in Allegheny County, Pennsylvania. https://core.ac.uk/download/12206720.pdf (accessed on 25th June 2025).

21. Cevallos, M., Dohoo, I., Egger, M., Erb, H. N., et al. (2016). Explanation and elaboration document for the STROBE-Vet statement: Strengthening the reporting of observational studies in epidemiology—Veterinary extension. https://core.ac.uk/download/76980915.pdf (accessed on 25th June 2025).

22. Chandler, T., English, C. L., Furmanek, S., Wiemken, T. L., et al. (2017). Most common statistical methodologies in recent clinical studies of community-acquired pneumonia. https://core.ac.uk/download/143836143.pdf (accessed on 25th June 2025).

23. Cooper, N. J., Lees, R., Owen, R. K., Quinn, T. J., et al. (2018). Network meta-analysis of diagnostic test accuracy studies identifies and ranks the optimal diagnostic tests and thresholds for healthcare policy and decision making. https://core.ac.uk/download/153572328.pdf (accessed on 25th June 2025).

24. Cranor, C. F. (1990). Scientific conventions, ethics and legal institutions. https://core.ac.uk/download/72056943.pdf (accessed on 25th June 2025).

25. Danon, L., Ford, A. P., House, T. A., Jewell, C. P., et al. (2010). Networks and the epidemiology of infectious disease. https://core.ac.uk/download/1381886.pdf (accessed on 25th June 2025).

26. Henauw De , S., De Vriendt, T., Huybrechts, I., Michels, N., et al. (2012). Children's body composition and stress, the ChiBS study: Aims, design, methods, population and participation characteristics. https://core.ac.uk/download/55802904.pdf (accessed on 25th June 2025).

27. Desvaux, S., Goutard, F., & Thonnat, J. (2009). *FAO Training Workshop On "Epidemiology, Surveillance, Outbreaks Investigation and Training Engineering in Epidemiological Field," U Choice Hotel, Luning–China, 29th June–9th July 2009: Mission Report.* http://agritrop.cirad.fr/553694/1/document_553694.pdf (accessed on 25th June 2025).

28. Ersbøll, A. K., O'Connor, A. M., Waldner, C., Pearl, D. L., Pfeiffer, D. U., Dohoo, I. R., Erb, H. N., et al. (2016). Methods and processes of developing the Strengthening the Reporting of Observational Studies in Epidemiology–Veterinary (STROBE-Vet) Statement. https://core.ac.uk/download/76980914.pdf (accessed on 25th June 2025).

29. Gerstman, B. B. (1995). Student evaluations of teaching effectiveness: The interpretation of observational data and the principle of faute de mieux. https://core.ac.uk/download/70425939.pdf (accessed on 25th June 2025).

30. Göke, B., Kolligs, F. T., Lamerz, R., Nagel, D., et al. (2012). Prognosis of patients with hepatocellular carcinoma: Validation and ranking of established staging-systems in a large western HCC-cohort. https://core.ac.uk/download/12175583.pdf (accessed on 25th June 2025).

31. Held, L., Höhle, M., & Paul, M. (2007). Statistical approaches to the surveillance of infectious diseases for veterinary public health. https://core.ac.uk/download/12163041.pdf (accessed on 25th June 2025).

32. Hentschel, J. (2025). Distinguishing between types of data and methods of collecting them. https://core.ac.uk/download/pdf/6521437.pdf (accessed on 25th June 2025).

33. Kang, H., Keele, L., & Peck, L. (2018). Inference for instrumental variables: A randomization inference approach. http://arxiv.org/abs/1606.04146 (accessed on 25th June 2025).

34. Kang, Y. P., Kim, H. M., Kwon, S. W., NGHI, D., et al. (2020). Toward a standardized strategy of clinical metabolomics for the advancement of precision medicine. https://core.ac.uk/download/288117835.pdf (accessed on 25th June 2025).

35. Leonardi-Bee, J., Lim, W. S., Nguyen-Van-Tam, J. S., Rodrigo, C., et al. (2015). Effect of corticosteroid therapy on influenza-related mortality: A systematic review and meta-analysis. https://core.ac.uk/download/80688904.pdf (accessed on 25th June 2025).

36. Lewnard, J. A., & Reingold, A. L. (2019). Emerging challenges and opportunities in infectious disease epidemiology. https://core.ac.uk/download/323082106.pdf (accessed on 25th June 2025).

37. Molanes, E. M., & Romera, R. (2008). Copulas in finance and insurance. https://core.ac.uk/download/29428412.pdf (accessed on 25th June 2025).

38. N/A. (2025). *Curr Environ Health Rep.* https://core.ac.uk/download/153363885.pdf (accessed on 25th June 2025).

39. Preiss, D., Rankin, N. J., Sattar, N., Welsh, P., et al. (2016). Applying metabolomics to cardiometabolic intervention studies and trials: Past experiences and a roadmap for the future. https://core.ac.uk/download/46567783.pdf (accessed on 25th June 2025).

40. Reidpath, D. D., & Soyiri, I. N. (2012). Semi structured black-box prediction: Proposed approach for asthma admissions in London. https://core.ac.uk/download/200297017.pdf (accessed on 25th June 2025).

41. Rubin, D. B., & Waterman, R. P. (2006). Estimating the causal effects of marketing interventions using propensity score methodology. http://arxiv.org/abs/math/0609201 (accessed on 25th June 2025).

42. Steen, J., & Vansteelandt, S. (2018). Graphical models for mediation analysis. http://arxiv.org/abs/1801.06069 (accessed on 25th June 2025).

43. Sullivan, K. L. (2017). *EPID 7134–Epidemiologic Methods II*. https://core.ac.uk/download/229148032.pdf (accessed on 25th June 2025).
44. Wang, B. (2002). Estimation of standardized mortality ratio in epidemiological studies. https://core.ac.uk/download/217047159.pdf (accessed on 25th June 2025).
45. Ye, Z., Liu, H., Shi, L., & Ke, X. (2025). Investigating causal associations between pork intake and multiple sclerosis using Mendelian randomization: Insights from large-scale GWAS data in European populations. *Nutrition and Health*. https://www.semanticscholar.org/paper/eea2e01d1d896cd5ef40ea71ecfbf3325af44ae5 (accessed on 25th June 2025).
46. Younce, L. (2018). The shape of disease: Applying geometric data analysis and other methods to time series survey data. https://core.ac.uk/download/616453167.pdf (accessed on 25th June 2025).

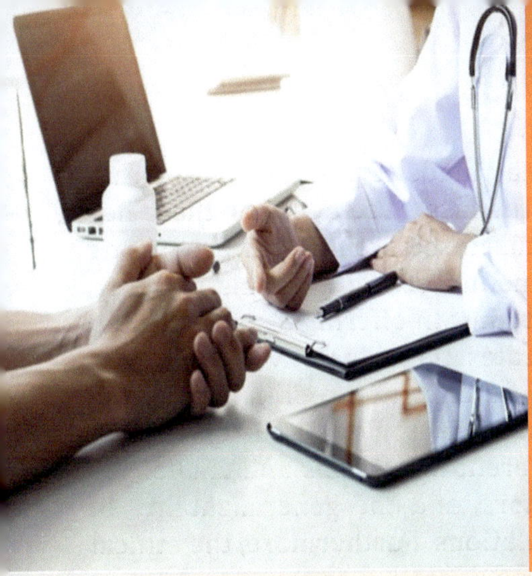

Chapter 9

PROGNOSIS STUDIES

Contents

Introduction

Prognosis studies are a standard of clinical epidemiology that are dedicated to identifying the likely consequences of illness or health conditions in groups of patients. The studies aim to answer significant clinical questions, such as survival and the likelihood of recovery. By applying observational data and statistical modeling, prognosis studies provide extremely valuable information that informs clinicians to make correct decisions for patients. The generalizability of these studies goes beyond immediate healthcare use, extending to public health guidelines and resource allocation. As medicine progresses toward complex health conditions, prognostic understanding becomes the top priority for the development of patient care and optimized outcomes. Prognosis research offers such a system that integrates empirical evidence with clinical practice, distilling greater insight into disease course over the period. The evolution of prognosis research over time parallels the overall history of clinical epidemiology and evidence-based medicine, more particularly as championed in the Hippocratic school of thought. The triumph of rationalism in this discipline has made it possible to open up doors for rational methods of analyzing outcomes of health. Over the last three decades, there has been a dramatic advancement in research in prognosis that has raised the accuracy of prognostic models, allowing clinicians to risk-stratify and individualize treatments accordingly. This merging, along with big data sets, contributes to the strength of prognosis studies in offering a sophisticated understanding of disease outcomes. This advancement demonstrates the interactive connection between clinical practice and science, making prognosis studies a fundamental tool in addressing contemporary health challenges and improving patient-centered care (Newton et al., 2001). Though their utility cannot be discounted, prognosis studies also have inherent limitations and challenges worthy of a precise assessment. Selection bias, confounding factors, and the generalizability of findings can affect the utility of prognosis models for different populations. Furthermore, the ethical effects of the communication of prognosis to patients need careful consideration so that patients are given accurate yet compassionate information regarding their health status. The ongoing controversy of the profession underscores the need for firm methodology and open transparency in prognosis research, reasserting a commitment to both scientific integrity and patient self-determination. As the healthcare environment continues to evolve, the role of prognosis studies remains at the forefront in guiding clinical decision-making and empowering patients through informed decisions on their health course (Black et al., 2015) (Figure 9.1).

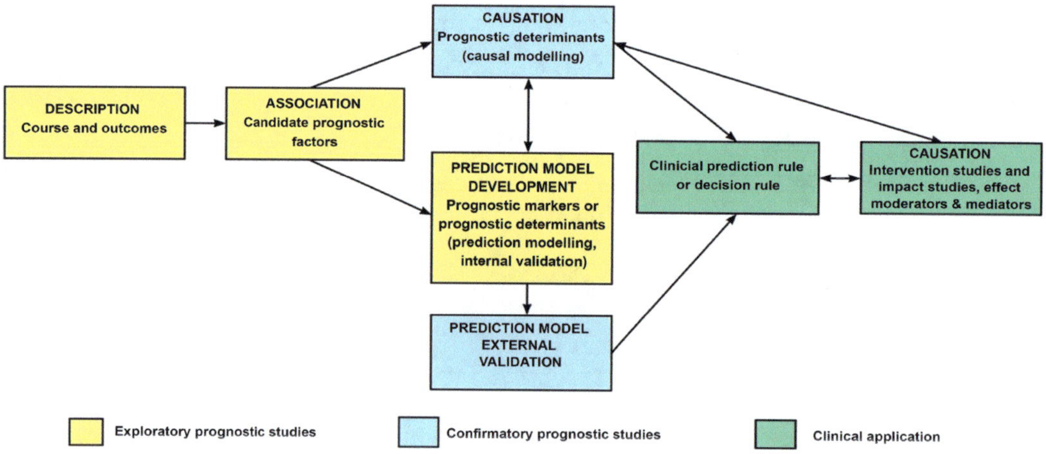

Figure 9.1. Prognostic research conceptual framework.

Source: https://media.springernature.com/full/springer-static/image/art%3A10.1186%2Fs12874-020-01050-7/MediaObjects/12874_2020_1050_Fig1_HTML.png?as=webp.

Definition of Prognosis in Clinical Epidemiology

Prognosis in clinical epidemiology is a fundamental template to describe the future evolution of diseases and conditions over time in specified populations. It entails predictions about the likely course and outcomes of a disease, including recovery, complications, and death. The predictive role serves to inform clinical decision-making, patient management, and optimal resource allocation in healthcare. Prognostic research frequently utilizes a variety of methodologies, including survival analysis and cohort studies, to evaluate the relevant patient characteristics, disease severity, and treatment effects that may influence outcomes. Prognosis not only assists clinicians in predicting the future state of patients' health but also allows patients to make informed decisions regarding their care options. Prognostic information finally intersects with clinical practice to maximize patient outcomes, particularly when faced with chronic or life-threatening conditions. Proper definition and measurement of prognosis are intrinsically connected to the concept of epidemiological measures, which lends meaning to understanding disease impact on populations. In clinical epidemiology, prognostic assessments rely on evidence derived from information that presents the likelihood of specific outcomes using specified health parameters and social determinants. Age, gender, comorbidities, and environmental contexts dictate fundamental roles in prognostic prediction. Further, the evolving nature of diseases, as shown in existing studies, calls for continued revisions of existing definitions and prognostic models to reflect real-world complexity consistently. For instance, variable geographical contexts can offer variable data on disease outcomes, which makes it necessary to re-evaluate consensual definitions to enhance diagnostics and the effectiveness of treatment. Defining prognosis in this regard, thus, must be flexible and sensitive to new emerging evidence. Clinical epidemiology is similarly interested in the proper utilization of prognostic tools to enhance patient care. One of the ways in which prognosis evaluation can be enhanced is through interdisciplinarity, wherein various medical specializations collaborate to develop prognostic models and criteria. For example, in acute respiratory distress syndrome (ARDS), a condition with high mortality and difficult management, the coming together of disparate clinical data has led to a good understanding of epidemiological patterns. Recent evidence has indicated ARDS to be frequently underdiagnosed, suggesting the necessity for urgent changes in its classification and treatment guidelines. Such constant evolution within definitions and prognostic indicators is required to facilitate better recognition of conditions like ARDS so that interventions can be initiated by health care providers to optimize patient outcomes. By directing prognosis research towards emerging clinical evidence, the application of clinical epidemiology can significantly maximize the care pathways provided to patients.

Importance of Prognosis Studies in Healthcare

Prognosis research is a critical element of the health care setting by enabling clinicians to anticipate probable health outcomes of their patients. Such a capability is naturally necessary for guiding treatment choice and enhancing the quality of care received by patients. Through knowledge of likely paths of various diseases, health care providers are capable of tailoring interventions based on individual needs, thus optimizing therapeutic intervention. Besides, prognosis research helps risk-stratify patients so that resources can be allocated to those in the highest need. As shown through current developments in clinical research, incorporating prognosis in clinical practice fosters more personalized medicine because it reflects significant developments in research in prognosis that further underscore its role in modern health care (Abrams et al., 2013). Moreover, clinical epidemiology has made prognosis studies more pivotal in guiding public health policy as well as deciding on resource distribution. Incorporating prognosis studies within the overall framework of healthcare enables policymakers to prepare for healthcare needs in advance and distribute resources effectively. Researchers are able to provide key data on the occurrence, course, and outcome of diseases using statistical models and long-term studies, which are very important to decision-makers. This model, based on evidence, not only helps in the development of preventive strategies but also guides the construction of healthcare guidelines. As the intricate nature of health conditions is evolving through time, knowledge and dissemination of prognostic determinants are becoming indispensable components to improve outcomes across populations (Newton et al., 2001). In addition, the ethical issue of prognosis studies cannot be underestimated since they are quite central to informed consent and shared decision-making between patients and providers. The fact that prognosis information empowers patients so that they may select the alternatives consistent with their values and priorities about their treatment is paradigmatic. Such openness cultivates trust and enhances the patient-provider relationship, which is central to successful healthcare delivery. Besides, as prognosis research advances, it leads to critical exploration into healthcare access and disparities, which creates a cry for more research in order to ensure equal access to prognostic data across the population. In effect, the integration of prognosis research not only enhances clinical care but also deepens the ethical underpinnings of contemporary healthcare provision (Abrams et al., 2013) (Figure 9.2).

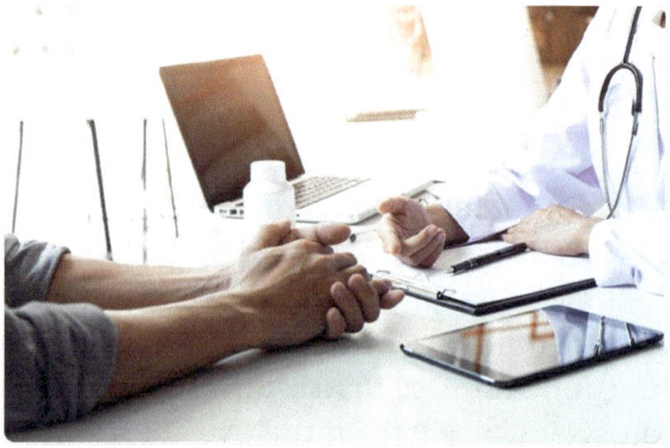

Figure 9.2. Importance of prognosis in healthcare.

Source: https://www.news-medical.net/image-handler/ts/20211022093005/ri/673/picture/2021/10/shutterstock_619483583.jpg.

Overview of the Methodology Used in Prognosis Research

The methodological design for prognosis research is multifaceted, utilizing a battery of approaches to assess future health outcomes. At its core, prognosis research seeks to delineate expected disease course and patient recovery paths in relation to pertinent clinical and demographic factors. Cohort studies are particularly prevalent in this application since they enable longitudinal observation of patient populations over extended periods. Through systematically amassing data on patient demographics, treatment outcomes, and results, scientists can identify patterns that inform decision-making in the clinic. Crucially, the approach does not merely reflect current practices but seeks to understand future consequences of these practices, enhancing the quality of care that patients receive. Such an integrated design is in accord with the objective of prognosis research, which is to provide actionable information on disease progression and management strategies in clinical epidemiology. Another critical component of prognosis research methodology is the application of statistical models for the analysis of complex data sets. Such models, for example, Cox proportional hazards models or regression analyses, enable researchers to quantify associations between various prognostic factors and health outcomes. This statistical accuracy is what differentiates causation and correlation, providing a clearer description of the ways in which various factors influence prognosis. Further, the addition of machine learning techniques in more recent research has optimized traditional methods by presenting personalized risk assessment through large data sets. The application of these sophisticated statistical tools underlines the dynamic nature of prognosis research with continuous developments to enhance predictive ability in patients. As healthcare becomes increasingly dependent on data, the application of sophisticated statistical models has the potential to understand disease trajectories better, ultimately enhancing patient treatment and care. Furthermore, the dynamic recurring process of prognosis research strategy specifically emphasizes the importance of validation and replication in deriving effective prognostic tools. Effective prognosis studies not only create models for prediction but also rigorously test them to confirm if these models are transplantable across populations of patients and practice settings. This methodological aspect ensures results are not confined to theoretical constructs but are grounded in the practical application. External validation cohorts are fundamental to this, trialing the usability of the prognostic models that have been developed. Adhering to methodological guidelines that emphasize open reporting of results, scientists contribute to a heightened awareness of the prognosis of disease. These practices are in line with the established traditions of prognosis studies that underscore the interconnectedness of knowing the future and present diagnostic and treatment procedures, hence consolidating the position of prognosis studies within clinical epidemiology (Abrams et al., 2013) (Figure 9.3).

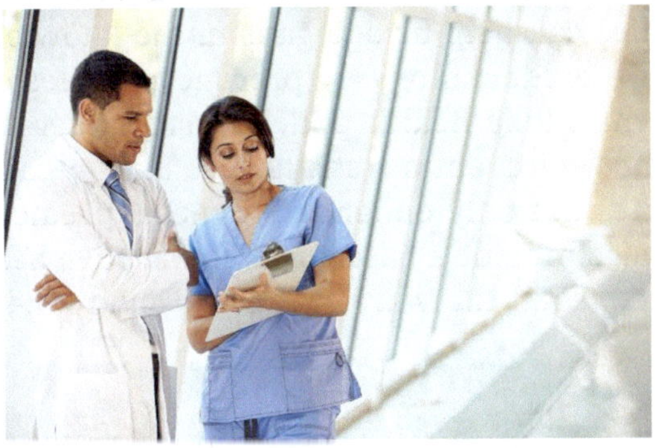

Figure 9.3. Prognosis research.

Source: https://elevate.eu/wp-content/uploads/2022/08/Systematic-Reviews-and-Meta-Analysis-of-Prognosis-Research.jpeg.

9.1. Types of Prognosis Studies

Prognosis studies form a crucial part of clinical epidemiology by facilitating the prediction of health outcomes according to patient characteristics and disease environments. Of the prognosis study designs, cohort studies are most useful as they can follow groups over time and establish the relationship between risk factors and subsequent health outcomes. This longitudinal approach allows scientists to capture the dynamic path of diseases and provide clues regarding the natural history of disease. Through the careful choice of cohorts based on specific variables, scientists are able to identify trends and associations that add to our understanding of the disease course. Cohort studies have the benefit that they can yield high-quality prognosis evidence, but at a price of requiring large resources and lengthy follow-up, both of which are possible limiting factors within certain clinical settings. Case-control studies are also highly conspicuous forms of study of prognosis and are particularly suited to investigating rare diseases or outcomes. In this design, cases are contrasted with controls with no such condition, examining past exposures to potential risk factors. The retrospective design allows detection of an association that can inform prognosis, especially in circumstances where cohort studies would be impractical due to time constraints or the condition being rare. While case-control studies are efficient and cost-effective, there are also built-in biases like recall bias and selection bias, which can undermine the validity of the outcome. Despite the limitations, case-control studies are a valuable tool for epidemiologists who wish to shed light on factors that influence disease outcomes, particularly when these cannot be directly observed over time. Integrative approaches to prognosis studies are also becoming popular, particularly in the application of multi-omics data. This is a shift in tactic in which genomic, proteomic, metabolomic, and other types of molecular profiles are combined to create a composite picture of disease pathophysiology. These multi-dimensional data have the ability to predict biomarkers more specifically associated with disease prognosis that can enhance the precision of predictions in the clinic. The addition of gender medicine further strengthens such research, recognizing the contribution that biological and cultural determinants can have on influencing disease outcomes and treatment effects. As researchers proceed with developing such integrative strategies, they are in a position to transform prognostic ability and improve personalized care in clinical practice. The novelty of these integrative approaches and the promise of personalized medicine suggest a rosy future in the epidemiological context of prognosis studies in clinical epidemiology (Argano et al., 2019; de Gomes et al., 2017).

9.1.1. Cohort Studies and Their Significance

Within the field of clinical epidemiology, the cohort study is a key study design that enables investigators to evaluate the effect of various risk factors on the outcome of disease over time. Through the monitoring of cohorts of people with a shared characteristic or exposure, it is possible to measure the natural history of diseases, for example, oral squamous cell carcinoma or hepatocellular carcinoma. These investigations form the foundation for causal process determination, where temporal relationships between cause and effect are a prerequisite. As in most research, the ability to pre-estimate prognosis to a significant degree is highly reliant on thorough examination of demographic factors, clinical factors, and aetiology; hence, cohort studies remain increasingly pertinent in cancer research, for instance, studying survival levels among cohorts with HCC (Göke et al., 2012). Furthermore, the utility of cohort studies extends beyond mere associations, given that they are also essential in validating existing medical paradigms and developing new prognostic models. An illustration is in the case of prognostic staging systems for HCC, where cohort studies have been used to examine whether the models can forecast patient survival. A number of staging systems in research demonstrate how these systems can effectively stratify patients and guide therapy decision-making. The potential to use cohort data in multicentric trials increases the robustness of findings, encouraging generalizability across broad populations. As noted, differential variables such as bilirubin and tumor node number remain significant prognostic variables, cementing the role of cohort studies in defining patient-based treatment regimens (Göke et al., 2012). Cohort studies also facilitate the evaluation of preventive treatments and screening regimens in clinical epidemiology. Even though there is a low incidence of oral cancer in some populations, the trend needs preventive measures for the promotion of early diagnosis and treatment. Current literature demonstrates that although there are low-cost and simple visual screening tests available for oral cancer, definitive evidence proving effectiveness is still lacking, pointing towards the necessity of conducting cohort-based research of high standard. These studies can help bridge gaps in the knowledge of the epidemiology of precancerous lesions, inform public health policies, and underscore primary prevention strategies. Lastly, cohort studies not only enhance prognosis prediction but also provide a basis for breakthrough health strategies in the war on cancer (Figure 9.4).

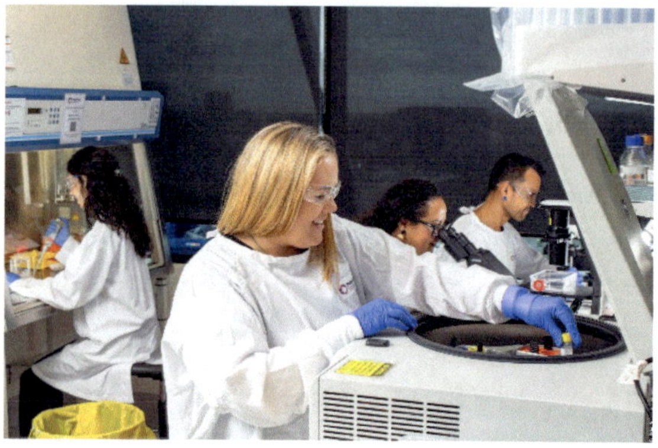

Figure 9.4. Cohort studies.

Source: https://www.petermac.org/images/Research%20Labs/DJ3_2873_V2_FS_BrAf.jpg.

9.1.2. Case-Control Studies in Prognosis

Case-control studies are the core of the prognosis domain in clinical epidemiology because they enable researchers to examine the correlations among several risk factors and disease outcomes. Unlike cohort studies involving the follow-up of study subjects over time, case-control studies examine already present cases of a certain condition compared with controls without the condition. This retrospective design allows effective investigation of prognostic variables, particularly when the disease of interest is rare or the outcome is long in developing. The greatest advantage of such studies is that they are able to assess multiple exposures or risk factors simultaneously and thus enhance our knowledge of disease etiology. Conversely, historical data can be subject to biases, such as recall bias, which must be critically evaluated in order for the results to be valid. Moreover, case-control studies assist in developing prognostic models for clinical decision-making. By identifying and investigating the parameters that determine the course of disease, investigators can derive survival rate prediction models and guide treatment regimes. For example, in cancer of the mouth, where the natural history of the condition remains poorly elucidated, case-control studies could account for the associations between lifestyle, genetic susceptibility, and disease prognosis.

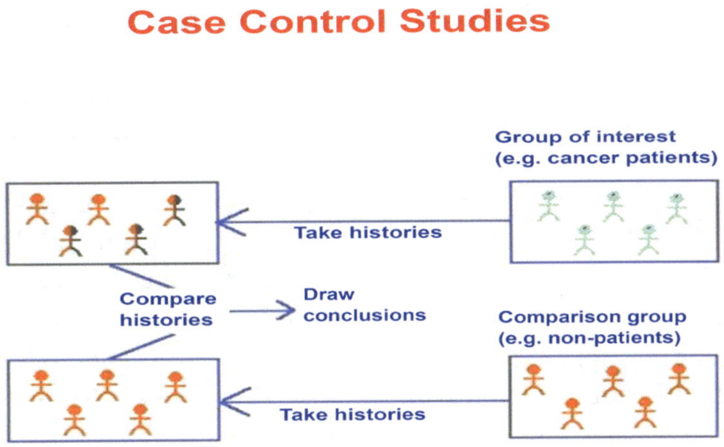

Figure 9.5. Case control studies.

Source: https://howmed.net/wp-content/uploads/2013/07/Case-control-studies-1.jpg.

These could be valuable for developing interventions and improved patient management plans. Despite the potential benefits, the lack of longitudinal information and the inherent challenges of establishing causation within case-control studies may limit the generalizability of prognostic models, warranting careful interpretation of findings to inform clinical practice. In some settings, such as breast cancer prognosis, integration of case-control studies with advanced statistical methods yields profound insights into genetic and biological determinants. By means of a network-based approach, researchers can analyze complex sets of data and reveal associations between genetic variations and patient outcomes. This kind of versatility is valuable because of the intricacy of cancer prognostic factors. The ability of case-control studies to integrate prognostic influences between groups of genes has proven highly useful, pinpointing biological pathways most crucial for disease onset and survival. For instance, such studies have identified key gene modules involved in survival prognosis in estrogen receptor-negative and positive breast cancer patients. As the field advances, the case-control methodology will be incorporated with emerging technologies to better understand prognosis in a multitude of disorders leading to improved patient outcome and treatment targeting (Rodrigues et al., 1998; Abraham et al., 2020) (Figure 9.5).

9.1.3. Randomized Controlled Trials and Prognosis

Randomized controlled trials (RCTs) are often automatically hailed as the gold standard for clinical research, particularly in clinical epidemiology and prognosis studies. By random assignment to control or treatment groups, RCTs minimize biases that otherwise distort the interpretation of health outcome results. Such methodological rigor allows researchers to draw more valid inferences about the effectiveness of interventions, providing a crucial basis for evidence-based medicine.

The RCT lessons provide critical considerations for shedding light on disease courses, educating health professionals on potential patient experiences, and guiding individualized patient care management. Its historical origin was rooted in the rationalist school of the Hippocratic corpus, wherein empirical verification of medical intervention plays a central role, further establishing the positions of RCTs in modern prognosis (Newton et al., 2001). In the context of prognosis research, RCTs not only study the efficacy of specific interventions but also quantify the overall impacts of such interventions on population health. Through the analysis of heterogeneous cohorts, RCTs can account for how age, gender, and comorbidities influence prognosis, thereby enhancing personalized medicine. This is very relevant in the development of healthcare policies, as evidence gained from RCTs is an important aspect of devising guidelines that optimize outcomes for patients across various populations. The evidence-based healthcare movement advocates for the incorporation of research results into clinical practice, which can be utilized to bridge knowledge gaps regarding prognosis and effectiveness of treatment (Guyatt et al., 1998).

Thus, RCTs are a core link between clinical research and real-world use of healthcare, founded on the need to insist upon rigorous evidence for decision-making. Further, the policymaker and clinician become increasingly important with the evolving picture of healthcare. RCTs not only provide empirical evidence for clinical decision-making but also form the backbone of the policy-making process with regard to the manner in which healthcare systems ought to allocate resources and implement practices according to research. Policymakers, therefore, have the responsibility of making sure that the application of such findings leads to efficient healthcare delivery, and hence the need for close working relationships among researchers, clinicians, and health authorities.

Through the creation of a healthcare climate that values evidence-based practices, the findings from RCTs can contribute considerably to patient outcomes and public health programs. As the call for accountability and openness in healthcare grows, the value of good prognosis research through RCTs remains priceless in delineating the intricacies of modern-day healthcare (Guyatt et al., 1998) (Figure 9.6).

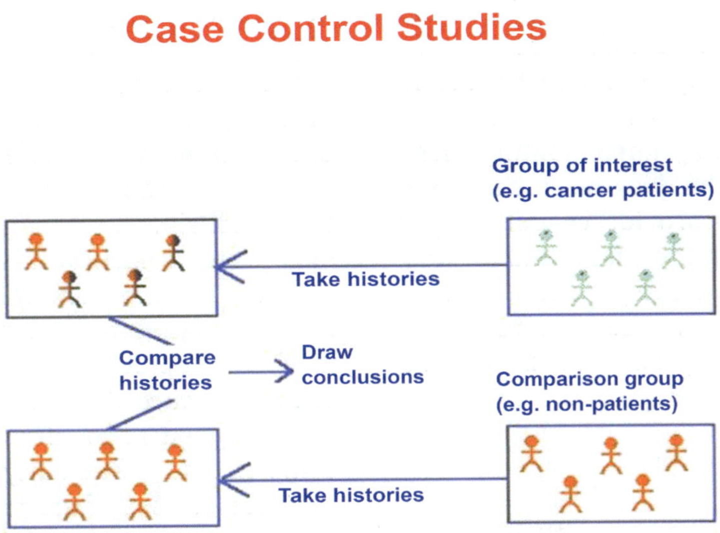

Figure 9.6. Randomized controlled trials.

Source: https://howmed.net/wp-content/uploads/2013/07/randomized-controlled-trials.jpg.

9.2. Methodological Approaches

In clinical epidemiology, methodological approaches used in studies of prognosis play an important role in deciding whether the findings are reliable and generalizable. Prognosis studies usually utilize numerous varied research designs, including cohort and case-control studies, to quantify the outcomes of health conditions over the long term. The selection of an ideal design is pivotal to conducting quality prognosis research because it not only influences the result of the data derived but also the relationships between prognostic variables and outcomes. Abrams et al. (2013) emphasize the need to understand the future consequences in alignment with current diagnosis and treatment protocols, thereby establishing the need for adequate methodological frameworks. By adopting robust methodologies, researchers can ensure that the findings are valid and can adequately inform clinical decision-making and public health policy. Moreover, systematic review procedures in prognosis studies are essential for the synthesis of evidence and understanding prognostic factors for clinical outcomes. With their pursuit of systematic assessment, research can have a number of steps, from determining core areas to developing precise questions to perform systematic evidence searches. Methodological guidance, as mentioned in de Gomes et al. (2017), becomes extremely important in undertaking these systematic reviews to ensure that evidence is evaluated utilizing quality appraisal tools suitable for several study designs. This systematic approach facilitates the generation of high-quality evidence required to foster clinical understanding of disease progression and outcome prediction. By systematic review and grading of the evidence, scientists present a robust and merit-worthy body of evidence accessible to guide clinicians toward making informed decisions for patient care. Finally, integrating new statistical approaches in prognosis studies enhances the methodological robustness and analytical richness. Use of sophisticated statistical models allows researchers to adjust for potential confounders and assess causal relationships with greater accuracy. Accuracy is critical in the identification of risk factors influencing patient outcomes.

As the methodological strategies offered by Abrams et al. (2013) and de Gomes et al. (2017) indicate, emphasis on open and reproducible methods adds further credibility to evidence in prognosis research. By implementing these advanced statistical techniques, researchers will be well positioned to provide cogent insight into the prognosis of most diseases and thereby enhance clinical practice and patient outcomes. As clinical epidemiology also increases, the acceptance of various approaches will continue to be instrumental in shaping the future of prognosis research.

9.2.1. Data Collection Techniques in Prognosis Studies

Data collection techniques are an important aspect of prognosis research in clinical epidemiology because they serve as the foundation for effective analysis and interpretation of the outcomes of patients. There are numerous varying methods ranging from observational studies to clinical trials, each with strengths and limitations. Observational designs, such as cohort studies, involve following a cohort of patients longitudinally in order to assess the progression of disease after controlling for a number of risk factors. This approach allows researchers to collect data on true circumstances, rendering their findings more generalizable. Detailed protocols are vital to facilitate standardization and reliability of data collection, especially while dealing with complicated or multidimensional health conditions that may encompass diverse data points and broad-based measurements, thereby encouraging more accurate prognostic analysis. The ethical guidelines for the methods used in data collection are also very important. As prognosis studies would generally involve vulnerable groups, stringent compliance with ethical guidelines is essential. This entails obtaining informed consent from the participants and ensuring researchers disclose the purposes of the study before embarking on it, as indicated in Gonzalez et al. (2006). Failure to report ethical approval and consent implies undermining the authenticity of research findings. In the absence of an open ethical framework, the resultant data will be vulnerable, with consequences limiting its scientific acceptance. Therefore, the establishment of high ethical standards not only protects participants but also strengthens the validity and generalizability of prognosis research, enabling successful advancement in clinical epidemiology. New data collection strategies, such as network-based approaches, have stepped in to fill the void in addressing complex data, particularly in cancer studies. For instance, studies of the genetic determinants of breast cancer outcomes illustrate the utility of integrating large variants across populations of patients, as exemplified in Abraham et al. (2020).

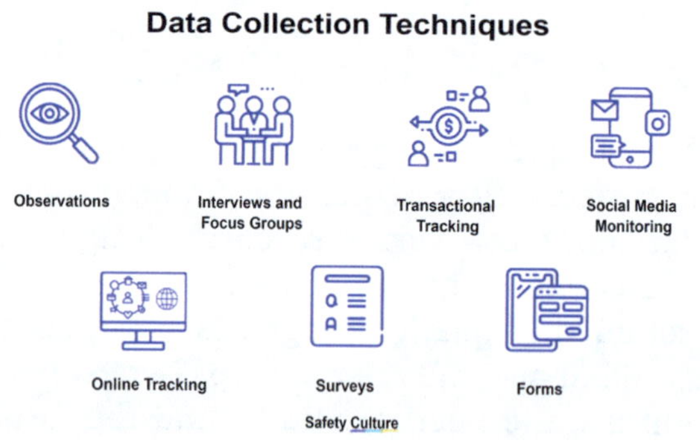

Figure 9.7. Data collection methods and techniques.

Source: https://safetyculture.com/_next/image/?url=https%3A%2F%2Fwp-website.safetyculture.com%2Fwp-content%2Fuploads%2Fsites%2F3%2F2023%2F12%2F7-Data-Collection-Techniques.png&w=1920&q=75.

Such approaches can reveal gene modules with survival outcomes, facilitating enhanced understanding of the biological basis of heterogeneous presentations of disease. These approaches are prime examples of the integration of computational methods with traditional epidemiologic approaches to enable a greater understanding of patient prognosis. As methods of data collection continue to advance, the integration of new paradigms of analysis will ever more result in new solutions for improving prognostic effectiveness and accuracy, greatly advancing the field of clinical epidemiology (Figure 9.7).

9.2.2. Statistical Analysis Methods Used

Prognostic clinical epidemiology relies heavily on sound statistical analysis methods to ensure the validity and reliability of the results. Of all the methods, survival analysis is particularly important in that it allows researchers to analyze the time to the occurrence of the event, e.g., death or disease recurrence. Techniques such as the Kaplan-Meier estimator and Cox proportional hazards regression are used widely to estimate the probability of survival and to identify potential prognostic variables. The techniques facilitate better comprehension of how various covariates, for example, age, gender, or treatment regimens, might influence patient outcomes. Moreover, they enable adjustment for confounding variables, which greatly matters when trying to draw valid conclusions from clinical data. Through their correct application of these statistical techniques, researchers are able to make significant contributions toward disease course knowledge and intervention impact, which in turn contributes toward ultimately improving clinical decision-making and patient outcomes. Another extremely critical aspect of statistical analysis in prognosis research is using multivariable models, by which one can investigate multiple predictors simultaneously. This technique is useful as it enhances the study's capacity to identify statistically significant associations with control of possible confounders. Logistic regression is often applied to binary responses, while linear regression can be used for continuous outcome variables. Furthermore, advanced techniques such as machine learning are increasingly being used to handle complex datasets, especially when traditional techniques may not be adequate due to underpowered analyses. For instance, studies examining genetic risk factors for prognosis in breast cancer have applied network-based approaches to study large and complex data sets, such as those found in genome-wide association studies, to identify important gene modules associated with different breast cancer phenotypes' survival rates (Abraham et al., 2020). Such methodological advancement emphasizes the importance of using rigorous statistical methods in prognosis studies in an effort to make meaningful inferences based on clinical data. The moral right of statistical analysis in clinical epidemiology cannot be overlooked. For instance, it is essential that researchers incorporate transparent reporting of ethical approval and consent in their study designs to safeguard the rights and well-being of research participants.

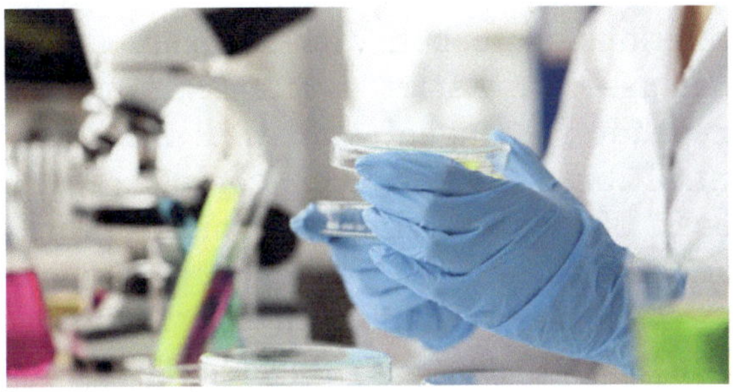

Figure 9.8. Statistical methods.

Source: https://llri.in/wp-content/uploads/2024/06/39-1024x536.png.

Research evidence shows that there has been a significant improvement over time regarding transparency in reporting ethical regulations, particularly in RCTs (Gonzalez et al., 2006). However, discrepancies are present in most study designs, as there is a notable percentage of manuscripts that lack important ethical information. Such transparency issues might undermine the validity of conclusions and can influence the generalizability of the studies. Consequently, the establishment of sound statistical practice and sound ethical guidelines is imperative in an effort to advance the integrity of clinical epidemiology prognosis research so that the knowledge generated will be meaningful in contribution to public health as well as clinical care (Figure 9.8).

9.2.3. Challenges in Methodology and Data Interpretation

Prognostic clinical epidemiology researches present difficulties that are inherently rooted in methodological rigor and appropriate interpretation of data. One of the more salient methodological difficulties is that of outcome selection and definition, which may be utterly variant between studies. Researchers must then decide on outcomes that are significant and worth studying, a process bias that can be biased if not clearly defined. Furthermore, the probability of confounders—variables with a relationship to both the exposure and the outcome—can distort causal relations. This necessitates stringent statistical methods to control for these variables, complicating the process of data analysis. Employment of various modeling techniques, while necessary, can also introduce variability in conclusions and findings, which makes synthesis across clinical studies even more difficult, as noted in more recent research (Alnabulsi et al., 2016). Data analysis in prognosis research is likewise not without problems, particularly regarding the generalizability of the findings. Research is typically conducted on selected populations, and the findings may not be generalizable to broader or other patient populations. This proviso challenges the degree to which the conclusions drawn may affect clinical practice in a heterogeneous setting. Patient heterogeneity, co-morbidities, and treatment heterogeneity also make extrapolation more difficult. To make matters more complicated, there also tends to be non-standardized definitions and measurement procedures across studies, and this can lead to inconsistencies and confusion over the data's implications. This lack of homogeneity enhances the risk of misinterpretation of results, undermining the validity of prognostic tools and models (Kitsiou et al., 2013). In addition to this, multicenter and multinational data create unique methodology and interpretation issues. Differences in local processes, patient populations, and health care systems may contribute to heterogeneity of data, and therefore, pooling of data for analysis may be difficult. Meta-analyses will try to cut across this by pooling evidence from various studies; methodological disparities, however, can lead to differences in findings. In addition, variability of data between centers can inject bias and yield an unbalanced overall assessment of prognosis. Hence, good governance of data and maintaining methodological stringency are necessary to overcome these problems. Without these considerations, the progress in prognostic research in clinical epidemiology would be jeopardized to a great extent, limiting the efficacy of interventions based on such studies (Alnabulsi et al., 2016).

9.3. Clinical Applications of Prognosis Studies

Clinical applications of prognosis studies form the core of effective patient care management and decision-making in health settings. Prognosis studies enable clinicians to predict outcomes in patients based on prognostic factors, such as demographics, clinical presentation, and comorbidity. Clinicians are hence able to tailor interventions by recognizing those at a higher risk of poor outcomes. For instance, in oncology, prognosis research can guide treatment based on the estimation of all-cause survival probabilities and identification of patients who are likely to benefit from more aggressive treatments. Secondly, the implementation of the findings into practice needs constant validation across cohorts, thus expanding the utility of prognosis into diverse disease environments. This underscores the imperative for integration of high-quality data from prognosis research into clinical guidelines for better patient outcomes. Furthermore, perhaps one of the most important aspects of prognostic studies is that they can improve patient communication and shared decision-making. If clinicians give their patients a clear prognosis, then patients are better able to make informed decisions regarding potential treatments, risks, and benefits. This type of communication enables a patient-centered approach to treatment so that patients can take into account their values and preferences when selecting their care. Evidence has shown that effective prognostic communication can reduce anxiety and uncertainty for patients, thus promoting greater care satisfaction and improved treatment adherence. As seen in various clinical situations, the integration of prognosis research into practice not only enhances care interaction quality between providers and patients but also promotes a collaborative setting in which patients are empowered to be engaged in their healthcare decisions. In addition to enhancing outcomes for individual patients, prognosis studies also have major applications in public health policy and resource allocation. By determining populations with increased risk for adverse health outcomes, such studies enable health providers to implement targeted prevention and intervention activities. For example, an understanding of chronic disease prognostic factors can inform planning for community health interventions to reduce risk factors, e.g., smoking reduction campaigns or lifestyle changes initiatives. Furthermore, prognosis research is also relevant to policy because it can provide evidence to inform funding decisions for healthcare, planning the healthcare workforce, and planning health services. By recognizing individual and population-level needs, prognosis research is a cornerstone not only in clinical epidemiology but also towards the development of a more efficient and equitable healthcare system overall (Gonzalez et al., 2006; Alnabulsi et al., 2016) (Figure 9.9).

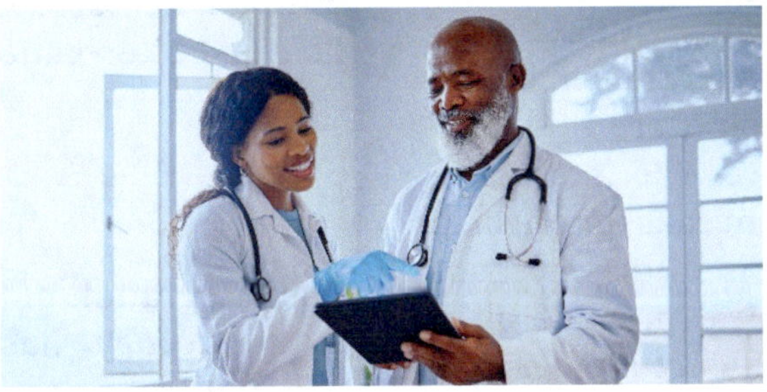

Figure 9.9. Clinical applications of prognosis studies.

Source: https://trubridge.com/wp-content/uploads/2024/02/TB-ClinicalApplications-2400x1200min.jpg.

9.3.1. Role in Patient Management and Treatment Decisions

The incorporation of prognosis studies within clinical epidemiology is critical to patient care management and treatment planning. By shedding light on anticipated disease courses, these studies equip clinicians with the ability to individualize care approaches focused on maximizing patient outcomes. For example, knowing the possible course of a condition can impact treatment directly, making intervention timely and relevant. This tailored approach not only fosters a heightened level of interaction between patients and health care providers but also ensures patient compliance with treatment protocols because the individual is more likely to engage when they are aware of how some treatments may influence their future. Prognosis-clinical decision-making association is evidence of the change in the center of medical practice, in harmony with the legacy that puts emphasis on rational empiricism in clinical education and in patient care (Newton et al., 2001). Additionally, prognosis research has a central role to play in refining clinical guidelines, which are critical tools that inform healthcare practice. These suggestions are generally based on an integration of research in prognosis, simplifying complex information into effective guidance. Through the uncertainty of patient prognosis, clinicians can make decisions more quickly with access to sound, evidence-based prognosis information. Particularly, studies that clarify future prognosis against current standards of diagnosis enable clinicians to decide on what interventions are most likely to yield beneficial results (Abrams et al., 2013). This systematic framework, grounded in prognosis research, not only enhances the quality of care provided but also allows efficient resource utilization in health systems, providing an environment where both patient and provider choices are guided by the highest order of evidence. The interactive process of patient management calls for ongoing discussion based on prognosis studies because patient conditions and clinical practice alike keep evolving. Where new evidence is emergent, it is critical that healthcare professionals continually update and refine their treatment plans according to the latest prognostic data. This adaptability enhances resilience in healthcare practice so that it remains sensitive to patient needs as well as novel evidence. An additional benefit of prognosis research is that it has the potential to contribute significantly to inter-professional communication, bridging gaps between specialists and generalists. With aligned action informed by research on prognosis, health care teams can create an extensive model of patient management that not only manages existing clinical problems but also anticipates and prepares for potential future challenges, ultimately creating an anticipatory model of care that optimizes population health (Newton et al., 2001) (Figure 9.10).

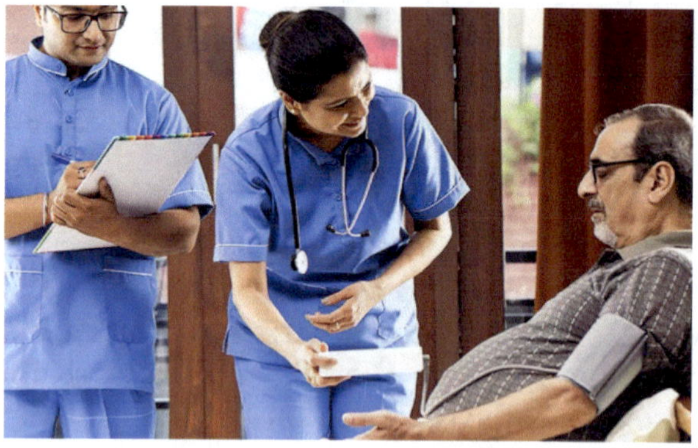

Figure 9.10. Empowering nursing staff through advanced clinical decision support systems (CDSS) to deliver better patient care.

Source: https://etimg.etb2bimg.com/thumb/msid-94263780,imgsize-64172,width-1200,height=765,overlay-ethealth/industry/empowering-nursing-staff-through-advanced-clinical-decision-support-systems-cdss-to-deliver-better-patient-care.jpg.

9.3.2. Impact on Public Health Policies

The integration of prognosis studies in clinical epidemiology has significant implications for public health policy, particularly in the area of guiding preventive interventions and therapeutic care. By providing data on the potential results of diseases under current health interventions, prognosis studies supply policymakers with crucial information that they can utilize to maximize resources. For instance, the understanding of the long-term impacts of chronic conditions enables policymakers to create intervention programs aimed at high-risk populations. This knowledge enhances the ability of public health systems to provide evidence-based interventions, thus preventing disease occurrence and burden and optimizing overall health outcomes. Associating prognosis with health policies exemplifies the pivotal role of research in rendering public health interventions relevant and science-driven, thereby maximizing their effectiveness and efficiency in addressing community health problems. Furthermore, the ethical implications of prognosis research significantly influence public health policies, particularly with regard to patient consent and participant protection. Informed consent and ethical approval are the pillars of research on human subjects, yet these research components are all too often underdocumented in published articles, as evidenced by criticism for unethical compliance across various journals (Gonzalez et al., 2006). Public mistrust and hindrance to translating research findings into applied health policy may be caused by such inconsistency in reporting. By strict compliance with ethical principles and transparency of the research process, public health institutions can cultivate community trust and involvement that are critical to the success of health interventions. Prognosis research actually emphasizes compassion reporting as a key component of policy-making in health matters, and hence enhancing their legitimacy and popular acceptability. The predictions of prognosis have implications even further into the field of health equity, informing policymakers about disparities in health outcomes among different populations. Being aware that socio-economic status, genetics, and access to healthcare contribute to prognosis differences enables public health policymakers to develop interventions to address these disparities. By utilizing outcomes from prognosis studies, policymakers are able to develop specific interventions to enhance health outcomes among marginalized populations, thus striving for health equity. This is not only an efficient way to make public health programs more effective but also serves to align with overall societal objectives of equity and justice in healthcare. With evolving methods in studies of prognosis, their results can serve as policy guidelines in formulating health policies that can improve the health of various populations to make the healthcare system as a whole equitable (Abrams et al., 2013) (Figure 9.11).

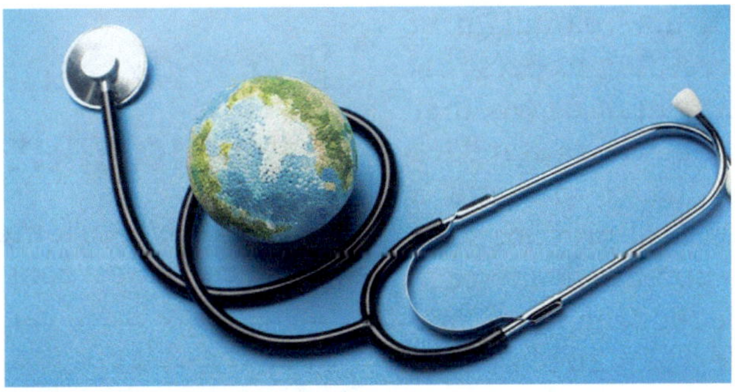

Figure 9.11. The global impact of public health policies.

Source: https://assets.everspringpartners.com/dims4/default/986c3d1/2147483647/strip/true/crop/952x500+144+0/resize/1200x630!/quality/90/?url=http%3A%2F%2Feverspring-brightspot.s3.us-east-1.amazonaws.com%2Ff4%2Fb9%2F6a40c4c647d5b3038a8ec72b55ff%2Fkent-bsph-blog-global-impact-public-health-policies.jpg.

9.3.3. Use in Risk Stratification and Patient Counseling

In the field of clinical epidemiology, risk stratification is responsible for personalizing patient counseling and management. With the stratification of patients in relation to their own risk factors, healthcare providers can offer personalized advice that is relevant to each patient's own disease profile. Personalized treatment not only raises the level of participation of patients but also compliance with management strategies, particularly with chronic diseases such as chronic kidney disease (CKD). For example, a study developed a Short Sodium Knowledge Survey (SSKS) to identify areas of dietary sodium knowledge deficit in pre-dialysis CKD patients. The tool assessed that an overwhelming majority of the patients were unaware of their sodium intake requirements, particularly among some groups of the population, and highlighted the need for individualized counseling interventions to improve dietary adherence and patient outcomes (Anderson et al., 2015). Moreover, risk stratification extends beyond the treatment of chronic diseases to preventive interventions in cancer screening. The controversy of breast cancer screening is exemplified by the conflict generated from adopting a one-size-fits-all school of thought. Current practices do not acknowledge heterogeneity of cancer risk among women and thus deny the screening protocols the highest benefit possible. The WISDOM Study promotes a new paradigm of individualized screening according to personal risk factors. Through investigation of whether risk-based screening is as effective as standard methods, this research aims to provide a framework for informing clinical practice with tailored guidelines that can potentially increase early detection rates and reduce inappropriate intervention (Esserman et al., 2017). This realignment in screening methods places the emphasis on the adoption of risk stratification to optimize patient outcomes. Lastly, the use of risk stratification in patient counseling can significantly affect treatment compliance and health outcomes. By providing physicians with an idea of the unique characteristics and needs of patients, risk assessment tools like the SSKS and recent studies like WISDOM enable practitioners to provide more effective and tailored treatment. In doing so, they exclude patient knowledge and understanding variation and lay the groundwork for improved health literacy and outcomes. With further development of clinical epidemiology, embracing individualized approaches on the basis of risk stratification will be paramount to advancing patient-focused care and optimizing healthcare interventions within diverse populations (Figure 9.12).

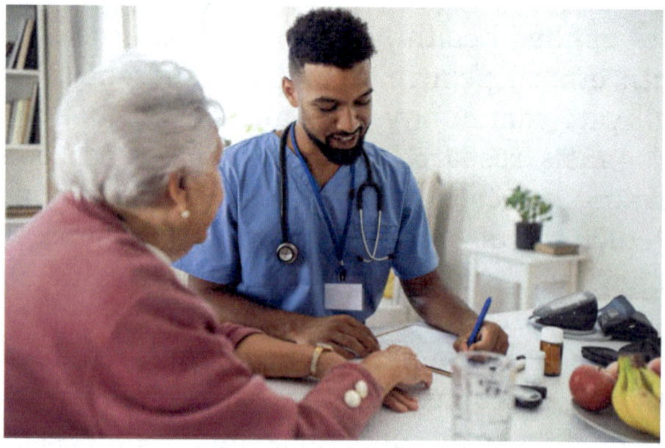

Figure 9.12. Risk stratification.

Source: https://genomind.com/wp-content/uploads/2022/10/risk-stratification-pop-health-1030x687.jpg.

9.4. Ethical Considerations

In prognosis-oriented clinical epidemiology research, ethical consideration is most relevant, particularly when conducting research involving human subjects. One aspect of the ethics of research is securing ethical clearance by a proper committee, as quoted in the literature. Failure to explicitly report ethics clearance and patient consent has been reported as a common issue, with significant gaps described in all research designs. Notably, a study found that nearly 31% of the manuscripts did not mention ethical approval, and 47% didn't mention patient consent, undermining the integrity of the research process itself and the allowance for safeguards put in place to protect participants (Gonzalez et al., 2006). Such statistics demonstrate that despite increased measures to recognize the need for ethics standards, an overreaching need for accountability and transparency is present in medical research. The therapeutic choices in patients with poor prognoses, as in head and neck squamous cell carcinoma (HNSCC), are highly problematic from an ethical point of view. With a survival rate of around 30% and the expense of treatment close to €62,500 per year, the justification for aggressive treatment modalities comes into question. Ethical frameworks must balance whether it is ethically appropriate to pursue treatment that has significant potential to help alleviate tremendous physical and psychological burdens with no guarantees of significant survival benefits (Xuereb et al., 2015). Furthermore, these decisions are typically made even harder because of the difficulties inherent in informed consent, with patients often not being adequately informed about the consequences of their treatment options. Healthcare professionals dealing with HNSCC patients have seen that treatment options are heavily influenced by quality of life, age, and social factors, a testament to the richness in clinical care's ethical environment.

Moreover, ethical issues not only include individual decisions in treatment but also encompass broader healthcare rationing issues within the health system. Limited resources distribution means difficult decisions regarding the kinds of patients to treat, especially with low predicted survival. Under conditions of limited healthcare spending, ethical considerations must inform decision-making to reconcile patient autonomy with access to care (Xuereb et al., 2015). This is a particularly highlighted issue in prognosis studies because the findings may have substantial effects on public health policy and resource distribution. The ethical implications of these choices necessitate an integrated effort to engage healthcare professionals, policymakers, and patients in dialogue reconciling moral imperatives with practical requirements, ultimately toward a healthcare system balancing efficacy and compassion (Figure 9.13).

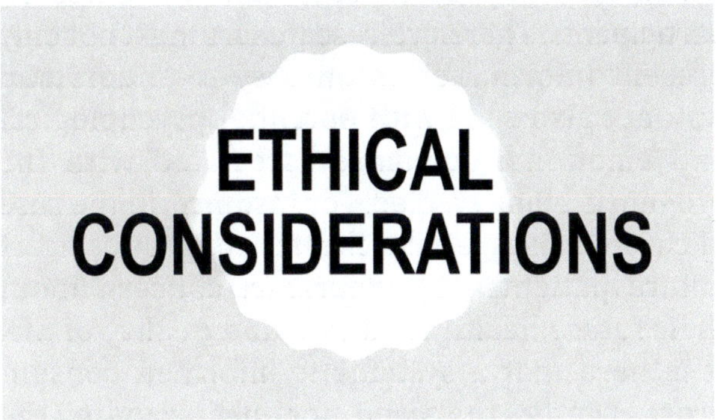

Figure 9.13. Ethical considerations.

Source: https://yoursmartclass.com/wp-content/uploads/2021/06/image-1.jpg.

9.4.1. Informed Consent in Prognosis Research

In clinical epidemiology studies of prognosis, informed consent is a fundamental ethical mandate that safeguards the participants' autonomy and interests. The act of obtaining informed consent is more than a legal formality but a fundamental element that empowers individuals to make well-informed decisions regarding participation in research. This process requires researchers to present relevant information regarding the study purpose, potential risks, and benefits in understandable ways. From this, researchers establish transparency and credibility so participants can make informed decisions and understand the consequences of their participation. In prognosis research, where outcomes can have significant implications for practice, it is essential that volunteers are made to feel secure and fully informed of the possible application of their data, so that their contribution is voluntary and informed. In addition, the nuances of informed consent are of greater specific significance in the field of prognosis research, particularly in light of uncertainty about future health pathways. Prognosis research usually works with the collection of intimate information and the prediction of various courses of health, which may impose considerable outcomes on participants. Therefore, researchers must not only present information in an easy-to-understand way but also cope with potential psychological and emotional outcomes associated with the prognosis being studied. For instance, in the case of chronic diseases like chronic congestive heart failure, patients may experience concern about their future health condition and quality of life. It is here that a systematic informed consent process enters the scene, not only providing the legally appropriate ground but also emotional support through empathetic communication. This is in accordance with principles of ethics in clinical research for limiting excessive distress and a cure integrated. Lastly, informed consent in studies of prognosis must be adaptive and iterative as it does not cease at the moment when initial consent has been given.

Since participants' understanding may change, there should be measures put in place by the researchers to revisit consent during the study period. This is especially the case in longitudinal studies, as participants might have changes in their health condition or new therapies that could alter their desire to remain in the study. Enhancing the informed consent process in such a manner promotes a dynamic collaboration between researchers and participants aimed at continuous discussion of risks, benefits, and fresh findings that could be identified. Such an approach not only ensures high ethical standards but also enhances the research process by engaging participants actively and being kept informed along the way, therefore providing strengthened and ethically enhanced prognosis studies in clinical epidemiology, as in a number of health interventions (Steptoe et al., 2007; Adragao et al., 2015) (Figure 9.14).

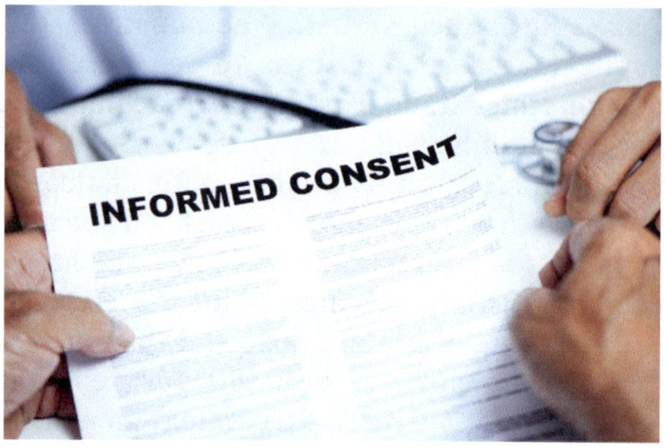

Figure 9.14. Informed consent.

Source: https://depts.washington.edu/bhdept/sites/default/files/InformedConsent.png.

9.4.2. Confidentiality and Data Protection Issues

Of late, the growing importance of confidentiality and data protection concerns in clinical epidemiology has come into greater prominence. As research depends much on patient information for prognostic analyses, maintaining the integrity and confidentiality of sensitive data is essential. With rapid advancements in technology, healthcare organizations are likely to face challenges in managing volumes of health data in a secure manner. Comprehensive and economically viable utilization of technological tools is essential so that patient data can be safeguarded while effective research outputs are facilitated. In response, organizations must take steps to enhance the handling of data and follow standards of ethics applied in processing patient data, as highlighted by trends in the digital health industry (Karakkamandapam et al., 2010). The ethical issues related to data confidentiality are even more pronounced in the context of applications of machine learning and artificial intelligence in clinical epidemiology. While these technologies will be the key to revolutionizing prognosis research by providing sophisticated data analysis, they are also responsible for bringing significant concerns regarding patient privacy and autonomy. With machine learning models integrated into clinical decision-making, there exists an inherent fear of the risk of misuse or data breaches that would infringe on patient rights. In addition, machine-based recommendations that differ from clinician judgment can lead to ethical concerns regarding the decisions on treatment made in the best interest of patients, demonstrating the need for end-to-end ethical regulations to protect patient interests as well (Alabi et al., 2020).

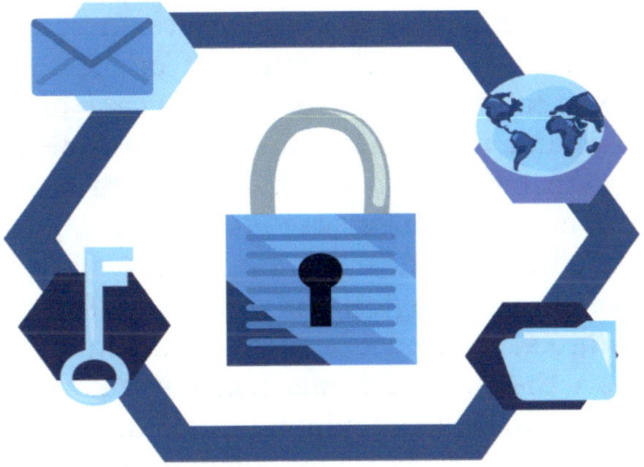

Figure 9.15. Maintain data integrity by confirming technologies have detection of corruption and restoration of accurate original data capabilities.

Source: https://www.ripplescience.com/wp-content/uploads/2022/06/Screen-Shot-2022-06-01-at-3.10.14-PM.png.

For such concerns regarding data confidentiality and protection, healthcare organizations will need to undertake developing in-depth protocols that incorporate the technological as well as ethical considerations. Multi-stakeholder collaboration between data scientists, ethicists, clinicians, and legal professionals is essential to developing a robust framework that safeguards patient data within the expanding ambit of clinical epidemiology. Such cooperation can assist in fostering uniform methods that not only align with relevant regulations but also increase patient and healthcare professional trust and transparency. Ultimately, by openly confronting such concerns, the profession can gain from technological advancements while making patient confidentiality a central feature of prognosis research (Karakkamandapam et al., 2010; Alabi et al., 2020) (Figure 9.15).

9.4.3. Ethical Dilemmas in Communicating Prognosis to Patients

It is necessary to manage the ethical dilemma in reporting prognosis to patients, particularly in the context of progressive illnesses such as dementia and mild cognitive impairment. Such illnesses pose unique challenges, as clinicians are often stuck between being open and honest with diagnoses regarding the disease's course while not wishing to needlessly disturb patients. These challenges are further complicated by varying patient preferences to be informed about prognosis. While there will be individuals who will want a clear understanding to enable them to make careful choices about their own care, there will be others who would rather have a more positive story to help them adjust to their condition. Communication of prognosis must therefore be individualized to patient preference, highlighting the importance of healthcare professionals weighing not only clinical information but also affective and psychological readiness in their patients to result in a more personalized approach to disclosure of prognosis. Additionally, medical practitioners have the ethical responsibility of informing patients adequately about the choices of palliative care as they present with life-limiting illnesses. From empirical evidence, it is evident that there are many patients who have advanced dementia and do not access required palliative care services, despite evident proof of its advantage in end-of-life situations (Aslanpour et al., 2019). Barriers such as poor training among healthcare professionals and poor coordination between care settings are responsible for this gap in care. Clinicians, therefore, must be capable of discussing prognosis and modifying treatment plans in accordance with palliative principles, facilitating early intervention and cohesive supportive care. This requires healthcare professionals to contend with their own limitations and prejudices in ensuring the empathetic and ethical communication of prognostic information aligns with consensually agreed palliative care standards. Finally, ethical challenges in the disclosure of prognosis are also promoted by the dynamic evolution of diagnostic technologies and interventions, especially in neurodegenerative illnesses. Research like ABIDE is an advancement toward increasing biomarkers' incorporation into practice to improve decision-making regarding mild cognitive impairment (Barkhof et al., 2017).

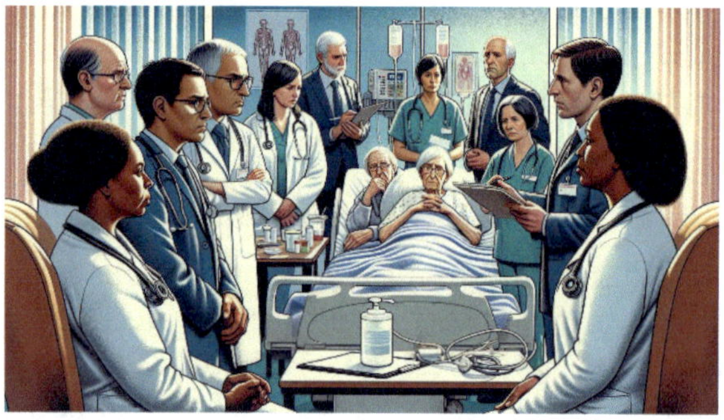

Figure 9.16. End-of-life care ethical issues.

Source: https://cdn.growtha.dev/6516de5dbcce181d2bd88c56/662295c74028c1f984d5511d_1713539613946x540498236896064450.jpg.

However, as tests become more prevalent, clinicians must then deal with the ethical implications of delivering complex information regarding the meaning of test results. These conversations need clarity regarding the uncertainty of prognosis as well as potential impacts on patients' futures. Clinicians must execute the fine art of fostering hope without sacrificing patients' understanding of their conditions, and therefore, good communication strategies are an essential component of fostering ethical involvement in prognosis studies (Figure 9.16).

9.5. Future Directions in Prognosis Research

With advancing research in prognosis, the future direction needs to emphasize the integration of newer technological strategies, including those in genomics and epigenomics. Increasing awareness of the sophistication of biological systems, as illustrated by the concept of the CpG island methylator phenotype (CIMP), is a promising area to be explored further. This phenomenon, since its identification, has contributed significantly to our understanding of the epidemiological and prognostic features of colorectal cancer. A joint research initiative to explore the epigenetic mechanisms that lead to tumorigenesis could generate new diagnostics and therapies, complementing traditional prognosis models and establishing a more individualized practice for the management of patients. The use of high-end technologies that map the human methylome in cancer and normal tissues is a significant advancement to unravel intricate disease processes and improve prognostic abilities, with the hope of better patient outcomes (Curtin et al., 2011). Beyond molecular advancements, subsequent studies need to focus on multi-dimensional prognostic factors to enhance the predictive power of prognosis studies. The prognostic risk factor serum alpha-fetoprotein (AFP) itself, for instance, has demonstrated potential as a marker of risk in hepatocellular carcinoma (HCC), with research linking high AFP levels with positive FGF19 expression in a strong correlation. Such findings point to a critical correlation reinforcing the utility of combining clinical factors and molecular profiling. Future research must not only replicate these promising results but also expand on the biological pathways being explored. By taking an integrated approach to evaluating clinical data as well as molecular markers, investigators may develop more sophisticated prognostic models that, in the long term, enable tailored treatment strategies that can be reconciled with individual patient risk profiles (Clifford et al., 2017). Lastly, the research on the future of prognosis must also consider the ethical aspects and concerns of emerging predictive technologies. With personalized medicine on the rise, it is crucial that such innovations are available and fair to diverse populations. Furthermore, researchers and clinicians must also take into consideration the potential psychological impact of prognostic information on patients and their families. As our understanding of disease trajectories grows, so too should research focus on how to discuss the effects of prognostic information. Drawing in multidisciplinary teams of ethicists, psychologists, and sociologists can help break down the challenges related to available prognostic tools. This collaborative model will not only make prognosis studies more robust in validity but also foster trust and transparency in the clinician-patient relationship, paving the way for more responsible and empathetic applications of new prognostic knowledge.

9.5.1. Advances in Technology and Data Analytics

The integration of technological innovations and data analysis has significantly transformed the status of prognosis studies in clinical epidemiology. With the union of large data sets and sophisticated algorithms, researchers have been able to evaluate immense amounts of data that were unimaginable in the past. For example, in studies of the less common diseases like amyotrophic lateral sclerosis (ALS), the availability of vast data repositories such as the Pooled Resources Open-Access Clinical Trials (PRO-ACT) database facilitates advanced analyses across heterogeneous patient populations. Technology like this not only facilitates a more complete understanding of disease presence and pathology but also a more convenient identification of trends that may be applied to influence practice in the future. Therefore, the more technologically driven methods then redefine the capabilities of clinical researchers to alter the trajectory of disease, even in situations where the traditional methods have been met with partial success (Mathew et al., 2019). Moreover, machine learning and artificial intelligence in data analytics also hold unparalleled promise for prognosis studies. When health data grow exponentially, computer-based data mining algorithms become the need of the hour to release meaningful insights that are capable of affecting patient care. Machine learning classifiers can analyze sophisticated data, identify risk markers, and predict at a fast rate, allowing clinicians to tailor interventions more accurately. The metabolomics approach detailed in recent literature highlights this shift, focusing on the need to integrate multi-omics approaches for an integrated understanding of disease. With the aid of advanced computational resources, researchers can resolve the inherent problems of metabolomics studies, including the difficulties posed by logistical and analytical flaws, ultimately guaranteeing the solidity and usability of clinical findings (Kang et al., 2020). Apart from improving data analysis techniques, technological advancements in communications have been instrumental in epidemiological studies. Cyber facilities allow for real-time sharing of data, facilitating collaborative efforts by researchers regardless of location. This collaboration not only leads to a deeper data pool but also introduces diversity in research focus, which ultimately elevates the overall quality of clinical studies. Moreover, online survey facilitation and data collection tools enable one to tap into a broader demographic, paving the way for exploration of population-based trends that have been hitherto underrepresented. The efficiency of these technological tools is evident from their application in ALS studies, where scientists used social media and websites to gain patient data successfully. These innovations ultimately form the basis for a more precise and contextualized approach to prognosis studies in clinical epidemiology, advocating for the accommodation of technological advancement (Mathew et al., 2019) (Figure 9.17).

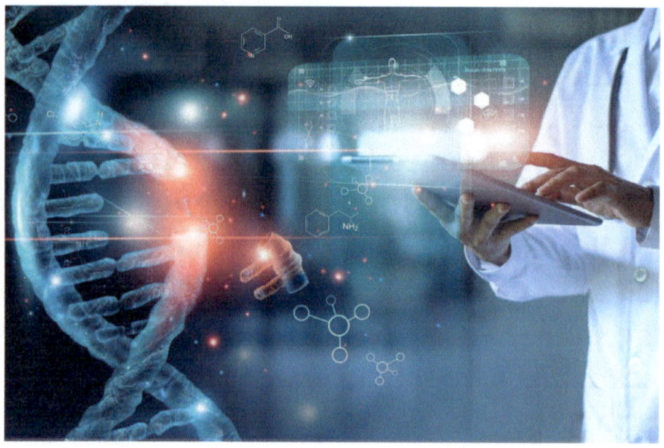

Figure 9.17. AI helps to diagnose rare genetic diseases.

Source: https://imageio.forbes.com/specials-images/imageserve/1150397417/DNA-molecule/0x0.jpg?format=jpg&crop=3656,2438,x670,y0,safe&width=960.

9.5.2. Integration of Artificial Intelligence in Prognosis Studies

Use of artificial intelligence (AI) in prognosis research is a paradigm shift in clinical epidemiology. The computational capability of AI to process intricate data allows more advanced insight into patient outcomes, particularly in conditions with numerous elements that may affect them, such as cancer. Machine learning and deep learning are AI methods that enhance the application of statistics by revealing patterns and relationships that may be missed in basic analyses. Such innovations also facilitate the development of predictive models that assist in clinical decision-making, thereby improving the overall accuracy of prognosis studies. According to the literature, incorporating AI methods can significantly improve the prognostic capability of such studies, thus making it possible for healthcare practitioners to individualize interventions more appropriately based on the patient's profile (Bacalbasa et al., 2024). Moreover, the use of AI in augmenting prognosis investigations is evidently apparent in the case of particular diseases, such as ovarian cancer. Early detection of complications and finding effective biomarkers represent the demand for advanced analysis techniques. Recent reviews identify that laboratory test examination and imaging procedures have been aided by implementations of AI, later enhancing diagnostic and prognostic precision (Bacalbasa et al., 2024).

Such advancements not only foster thorough observation of disease trends but also enable clinicians to consider the multi-factorial nature of patient conditions, leading to more specific therapeutic plans. Hence, integration of AI technologies is not only an augmentation of prevailing techniques but a driving force that pushes prognosis research into more adaptive and dynamic frameworks with the goal of improving patient care outcomes. Finally, the intersection of AI and prognosis science extends beyond general cancer applications to touch on some comorbidities. For instance, emerging research underscores the importance of pairing AI in the personalization of cancer treatments for patients presenting with underlying conditions, such as migraines. Through machine learning and predictive analytics, physicians can better assess how such comorbidities may impact treatment response and outcomes, providing a more streamlined pathway to personalized medicine. Although the potential advantages are evident, challenges with data convergence, clinical validation, and ethical considerations are still present. These challenges will have to be overcome in order for AI to fulfill its potential for enhancing prognosis research, thereby bridging the gap between theory-driven research and clinical practice (Figure 9.18).

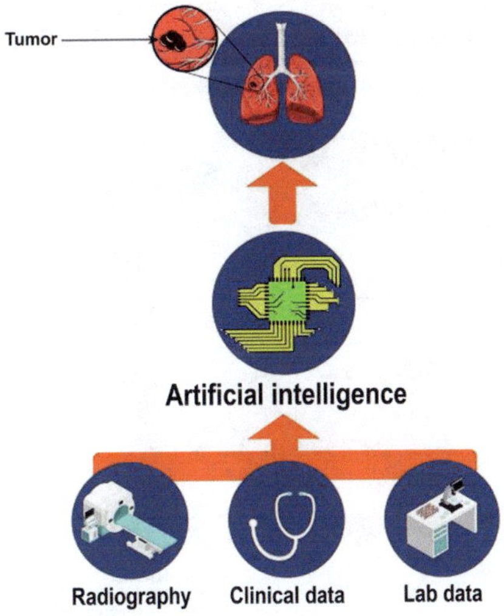

Figure 9.18. The integration of artificial intelligence (AI) with medical engineering, diagnostic, and screening techniques has provided significant advancements in the medical field.

Source: https://www.researchgate.net/publication/384160349/figure/fig2/AS:11431281279086218@1726818570769/The-integration-of-artificial-intelligence-AI-with-medical-engineering-diagnostic-and.png.

9.5.3. Potential for Personalized Medicine in Prognosis

Personalized medicine promises in prognosis is a new revolution in clinical epidemiology. The new strategy personalizes medical treatment based on patient-specific factors, including genetics, environment, and lifestyle. With the integration of personalized medicine in prognosis, medical care providers are able to aid in better forecasting ability for disease outcomes and more efficient patient management plans. This is most relevant to cancer, where identifying specific genetic markers will inform treatment and give an indication of likely disease progression, moving away from a one-for-all solution. This precision not only provides patients with more empowerment through better information but also produces a more proactive healthcare system in which personalized treatment can prevent side effects and improve overall quality of life. Further, the advent of predictive, preventive, and personalized medicine (PPPM) is revolutionizing the treatment of patients by healthcare professionals. As cited in recent studies, such a change in philosophy becomes feasible with more precise screening procedures, which are highly critical in the early diagnosis of diseases such as cancer. The ability to identify individuals who are at risk using genetic stratification makes targeted interventions feasible as well as improved prognostic outcomes.

Individual risk assessments and tailored treatment plans based on the specific biological mechanisms of disease can essentially change management styles in clinical practice. These elements enhance the efficacy of health care delivery by rendering the interventions reliant on knowledge of the patient's individual risk factors and biological responses (Bubnov et al., 2015). Despite the incredible advantages of personalized medicine, there are obstacles, particularly in data management and ethics concerning genetic information. Possibilities for abuse of genetic information, privacy issues, and consent requirements present massive obstacles to the widespread application of personalized practices. Thus, establishing guidelines on data protection and ethical protocols is the foundation of fostering trust between physicians and patients. Moreover, cost-benefit analyses must be thoroughly conducted in order to establish the economic feasibility of population screening programs. These considerations are highly significant as they directly contribute to establishing the practicability and acceptability of practices in personalized medicine within prognosis studies, hence establishing the extent to which such technologies can be best utilized in regular clinical practice (Minhat et al., 2004) (Figure 9.19).

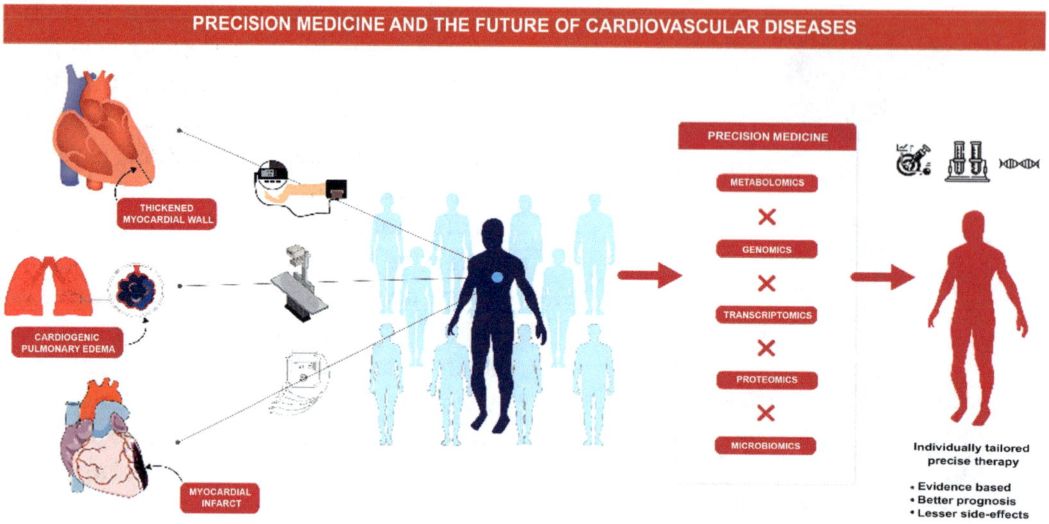

Figure 9.19. Precision medicine and the future of cardiovascular diseases.

Source: https://pub.mdpi-res.com/jcm/jcm-12-01799/article_deploy/html/images/jcm-12-01799-ag.png?1677483229.

Summary

In the final part of the discussion of prognosis studies in clinical epidemiology, the learning of disease courses and outcomes is of significance. Prognostic research is most essential since it informs clinicians and public health officials about the probability of outcomes for patients, hence decision-making. This aspect becomes more relevant, especially in fields like oncology, in which the prognosis of cancer can identify treatment regimens and the utilization of resources. As evident from recent data, oral squamous cell carcinoma, being a comparatively low-incidence cancer in the UK, exhibits a rising trend for incidence and mortality, and hence demands greater emphasis towards epidemiologic awareness and intervention strategies (Rodrigues et al., 1998). The severity of disease progression necessitates an efficient system for clinical prediction to integrate various factors affecting the outcome of patients in varying populations. In assessing the implications of prognosis studies, we must not downplay the ethical implications of clinical studies involving human subjects. This point reminds us of the importance of ethical guidelines in conducting and reporting medical research, particularly in prognosis studies that often dictate public health intervention. The demand for ethical clearance and informed consent is crucial and cannot be evaded, considering the reality that most studies do not report on these items appropriately. Unavailability of ethics reporting, not to say adequately reported ethics in most studies as described in most medical reviews, makes transparency and accountability in science challenging (Gonzalez et al., 2006). It is thus essential to strengthen the ethical underpinnings of prognosis studies in order to advance public confidence and ensure findings are well translated into practice without compromising participant well-being. Finally, effective communication of results from prognosis studies is paramount for maximizing their impact on clinical practice and policy making. Investigators must make surethat they communicate their findings not just accurately but also in a form that facilitates comprehension by practitioners and stakeholders. The educational potential of prognosis studies can be realized significantly by means of educational activities that provide healthcare professionals with the necessary information to comprehend and apply these data in real-world practice settings. In addition, the inclusion of prognosis study data in guidelines will facilitate the development of more individualized methods in patient care, especially when it comes to diseases like oral cancer, which has uncertainty still prevailing owing to the fact that it has not been well understood in terms of its natural history (Rodrigues et al., 1998). Finally, by strengthening the significance of prognosis studies and their ethical context, we can enhance clinical epidemiology's role towards public health and further enhance patient outcomes.

Prognostic research is crucial in clinical epidemiology because it assists in establishing factors that lead to patient outcomes. Among the key research findings in various prognosis studies is that numerous variables are likely to affect survival and recurrence rates among patients with diverse conditions. Psychological coping strategies have been explored as potential determinants of patient outcomes in cancer prognosis studies. Unfortunately, findings have largely been inconclusive. A meta-analysis of the interaction between coping styles and cancer survival observed that helplessness/hopelessness and fighting spirit were insignificantly correlated with survival in the majority of cases. This means that the psychological factors may not have a quantifiable effect on prognosis, and the evidence regarding how much the emotional and mental strategies contribute to clinical outcomes is dubious (Bell et al., 2002). Another essential area of research in prognosis studies is the ways in which demographic and clinical variables affect the outcomes of patients. Evidence shows that gender, age, and cancer type have significant influences on prognosis for cancers. For example, elderly patients may have differing survival patterns from young patients because of differing impacts of treatment and comorbidities. Similarly, presentation staging typically helps stratify the patients according to the severity of their disease in a way that makes subsequent intervention appropriately patterned. These findings reaffirm the importance of a multitemporal prognosis incorporating not only psychological but also biological and demographic variables to better inform predictions and maximize personalized management strategies for individual patients (Alnabulsi et al., 2016). Moreover, the literature documenting prognostic studies insists on methodological accuracy in study design so that proper inferences can be made. Most of the studies are bedeviled by the problem of small numbers of observations and failure to control for confounding variables, which can invalidate the observed association between prognostic factors and outcome. As noted from the systematic review of psychological coping styles, most studies presented non-robust data, and hence, the effect was the generation of publication bias that distorts the overall perception of patient prognosis. Subsequent studies on prognosis, therefore, must use larger sample sizes and more rigorous methodologies to ensure results are valid and applicable to clinical work. Through an improvement in the quality of evidence for prognosis research, clinical professionals are able to make better treatment decisions and enhance patient outcomes in the long run (Bell et al., 2002).

CLOSER LOOK

FUTURE IMPLICATIONS FOR RESEARCH AND HEALTHCARE DELIVERY

Looking ahead to the future of research and healthcare delivery in the context of studies of prognosis in clinical epidemiology, emphasis on the integration of prognostic data into clinical decision-making will be crucial. More understanding of future health status according to current diagnostic and treatment modalities will be needed if patient' care is to be improved. By developing a paradigm that explores the interconnectedness of diagnostic reliability, treatment efficacy, and predictive outcome, researchers are able to present clinicians with effective tools to predict patient development precisely. The justification for such synthesis is highlighted by the ongoing research impetus in data analysis, allowing increasingly advanced interpretations of prognostic data and results, and hence treatment individually. This approach not only enhances patient engagement but also shifts care practices to accommodate evolving clinical settings, as a response to the necessity of customized therapeutic interventions in diverse patient populations (Abrams et al., 2013).

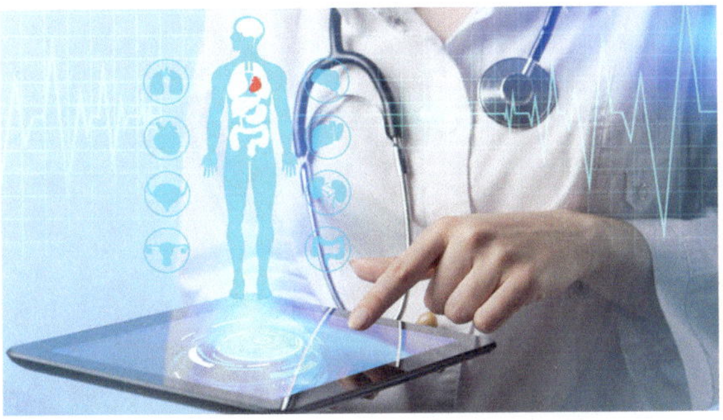

Figure 9.20. A doctor using a digital tablet integrated with virtual health monitoring and diagnostic tools.

Source: https://www.hhmglobal.com/wp-content/uploads/articles/37434/the-future-of-healthcare.jpg.

The second broad avenue of future implications is the integration of palliative care into the healthcare delivery model, particularly for those with chronic or life-limiting diseases like advanced dementia. Despite the global recognition of the necessity for PC, there are still existing barriers that restrict access for patients with illnesses that require balanced management strategies. As revealed through existing research, these include healthcare providers lacking the necessary skills and training to deliver PC and difficulty in recognizing the palliative elements of dementia (Aslanpour et al., 2019). These gaps can be bridged by targeted training programs and interprofessional collaboration, significantly enhancing the quality of care provided. Furthermore, the incorporation of prognostic studies into PC discussions will enable patients, family members, and physicians to engage more actively in advance care planning, ultimately towards ensuring care congruent with patient preference and needs. Incorporation of new prognostic research with pragmatic delivery of health care not only presents challenges but also great opportunities for innovation. Technological developments, such as artificial intelligence and machine learning, may facilitate the analysis of large amounts of health data and further refine prognostic models for real-time use in clinical practice. This innovation presents opportunities to create dynamic prognostic instruments that adapt based on patient response and treatment, maximizing care pathways. Researchers must accord prominence to collaborations with healthcare providers to engage in their application in practice, thus making them applicable to existing systems. By promoting a learning culture and adaptability, the prognosis studies of the future can significantly improve healthcare delivery, ultimately translating research results into real impacts for patients and healthcare providers (Figure 9.20).

References

1. Abraham, J., Andrulis, I. L., Anton-Culver, H., Arndt, V., et al. (2020). A network analysis to identify mediators of germline-driven differences in breast cancer prognosis. https://core.ac.uk/download/288432807.pdf (accessed on 25th June 2025).
2. Abrams, D., Altman, D. G., Briggs, A., Brunner, E., et al. (2013). Prognosis research strategy (PROGRESS) 1: A framework for researching clinical outcomes. https://core.ac.uk/download/16461730.pdf (accessed on 25th June 2025).
3. Adeleye, K., Boussios, S., et al. (2024). AI-guided cancer therapy for patients with coexisting migraines. https://core.ac.uk/download/630335354.pdf (accessed on 25th June 2025).
4. Adragao, T., Bover, J., Brandenburg, V., Covic, A., et al. (2015). Blueprint for a European calciphylaxis registry initiative: The European Calciphylaxis Network (EuCalNet). https://core.ac.uk/download/74320781.pdf (accessed on 25th June 2025).
5. Agabiti, N., Aloe Spiriti, M. A., Andriani, A., Breccia, M., et al. (2017). A population-based study on myelodysplastic syndromes in the Lazio Region (Italy), medical miscoding and 11-year mortality follow-up: The Gruppo Romano-Laziale Mielodisplasie experience of retrospective multicentric registry. https://core.ac.uk/download/127588182.pdf (accessed on 25th June 2025).
6. Alabi, R. O., Elmusrati, M., & Vartiainen, T. (2020). Machine learning for prognosis of oral cancer: What are the ethical challenges? https://core.ac.uk/download/347178568.pdf (accessed on 25th June 2025).
7. Albert, U., Apergis-Schoute, A., Brakoulias, V., Carmi, L., et al. (2019). Early intervention for obsessive compulsive disorder: An expert consensus statement. https://core.ac.uk/download/287581694.pdf (accessed on 25th June 2025).
8. Alnabulsi, A., & Murray, G. I. (2016). Integrative analysis of the colorectal cancer proteome: Potential clinical impact. https://core.ac.uk/download/131024645.pdf (accessed on 25th June 2025).
9. Anderson, C. A. M., Cavanaugh, K. L., Greene, J. H., Ikizler, T. A., et al. (2015). Results of a novel screening tool measuring dietary sodium knowledge in patients with chronic kidney disease. https://core.ac.uk/download/323065782.pdf (accessed on 25th June 2025).
10. Argano, V., Balistreri, C. R., Giarratana, R. M., Lio, D., et al. (2019). On the road to accurate biomarkers for cardiometabolic diseases by integrating precision and gender medicine approaches. https://core.ac.uk/download/268910274.pdf (accessed on 25th June 2025).
11. Aslanpour, Z., & Mataqi, M. (2019). Factors influencing palliative care in advanced dementia: A systematic review. https://core.ac.uk/download/287581724.pdf (accessed on 25th June 2025).
12. Bacalbasa, N., Balalau, C., Balescu, I., Bucur, S., et al. (2024). Artificial intelligence in ovarian cancers—from diagnosis to treatment: A literature review. https://core.ac.uk/download/624145776.pdf (accessed on 25th June 2025).
13. Barkhof, F., Batrla-Utermann, R., Biessels, G. J., Bouwman, F. H., et al. (2017). Alzheimer's biomarkers in daily practice (ABIDE) project: Rationale and design. https://core.ac.uk/download/79558589.pdf (accessed on 25th June 2025).

14. Bell, R., Hunter, D., & Petticrew, M. (2002). Influence of psychological coping on survival and recurrence in people with cancer: Systematic review. https://core.ac.uk/download/1592485.pdf (accessed on 25th June 2025).

15. Black, C., Fluck, N., Marks, A., Mitchell, M., et al. (2015). Long term prognosis after acute kidney injury (AKI): What is the role of baseline kidney function and recovery? A systematic review. https://core.ac.uk/download/29151088.pdf (accessed on 25th June 2025).

16. Xuereb Borg, H. K., Dimech, A., & Muscat, K. (2015). Local attitudes in the treatment of low-prognosis head and neck squamous cell carcinoma. https://core.ac.uk/download/46603095.pdf (accessed on 25th June 2025).

17. Bottlender, R., Jäger, M., Möller, H. J., Strauss, A., et al. (2004). Classification of functional psychoses and its implication for prognosis: Comparison between ICD-10 and DSM-IV. https://core.ac.uk/download/16432278.pdf (accessed on 25th June 2025).

18. Bubnov, R., Danesi, R., Desiderio, D. M., Grech, G., et al. (2015). EPMA position paper in cancer: Current overview and future perspectives. https://core.ac.uk/download/293881196.pdf (accessed on 25th June 2025).

19. Clifford, C. (2017). A cross-sectional analysis of the association between FGF19 tumor expression and serum AFP levels in advanced HCC patients. https://open.bu.edu/bitstream/2144/23745/5/Clifford_bu_0017N_12724.pdf (accessed on 25th June 2025).

20. Confalonieri, M., Fabiano, F., & Salton, F. (2017). Acute respiratory distress syndrome. https://core.ac.uk/download/141698214.pdf (accessed on 25th June 2025).

21. Consonni, D., Del Giovane, C., Emilia Romagna Registry for ALS Group, Fasano, A., et al. (2016). Amyotrophic lateral sclerosis: A comparison of two staging systems in a population-based study. https://core.ac.uk/download/80172306.pdf (accessed on 25th June 2025).

22. Curtin, K., Samowitz, W. S., & Slattery, M. L. (2011). CpG island methylation in colorectal cancer: Past, present and future. https://core.ac.uk/download/pdf/8561920.pdf (accessed on 25th June 2025).

23. Gomes de Carvalho, H., Eckmanns, T., Ellis, S., Forland, F., et al. (2017). PRECEPT: An evidence assessment framework for infectious disease epidemiology, prevention and control. https://core.ac.uk/download/293884153.pdf (accessed on 25th June 2025).

24. Erens, B., Fenton, K. A., Johnson, A. M., Macdowall, W., et al. (2002). Learning about sex: Results from Nasal 2000. https://core.ac.uk/download/1670453.pdf (accessed on 25th June 2025).

25. Esserman, L. J., & WISDOM Study and Athena Investigators. (2017). The WISDOM Study: Breaking the deadlock in the breast cancer screening debate. https://core.ac.uk/download/323063162.pdf (accessed on 25th June 2025).

26. Göke, B., Kolligs, F. T., Lamerz, R., Nagel, D., et al. (2012). Prognosis of patients with hepatocellular carcinoma: Validation and ranking of established staging-systems in a large western HCC-cohort. https://core.ac.uk/download/12175583.pdf (accessed on 25th June 2025).

27. Gonzalez, A., Hutchings, A., Plowman, R., Schroter, S., et al. (2006). Reporting ethics committee approval and patient consent by study design in five general medical journals. https://core.ac.uk (accessed on 25th June 2025).

28. Guyatt, G. H., Haines, A., & Sheldon, T. A. (1998). Getting research findings into practice:

When to act on the evidence. https://core.ac.uk/download/58135.pdf (accessed on 25th June 2025).

29. Kang, Y. P., Kim, H. M., Kwon, S. W., NGHI, N. T., et al. (2020). Toward a standardized strategy of clinical metabolomics for the advancement of precision medicine. https://core.ac.uk/download/288117835.pdf (accessed on 25th June 2025).

30. Karakkamandapam, S., Nair, N. S. K., & Sharma, P. S. V. N. (2010). Development of a cost-effective database software for psychiatric research: A study from tertiary care teaching hospital. https://core.ac.uk/download/pdf/14946.pdf (accessed on 25th June 2025).

31. Kitsiou, A., Caforio, A. L. P., Porta-Sanchez, A., Vahanian, A., Iung, B., Carrera, C., Szymanski, C., et al. (2013). *ESC Core Curriculum for The General Cardiologist (2013)*. https://core.ac.uk/download/55756305.pdf (accessed on 25th June 2025).

32. Mathew, V. (2019). Understanding disease heterogeneity and patient characteristics in patients with amyotrophic lateral sclerosis (ALS). https://core.ac.uk/download/305124977.pdf (accessed on 25th June 2025).

33. Minhat, N. (2004). *Pemilihan Kerjaya Di Kalangan Pelajar Aliran Perdagangan Sekolah Menengah Teknik: Satu Kajian Kes*. https://core.ac.uk/download/12007754.pdf (accessed on 25th June 2025).

34. Newton, W. (2001). Rationalism and empiricism in modern medicine. https://core.ac.uk/download/62568601.pdf (accessed on 25th June 2025).

35. Rodrigues, V. (1998). Oral cancer in the UK: To screen or not to screen. https://core.ac.uk/download/2778984.pdf (accessed on 25th June 2025).

36. Steptoe, A., Löwe, B., Ruo, B., Mathe, C., Opasich, C., Muth, C., Green, C. P., et al. (2007). Rationale, design and conduct of a randomized controlled trial evaluating a primary care-based complex intervention to improve the quality of life of heart failure patients: HICMan (Heidelberg Integrated Case Management): Study protocol. https://core.ac.uk/download/14500332.pdf (accessed on 25th June 2025).

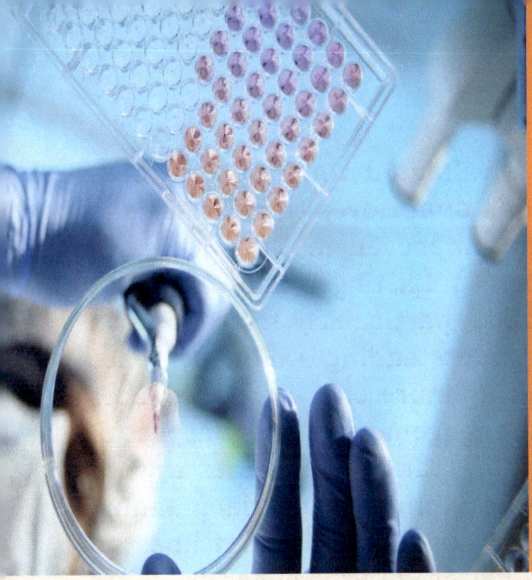

Chapter 10

CLINICAL TRIALS

Contents

Introduction

The conduct of clinical trials serves as a cornerstone in reinforcing the advancement of medical knowledge and treatment, particularly in cancer study development. Understanding the intricate processes of disease mechanisms requires rigorous methodologies to evaluate potential treatments. Clinical trials serve as formal investigations designed to measure the efficacy and safety of new interventions, ultimately enhancing evidence-based practice in healthcare. By observing patient responses to such interventions, scientists can make inferences not only impacting individual patients but also influencing healthcare policy and practice more broadly. Such importance in the development of reliable, valid biomarkers is underscored by the challenge presented by the complexity and heterogeneity of cancers, requiring proactive diagnostic approaches, as seen in the metabolomics results (López-López et al., 2024). An increasingly discussed topic among the clinical trials community is surrogate outcome validation, particularly for treatments of early-stage cancer. Although such endpoints will hasten new therapy approvals, they are mostly unvalidated compared to more conclusive endpoints such as overall survival. Consequently, there is doubt over the validity and reliability of such surrogate markers that have brought calls for improved methodologies in health technology assessment (HTA). Such enhancement is critical, as existing frameworks lack in capturing the nuances required in supporting surrogate endpoints, particularly for cancers in their early stages (Thorlund et al., 2024). Therefore, an in-depth understanding of how evidence progresses through stages of clinical evaluation is required, triggering more effective approaches that bridge gaps in the current research body. In addition, patient engagement is a key aspect of modern clinical trials, particularly in oncology studies. Understanding patients' attitudes toward treatment options and preferences related to outcomes can be a radical influence on trial planning and management. Including the patient voice in the assessment process not only provides richness to understanding what surrogate outcomes are important but also fits better with the generalizability of findings. This ongoing dialogue between researchers and patients is the foundation of more patient-centered, open care. By including real-world evidence within clinical trial approaches, researchers can make their assessments stronger and steer clear of biases in traditional methods. The increasing incorporation of patient experience, along with enhanced biomarker research and outcome validation, is a typical example of a comprehensive method needed for clinical trials' future (López-López et al., 2024; Thorlund et al., 2024) (Figure 10.1).

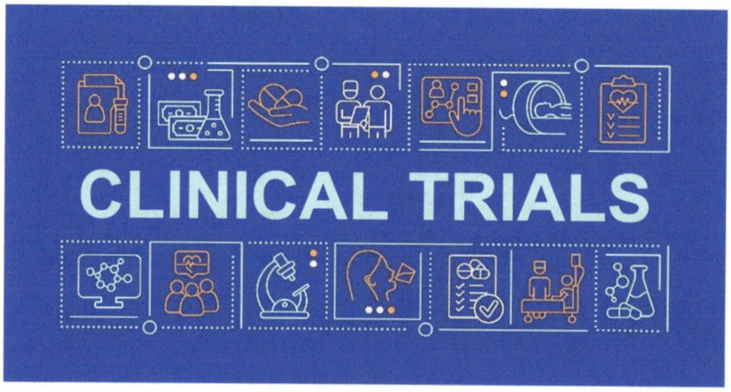

Figure 10.1. Clinical trials.

Source: https://www.news-medical.net/images/Article_Images/ImageForArticle_22414_16508973572704226.jpg.

Definition of Clinical Trials

The definition of clinical trials has a vital function in establishing a common understanding for the medical field, as it affects study design, regulation, and patient care. Clinical trials are systematic studies that establish the safety, effectiveness, and efficacy of emerging interventions ranging from drugs to devices. Clinical trials can involve human participants and implement strict protocols to ascertain their outcome. Lack of a common definition that has been accepted everywhere could be partly responsible for discrepancies about how various studies are defined and reported. For instance, a recent survey among oncology practitioners showed that differences in definition existed, and consequently, varying interpretations of what a clinical trial would be accepted, thus demanding the establishment of standardized definitions in this field (American

Medical Association Council on Scientific Affairs, Cassileth et al., 2008). Furthermore, the heterogeneity of clinical trial design complicates their definition, given that different approaches can be employed by researchers depending on their objectives and populations. The trials may be drug-effectiveness-only, or they may assess broader outcomes such as quality of life, cost-effectiveness, or longer-term safety. With the recent development of clinical research, there is greater flexibility for non-traditional studies like observational trials and pilot trials. They necessitate contemporary definitions and necessitate a more extended design point of view, which accommodates different study designs. By encouraging a general definition for clinical trials, the medical field would benefit from increased cooperation and exchange of data, and hence propel advancements in patient care and treatment practices (American Medical Association Council on Scientific Affairs, Cassileth et al., 2008). Apart from the variations in their approaches, clinical trials also face problems of classification of some studies, particularly in areas like complementary and alternative medicine.

From the professional survey, some studies, such as those evaluating non-conventional interventions, are typically read from a different angle, thus necessitating the clarification of definitions to enable them to be accepted and comprehended. The absence of a consistent framework can also hinder regulatory processes, complicating drug approval and the implementation of novel treatments. The heterogeneity underscores the imperative for researchers, clinicians, and policymakers to reach an agreement that accurately describes the evolving nature of clinical research. Therefore, it is important to set strict and commonly accepted clinical trial definitions, since they underlie quality measurements in patients' treatment and serve as drivers of innovation in medicine (Figure 10.2).

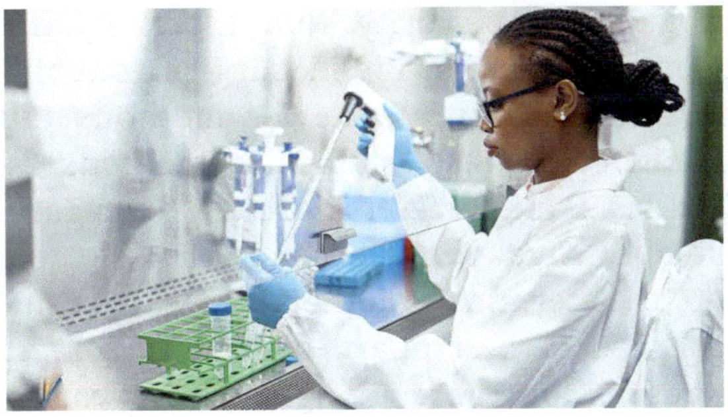

Figure 10.2. Understanding clinical trials.

Source: https://www.heart.org/en/-/media/Images/Health-Topics/Consumer-Healthcare/woman-working-in-lab.jpg?h=450&w=800&sc_lang=en.

Importance in Medical Research

The significance of medical research is effectively brought to the fore by the medium of clinical trials, which serve as a safeguard for evaluating new treatments. Clinical trials formally investigate the safety and efficacy of new treatments compared to established comparators. It is particularly relevant in areas such as oncology, where new treatments can potentially dramatically alter patient outcomes. For instance, trials may be found to demonstrate improvement in the surgical technique or reveal potentially less invasive techniques with decreased post-operative complications. Recruitment issues do arise in such research, but typically as a result of patient preference that swings towards familiar or traditional treatments. Research, such as the qualitative findings of the BOLERO trial, points towards how the pre-existing knowledge and patients' perception can play a vital role in their decision to participate in clinical trials, and hence clinicians and patients need more effective communication regarding trial participation and treatment choices. Also, the diversity of clinical trial designs, e.g., non-inferiority trials, extends the range of medical research by enabling comparison of new interventions with established ones without necessarily establishing superiority. Non-inferiority trials are especially relevant in surgical oncology, where the benefits of newer methods must be weighed against established methods with actual risks like greater morbidity or rigorous post-operative convalescence. These trials seek to determine whether a new treatment is as good as a standard treatment, a matter of great importance in light of the variable consequences for patient quality of life. For all their potential value, though, many surgeons remain insufficiently informed about the design and objectives of non-inferiority trials, and this could delay progress in evaluating newer therapeutic methods.

Emphasizing the importance of such trials can lead to increased awareness and increased involvement by clinicians and researchers. Beyond patient-specific therapies, the value of medical research in clinical trials extends to the broader public health context. Gains from these trials translate into regulator and health policy decision-making and evidence-based medicine. For example, precise trial information can lead to updated treatment regimens, influencing the manner in which different conditions are addressed in clinical practice.

Continuously, therapeutic approaches are monitored and adjusted on the basis of trial findings to enable constant patient care refinement. Second, an understanding of patient-centered factors, such as those established in the BOLERO study, can enable more effective collaboration between patients and healthcare professionals, and thus enhance the rate of recruitment and ensure that trials reflect the heterogeneity of patient experiences and decision-making. In this context, the utilization of knowledge that has been accumulated in clinical trials is an important component of facilitating medical research in general (Figure 10.3).

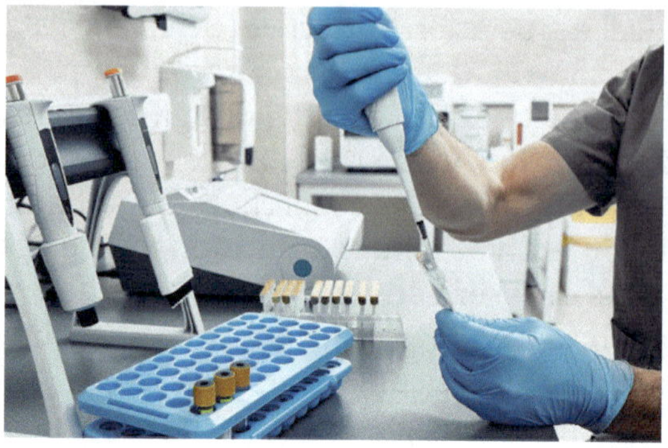

Figure 10.3. The importance of clinical research.

Source: https://attraxcdnprod1-freshed3dgayb7c3.z01.azurefd.net/1481126/e40ce6f4-d08e-41da-9b68-65e34e789e42/2025.5.21.13180/img/4585c918-92ab-4452-375f-08dbe11c8eb3.

10.1. History of Clinical Trials

The history of clinical trials is inextricably linked with the evolution of methods of medical research and ethics. The process has its roots in ancient times when treatment effects were investigated through empirical means. However, it was only in the 20th century that clinical trials as we employ them today began to take shape. The onset of randomized controlled trials (RCTs) during this period was a significant achievement in medical research. The trials brought a formal method to establish the efficacy of novel interventions while controlling bias, thereby ensuring the highest possible validity of findings. With further development, the need for adequate measures to protect participants became increasingly clear, and procedures were made to ensure the protection of participants as well as to maintain the data integrity of the research. This resulted in the establishment of institutional review boards (IRBs) and regulations governing the conduct of clinical trials. Clinical trials have increased in complexity and scope in the modern era. New technology, such as genomics and biostatistics, has transformed trial design and conduct, allowing for the targeting of therapies to specific patient populations with greater precision. For instance, the molecular profiling technologies enabled research with consideration of individual genetic makeups, considerably contributing to personalized medicine. Moreover, international collaboration and regulation have facilitated multi-center trials, which have improved the generalizability of results. The advance also comes with problems, for example, ensuring that patients are clearly informed regarding health risks and uncertainties of trial participation. As highlighted by the contest among health workers with the burden of balancing individual patient need within the context of broader public health interests, tension within clinical practice is noted to be influenced by outcomes of clinical trials (Alaszewski et al., 2005).

History in clinical trials sheds light as much on the development of methodologies as on the ethical dilemmas that researchers face. Particularly in oncology and the diseases of glioma, significant advances in genetic and epigenetic research have come along with the creation of collaborative projects such as the Glioma Longitudinal Analysis Consortium (GLASS). The collective endeavor aims to systematically document the changes that occur in gliomas longitudinally and address significant knowledge gaps that exist within the literature (Consortium, 2018). These measures highlight the importance of ongoing clinical trials in determining the direction of the disease process and the development of targeted therapies. Finally, the history of clinical trials is one of tension between scientific advancement and ethics guiding the evolution of medical research to meet the complex needs of patient care and population health (Figure 10.4).

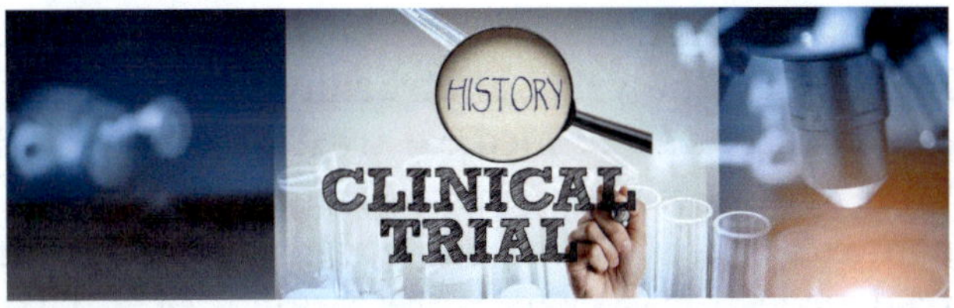

Figure 10.4. History of clinical trials.

Source: https://www.sciencepharma.com/wp-content/uploads/2024/01/Kopia-%E2%80%93-baner_www_szablon3-scaled.jpg.

10.1.1. Early Examples of Clinical Trials

The origin of clinical trials was in ancient times during the period of ancient civilization, when, in its crude form, experimentation was utilized for determining the efficacy of medicinal therapy. One such example comes from ancient Greek times, and in particular, Hippocrates, who is renowned as the father of medicine. He believed that patients should be observed in an orderly fashion and the results of treatment were to be tried through empiricism, setting aside the canvas for future clinical practices. This practice centered on the reporting of outcomes and conclusions drawn from variable responses of patients, laying the groundwork for the formalized methods of today's clinical trials. Although these practices were less stringent and less ethical than those done today, they were important to the development of a culture of inquiry and evidence-based decision-making that would be radically altered in centuries to come. The 18th and 19th centuries were the era of evolution for clinical trials growth, with the development of extensive systematic methodologies during the practice of medicine. James Lind's contribution during the 1740s is often cited as one of the earliest controlled clinical trials. Lind's experiment on scurvy among sailors demonstrated the requirement of controlled experimentation, where sailors were given different diets and subsequently given these diets to observe their effectiveness. This straightforward method not only provided robust evidence for the efficacy of citrus fruit but also highlighted the value of structured trials in informing health interventions. His work promoted a deeper scrutiny of medical treatments and led to further investigation, ultimately informing the underlying principles necessary for modern clinical trial design and use. In more contemporary contexts, the evolution of statistical methods and the influence of ethical factors have made clinical trial procedures even more refined. Group sequential designs were a major leap ahead in this context, which emphasized the adaptation of trial methodologies that could adapt to data that accrue with time. This design is particularly relevant to discrete outcome modeling, such as the number of exacerbations of chronic conditions, in order to be more responsive and flexible in trial conduct. By analyzing data increments and making timely decisions on continuing or modifying trials, today's clinical scientists embody ideas contained in experimental design procedures in infancy and integrate rigorous statistical frameworks to ensure uniform and accurate conclusions from their studies (Friede et al., 2018). Through all these advances, initial trials have therefore impacted study protocols of today and have established themselves as important mechanisms in modern medicine (Figure 10.5).

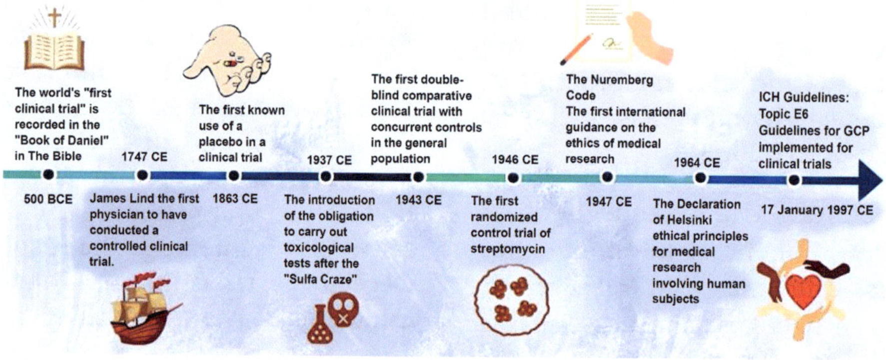

Figure 10.5. Origins of clinical trials.

Source: https://www.sciencepharma.com/wp-content/uploads/2024/01/Historia-BK-grafika5.jpg.

10.1.2. Development of Ethical Standards

The development of ethical standards in clinical trials has emerged as a prominent character in medical research, largely influencing practice and policy. Because clinical trials are done on human beings, ethics must prevail, particularly in informed consent issues, protection of vulnerable populations, and integrity in the research process. The saga of unethical practice, as that of the Tuskegee Syphilis Study, highlighted the need for stringent ethical standards. In response, organizations such as the Declaration of Helsinki and the Belmont Report have created core principles aimed at protecting participant rights and welfare as well as furthering scientific research. Respect for persons, beneficence, and justice are highlighted by these standards as the elements of a framework that supports ethical clinical trial practices today. Without those guidelines, opportunities for exploitation and injury would grow notably, and public confidence in medicine as well as medical research and therapeutic progress would erode. Furthermore, ethical needs must be incorporated in response to the complexities of employing a placebo in clinical trials. The placebo effect is capable of influencing treatment efficacy enormously by taking advantage of patients' psychological and physiologic responses to perceived medical interventions. While placebo-controlled clinical trials are helpful in separating the efficacy of new treatments, ethical issues entail withholding effective therapies from control group patients. Researchers must navigate these ethical waters carefully to ensure participant autonomy and trust, and ensure there is transparency in the trial process. Ethical integration also requires the building of robust communication channels through which patients can become aware of their involvement in such trials. Balancing scientific need with moral obligation remains a core dilemma in the field of clinical trials, necessitating ongoing discussion among scientists, ethics committees, and regulatory bodies (Adadzi et al., 2024).

Even having ethical procedures also presents unique challenges in LMICs, where poor infrastructure and resources limit compliance with agreed-upon protocols. The imbalance in the availability of trained personnel, ethics committees, and research funding is a primary obstacle to attaining ethical standards among these nations. Global health programs must address the challenges by engendering collaborative efforts toward facilitating stronger ethical practices for clinical trials within LMICs.

These should include training programs designed to orient healthcare professionals toward international ethical standards and how these can be delineated within the local context. In addition, advocacy to obtain additional funding and infrastructural support is necessary to establish efficient regulatory agencies to oversee clinical trials. Providing the ethical integrity of research conducted in LMICs, the global community can promote medical science innovations equitably and culturally sensitive, finally benefiting the patients enrolled in the trials (N/A, 2024) (Figure 10.6).

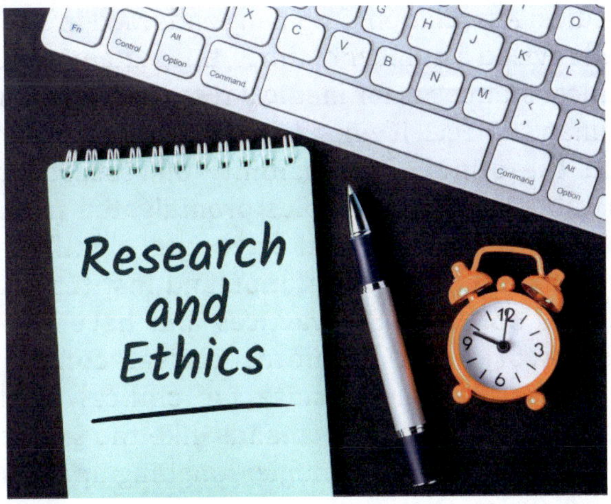

Figure 10.6. Evolution of the ethical and regulatory framework.

Source: https://www.sciencepharma.com/wp-content/uploads/2024/01/Kopia-%E2%80%93-grafika2_www_szablon-3.jpg.

10.1.3. Milestones in Clinical Trial Legislation

The journey towards sound clinical trial regulation has been marked by significant milestones that have shaped the landscape of medical research. Some key legislations have arrived as a response to ethical concerns and demands for increased regulation in the conduct of clinical trials. For instance, the establishment of the U.S. Food and Drug Administration (FDA) in 1906 laid the groundwork for regulating drug safety, which would become increasingly more stringent standards of clinical trials. The Kefauver-Harris Amendment of 1962, enacted following the thalidomide tragedy, emphasized the need to prove both safety and efficacy before drugs could be marketed. Those landmarks express a renewed commitment to protecting participants and upholding scientific integrity in the research process, with implications ringing through global health disciplines and affirming the ongoing evolution of clinical trial regulation. Globally, another milestone in clinical trial law is the Declaration of Helsinki, written by the World

Medical Association. Originally endorsed in 1964 and revised a number of times, this statement set ethical standards for medical research involving human subjects. It emphasized informed consent and the ethical responsibility of researchers to subjects. The principles promulgated in the Declaration of Helsinki have had significant effects on national legislation and institutional review board (IRB) practices and have set a framework that promotes ethical conduct. Moreover, as the climate for clinical trials evolves to meet new demands, like the growth of digital health technologies, ongoing updating of such international guidelines will remain vital. Thus, milestones like the Declaration of Helsinki not just recognise past milestones but also point to the need for a visionary process that addresses new emerging ethical challenges in clinical research.

The clinical trials regulatory landscape has grown more complex, especially in nations such as India, where growth potential was confronted with enormous challenges. After a growth phase between 2005 and 2010, the Indian clinical trials industry suffered a significant decline as a result of a variety of factors, such as regulatory holdups and increasing scrutiny by the media and public activists, as described in recent literature. This development highlights the imperative for legislative change and implementation of strict regulations to assist in neutralizing obstacles to research progress. Calls for fundamental transformation of the regulatory climate as a whole, and for targeted steps encompassing training, public sensitization, and ethical principles, are essential moves towards shaping a more propitious environment for clinical trials. Addressing such challenges will ensure that the advancements in clinical research achieve their maximum potential, ultimately benefiting both society and the scientific community (Bennett et al., 2007; Burt et al., 2014) (Figure 10.7).

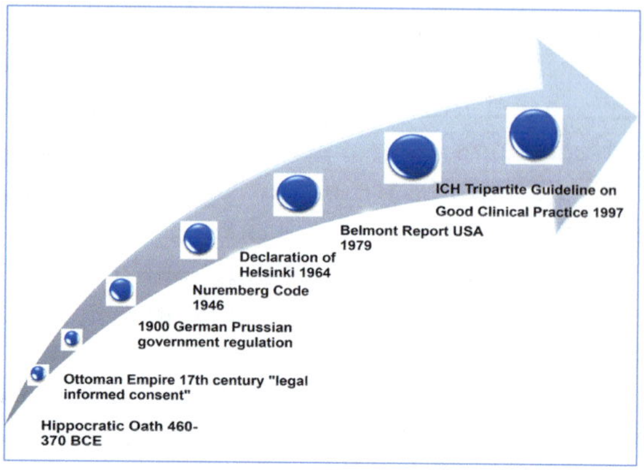

Figure 10.7. Milestones of important documents in clinical research.

Source: https://www.researchgate.net/profile/Ferdinand-Hundt/publication/235368588/figure/fig3/AS:669694482726929@1536679015456/Milestones-of-important-documents-in-clinical-research-own-illustration.ppm.

10.2. Types of Clinical Trials

Clinical trials are divided into various categories, each of which is designed to provide answers to particular research questions and objectives in the field of medicine. The most common categories are interventional, observational, and prevention trials. Interventional trials, also referred to as clinical studies, actively evaluate the effect of medical treatment, i.e., therapies, drugs, or devices, on health outcomes. In contrast, observational trials gather data without intervening on participants' treatment or behavior; however, researchers observe events in real life to see if there is a trend or correlation or not. Prevention trials deal with only those means by which diseases or conditions are prevented from happening and whether lifestyle changes, drugs, or vaccines work. Each type of trial is crucial to advance medical science on the basis of empirical data that guide clinical and regulatory decisions. Of the interventional trials, RCTs are particularly critical due to their methodological robustness. RCTs randomize participants into an experimental or a control group, thereby lowering biases and ensuring that one separates the effects of the intervention from other causes. This systematic approach is essential in developing and testing new treatments or drugs, as it allows researchers to draw strong conclusions about safety and efficacy. The results of an RCT can lead to profound developments in personalized medicine, especially in conditions like cancer, where responses to treatment could be extremely heterogeneous in patients based on biological and genetic factors. Here, there is a growing tendency toward precision medicine where molecular targeting approaches are engineered specifically using genomic information, and therefore, it becomes very important to have well-planned clinical trials, like those described in Baianu (2012). Observational trials are an essential source of data for clinical research that provides information regarding treatment and patient outcomes within the real-world clinical setting. They are most often employed to identify side effects or the effectiveness of interventions after their approval for general application. For example, advances in immunotherapy have spurred increases in observational studies aiming to find biomarkers and responses to treatment in large numbers of patient populations. With the use of technologies such as mass cytometry (CyTOF), it has become viable to conduct comprehensive immunophenotypic analyses, hence increasing the prospect of tailored treatment regimens based on response to therapy at an individual level. Such trials enhance the ability to translate laboratory findings to real-world applications, which finally translates to improved patient care and outcomes in conditions like cancer treatment, which calls for personalization, as observed in Amir et al. (2019) (Figure 10.8).

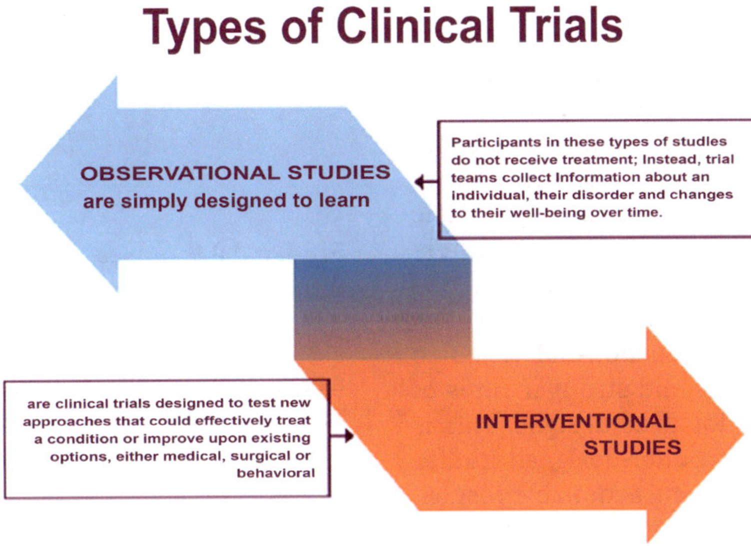

Figure 10.8. Types of clinical trials.

Source: https://www.bleeding.org/sites/default/files/image/CT%20Kit_Types%20of%20Clinical%20 Trials.png.

10.2.1. Interventional Trials

Interventional trials, which are an integral component of clinical research, are applied to evaluate the effect of various interventions on specific health outcomes. Interventional trials apply experimental study methods that often include random assignment of participants to compare the efficacy of new treatments against current standards or placebos. The relevance of such trials lies in their ability to establish cause-and-effect relations between interventions and outcomes and thus generate robust evidence to guide clinical practice. A study on emergency medicine (EM) interventional trials highlighted that although EM studies have fewer total trials compared to non-EM studies, EM trials are found to be better in quality compared to their counterparts, with higher randomization and methods of blinding. This outcome emphasizes the significance of interventional trials in generating valid and actionable health data critical in the improvement of patient care and outcomes (Calvocoressi et al., 2020). The study design of interventional trials can vary significantly based on the area of study and the specific research question posed. In the context of emergency medicine, for example, researchers have documented a highly impressive number of trials across medical, surgical, and psychiatric illnesses, all consistent with an extremely broad array of research interests within this subspecialty. Perhaps most surprisingly, EM trials are more likely than non-EM trials to have larger sample sizes and stronger rates of using rigorous methodological designs. This is significant, as larger and better-designed studies yield more generalizable and actionable results. The balance between quality trials and funding sources is also dramatic. While many EM studies struggle to obtain federal or industry funding, their methodological soundness bodes well for research in the emergency setting (Calvocoressi et al., 2020). Furthermore, intervention trials play an important role in narrowing health disparities among ethnic and racial populations, and among older ethnic and racial minorities, who are often underrepresented in medical research. For instance, a just-conducted intervention developed within community settings to engage older African Americans in clinical research demonstrated the value of targeted outreach and education. By providing directed information about the role of clinical trials, the effort moved toward boosting rates of participation in a population that tends to be open to disparities in clinical research participation. This strategy not only spotlights interventional designs as effective means of measuring medical interventions, but also as agents toward increased representation and inclusion in clinical trials, ultimately producing research results better reflective of diverse populations (Figure 10.9).

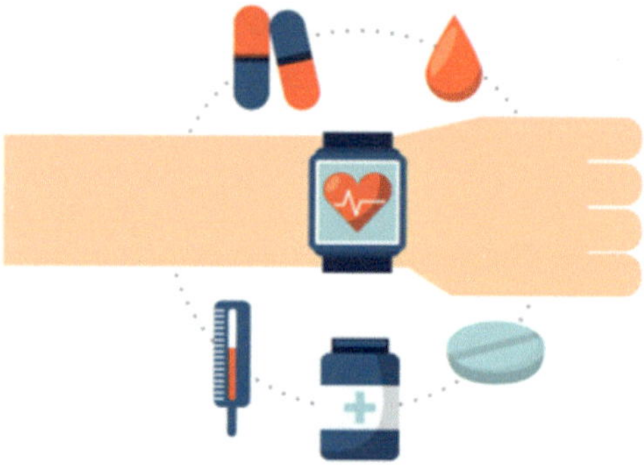

Figure 10.9. Assessing the value of wearables in interventional clinical trials.

Source: https://vertassets.blob.core.windows.net/image/47ebfee2/47ebfee2-266b-4165-ac9d-b4d3a9f931a2/375_250-health_wearable_smart_watch_istock_953701992_450x300.png.

10.2.2. Observational Trials

Observational trials play a critical role in the field of clinical investigation, particularly in understanding outcomes under real-life conditions. Unlike randomized controlled trials (RCTs) with strict inclusion and therapy administration criteria, observational studies allow scientists to gather information in a more natural setting. This offers the benefit of examining a greater population of patients as well as various treatment modalities without the ethical and logistical constraints of RCTs. Observational trials focus more on long-term health conditions and disease development and, therefore, are particularly valuable to establish trends and identify potential therapeutic effects that do not become obvious under conditions of intense control. The density of data obtained in such trials can enhance the generalizability of findings to the general population, thereby informing clinical practice and health policy. Secondly, methodological rigor in their assessment is required to ensure the validity of evidence generated from observational trials. Researchers must carefully examine potential biases and confounding factors, which are key elements that influence the outcomes. To this end, robust frameworks and assessment instruments specially designed to review the quality of observational studies are paramount. For instance, a systematic review has introduced varying instruments for assessing methodological quality in mixed study designs, including cohort and case-control studies. Systematically assessing the validity of observational studies based on these set criteria, clinicians can better identify credible studies from those that can manipulate evidence due to their methodological flaws. This commitment to critical appraisal is also seen in articles emphasizing the need for sound evaluation of trial quality, such that evidence from such trials contributes to the universe of medical knowledge in a meaningful way (Ma et al., 2020). Observational trials are increasingly influencing clinical practice guidelines and treatment algorithms due to the growing emphasis on evidence-based practice. The findings of these trials not only contribute to the robustness of the database of current evidence but also hint at the nuances of patient-centric approaches in medicine. For instance, societal organizations like the Society for Cardiovascular Angiography and Interventions have updated their guidelines based on varying forms of evidence, such as observational data and RCTs, to offer clinicians sufficient information upon which to base a decision for treatment. Individual recommendations are more likely to be generated from large cohort trials, which can make conclusions about long-term effectiveness, safety, and real-world outcomes that RCTs cannot observe due to more restricted inclusion criteria. Hence, observational trials play a vital role in shaping wise clinical practice, driving the evolution of treatment recommendations toward conforming with contemporary evidence (Dmitriy et al., 2018) (Figure 10.10).

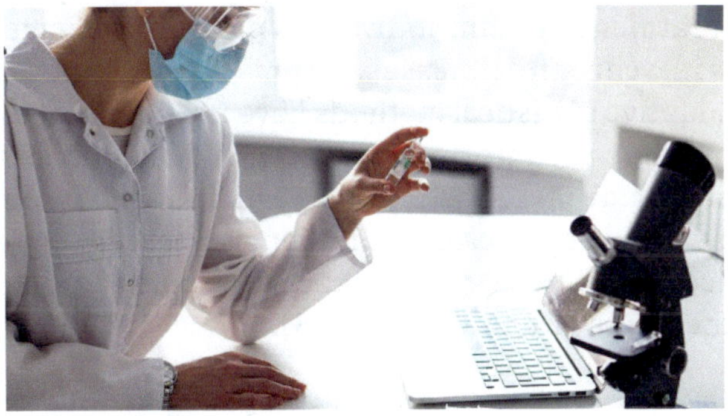

Figure 10.10. Observational study design.

Source: https://scientific-publishing.webshop.elsevier.com/wp-content/uploads/2021/09/2020-30-Observational-Study-1200x675.jpg.

10.2.3. Adaptive Trials

Adaptive trials represent a significant development in clinical trial design and execution, where the ability exists to modify elements of the trial in progress. This flexibility is in contrast to fixed-design trials, in which every one of them uses a predetermined pattern from initiation through completion. The adaptive design has the potential to improve trial efficiency with the utilization of early interim results to make highly informed decisions regarding the continuation, modification, or termination of a trial. Adaptability not only minimizes participants' exposure to ineffective treatment but also conserves resources, and ultimately results in a more effective drug development process. By combining adaptive strategies, researchers are able to facilitate the selection of the most effective therapies while solving the ethical issues of patient engagement in clinical trials. One main advantage of adaptive trials is that they can adapt treatment strategies, making therapy more specific. Patient-specific data can make treatment regimens more individualized to better align clinical outcomes with individual patient profiles. This is particularly noteworthy within the framework of single-patient trials, where the goal is to identify the efficacy of treatments within individual patients afflicted with chronic illnesses. From the literature, adaptive statistical methods have the potential to improve the informational return of such trials alongside a reduction in participant burden and thereby increase the generalizability and acceptability of personalized therapies within the clinic (Duan et al., 2013).

The potential for tailoring treatments to interim results provides an opportunity for clinicians to enhance patient outcomes through more focused therapeutic interventions that take into account variability. Second, the development of new methodologies to which adaptive trials are associated may help shift the paradigm in comparative effectiveness research. An understanding of treatment performance dynamics through adaptive designs holds the promise of delivering benefits that are novel in an environment with resource constraints, as evidenced by several optimal design approaches highlighted in contemporary literature (Ryeznik et al., 2019). These approaches allow for the concurrent evaluation of multiple treatment arms with flexibility over drug development intricacies. Adaptive trial application not only addresses the issues of traditional trial designs, but it also maximizes the overall quality of clinical evidence generated. Thus, adaptive trials are becoming an essential part of modern clinical research, unfolding possibilities for more efficient and patient-oriented approaches to therapeutic evaluation (Figure 10.11).

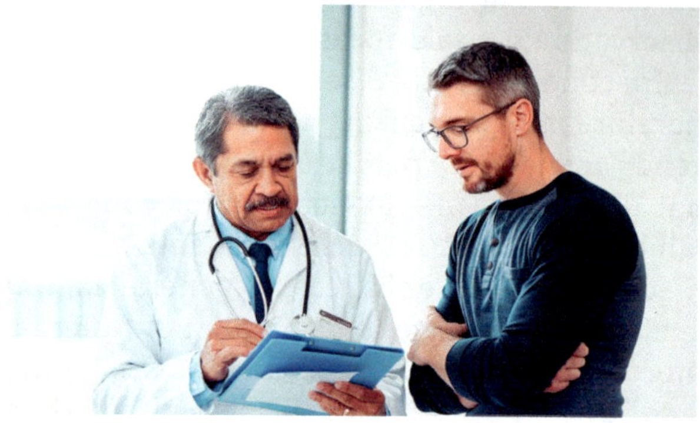

Figure 10.11. Adaptive clinical trial design.

Source: https://www.allucent.com/wp-content/uploads/2020/02/What-are-Adaptive-Clin-Trial-Designs.webp.

10.3. Phases of Clinical Trials

Clinical trial designs are typically divided into four distinct phases, each charged with answering specific aims and questions regarding the safety and efficacy of new interventions. Phase I trials predominantly focus on safety, utilizing a small group of healthy volunteers or patients. The point here is to assess pharmacokinetics and pharmacodynamics, i.e., how the drug is metabolized in the body and its immediate effects. These tests also define optimal levels of dosage and any adverse effects that may arise from treatment. By this cautious examination, researchers ensure that any potential harms are understood prior to proceeding with the next phase. This baseline level is significant, as information gathered here becomes the foundation upon which additional phases are created, offering a more accurate estimation of treatment as it is being delivered to a growing population (Bandura et al., 2007). Entering Phase II, the focus shifts to efficacy, as participant samples grow in size, and target participants with the target condition are recruited. This stage focuses on determining whether the treatment has the expected effects when administered to those directly impacted by the disease. Phase II studies also examine the best regimen of dosage while still observing safety. Significantly, Phase II trials are frequently separated into exploratory and confirmatory phases, allowing scientists to collect initial data on treatment efficacy and guide further development decisions. The outcome of these trials is of utmost importance since they can confirm or refute the progression of the drug to Phase III trials, where rigorous comparison with existing therapy or placebo takes place. This phase also further establishes the therapeutic advantage of the new intervention (Curley et al., 2017). Phase III trials are essential to the clinical trial process, the final stage of testing prior to a regulatory approval of a treatment. With a representative population across a range of sites, Phase III trials compare effectiveness and side effects in detail to offer conclusive evidence of the treatment's superiority over current standards. Phase III trial data robustness directly influences drug approval by regulatory agencies, and hence, high levels of scientific integrity and ethics are essential. Proper implementation of this phase also generally leads to Phase IV, which is the post-marketing surveillance phase. This phase continues to monitor the long-term effect and safety of the medication once it is available to members of the public, thereby providing continuous information about its real use and effectiveness once brought into the healthcare system (Bandura et al., 2007) (Figure 10.12).

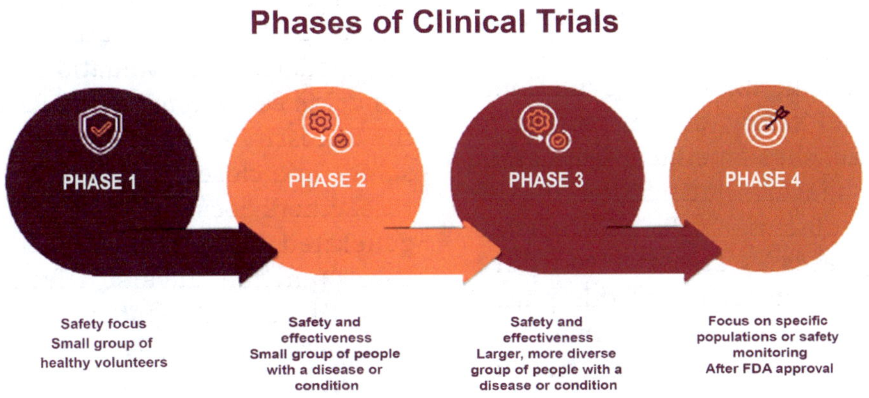

Figure 10.12. Phases of clinical trials.

Source: https://www.bleeding.org/sites/default/files/image/CT%20Kit_Phases%20of%20Clinical%20Trials.png.

10.3.1. Phase I: Safety and Dosage

The initial phase of clinical trials, often referred to as Phase I, is primarily used to identify the safety and dosage of newly introduced drug agents. It is a significant phase because it is applied in establishing the tolerability of a drug in human subjects, yielding information on possible adverse effects that may result. The typical cohort for Phase I trials is small, usually involving 20 to 100 normal volunteers or patients who have no other treatment options. In Phase I, researchers administer rising doses of the drug to determine how it is metabolized and released from the body and to watch for any harmful reactions. The challenge is not to assess therapeutic efficacy but to create a safety profile that will inform subsequent phases of clinical development. Further, Phase I trials play a significant role in the monitoring of the pharmacokinetics and pharmacodynamics of the drug. Since these experiments are conducted to compare the various dosing regimens, they provide critical information about how the drug behaves over time in the body. Particular interest is dosing considerations in pediatric and special populations, such as those with HIV infection. For example, the pharmacokinetic factors may differ significantly due to the ongoing maturation of organ systems. This includes age-related variation in immunologic markers, a factor recognized in children's practice where the unique needs of HIV-infected infants and children are listed (Therapy A and Management M of Children H. I et al., 2003). These differences in dosing needs are necessary to effectively navigate the complexities of drug administration in different populations. Beyond dosage and safety, documentation in Phase I trials establishes an ethical foundation for subsequent phases. Notification of the patient regarding potential risks and benefits in subsequent phases is required to afford openness regarding the results of this phase. The regulating agencies usually insist on extensive data regarding adverse event profiles prior to approving transition to Phase II trials. This multidimensional approach also includes participant feedback on tolerability, enhancing the ethical design of clinical trials even more. The experience of trials for delayed-release dimethyl fumarate (DMF) in relapsing multiple sclerosis treatment, for instance, emphasizes the sophistication of safety evaluations. The DEFINE and CONFIRM trials illustrated controlling side effects while establishing DMF's therapeutic potential (Pontecorvo et al., 2016). Such emphasis on Phase I safety and dose assessment is essential to prudent and wise clinical advancement (Figure 10.13).

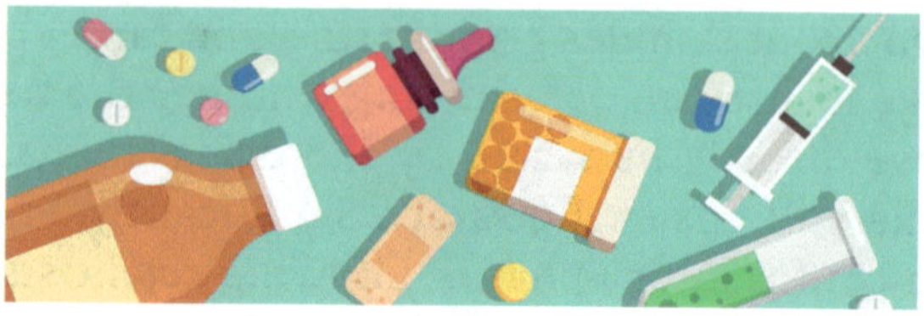

Figure 10.13. Phase 1 clinical trials.

Source: https://www.quanticate.com/hs-fs/hubfs/Phase%201%20Clinical%20Trial%20Designs.jpg?width=3508&name=Phase%201%20Clinical%20Trial%20Designs.jpg.

10.3.2. Phase II: Efficacy and Side Effects

The validity of a clinical treatment is strictly tested in Phase II trials, the succeeding phase following the outcome of Phase I. Scientists in this case seek to ascertain both therapeutic worth and a more defined profile of adverse effects that are associated with a treatment. For instance, the evaluation of an autologous dendritic cell vaccine for SARS-CoV-2 indicated the necessity of proving efficacy equated with safety. In a closely followed-up one-year study, researchers documented that, while this vaccine generated high-grade response in T-cell and B-cell function, adverse effects were noted as well. Of particular interest, during the Phase II trial, approximately 16.54% of participants experienced non-COVID adverse effects, while moderate to severe COVID-19 risk was limited to 4.31% of such individuals (Ramadhani et al., 2023). These findings highlight the dual responsibility of Phase II studies to prove both efficacy and safety. Phase II studies are also a critical crossroads in optimizing dosage and treatment regimens from earlier studies. This optimization is crucial to maximizing therapeutic effects while avoiding side effects. For skin fibrosis studies, for example, LED-red light therapy is explored for its potential in minimizing post-operative scarring. Phase II design involved multiple treatment groups, allowing comparative assessment of various dosages of LED therapy. Phase I trials initially established safety parameters that served as the basis for large-scale testing of therapeutic efficacy. The systematic strategy aims to help dispel uncertainty regarding the degree to which fibrosis can be lessened by LED therapy and whether it is well tolerated. Lastly, rigorous scrutiny of side effects within such trials is required to establish an effective clinical protocol (Heilman et al., 2019). What is gained in Phase II trials not only makes subsequent clinical practice, but also encourages innovation in some therapeutic areas. At the completion of Phase II, scientists focus on refining the effectiveness of treatments while still keeping a close eye out for side effects. With the dendritic cell vaccine, both the elicited immune response and the side effects yield dual confirmation: of the vaccine's effectiveness and of the safety of participants in the course of the therapeutic intervention.

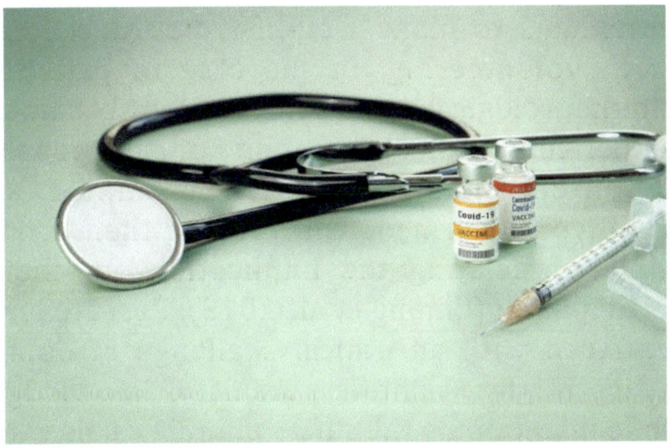

Figure 10.14. Phase 2 of clinical trials.

Source: https://dbgp98ysvt3y0.cloudfront.net/blog/UMeDJJfb7nPsWcEYTmqtLvr5iPPKdDYbRDjdVePF.jpg.

In a parallel manner, in the LED-red light trial, concurrent evaluation of the scar pliability relative to the control sites provides a definitive sign of the therapy's efficacy while systematically recording side effects, thereby contributing to greater knowledge in dermatological applications. Double-blinded design integrated into Phase II trials ensures that new therapies go into Phase III with the amount of rigor they need to have, with the capacity to expose higher numbers subsequently to establish safety and efficacy (Ramadhani et al., 2023; Heilman et al., 2019) (Figure 10.14).

10.3.3. Phase III: Confirmation and Comparison

Phase III is the core when it comes to the setting of efficacy and safety of a treatment approach in the case of clinical trials. Due to the promising results on earlier phases, Phase III trials are designed to verify the advantages of the treatment through the use of strict comparison with the normal treatment or the placebo controls. This confirmation is critical, particularly in situations where there are limited available treatments, such as the advanced pancreatic cancer. For instance, a trial examining oral capecitabine in patients who had failed gemcitabine treatment did find that although there were no partial or complete responses, 39% of evaluable patients had stable disease with the treatment (Boeck et al., 2007). This highlights the importance of proper statistical analysis in Phase III trials, where a larger number of patients and more diverse participants contribute to the validity of the conclusions. Comparison in Phase III trials not only includes the determination of effectiveness but also includes close examination of treatment-related toxicities and adverse reactions. Researchers must be extremely certain that the advantages overrule the risks, if any, for the patients and present a clear view of the range of therapy. As an example, the capecitabine trial showed overwhelming toxicities like hand-foot syndrome and anemia, which occurred to a significant extent (Boeck et al., 2007). This phase is an important part of the drug development process since the data it generates assists regulatory bodies in making informed decisions on drug approval and eventual use in the clinic. Furthermore, the comparative data from such trials inform best practices, guiding clinicians in their therapeutic decisions and potentially influencing updates to clinical guidelines. Phase III trial outcomes often have broader implications for treatment models in specific diseases. A useful case in point is provided by a national German survey of pancreatic cancer treatments, which found discrepancies between adherence to the then-prevailing clinical guidelines among doctors. Such results highlight a fundamental gap in research versus clinical utilization knowledge and necessitate continuing education as well as a reevaluation of treatment plans. As the landscape of Phase III trials evolves, becoming intimate with the nuances of confirmation and comparison will be key. Not only do these trials lay the ground for new therapy, but they also establish standards that ensure patient safety and optimize care outcomes in the real-world setting (Figure 10.15).

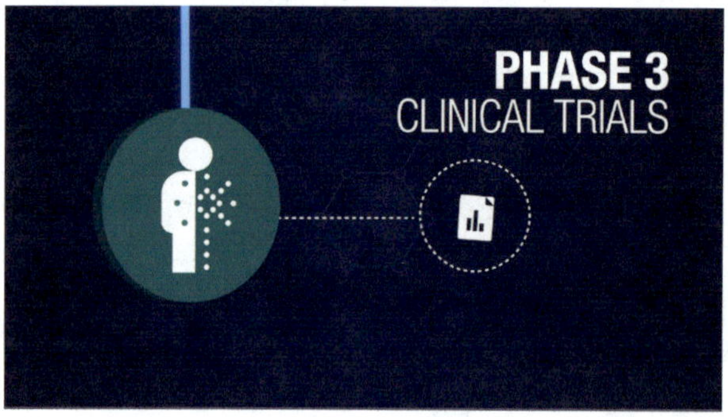

Figure 10.15. Phase III clinical trials.

Source: https://i.ytimg.com/vi/iWqQiJeP5ac/maxresdefault.jpg.

10.4. Ethical Considerations

The ethical aspects of clinical trials are multifaceted and integral to the integrity of research involving human subjects. Safeguarding the safety and well-being of participants is of utmost concern, which necessitates a strong understanding of guiding ethical principles applicable to clinical studies. Mandates for safeguarding subjects have been established by regulatory bodies, but their application in practice must ensue with subtle professional judgment on the part of clinicians and researchers. For instance, the ethical obligation of informed consent is essential but becomes complicated in the case of vulnerable populations, such as children or individuals with compromised capacity to consent. These issues emphasize collaboration among all concerned to scrutinize every detail of a clinical trial with respect to ethical standards and prioritize the rights and well-being of the participants during research, as noted in the International Myopia Institute's results for myopia control treatment (Drove et al., 2019). Informed consent is an overriding principle in clinical trials both legally and ethically, in that it honors participants' autonomy. It involves researchers being very clear about potential risks and benefits, allowing individuals to make well-informed decisions about volunteering. In the case of patients with neurological conditions, consent becomes further complicated. The ability of such people to consent should be closely examined, as cognitive impairment will prevent them from fully appreciating the implications of their participation (Chiong et al., 2018). Researchers are faced with an ethical challenge of doing justice to the scientific pursuit of knowledge while maintaining the safety of individuals who cannot give informed consent. This necessitates ongoing training and directions of researchers to offer to participants that they are treated with dignity and respect without compromising the integrity of the study. Moreover, ethical concerns extend beyond consent and protection of the participants to the extent of researchers' roles in reporting results and being open. Adequate reporting of trial results not only matters for the creation of medical knowledge but also for establishing public confidence in the research endeavor. Ethical misconduct, such as selective reporting or data falsification, can cause severe harm, discrediting the credibility of clinical research as a whole. During treatment development and promotion, as per the International Myopia Institute report, it is the responsibility of stakeholders to provide accurate and comprehensive information to clinicians and patients (Drove et al., 2019). It is not only through this ethical platform that protection of participants is guaranteed, but also the values of scientific research are maintained, so clinical trials are designed to improve the healthcare setting without compromising ethical principles (Figure 10.16).

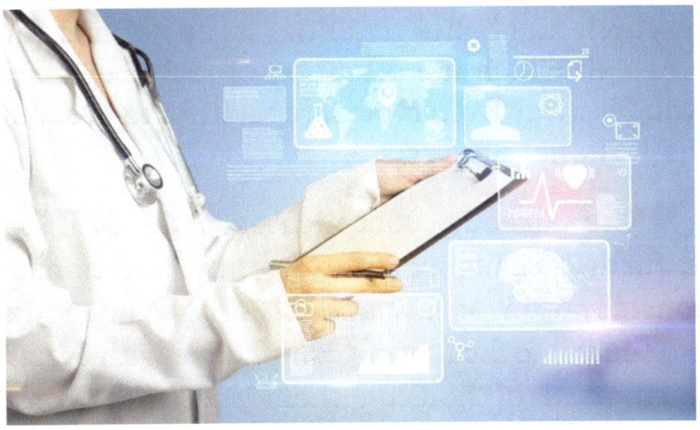

Figure 10.16. Regulations and ethics of clinical trials.

Source: https://www.news-medical.net/images/Article_Images/ImageForArticle_22878_16581465461381942.jpg.

10.4.1. Informed Consent

Informed consent is a principle of ethical conduct in clinical trials, ensuring participants have a clear understanding of the risks and benefits of their involvement. This is particularly challenging when dealing with vulnerable populations such as children who do not possess the capacity to provide informed consent independently. Researchers should then decompose technical information into something they can comprehend while safeguarding participants' rights. This commonly involves caregivers or guardians who must navigate the ethical landscape to make decisions on behalf of children, further complicating consent. The interest in protecting vulnerable populations and advancing medicine demands a systematic method of informed consent, with an emphasis on transparency and understanding to maintain clinical research integrity. The ethical perspective concerning informed consent exceeds mere adherence to regulatory requirements. The intricate nature of the process of consent involves not only asking permission but also fostering a culture of respect and trust among participants and researchers. For trials involving children, this is compounded by the fact that children cannot make independent, informed decisions, which puts in doubt the representations and advocacy. Ethical principles advocate for the inclusion of information commensurate with the age to facilitate effective communication, empowering the children and their guardians. By emphasizing education and comprehension, the process of informed consent can be a foundation for ethical research practice and ensure that participants are actively engaged with their treatment plans, ultimately providing better results in clinical trials as well as enhancing participant autonomy. Moreover, the lack of novel treatments for children is an acute concern directly linked with issues in informed consent. As some discussions of the pharmaceutical innovation process have noted, barriers such as monetary incentives as well as moral dilemmas inhibit children's drug development (Entorf et al., 2004). Because children are commonly incapable of consenting on their own behalf, this limitation may deter scientists from conducting trials that ultimately benefit this population. The ethical requirement to protect children cannot be overemphasized, but has to be, however, balanced against efforts towards developing effective treatments. Overcoming such challenges requires a re-evaluation of existing practices and incentives in clinical trials so that pediatric subjects are not only kept safe but also benefit from important progress in medicine (Entorf et al., 2004) (Figure 10.17).

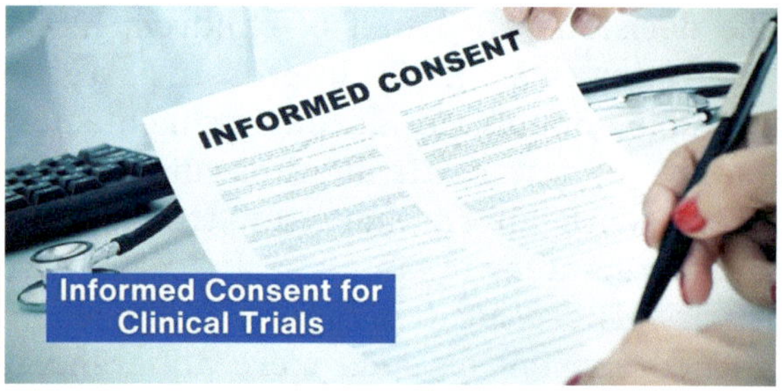

Figure 10.17. Informed consent for clinical trials.

Source: https://www.news-medical.net/image-handler/ts/20220518011117/ri/950/src/images/Article_Images/ImageForArticle_22535_16528938764304702.jpg.

10.4.2. Institutional Review Boards (IRBs)

The role of IRBs in clinical research is primarily to safeguard the rights and well-being of human participants in research. Formed as a response to historical ethical misconduct in medical research, IRBs have an obligation to scrutinize research protocols to ascertain compliance with ethics and regulatory requirements. Their scrutiny is critical in guaranteeing ethical practice, enabling informed consent, and minimizing the probability of harm to participants. However, in maintaining their protective goals, there is prevailing contention as to whether IRBs are adequate in explaining the complexity of contemporary research approaches. The critics argue that the strictness of IRB procedures is responsible for inefficiencies and inhibits the development of valuable clinical trials, thus ruining the very goals they seek to fulfill. This tension emphasizes the need for an equilibrium reaction that respects participant safety but also encourages creative research activity. As IRBs evolve, issues have appeared that seriously question their operational scope and effectiveness. IRBs, according to some researchers, are diminishing research autonomy, particularly by applying overly restrictive guidelines that threaten academic freedom and methodological creativity. There have been reported cases in which the IRB's fear of qualitative research led to misinterpretation of the nature and purpose of such research. Such misconceptions might result in censorship, preventing researchers from pursuing important, often neglected topics. The fear that IRBs would inadvertently narrow the boundaries of research is, as such, contrary to their intended function of protecting subjects, and reevaluating their methodology and application in light of new paradigms of research is an imperative. This research highlights potential issues of mission creep, in which the attention of IRBs begins to wander away from ethical regulation to broader institutional interests.

The already complicated role of IRBs is further made complex by the addition of consideration of law and liability. While IRBs are central to facilitating compliance with ethics, the notion of holding them accountable for failing to protect human subjects has become increasingly evocative in the imagination of legal specialists. There is the suggestion that IRBs can be held to account for negligence in cases where their conduct causes injury to clinical trial participants. Considerations of IRB accountability raise important questions about the effects of excessive expansion of their legal duties. Though such accountability could be a spur to more rigid adherence to ethical standards, it will also have the potential to instill fear in researchers that would translate into heightened caution and chill clinical trial innovation. Balancing the ethical mandate of IRBs with their functional limitations is a challenge that needs to be taken very seriously and reformed in order to ensure that they fulfill their desired function without compromising the integrity of the research process (Noah et al., 2004; Jacob et al., 2014) (Figure 10.18).

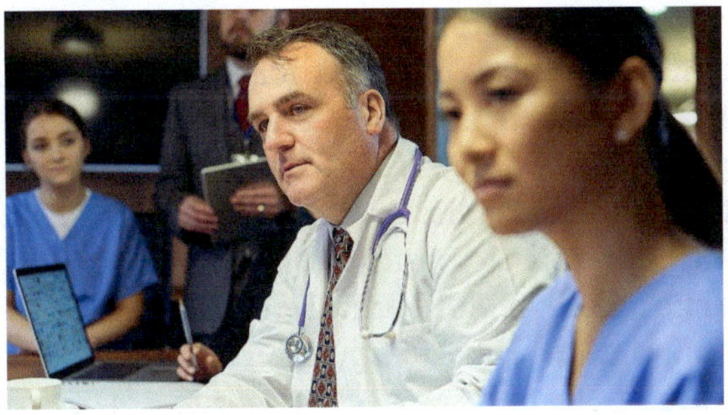

Figure 10.18. Institutional review boards (IRBs).

Source: https://www.ncbionetwork.org/sites/default/files/styles/1280x720/public/1280x720-images/reviewboard_preview.jpg?itok=usbCZ1ou.

10.4.3. Patient Safety and Rights

In clinical trials, the patients' rights and safety are a basic issue that must be carefully safeguarded during the performance of research. Safeguarding participants from harm is of crucial significance because their involvement in trials is, by definition, linked to the exploration of unknown effects and risks of experimental therapies. Ethical concerns mandate the implementation of informed consent procedures, which protect participants by allowing them to have complete knowledge of the implications and possible hazards surrounding their participation. In the long run, conformity with these ethical principles not only maintains individual autonomy but also maximizes public confidence in the clinical research system. For instance, in the context of evolving legislation regarding sharing data, as is the case in Sethi et al. (2014), it is critical to examine if legislative frameworks facilitate safe and informed participation in different groups. Clinical trials also often tread a delicate balance between the rights of patients and the interests of public health. Research conduct decisions need to balance the possibility of benefit to society against the ethical treatment of participants. Particularly, sensitive issues such as fetal tissue research involve significant ethical concerns, especially considering the implications for women's health and reproductive rights. As discussed in Halabi et al. (2017), such situations necessitate judicious consideration to ensure women's rights are upheld while also addressing urgent public health problems. The ongoing controversy over the legal and ethical guidelines underpinning such a study is critical to the refining of policies that promote patient rights and inspire innovation in therapy. Protection and sharing of data within clinical trials have a profound bearing on patient safety and rights as well. As demand for solid pharmacoepidemiological studies increases, legislative controls are a significant obstacle to the freedom to optimize patient safety through effective data sharing. Current and future regulations must be evaluated to allow greater re-use of health data, as defended in Sethi et al. (2014). Enabling broader access to clinical information significantly improves patient benefits by ensuring that researchers have the opportunity to thoroughly investigate safety trends and dangers across diverse populations. As such, establishing a culture that fosters sharing of data while duly protecting individual rights is key to the advancement of safe, effective medical interventions within clinical trials (Figure 10.19).

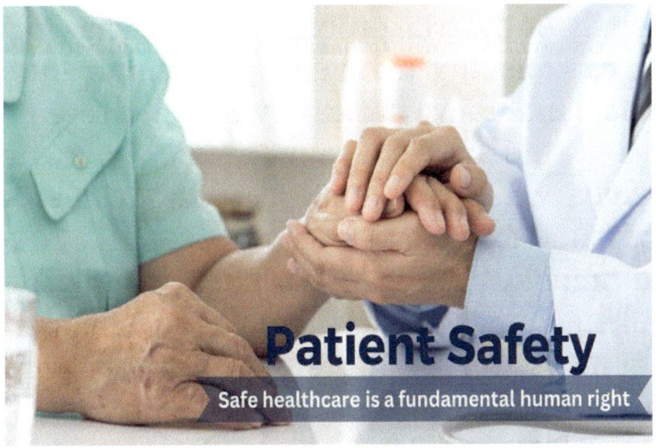

Figure 10.19. Patient safety.

Source: https://www.worldpatientsalliance.org/wp-content/uploads/patientsafety1.jpg.

10.5. Recruitment and Retention of Participants

Recruitment and participation retention are critical components to the success of clinical trials due to their profound impact on the validity and representativeness of study results. Effective recruitment strategies are required to achieve diverse participant groups that reflect the population under investigation accurately. Multiple methods can be employed for recruitment, such as through the utilization of online marketing campaigns and research registries, which have proven efficacious in generating interest and participating in trials (Blazeby et al., 2018). Moreover, establishing an accommodating environment at trial sites can enhance recruitment, as observed by practices enabling rapport development between research staff and prospective participants. This dynamic not only encourages enrollment but also lays the groundwork for sustained commitment throughout the trial, critical to participant retention. Efforts at retention, although equally critical, are often less prioritized in clinical trial design and implementation. Effective retention lies in sustained communication and the development of positive participant relationships throughout the trial process. Research has found that establishing trust and providing value to participants can significantly enhance retention rates, as individuals are more likely to remain engaged when they believe their involvement is of value and worth it (Blazeby et al., 2018). Additionally, trial teams should be cognizant of challenges that could affect participants, such as time issues or life situations that would render it challenging for them to fully engage. By anticipating these issues and acting aggressively upon them, researchers can develop participant-specific retention strategies that are optimal for the needs of the participants and ensure long-term participation and data quality. There remains insufficient research on methods of retention despite its identification as a priority area of research, and an entrenched need exists for intensive measures to address the issue within clinical trials. Creative approaches, such as utilizing participant feedback and exploring alternative forms of communication, have been promising for enhancing retention (Agarwal et al., 2025). Among the determinants of retention is trial staff support, whose dedication and interpersonal skills can have a great influence on participant experiences. Second, sponsor recognition of the significance of retention activities will be capable of determining shared aims for clinical researchers and trial staff, such that adequate resources are allocated to these activities. With recruitment and retention provided for in a holistic manner, clinical trials have the best chance of maximizing participant engagement, ultimately leading to stronger and more meaningful research conclusions (Figure 10.20).

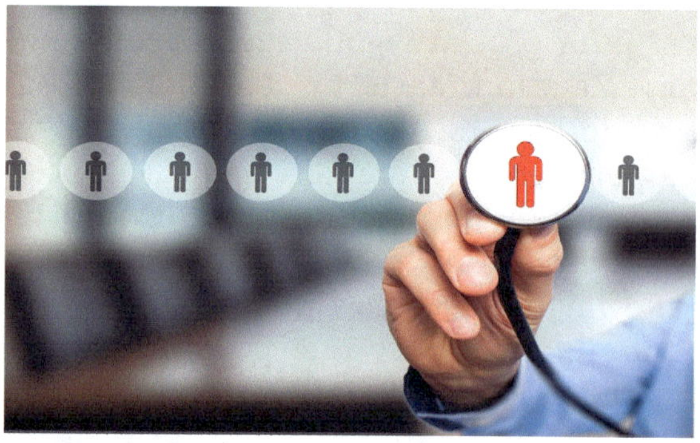

Figure 10.20. Clinical trial patient recruitment and retention.

Source: https://www.healthchek.in/images/blogs/98540094.jpg.

10.5.1. Strategies for Recruitment

Effective recruitment is key to the effective conduct of clinical trials, especially in enrolling ever more diverse populations of patients. Putting a high value on personal contact and face-to-face communication over traditional mass marketing is one striking approach. A trial testing the recruitment of participants into a trial of the yellow fever vaccine has reported that participants are more likely to be recruited upon invitation and that odds are 2.433 for personally invited participants compared to those who have been told about the study through advertising (Edupuganti et al., 2013). This underlines the importance of building rapport and trust with communities and can significantly boost the rates of enrollment. Market-specific recruitment not only increases outreach effectiveness but also supports a feeling of ownership and investment on the part of potential participants, ultimately resulting in more robust data and outcomes in clinical studies. An additional means of increasing recruitment within clinical trials is the utilization of community-based collaborations, particularly with religious-based groups. By collaborating with established community organizations, information regarding clinical trials and their paramount importance in the diminution of health disparities can be conveyed effectively. For instance, a cluster-randomized trial demonstrated that church-based education sessions were sufficient to enhance older African Americans' willingness to participate in clinical research (Anderson et al., 2015). This intervention not only educated potential participants but also leveraged the social cohesion and trust that exist in such communities. By framing discussions around clinical trials in culturally relevant settings, researchers can overcome barriers to participation, thereby enhancing demographic representation and maximizing clinical results' generalizability across populations. Further, using continuous engagement tactics like periodic updates and newsletters can greatly enhance recruitment and participation retention in clinical trials. Regular communication maintains the participants engaged and interested for the entire duration of the trial while keeping them updated on any meaningful news. Using more than one platform for communication, such as digital media and postal service, caters to different preferences and maximizes reach for information. By emphasizing the value of participant involvement in research and its potential beneficial effects within their own communities, researchers can build long-term interest in clinical trials. Such an all-encompassing approach not only increases early enrollment rates but also maintains long-term involvement, which is critical to the quality and success of clinical research efforts (Figure 10.21).

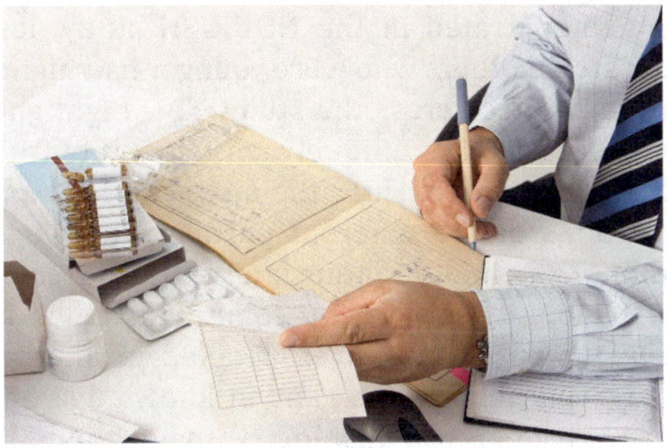

Figure 10.21. Recruitment strategies for clinical trials.

Source: https://iprocess.net/wp-content/uploads/2022/10/Clinical-Trial-Recruitment.jpg.

10.5.2. Challenges in Participant Retention

Participant dropout in trials is a significant problem that compromises the validity and reliability of the research outcome. Huge dropout numbers can lead to biased data and weak statistical power, eventually affecting the generalizability of the results. For instance, in the NOURISH RCT, where a community-level intervention in first-time mothers was being tested, nearly 21% of potential participants were retained at the end of the trial, a demonstration of the multifaceted dynamics at play with participant follow-up. Factors that contribute to participant attrition include personal problems, feelings of burden of study participation, and not having suitable support systems. Successful retention measures must therefore address these factors to optimize longer-term participation by participants, so that the trial achieves its intended goals while minimizing wastage of resources unnecessarily. The demographic determinants of participant retention cannot be overlooked, either. Research has identified certain groups, principally young individuals and the less educated, who are most susceptible to clinical trial dropout. As demonstrated in the NOURISH study, less educated mothers who were younger had higher dropout rates across the study. This highlights the necessity for uniquely targeted retention strategies that consider the distinct needs and situations of the different participant groups. Additionally, implementing interventions created in collaboration with the community, such as religious-based initiatives detailed in another study, can help bridge gaps in knowledge and trust. Through establishing stronger bonds by culturally relevant outreach and education, researchers may be able to enhance retention rates among underrepresented populations. Additionally, procedural measures such as increased communication and facilitation can contribute significantly to enhancing participant retention. For clinical trials, participant engagement over the study period is critical. The application of mobile communication aids, i.e., text message reminders, and the offer of alternatives such as home visits to reduce participant burden may prove to be helpful. According to Daniels et al. (2012), effective retention activities in studies have also involved active calling and education programs that are geared towards involving participants and keeping them informed. Similarly, the benefits of public involvement in research contexts, as noted in Anderson et al. (2015), play a role in heightening awareness of participation among selected demographic groups, hence encouraging ongoing participation. Hence, an integrated strategy that involves the above measures has the capability to improve retention outcomes, eventually boosting the integrity of clinical trial research (Figure 10.22).

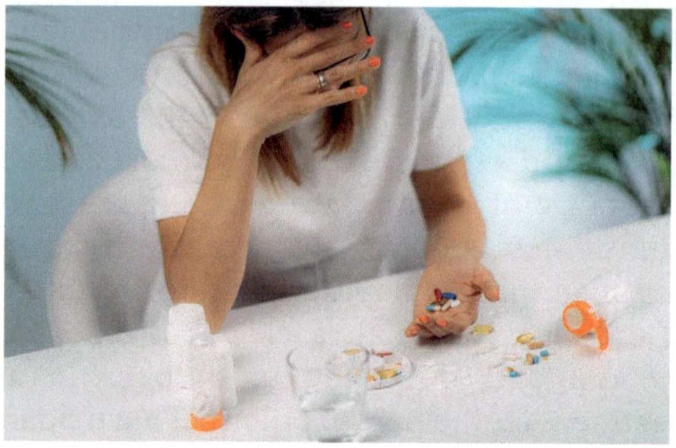

Figure 10.22. Enhancing participant retention in clinical trials.

Source: https://www.anjusoftware.com/wp-content/uploads/2023/01/trial-participant-retention.webp.

10.5.3. Importance of Diversity in Clinical Trials

Diversity of clinical trials is required for a myriad of reasons, with the majority of concern for accuracy and relevance of research findings. Since clinical trial participants are representative of a wide range of demographics—like race, ethnicity, age, and socioeconomic status—results of studies are also likely to be representative of actual efficacy and safety in the general population. This is critically vital since biological responses to therapy can vary significantly between different demographic groups. Inadequate representation can lead to incorrect conclusions about a drug's effectiveness, potentially harming certain populations and denying access to potentially life-saving therapy. Highlighted by recent studies, it remains too low to include diverse patients, particularly in areas like oncology, which strongly voices the need to make far-reaching changes toward more inclusion in trial design (Bandyopadhyay et al., 2024). Obstacles to diversity in clinical trials have been well reported, and correcting these issues is an ongoing challenge. Institutional mistrust, logistical issues, and cultural factors all generally keep minority groups away from clinical research. Effective recruitment, then, must utilize community outreach and culturally appropriate methods to traverse these obstacles and establish researcher trust with underserved populations. It has been demonstrated through studies that the application of strong Institutional Review Board (IRB) guidelines requiring diversity rules can significantly improve minority representation in clinical trials.

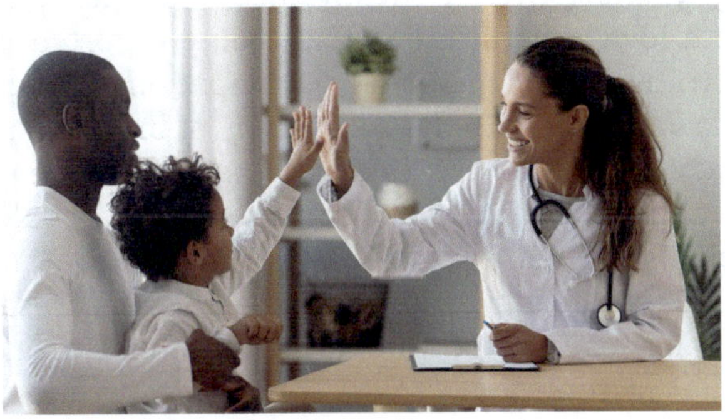

Figure 10.23. The importance of patient diversity in clinical trials.

Source: https://www.ppd.com/wp-content/uploads/2021/12/diversity-clinical-trials-blog-shutterstock_1463202674.jpg.

Strengthening outreach through active community partnerships and open dialogue can further ensure that trials are perceived as not exclusionary but inclusive steps towards better health outcomes among diverse populations (Cameron et al., 2011). A complete understanding of the worth of diversity in clinical trials goes beyond rates of recruitment; it involves the ethical obligation to conduct research that is sensitive to and respectful of the unique health issues of diverse populations. It requires a collaboration among stakeholders like clinicians, researchers, and community organizations, all of whom are committed to dismantling barriers to participation. Through multiple-level collaborations, the stakeholders have an opportunity to share ideas and resources that help maintain equitable practices along the research process. Through such alliances, not only is clinical data quality improved but also patient outcomes and confidence in the healthcare system in general. Lastly, having diversity in clinical trials is important, not just because it is a matter of access but because it is integral to the integrity and scientific soundness of medical research (Bandyopadhyay et al., 2024) (Figure 10.23).

Summary

In summarizing a review of clinical trials, there is a clear need to value their threefold contribution to the generation of medical knowledge and improvement of patient care. The conduct of clinical trials has the tendency to shed light on key questions regarding the potential of complex interventions in real-world healthcare practices. For instance, the application of the Normalization Process Model demonstrates that successful clinical trials must acknowledge not only the effectiveness of intervention but also how an intervention would be integrated into existing healthcare systems. Context and pragmatics focus is essential since it makes evaluators aware of how interventions are embedded in routine service practices, thus influencing patient outcomes. These factors not only enhance the validity of trial results but also enable the translation of findings into valuable clinical practice, thus realizing the ultimate aim of the trials to promote patient health outcomes (Nezu et al., 2007). Furthermore, the imbalances in recruitment between specific demographic groups prove to be significant problems that still exist in the field of clinical trials. Specifically, studies have indicated that adolescents and young adults (AYAs) typically face obstacles that block their recruitment into cancer clinical trials, with lower recruitment rates being reported in community sites. Efforts by the National Cancer Institute to enhance trial participation through community outreach have returned mixed results, bearing witness to the complexity of broadening access among diverse populations. It is then necessary to unravel the causes of such disparities, which may be socioeconomic in origin, care access, and patient attitudes towards clinical trials. By addressing these factors, researchers can develop targeted efforts that would propel AYA engagement, particularly among minorities, and thus guarantee inclusiveness and equity in clinical research (Blanke et al., 2020). In summary, the bringing together of an analysis of clinical trials brings to the fore the significance of both contextual factors and demographic considerations in guiding research outcomes. Through the integration of learning from implementation models such as the Normalization Process Model and overcoming challenges faced by underrepresented groups, clinical trial practice can move toward improved and equitable practice. The results of previous and ongoing trials constitute a blueprint for future research activity, with emphasis on systematic refinement in methodology and attempts at outreach. With increasing progression in clinical trials, the commitment towards greater participant diversity and pragmatic implementation of interventions will be part of promoting healthcare development accessible and beneficial to all (Nezu et al., 2007; Blanke et al., 2020).

Clinical trials are a key part of medical research, being the major vehicle for assessing the safety and effectiveness of new treatments before they are available in the market. Synthesis and reporting of results, particularly through generalist summarizations addressed to the public, are crucial in the conduct of clinical trials. The value of readable and clear lay summaries has also been emphasized with the introduction of European legislation mandating such reports. Such summaries must accurately capture the content of the trial, its objectives, methodology, and key findings in order to make the key points accessible to a range of different audiences regardless of their health literacy. By means of user testing, researchers can refine these summaries to maximum readability and acceptability within the context of public knowledge, rectifying any errors or cryptic details noted as needed from user testing results (Sless et al., 2018). The process of building consensus statements in clinical research also illustrates the necessity for establishing the most important concepts and parameters involved with a given medical condition. For instance, in acute renal failure (ARF), a diverse line of definitions has created confusion in the literature and hampered the comparison and interpretation of research. Systematic reviews and consensus conferences have enabled the identification of key questions, followed by consensus recommendations that provide standardized definitions and clinical endpoints. This collaborative approach facilitates an extensive examination of various methodologies and outcomes, which can enhance the collective validity of clinical trials. Through these foundations, researchers can be confident that future trials will be designed with precision and clarity, eventually maximizing their utilization and significance to patient care (Bellomo et al., 2004). Finally, the overwhelming implication of these debates surrounding clinical trials is the need for transparency of communication and consensus-building among research communities. Ensuring that outcomes from trials are not only scientifically sound but also comprehensible to lay audiences lies at the center of building public confidence and understanding in clinical research efforts. Better communication strategies may also ensure participation in upcoming studies because interested individuals will be better assured of participating in studies whose reasons and potential gains are explained in detail. As clinical trials continue to advance in complexity, so does the call for clear language, well-defined objectives, and specific lay summaries, affirming their place in facilitating medical science and patient care (Sless et al., 2018; Bellomo et al., 2004).

CLOSER LOOK

FUTURE DIRECTIONS IN CLINICAL TRIALS

As clinical practice continues to evolve, the incorporation of advanced technologies is a promising indication of a trend towards improved efficiency and efficacy in practice. The convergence of digital technologies, such as electronic health records and wearable tech, provides an arena for data generation in real time and patient monitoring remotely. With this development, varied participant populations can be enrolled, and treatment efficacy can be identified more accurately across populations. Through widening the scope of inclusion, clinical trials can achieve a higher degree of generalizability of the outcomes, ultimately contributing to the development of personalized medicine. In addition to this, these advances in technology may end up generating cost savings without sacrificing the validity and integrity of clinical trials. As modern trials require fewer resources and less time, the ability to accelerate drug development and access to the market is significant.

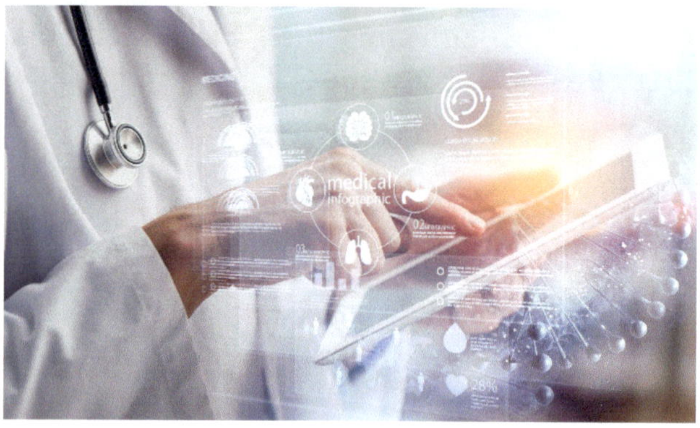

Figure 10.24. Healthcare professional interacting with digital medical infographics on a tablet for clinical data analysis.

Source: https://ft.com/partnercontent/images/medidata/hero-clinicaltrials.jpg

At the same time, the creation of regulatory guidelines specific to clinical trials plays a vital role in encouraging innovation while ensuring patient safety. Regulatory bodies are increasingly recognizing the significance of adaptive trial designs, wherein trial procedures can be modified on the basis of intermediate results. This flexibility can increase the learning capability from trials and improve their overall efficiency. Furthermore, collaboration between actors such as researchers, businesspeople, and regulators is vital to create an environment that fosters innovation. This collaboration can drive more significant breakthroughs in methods, particularly in areas such as artificial intelligence and machine learning, which have enormous potential in handling humongous datasets at velocity. Upcoming clinical trials will likely be structured on the framework of a synergistic strategy specifically aligned to quickly address changing patient needs and treatment trends. Further, the ethical principles underlying clinical trials are set to be redirected in the next several years due to increased public sensitivity and demands for transparency. Issues of informed consent and subject autonomy are ever more at center stage, and these issues must be carefully weighed in trial planning. Engage patients in the co-designing of studies in order to establish trust and allow them to feel heard in the research. With increased participative clinical trials, new models, such as decentralized trials, will facilitate increased accessibility and ease of use for participants. This not only improves the participant experience, but it could also result in improved quality data and greater retention rates. The recognition of the need for ethical standards will be key to defining the clinical research model of the future as a more patient-centered model that is constructed around shared decision-making and collaboration in the development of new interventions and treatments (Figure 10.24).

The Impact of Clinical Trials on Healthcare Advancements:

Clinical trials are the pillars of medical innovations, enabling controlled evaluation of new interventions and their influence on human health. In addition to enabling evaluation of safety and efficacy for prospective treatments, trials also contribute to improved insight into disease mechanisms. Through evidence that informs clinical practice, trials can potentially achieve significant improvements in patient outcomes. The voluminous data gathered by these studies find important use in the development of personalized medicine strategies, thus ultimately allowing healthcare professionals to tailor treatments according to individual patient needs. Secondly, the transition from paper-based data processing to computerized systems has allowed for improved collection and analysis of such data sets. With the records going digital, the harmonization of trial data with electronic health records raises the chances of new clinical insights (Arcuri et al., 2018). Interactivity between various stakeholders, such as academic centers, industry sponsors, and patient advocacy groups, is central to the successful execution of clinical trials and their interpretation. This multistakeholder research includes different perspectives, in the end enhancing research and adding to the relevance of trial outcomes. But for such collaborations to be maximally harnessed, there must be concise and uniform policy standards. The policies are supposed to address the complexities of synchronizing different stakeholder priorities and expectations without compromising the integrity of the research process. This pressure for collective action highlights the importance of processes that facilitate communication and cooperation between stakeholders, which together manage science development with patient-focused care (Abbracchio et al., 2018). With the advancement of such alliances, the impact of clinical trials can be scaled to deliver epoch-making improvements in healthcare. Additionally, the advancements in clinical trials have motivated new therapies and healthcare systems to enhance delivery. With every new treatment and intervention being tested and established with rigorous trials, they generally pave the way for better management strategies for various diseases. This practice of testing and optimizing has led to major progress in the areas of oncology, cardiology, and neurology and has impacted millions of lives worldwide. Clinical trials also reiterate how it is essential to maintain ethical standards so that the patient's safety is always paramount in conducting research. The emphasis on ethical practice serves not only to safeguard participants in trials but also to foster public trust in the research enterprise, critical to sustained recruitment of diverse populations in future trials. As the health care environment continues to evolve, the future of the role of clinical trials will assuredly remain at the forefront of propelling innovation and improving population health outcomes.

References

1. Abbracchio, M. P., Andreaus, M., Battaglia, M. A., Costa, A., et al. (2018). Steps towards collective sustainability in biomedical research. https://core.ac.uk/download/160052033.pdf (accessed on 25th June 2025).
2. Adadzi, J., Anderson II, J., Azi, C. I., Carsrud, A., et al. (2024). Balancing placebo uses with evidence-based treatments: The placebo effect in clinical practice and research. https://core.ac.uk/download/621451779.pdf (accessed on 25th June 2025).
3. Adamina, M., Fueglistaler, P., & Guller, U. (2018). Non-inferiority trials in surgical oncology. https://core.ac.uk/download/159150935.pdf (accessed on 25th June 2025).
4. Agarwal, V., Allgar, V., Allison, J., Bartlett, M., Bartolomeu-Pires, S., Boey, T., Carroll, C. B., et al. (2025). Improving recruitment and retention of people with Parkinson's disease to clinical studies: A scoping review. https://core.ac.uk/download/653315841.pdf (accessed on 25th June 2025).
5. Alaszewski, A., Armstrong, A., Ballard, K., Birke, L., Blaxter, M., Byrne, P., et al. (2005). Health professionals, their medical interventions and uncertainty: A study focusing on women at midlife. https://core.ac.uk/download/49213.pdf (accessed on 25th June 2025).
6. American Medical Association Council on Scientific Affairs, Cassileth, B. R., Kowaleski, B., Sackett, D., Wright, J. R., Sussman, J., Corrie, P., et al. (2008). What constitutes a "clinical trial"?: A survey of oncology professionals. https://core.ac.uk/download/pdf/7951237.pdf (accessed on 25th June 2025).
7. Amir, E. A. D., Babdor, J., Bendall, S. C., Gherardini, P., et al. (2019). Comprehensive immune monitoring of clinical trials to advance human immunotherapy. https://core.ac.uk/download/323074393.pdf (accessed on 25th June 2025).
8. Anderson, A. M., Archibald, M., Boggavarapu, S., Bolton, G., et al. (2015). Delivering a "dose of hope": A faith-based program to increase older African Americans' participation in clinical trials. https://core.ac.uk/download/215453357.pdf (accessed on 25th June 2025).
9. Anisimov, V. V. (2016). Discussion on the paper "Real-time prediction of clinical trial enrollment and event counts: A review," by D. F. Heitjan, Z. Ge, and G. S. Ying. https://core.ac.uk/download/78908347.pdf (accessed on 25th June 2025).
10. Antiretroviral Therapy and Medical Management of HIV-Infected Children, ATMMHC, Health Resources and Services Administration, HRSA, National Institutes of Health, NIH, National Pediatric and Family HIV Resource Center, et al. (2003). *Guidelines for the Use of Antiretroviral Agents in Pediatric HIV Infection*. https://core.ac.uk/download/pdf/11307015.pdf (accessed on 25th June 2025).
11. Arcuri, A., Rector, A. L., Wood, A. M., Glas, A. S., Kulis, B., Cortes, C., Sammut, C., et al. (2018). Beyond volume: The impact of complex healthcare data on the machine learning pipeline. http://arxiv.org/abs/1706.01513 (accessed on 25th June 2025).
12. Babbs, C. F. (2017). Meta-analysis of studies on CPR: A better route to new practice guidelines. https://core.ac.uk/download/77955506.pdf (accessed on 25th June 2025).
13. Baianu, I. C. (2012). Cancer clinical trials optimization and pharmacogenomics. https://core.ac.uk/download/pdf/1570002.pdf (accessed on 25th June 2025).

14. Bandura, A., Walker, A., Oxman, A. D., Walker, A. E., Lee, A. J., Del Mar, C. B., Armitage, C. J., et al. (2007). Translating clinicians' beliefs into implementation interventions (TRACII): A protocol for an intervention modeling experiment to change clinicians' intentions to implement evidence-based practice. https://core.ac.uk/download/177041.pdf (accessed on 25th June 2025).

15. Bandyopadhyay, S., Ghosh, M., Gunjan, G., Kulal, S., et al. (2024). Scientific validity and fair subject selection: An empirical analysis of recruitment practices in clinical trials. https://core.ac.uk/download/640070102.pdf (accessed on 25th June 2025).

16. Barnes, N. L., Blazeby, J. M., Branford, O. A., Breast Reconstruction Research Collaborative, et al. (2016). The iBRA (implant breast reconstruction evaluation) study: Protocol for a prospective multi-center cohort study to inform the feasibility, design and conduct of a pragmatic randomized clinical trial comparing new techniques of implant-based breast reconstruction. https://core.ac.uk/download/77021807.pdf (accessed on 25th June 2025).

17. Bellomo, R., Kellum, J. A., Mehta, R. L., Palevsky, P., et al. (2004). Acute renal failure–Definition, outcome measures, animal models, fluid therapy and information technology needs: The Second International Consensus Conference of the Acute Dialysis Quality Initiative (ADQI) Group. https://core.ac.uk/download/pdf/3543445.pdf (accessed on 25th June 2025).

18. Bennett, A. B., Fernandez, C., Graff, G. D., Kowalski, S., et al. (2007). *Intellectual Property Management in Health and Agricultural Innovation: Executive Guide*. https://core.ac.uk/download/72056336.pdf (accessed on 25th June 2025).

19. Bergan, R., Dickson, D., Johnson, J., Kurzrock, R., et al. (2020). The Master Observational Trial: A new class of master protocol to advance precision medicine. https://core.ac.uk/download/286729252.pdf (accessed on 25th June 2025).

20. Bishara, S., Clark, C., Egger, M., Hagg, U., Lewis, S., Peck, S., et al. (2008). Open versus closed surgical exposure of canine teeth that are displaced in the roof of the mouth. https://core.ac.uk/download/13505003.pdf (accessed on 25th June 2025).

21. Blanke, C., Budd, T., Freyer, D. R., Johnson, R. H., et al. (2020). Enrollment of adolescents and young adults onto SWOG Cancer Research Network clinical trials: A comparative analysis by treatment site and era. https://core.ac.uk/download/323070093.pdf (accessed on 25th June 2025).

22. Blazeby, J., Clarke, M., Clement, C., Daykin, A., et al. (2018). 'Recruitment, recruitment, recruitment'–The need for more focus on retention: A qualitative study of five trials. https://core.ac.uk/download/146502063.pdf (accessed on 25th June 2025).

23. Bobes, J., Cuijpers, P., & Dal Ré, R. (2017). Why prudence is needed when interpreting articles reporting clinical trial results in mental health. https://core.ac.uk/download/pdf/85166707.pdf (accessed on 25th June 2025).

24. Boeck, S., Bruns, C. J., Golf, A., Haas, M., et al. (2007). Oral capecitabine in gemcitabine-pretreated patients with advanced pancreatic cancer. https://core.ac.uk/download/16432403.pdf (accessed on 25th June 2025).

25. Boeck, S., Bruns, C. J., Heinemann, V., Jauch, K. W., et al. (2009). Current oncological treatment of patients with pancreatic cancer in Germany: Results from a national survey on behalf of the Arbeitsgemeinschaft Internistische Onkologie and the Chirurgische Arbeitsgemeinschaft Onkologie of the Germany Cancer Society. https://core.ac.uk/download/16432402.pdf

26. Burt, T., Dhillon, S., Manchanda, M., Mittal, S., et al. (2014). Clinical research environment in India: Challenges and proposed solutions. https://core.ac.uk/download/pdf/37750634.pdf (accessed on 25th June 2025).

27. Calvocoressi, L., Carroll, M., Dziura, J., Johnson, S., et al. (2020). Quality and publication of emergency medicine trials registered in ClinicalTrials.gov. https://core.ac.uk/download/287622009.pdf (accessed on 25th June 2025).

28. Cameron, M., Carr, W., Chelf, J. H., Elliott, J., Ely, M., Fearon, K. C. H., Poland, F., et al. (2011). Multidimensional collaboration; reflections on action research in a clinical context. https://core.ac.uk/download/2780307.pdf (accessed on 25th June 2025).

29. Carné Cladellas, X., Dal-Ré, R., Demotes-Mainard, J., Gluud, C., et al. (2011). Disclosure of investigators' recruitment performance in multicenter clinical trials: A further step for research transparency. https://core.ac.uk/download/43553092.pdf (accessed on 25th June 2025).

30. Casbard, A. C., Griffiths, G., Harrop, E., Kelly, J., et al. (2016). Why do patients decline surgical trials? Findings from a qualitative interview study embedded in the Cancer Research UK BOLERO trial (Bladder cancer: Open versus Laparoscopic or Robotic cystectomy). https://core.ac.uk/download/42530335.pdf (accessed on 25th June 2025).

31. Chiong, W., & Vaishnav, N. H. (2018). Informed consent for the human research subject with a neurologic disorder. https://core.ac.uk/download/286362450.pdf (accessed on 25th June 2025).

32. Curley, K., & Duong, N. (2017). Exosome membrane bound TNF-receptor for the treatment of rheumatoid arthritis. https://core.ac.uk/download/84118681.pdf (accessed on 25th June 2025).

33. Daniels, L., Magarey, A., Mallan, K., Mihrshahi, S., et al. (2012). Recruiting and engaging new mothers in nutrition research studies: Lessons from the Australian NOURISH randomized controlled trial. https://core.ac.uk/download/10915590.pdf (accessed on 25th June 2025).

34. Dautenhahn, K., Koay, K. L., Walters, M. L., Woods, S., et al. (2006). Comparing human-robot interaction scenarios using live and video-based methods: Towards a novel methodological approach. https://core.ac.uk/download/1642708.pdf (accessed on 25th June 2025).

35. Drove, B., Gifford, K. L., Gonzalez-Meijome, J. M., Gray, S., et al. (2019). IMI–Industry guidelines and ethical considerations for myopia control report. https://core.ac.uk/download/293867276.pdf (accessed on 25th June 2025).

36. Duan, N., Kravitz, R. L., & Schmid, C. H. (2013). Single-patient (n-of-1) trials: A pragmatic clinical decision methodology for patient-centered comparative effectiveness research. https://core.ac.uk/download/pdf/82183878.pdf (accessed on 25th June 2025).

37. Edupuganti, S., Frew, P. M., Keyserling, H. L., Lu, X., et al. (2013). Enrollment in YFV vaccine trial: An evaluation of recruitment outcomes associated with a randomized controlled double-blind trial of a live attenuated yellow fever vaccine. https://digitalscholarship.unlv.edu/cgi/viewcontent.cgi?article=1400&context=env_occ_health_fac_articles (accessed on 25th June 2025).

38. Entorf, H., Fegert, J., & Kölch, M. (2004). Children in need of medical innovation. https://core.ac.uk/download/76650117.pdf (accessed on 25th June 2025).

39. Feldman, D. N., Armstrong, E. J., Aronow, H. D., Gigliotti, O., Jaff, M. R., Klein, A., Parikh, S.

A., et al. (2018). SCAI consensus guidelines for device selection in femoral-popliteal arterial interventions. *Catheterization and Cardiovascular Interventions, 92*, 124–140. https://doi.org/10.1002/ccd.27635 (accessed on 25th June 2025).

40. Friede, T., Glimm, E., Mütze, T., Schmidli, H., et al. (2018). Group sequential designs for negative binomial outcomes. http://arxiv.org/abs/1707.04612 (accessed on 25th June 2025).

41. GLASS Consortium. (2018). Glioma through the looking GLASS: Molecular evolution of diffuse gliomas and the Glioma Longitudinal Analysis Consortium. https://core.ac.uk/download/323072182.pdf (accessed on 25th June 2025).

42. Halabi, S. F. (2017). Zika, pregnancy, and the law. https://core.ac.uk/download/148340614.pdf (accessed on 25th June 2025).

43. Heilman, E., Isseroff, R. R., Jagdeo, J. R., Jakus, J., et al. (2019). A dose-ranging, parallel group, split-face, single-blind phase II study of light emitting diode-red light (LED-RL) for skin scarring prevention: Study protocol for a randomized controlled trial. https://core.ac.uk/download/323070347.pdf (accessed on 25th June 2025).

44. Henney, A., Morley-Fletcher, E., & Viceconti, M. (2016). *In silico* clinical trials: How computer simulation will transform the biomedical industry. https://core.ac.uk/download/42625081.pdf (accessed on 25th June 2025).

45. Jacob, S. A., Musoba, G. D., & Robinson, L. J. (2014). The institutional review board (IRB) and faculty: Does the IRB challenge faculty professionalism in the social sciences? https://core.ac.uk/download/51086981.pdf (accessed on 25th June 2025).

46. Kyte, D., Draper, H., Ives, J., Calvert, M., & Keeley, T. (2013). Inconsistencies in quality-of-life data collection in clinical trials: A potential source of bias? Interviews with research nurses and trialists. https://core.ac.uk/download/pdf/81213453.pdf (accessed on 25th June 2025).

47. Leatherman, S. M. (2016). *Adaptive Methods for Bayesian Time-to-Event Point-of-Care Clinical Trials*. https://open.bu.edu/bitstream/2144/14317/9/Leatherman_bu_0017E_10368.pdf (accessed on 25th June 2025).

48. López-López, Á., López-Gonzálvez, Á., & Barbas, C. (2024). Metabolomics for searching validated biomarkers in cancer studies: A decade in review. *Expert Review of Molecular Diagnostics, 24*, 601–626. https://www.semanticscholar.org/paper/f92a13589b91872146894cc02ba41d0e5c57665f (accessed on 25th June 2025).

49. Ma, L., Wang, X., Yang, Z., Huang, D., Weng, H., & Zeng, X. T. (2020). Methodological quality (risk of bias) assessment tools for primary and secondary medical studies: What are they and which is better? *Military Medical Research, 7*. https://doi.org/10.1186/s40779-020-00238-8 (accessed on 25th June 2025).

50. N/A. (2024). The application of medical ethics in the developing countries–A neurosurgical perspective. https://core.ac.uk/download/635798426.pdf (accessed on 25th June 2025).

51. Nezu, A., Oakley, A., Strauss, A., Blackwood, B., Flyvbjerg, B., Starfield, B., Dowrick, C., et al. (2007). Process evaluation for complex interventions in primary care: Understanding trials using the normalization process model. https://core.ac.uk/download/pdf/7672960.pdf (accessed on 25th June 2025).

52. Noah, B. A. (2004). Bioethical malpractice: Risk and responsibility in human research. https://core.ac.uk/download/56355361.pdf (accessed on 25th June 2025).

53. Parry, E. L., Peat, G., & Thomas, M. J. (2018). Defining acute flares in knee osteoarthritis: A systematic review. https://core.ac.uk/download/161128902.pdf (accessed on 25th June 2025).

54. Pontecorvo, S., & Prosperini, L. (2016). Dimethyl fumarate in the management of multiple sclerosis: Appropriate patient selection and special considerations. https://core.ac.uk/download/74319286.pdf (accessed on 25th June 2025).

55. Ramadhani, B. P., Sitepu, E. C., Lestari, E. S., Jonny, J., Yana, M. L., Sofro, M. A. U., et al. (2023). Safety and efficacy of dendritic cell vaccine for COVID-19 prevention after 1-year follow-up: Phase I and II clinical trial final result. https://core.ac.uk/download/568272595.pdf (accessed on 25th June 2025).

56. Ryeznik, Y., Sverdlov, O., & Wong, W. K. (2019). On optimal designs for clinical trials: An updated review. https://core.ac.uk/download/286729243.pdf (accessed on 25th June 2025).

57. Sethi, N. (2014). The promotion of data sharing in pharmacoepidemiology. https://core.ac.uk/download/28977826.pdf (accessed on 25th June 2025).

58. Sless, D., Way, D., Raynor, D. K., Harris, E., Philip, G., et al. (2018). Clinical trial results summary for laypersons: A user testing study. https://core.ac.uk/download/153570486.pdf (accessed on 25th June 2025).

59. Thorlund, K., Shephard, C., Machado, L., Bourgouin, T., Hudson, L., Ting, E., Dempster, W., et al. (2024). Adapting Health Technology Assessment agency standards for surrogate outcomes in early-stage cancer trials: What needs to happen? *Expert Review of Pharmacoeconomics & Outcomes Research, 24*, 331–342. https://www.semanticscholar.org/paper/be2ded7f8d6be5d270bbb70e8c4dd9a60e1cced3 (accessed on 25th June 2025).

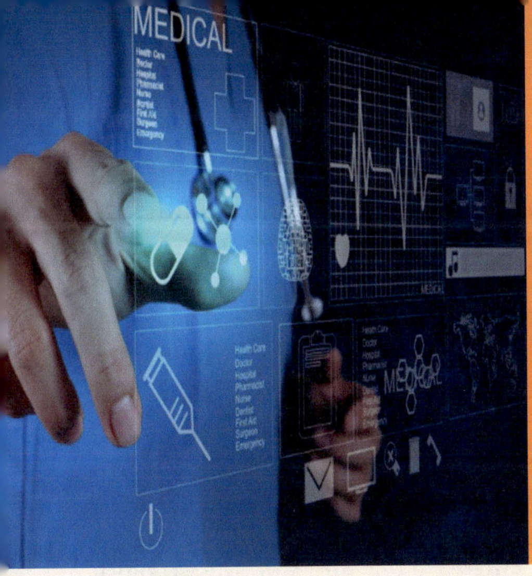

Chapter 11

EVIDENCE-BASED MEDICINE (EBM)

Contents

Introduction

Evidence-based medicine (EBM) is a paradigm shift in clinical practice, with decisions made based on the best available evidence. This approach seeks to integrate clinical experience, patient values, and current research to optimize outcomes for the patient. By integrating science into medicine, clinicians can decrease the risk of errors and enhance treatment effectiveness. At the heart of EBM practice is developing clinical questions and the systematic review of pertinent literature, which enables providers to stay abreast of medical advancements. This thorough approach not only helps develop evidence-based treatment plans but also helps foster an environment of ongoing learning in healthcare professionals. A fundamental component of EBM is to place priority on quality improvement and patient-centered care, which enhances the value of clinical outcomes. Leadership involvement in healthcare organizations is core to implementing EBM values, forming a culture where evidence-based practices are effective. This entails implementing practices that prioritize ongoing and team-based healing relationships, ultimately cultivating a setting where collaborative decision-making can prevail. For the implementation of these principles, the policies and workflows within healthcare systems must be modified accordingly to ensure that EBM is not a dream but something that is within the practitioner's and patient's reach. With progress in healthcare, the integration of quality improvement processes still remains essential for successful incorporation of EBM across settings and specialties (Wagner et al., 2012). In addition, the integration of EBM is problematic, particularly in balancing traditional and complementary medicine into the paradigm of evidence. The One-World Medicine concept recommends a subtle combination of traditional approaches to healing and contemporary medical science, respecting the possibilities of holistic therapy with rapport toward different populations of patients. In so doing, however, such integration necessitates adherence to strict requirements guaranteeing efficacy and safety in the context of respecting cultural practices. Legislative action, like the Nagoya Protocol, strives toward fair benefit-sharing of traditional knowledge, focusing on the importance of ethical practices in healthcare. Despite the progress in conjoining these models, systemic obstacles remain prevalent, particularly in the developing world, where infrastructures for healthcare are under strain (Abdelfatah et al., 2019). So, tackling these issues is very important for a fully holistic EBM model that brings together a range of healthcare practices in order to most effectively meet individuals with diverse backgrounds and healthcare requirements (Figure 11.1).

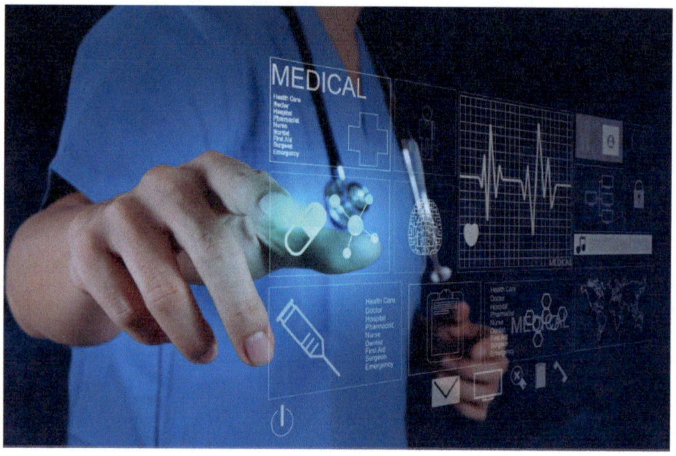

Figure 11.1. Evidence-based medicine.

Source: https://static.s4be.cochrane.org/app/uploads/2013/05/medical-doctor.jpg.

Definition of Evidence-Based Medicine

The origin of the definition of EBM stems from the drive to place clinical practice on scientific evidence, thereby enhancing patient outcomes. EBM is usually defined by the combination of best obtainable evidence, expertise in clinical practice, and patient values within decision-making in health care. The three form the basis for EBM, with the expectation that medical practitioners do not only rely on empirical evidence but also on the personal preferences and conditions of the individual patients. By anchoring treatment interventions in this paradigm, EBM aims to eliminate variability in medical practice that may be introduced by clinical judgment, and actually standardize procedures based on evidence-based findings. The requirement for continuous improvement of clinical practice through strict evidence assessment makes EBM a revolutionary methodology in contemporary medicine, with the additional advantages of increased accountability and efficiency in healthcare delivery. A crucial element of EBM is the process that underpins its adoption within medical education and practice. As noted within recent studies, medical schools are increasingly incorporating the principles of EBM into curricula in response to an increased trend towards empirically focused educational strategies. For instance, the development of applications like the Finding Information Framework application demonstrates how technology can be used to learn about EBM principles by providing students with the capacity to apply the evidence in a real-world setting (Liu et al., 2016). Additionally, this is an effort towards bridging the potential theoretical-practical knowledge gap in clinical practice. Therefore, EBM not only emphasizes the use of current evidence but also favors the acquisition of skills by future medical professionals in effectively handling and implementing such information, creating a culture of medical practice founded on life-long learning. In spite of the advancements associated with EBM, there are some problems inherent in its design that require critical examination. A specific issue involves the epistemological underpinnings of EBM, and in this instance, the emphasis on empiricism potentially at the expense of rationalism in clinical judgment (Webb et al., 2018). This practice could have the result of restricting the degree of clinical judgment and failing to resolve the issues regarding the cases of individual patients. This epistemic equilibrium has been the focus of contention in fostering the deliberate integration of empirical evidence along with the rational approach in medical education. The evaluation of historical views, as elaborated by Galen, allows for critical reflections towards combining these elements more harmoniously, suggesting that with a more critical understanding of EBM, medical practices would be made more robust. Thus, the establishment of an epistemically balanced practice can allow for better clinical outcomes and a fuller paradigm of evidence-based decision-making (Figure 11.2).

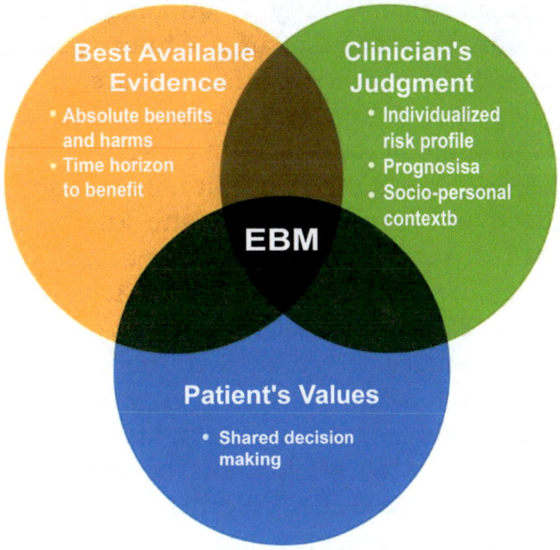

Figure 11.2. Evidence-based medicine framework for clinical decision making.

Source: https://www.researchgate.net/profile/Oanh-Nguyen-8/publication/312185769/figure/fig4/AS:710755242504192@1546468663074/Evidence-Based-Medicine-Framework-for-Clinical-Decision-Making-Adapted-from-a-conceptual.jpg.

Historical Development of EBM

The history of Evidence-Based Medicine (EBM) development through the ages goes back to significant alterations in the understanding and application of medical information. EBM is typically sourced from initiatives of doctors during the late 20th century to merge research evidence and clinical experience to best optimize patient outcomes. This concept was further encouraged with the establishment of the Evidence-Based Medicine Working Group in the early 1990s, which aimed at integrating individual clinical judgment with the best available external clinical evidence from systematic research. Significantly, this movement established a model of critical analysis of scientific literature, distinct from anecdotal methods otherwise predominant in the field. Last but not least, these efforts embodied the necessity of utilizing rigorous methods, the template of a clinical practice change that continues to this day. Moreover, the development of EBM was not only a paradigm change in medical practice, but also in medical education. Traditionally, medical education has focused on passing down static knowledge, rooted in procedural knowledge that can be contingent upon well-established techniques and guidelines accumulated over a period of several decades. However, with the increasing sophistication in healthcare as well as the application of data, the need for a more dynamic instructional strategy emerged. The alteration of training to include EBM precepts facilitated the enhancement of medical practitioners' critical thinking ability. By emphasizing the importance of staying in touch with new research findings and being sensitive to their clinical implications, teachers began nurturing a new generation of medical caregivers who could cope with the new situation of medical science. These developments highlighted an invaluable synergy between education and practice, eventually reflecting the altered needs of modern patient care within an era characterized by accelerated progress in medical research. Contemporary debates over the applicability of EBM also draw upon past settings for the integration of social sciences within medical education and practice. Scholarly researchers argue that the effectiveness of EBM can be enhanced by incorporating the wisdom of social science disciplines so that patient care is considered from a more integrated perspective. The argument is reflected in comparative analyses of hospitality management studies, which reveal potential scholarly gains from interdisciplinary research collaboration. By applying social science methods, healthcare professionals are able to better comprehend the patients' needs in their cultural and societal context. The identification of the key role played by context in medicine is parallel to the Ergonomic Education principles adopted in earlier studies, highlighting the educational models that embrace the intrinsic need for adaptation and learning among healthcare professionals. EBM's own historical evolution thus not only predicts clinical practice but also challenges educators and practitioners to consider critically how to prepare future generations for the challenges of medical decision-making in an increasingly evidence-based and complicated world (Barsky et al., 2014; Morrison et al., 2008).

Importance of EBM in Modern Healthcare

The integration of EBM into modern healthcare is absolutely essential, as it compels decisions to be made based on the best available evidence. By placing systematic findings of research at the forefront, EBM shifts the focus away from the typically heavily precedent- or anecdotal-based experience of more traditional practices and towards methods firmly based in scientific principle. Such orientation not only enhances the quality of patient care provided but also creates a culture of continuous improvement in healthcare systems. The continuous application of EBM principles leads to outcomes like reduced hospital stays, better diagnostics, and overall enhanced patient safety and satisfaction, demonstrating its foundational significance in contemporary medical practice. Finally, EBM's implementation offers healthcare workers a step-by-step method for evaluating treatments and interventions, which logically means connecting clinical practice with the ever-changing frontiers of medical science. In addition to improving clinical outcomes, EBM profoundly helps in the best allocation of healthcare resources. Increasing costs in the provision of care make it even more crucial to apply methods to optimize value while minimizing waste. EBM offers a structured method for evaluating the effectiveness and cost-utility of various medical interventions, which guides healthcare providers in making informed decisions that are desirable to patients and healthcare systems. For instance, effective utilization of laboratory medicine, as noted in Agarwal et al. (2013), generates the required knowledge that can enhance patient management and outcomes by considerable amounts. Through the integration of evidence-based guidelines with clinical practices, healthcare professionals can reduce the instances of unnecessary procedures and tests, thereby streamlining processes and reducing economic burdens on patients and healthcare systems, respectively.

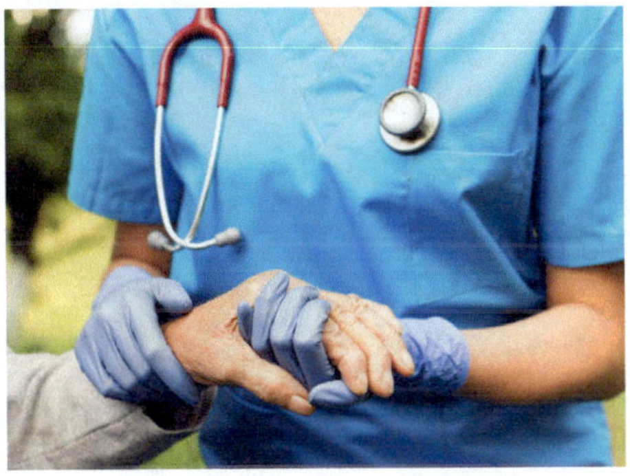

Figure 11.3. EBM: Role of Evidence-Based Medicine in improving quality of healthcare.

Source: https://etimg.etb2bimg.com/thumb/msid-66428983,width-1200,height-900,resizemode-4/.jpg.

Finally, the educational aspect of EBM must not be overlooked since it fosters learning cultures among healthcare professionals. Continuous education about the findings of ongoing research permits practitioners to remain proficient and familiarize themselves with the latest developments in clinical practice. Professionals are assisted by EBM in critically analyzing new literature and applying appropriate findings to practice, which is essential in an ever-evolving discipline. As highlighted by Miller et al. (2014), the application of expert opinion and rigorous evidence appraisal is imperative in medicine, especially owing to its complexity. Consequently, advocating for dedication to lifelong learning and evidence-based practice ensures that healthcare professionals are properly placed to deliver high-quality patient care, ultimately improving public health outcomes in a fast-changing medical landscape (Figure 11.3).

11.1. The Principles of Evidence-Based Medicine

The Evidence-Based Medicine (EBM) principles provide a firm basis to harmonize clinical experience with the latest applicable evidence based on systematic research. Essentially, EBM promotes the systematic application of the best current evidence in the making of clinical decisions, which involves critically evaluating the quality and relevance of research evidence. This systematic process keeps health care professionals from relying solely on tradition or anecdotal data; instead, they employ peer-reviewed information and evidence to guide their recommendations. Significantly, as noted, abandoning useless medical methods and minimizing the risks of untested methods are essential to improving patient health and constraining healthcare costs. This alludes to the importance of EBMs in abandoning ingrained routines supported by limited empirical evidence, thereby promoting a culture of consistent improvement in patient treatment and of the health care system in general (Ioannidis et al., 2014). Furthermore, the application of EBM principles is also accompanied by an understanding of the environment in which the evidence is being applied. The inclusion of social values and patient preferences is key to an integrative approach to health care. While EBM aims to bring medical practice together with scientific knowledge, clinical decisions must also persuade individual patient circumstances and cultural aspects. These flings open a patient-centered view, contrasting clinical protocols with patients' individual realities. Such an idea of integrative medicine, blending conventional practices with CAM, achieves this focus on individualism. The efficacy of CAM practices is doubtful as per EBM standards, yet their popularity shows that there is a rising demand for a system that balances tradition with rigorous evidence validation (Abdelfatah et al., 2019). Last but not least, the emerging medical environment necessitates a renewed critical analysis of the process of acquiring, evaluating, and applying evidence. The principles of EBM are fundamentally interested in evaluating the quality and relevance of evidence, a function that demands ongoing education and change among the users of healthcare. Healthcare providers must be skilled not only in understanding statistical findings but also in communicating them in a way that patients can understand. Professional development and research involvement are essential for guaranteeing high standards of care. As clinicians and researchers increasingly integrate different medical practices and paradigms, it is crucial to create an environment that fosters collaboration among a broader range of healthcare professionals. This helps ensure that the adoption of EBM ideas translates to evidence-informed and effective patient care that transcends the traditional (Ioannidis et al., 2014) (Figure 11.4).

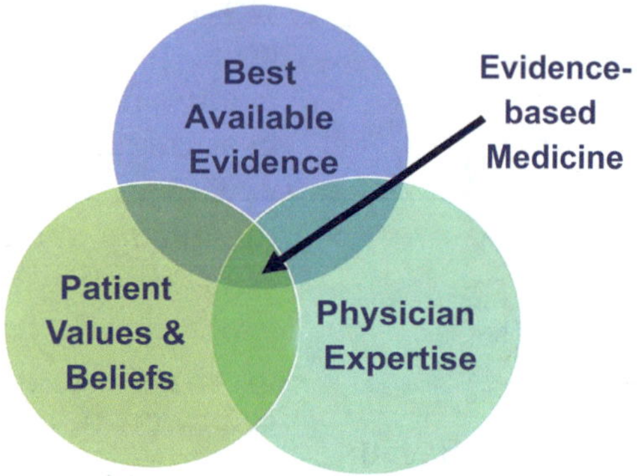

Figure 11.4. The core principles of evidence-based medicine.

Source: https://www.researchgate.net/publication/338203989/figure/fig2/AS:857796736200709@1581526087952/The-core-principles-of-evidence-based-medicine.ppm.

11.1.1. Integration of Clinical Expertise and Patient Values

Under the practice of EBM, the combination of clinical experience and patients' values is a fundamental principle. Clinical experience is what physicians acquire from education and experience that enables them to make decisions tailored to individual patients' requirements. This is not a repository of techniques but a sensitivity to the nuances of patient care gained through decades of practice. When combined with good research evidence, clinicians can leverage evidence so as to respect and respond to patients' values and beliefs in a way that guarantees an integrative mode of treatment. Thus, alignment of professional judgment with empirical evidence allows for individualized healthcare interventions that are not just beneficial from a clinical standpoint but also significant within patients' unique environments and interests. Patient values allow for a counterpart to EBM that stresses patients' own beliefs, expectations, and unique conditions need to be known. When these values are taken into consideration by clinicians, they establish a more participatory healthcare setting that empowers patients to engage in decision-making around their care. This collaboration is crucial in that it assists patients in making sense of detailed health information while ensuring that their opinions are valued in the development of their care pathway. Moreover, identification of patient values fosters patient adherence to therapy protocols, as individuals are more likely to follow plans that are congruent with their own values.

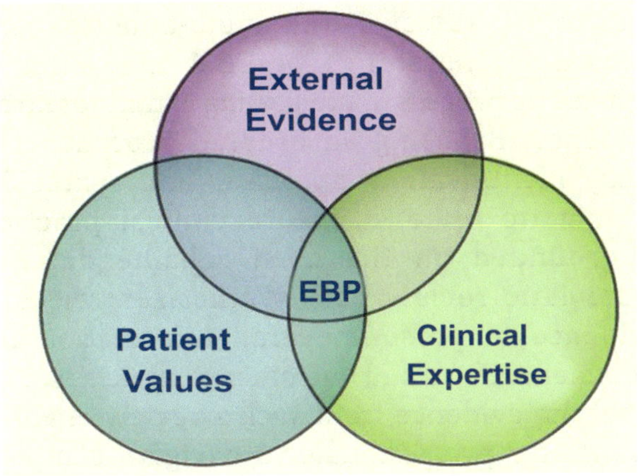

Figure 11.5. Integrate evidence with clinical expertise and patient preferences and values.

Source: https://www.ons.org/sites/default/files/styles/responsive_800w/public/2018-03/ebpVENN.PNG?itok=0Qj--OPd.

The end result is a synergistic relationship where clinical professionalism, under the direction of patient information, enhances overall well-being and patient satisfaction, demonstrating the intrinsic worth of the integrative process. The relevance of the integration of clinical knowledge and patient values cannot be overstated, particularly in evolving healthcare environments that increasingly emphasize individualized care. Research has highlighted that the best outcomes are not merely results of clinical guideline compliance but are the outcome of a contemplative process recognizing the complexity of individual human experiences. EBM attempts to reconcile empirical evidence with subjective factors, making the decision-making process better. Besides, tacit knowledge, the missing ingredient too often overlooked, complements formal clinical procedures, which allow medical practitioners to apply informed discretion in consideration of context, history, and the subtleties of interhuman communication (Thornton et al., 2006). Valuing this integration allows healthcare workers to make treatments scientifically sound and responsive to the experiential world of their patients, unlocking actual Evidence-Based Medicine potential (Mamo et al., 2023) (Figure 11.5).

11.1.2. Hierarchy of Evidence in Medical Research

Knowledge of the hierarchy of evidence is central to the practice of EBM. The hierarchy of evidence ranks studies by the soundness and reliability of their research methodology, from systematic reviews and meta-analyses at the highest level, followed by randomized controlled trials (RCTs), cohort studies, case-control studies, and finally expert opinion as the lowest level. This tiering allows clinicians to evaluate the quality of evidence as they make clinical judgments, thereby optimizing patient outcomes. Understanding the tiered hierarchy also assists researchers in identifying areas of weakness in the literature, which further encourages exploration and honing of better methodologies to direct practice in the clinical setting. Such a strong understanding of hierarchy, then, serves to close the gap between research findings and real-world applications in patient care. Systematic reviews and meta-analyses typically pool data from two or more studies to provide high-level estimates of therapeutic efficacy or safety. These are particularly valuable when individual studies provide contradictory results since they pool heterogeneous data to provide more definite answers. RCTs then follow as the criterion standard to establish cause-and-effect by reducing confounding factors through a random sample. But in fields like tumor pathology, normal hierarchies are difficult to apply due to the peculiar nature of evidence created within laboratory settings. Therefore, new structures, such as the Hierarchy of Research Evidence for Tumor Pathology, have been theorized to address the specific needs and peculiarities in this arena. These models stay current with evidence appraisal and are rigorously adequate for different specialties in medicine (Campbell et al., 2024).

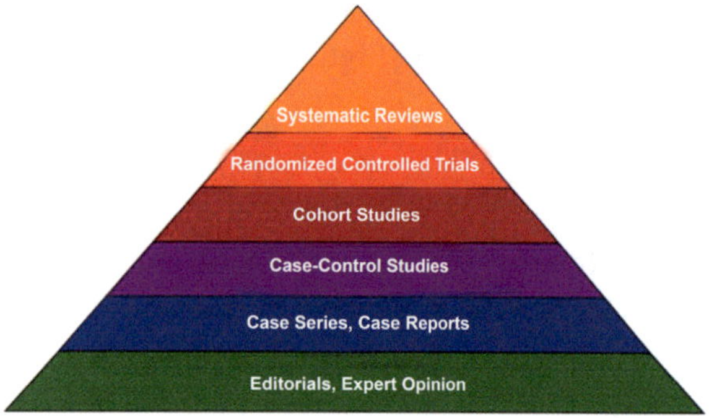

Figure 11.6. Hierarchy of evidence in medical research.

Source: https://www.physio-pedia.com/images/c/ce/Picture4.png.

In addition, the development of personal hierarchies reflects the significance of adaptability in incorporating the principles of EBM. For example, collaborative work recently yielded a new five-tiered model for tumor pathology that not only categorizes evidence types but also rates levels of confidence in conformity with pre-specified criteria. Such forward-thinking promotes enforcing the significance of maintaining context and methodological nuance during data assessment, particularly in discipline-specific fields (Campbell et al., 2024). By correlating these frameworks with dominant classification systems, such as the World Health Organization's, evidence-based practice may be enhanced to better address the varied needs of contemporary medical studies. Lastly, ongoing refinement of evidence hierarchies maintains a culture of critical assessment and evidence-based decision making, enhancing the foundations of EBM and the quality of care provided to patients (Figure 11.6).

11.1.3. The Role of Systematic Reviews and Meta-Analyses

Systematic reviews and meta-analyses are integral cornerstones of EBM that offer a systematic process of integrating extant research evidence. By using an ordered procedure of study identification, appraisal, and synthesis, systematic reviews ensure clinical practice is grounded on the most reliable data. A systematic review best synthesizes relevant evidence to present overall information on treatment effects and outcomes to clinicians. The resulting evidence from such a review enables healthcare professionals to navigate complex clinical settings, thus maximizing patient care. The effect of these reviews can nonetheless be undermined by widespread ignorance of their methods among clinicians, who might not value the significance of the systematic approach beneath in shaping clinical guidelines (Geusens et al., 2017). This knowledge gap not only limits the application of systematic reviews but also emphasizes the need for more training in the practices of EBM. Meta-analyses, often part of systematic reviews, continue to build the incorporation of research evidence further by aggregating evidence quantitatively from the included studies, thereby yielding a more robust analysis than qualitative reviews alone. These analyses allow researchers to combine results from a number of studies, observing patterns or trends difficult to discern within one study. For instance, in deciding the efficacy of varying treatments, meta-analyses allow one to observe directly the relative efficacy of varied therapies, which enhances the validity of clinical advice (Geusens et al., 2017). Moreover, the quantitative character of meta-analyses facilitates controlling for variability due to study design, sample size, and patient population, all of which can influence results. Aggregation to this extent becomes necessary to achieve the extensive generalizability of findings in clinical practice. Hence, meta-analyses are a necessary tool for clinicians and researchers in EBM to make evidence-based decisions based on the synthesis of large data. Apart from their use in individual patient care decision-making, systematic reviews and meta-analyses have an essential role in shaping public health policy and clinical guidelines through evidence-based recommendations. By offering an evidence base, these reviews compel policy-makers and health agencies towards practices that are supported by the best available current scientific evidence. Clinical medicine and public health professionals require the skill to critically appraise and apply the findings of systematic reviews and meta-analyses at a clinical level. This necessity justifies educational courses that provide healthcare professionals with the skills necessary to navigate complex data sets proficiently. Education programs on systematic review and meta-analysis techniques not only enhance understanding but also allow the translation of research evidence into effective practice guidelines in clinical medicine. Lastly, acquiring this competence facilitates the global application of evidence-based practices in healthcare and thereby improves patient outcomes on a wider scale (Figure 11.7).

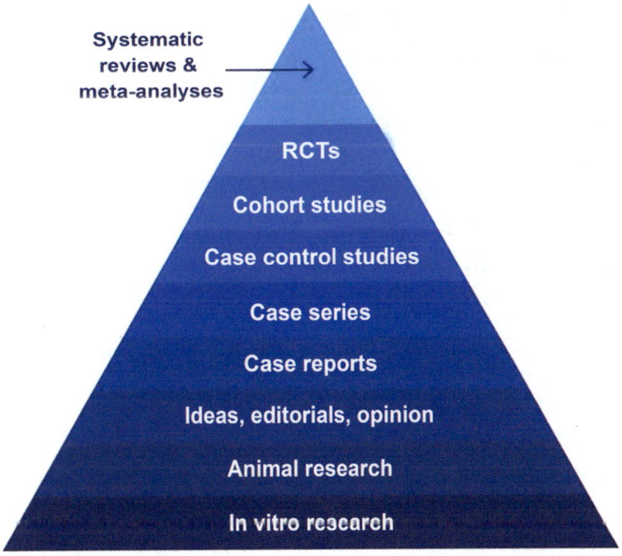

Figure 11.7. Quality of evidence ranking.

Source: https://digitalho.com/wp-content/uploads/2023/03/systematic-review-and-meta-analysis-03.jpg.

11.2. The Process of Implementing EBM

The application of EBM is a multifaceted process that involves the integration of scientific evidence with clinical expertise and patient values. This begins by establishing relevant clinical questions that arise in practice, which requires a common conversation among clinicians. Following the identification of a question, clinicians are then compelled to critically review current literature in order to search for evidence that can be applied to inform patient care. This literature search is not only a case of finding studies but also critically evaluating them for quality and relevance, thus making the evidence robust enough to guide clinical decisions. For clinical application, however, practitioners have preferred to borrow frameworks and guidance under which this evidence can be used to inform practical medical protocols, obtaining better quality of care for patients without losing artistic clinical judgment and patient preferences from the focus of medical practice. Following identification and evaluation of applicable evidence, the next critical phase in the process of implementing EBM is fitting and suitable adjustment of this information within a specific health care setting. This adjustment is crucial since clinical scenarios are quite diverse as a result of variations in patient populations, resources, and health organization policies. Engaging the stakeholders, including the administrators, the clinicians, and the patients, at this point results in a shared appreciation of the need for the adoption of specific EBM practices. To this end, community partnerships prove useful because they can provide the background familiarity with the immediate setting that will make the evidence more applicable. Appropriate communication about the value and importance of EBM is needed because it greatly contributes to the motivation of healthcare professionals to adopt new practices, as well as patients' outcomes, capturing the spirit of collaboration in overcoming potential obstacles to implementation. Lastly, the evaluation of the process of implementing EBM is pivotal in measuring effectiveness and sustainability. Systematic quality improvement frameworks need to be established for monitoring patient outcomes, adherence to evidence-based practice guidelines, and healthcare worker and patient satisfaction. Periodic assessment and feedback mechanisms are also necessary in identifying areas of potential improvement and demonstrating the impact of EBM on clinical care. The Consolidated Framework for Implementation Research is one such framework that can be used to drive these reviews by providing systematic measures for the implementation success. Such comprehensive evaluation plans not only ensure accountability but also inform subsequent projects aimed at enhancing the incorporation of EBM in daily clinical practice and consequently bring the potential to optimal levels for enhancing health outcomes and building a culture of evidence-based care in the healthcare system (Haire-Joshu et al., 2019; Aarons et al., 2016) (Figure 11.8).

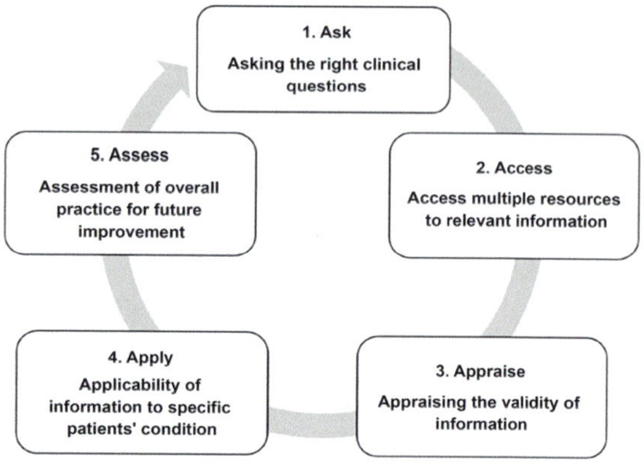

Figure 11.8. The 5-step guide to practice evidence-based medicine.

Source: https://www.researchgate.net/profile/Nor-Soleha-Mohd-Dali/publication/359777199/figure/fig1/AS:1143473147248640@1649636651236/The-5-step-guide-to-practice-evidence-based-medicine-adapted-from-Sackett-6.ppm.

11.2.1. Formulating Clinical Questions Using PICO

The PICO tool is a critical one when it comes to clinical question development in the context of EBM. It is an acronym for Patient, Intervention, Comparison, and Outcome, which efficiently helps healthcare providers arrange their questions to draw the most important information related to patient care. By succinctly describing each element, clinicians can narrow down literature searching so that it identifies the best literature corresponding to their precise issue. This systematic approach not only enhances the efficacy of literature searching but also enables critical appraisal of evidence. Moreover, by employing the PICO, health professionals are trained to identify knowledge gaps that exist, leading to more targeted research work that addresses real clinical requirements and thus improves patient outcomes (Gathoni et al., 2008). Incorporating the PICO strategy into clinical practice provides health professionals with the capacity to structure patient questions into targeted and useful research questions. For example, a clinician may be interested in understanding the effect of a new medication on a specific group of patients. Utilizing PICO, the clinician identifies the patient population of interest, the intervention being sought, an alternative intervention, and the desired health outcome. This clarity enhances not only the conduct of a thorough critique of the extant studies but also the preparation of valid research designs that can potentially yield significant information regarding therapeutic effects. The method encourages an environment in which the evidence can be carefully evaluated within the context of patient care, hence reinforcing the pillars of EBM (Mungra, 2010). Besides, the role of health information professionals is critical in enabling the use of the PICO framework. Through their skill in navigating the complex nature of medical literature, health information professionals can enable the understanding and use of PICO by healthcare practitioners. Under this setup, practitioners not only create well-structured clinical questions but also acquire high-quality evidence to support the same. Through collaboration with health information professionals, clinicians are able to become more proficient in EBM and hence deliver quality healthcare. Continuous professional development and learning in such areas is essential as they offer evidence for the capability of healthcare professionals to effectively cope with the amount of accessible medical information, and thereby end up delivering improved patient care results (Gathoni et al., 2008) (Figure 11.9).

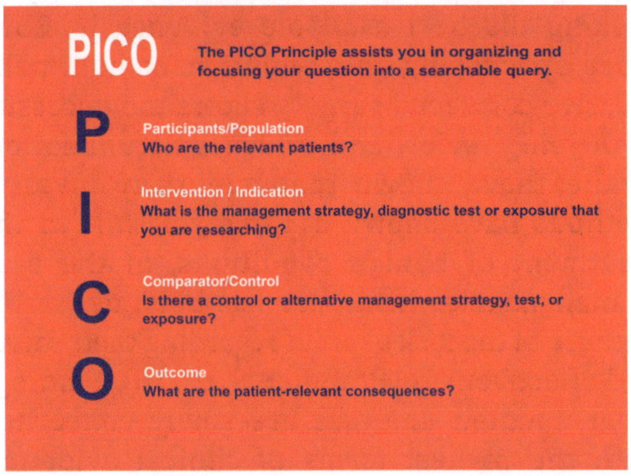

Figure 11.9. Evidence-informed practice: Clinical questions – PICO.

Source: https://s3.amazonaws.com/libapps/accounts/1925/images/EVIDENCE_INFORMED_PRACTICE__3_.jpg.

11.2.2. Searching for the Best Available Evidence

In the quest for optimal patient care, health and medical professionals are turning more to EBM as a basis for making treatment decisions. At the very center of EBM is the commitment to find the best available evidence in order to make treatment decisions. This entails a methodical process that not only surveys the current literature but also critically weighs the quality and relevance of the evidence. Technological and information management developments have made all this much more easily accessible, with practitioners being able to access large databases and systematic reviews in a few minutes. Including high-quality systematic literature reviews can provide clear indications of the effectiveness and safety of various therapeutic interventions, particularly in challenging cases where standard methods may be insufficient. However, while the amount of evidence can influence clinical practice, professionals are always obliged to consider how relevant that evidence is to particular patient contexts. In addition, the evolution of surgical techniques shows the necessity of seeking the best available evidence in EBM. More specifically, the evolution of minimally invasive colorectal surgery shows the necessity of ongoing review and evidence accumulation. Studies have shown that minimally invasive methods have shown a paradigm shift in the treatment of benign conditions, in the case of malignancies, their use has been debatable because of the lack of proof regarding their safety and effectiveness (Braun et al., 2016). Findings from updated analyses are solely concerned with the highest forms of clinical evidence, providing a lacuna in understanding the clinical limits of such surgical procedures (Braun et al., 2016). As this area of medicine continues to evolve, further research through controlled trials and objective review will be essential in establishing the role of minimally invasive methods in oncologic patient care. Along with technical advances in surgery, also threatening the evidence-based practice environment is the area of complementary therapy, affording the need for strong study. An organized review of acupuncture exhibits a substantial number of reviews with conflicting results, and often the limitations of clinical trials within this subject. The reviews show a common pattern: the incorporation of insufficiently powered studies as well as patient choice, intervention, and outcome diversity creates difficulty in drawing firm conclusions on the effectiveness of acupunctures (Lee et al., 2001). Therefore, the pressing demand for maximally powered larger clinical trials is highlighted, which would further clarify complementary therapies in EBM. This also emphasizes that identifying the best evidence is not an intellectual exercise but a critical action that has significant implications for patient safety and efficacy of treatments in different therapeutic domains.

11.2.3. Appraising the Quality of Evidence

Assessment of evidence quality is the cornerstone of EBM, enabling clinicians to formulate evidence-based decisions that enhance patient care. Central to this practice is the creation of hierarchies of evidence that inform the determination of the most valid study findings. Various organizations, such as the Cochrane Collaboration and the US Preventive Services Task Force, have institutionally systematized these hierarchies to classify research designs. Randomized Controlled Trials (RCTs) tend to sit atop most hierarchies due to their methodological quality and ability to limit bias. However, as highlighted in recent philosophical discussions, these hierarchies also present some assumptions that limit their ease of application in real-world clinical settings. Clinicians engaged in the pragmatics of evidence appraisal in EBM (Blunt et al., 2015) need to understand these hierarchies' significance and impact. Although evidence hierarchies are sequentially written down, the usefulness of these frameworks may theoretically be undermined by their inevitable shortcomings. For instance, conditional hierarchies like GRADE may not appropriately manage significant nuances, such as heterogeneity in treatment effects across groups or the sophistication of clinical decision-making. There is a serious issue here because the sole reliance on high-quality average treatment information can misguide clinicians. Further, it has been pointed out that even among nursing students, trust in EBP knowledge varies and that few of them are confident about their capability to carry out research. This evidence points towards the importance of an extended strategy for evidence appraisal that accommodates patient individuality of context and clinical variation while boosting confidence in practicing EBP (Tolentino et al., 2009). Lastly, evidence quality must be determined using a critical assessment of current hierarchies and their philosophical underpinnings. With the momentum of the EBM movement, it seems increasingly that rigid adherence to accepted frameworks may run contrary to the incorporation of practical lessons learned from real clinical cases. A robust appraisal process should encourage flexibility so that alternative forms of evidence can be included, beyond those accepted in accepted hierarchies. Such a shift would enable healthcare providers to critically consider evidence, elevating the practice of EBM to a higher level of understanding that is better equipped to handle the intricacies of therapy and patient care. Shying away from oversimplified hierarchies and exploring other evaluation tools, the discipline can become a more sophisticated methodologically and ultimately produce better health outcomes (Blunt et al., 2015) (Figure 11.10).

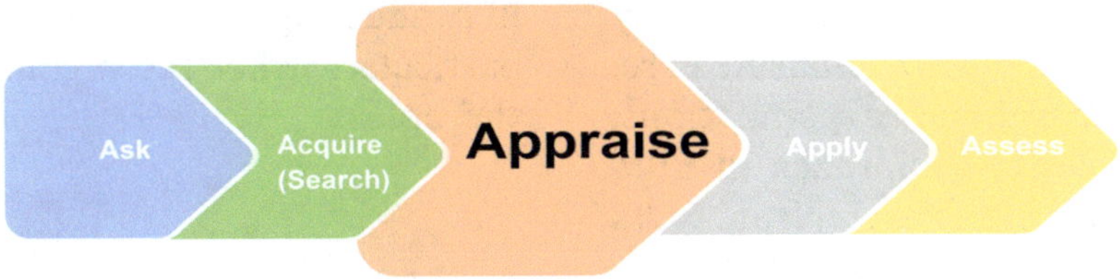

Figure 11.10. Appraise – evidence-based practice.

Source: https://libapps-au.s3-ap-southeast-2.amazonaws.com/accounts/27461/images/EBP_Appraise_Banner.PNG.

11.3. Types of Evidence in EBM

The EBM scenario is marked by various types of evidence that channel into proper decision-making in healthcare. At the helm are RCTs, which are the preferred yardstick due to their strict design to minimize bias. RCTs provide quantitative data that strongly influence clinical guidelines and recommendations and lead to uniform practices. Second, systematic reviews and meta-analyses synthesize data from multiple studies to produce a comprehensive overview of treatment outcomes. The hierarchical process of evidence ensures that clinicians are presented with high-quality data to make informed decisions. However, EBM also recognizes the place of qualitative research, noting the importance of understanding patient values and experiences, which can have a key influence on clinical outcomes as well as on patient satisfaction. Therefore, synthesizing different types of evidence becomes essential in creating a comprehensive practice of patient care. Apart from numeric data, qualitative evidence plays a critical role in addressing the gap in understanding patient needs and treatment scenarios in EBM. Qualitative studies, possibly through interviews and focus groups, investigate patients' perceptions of their conditions and of the healthcare system. Such results can help illuminate the ways that individuals perceive the effectiveness of intervention or barriers to receiving care. In the case of non-conventional medicines (NCMs), for instance, it is certain that many patients already habitually employ these as methods of dealing with health issues, and this draws attention to the necessity for clinicians to recognize these choices in terms of patients' everyday lives. From Bukonda et al. (2013), effective NCMs can provide a means of guaranteeing patient rights to health and healing. By identifying qualitative evidence, clinicians ensure that not only are the treatment plans of patients evidence-based, but also that patient values and expectations are aligned with them. Furthermore, the ethical dimension of EBM must not be left out in the establishment of the types of evidence employed in practice. Utilization of varying types of evidence should align with ethical standards that value patient autonomy and informed consent. As highlighted in Autrique et al. (2010), evidence-based practice ought to critically evaluate not only the effectiveness of interventions but also the extent to which they affect social justice, equity, and the maintenance of human rights in healthcare. This introduces the need to study the challenges posed by disparities in receiving evidence-based care, particularly among marginalized populations. Therefore, a comprehensive approach in EBM that addresses all types of evidence, from RCTs to qualitative evidence and ethical standards, ensures an optimal perception of patient care. The diversified strategy allows health professionals to address the complexities of particular patient situations while maintaining ethical specifications and ultimately achieving enhanced quality of care.

11.3.1. Randomized Controlled Trials (RCTs)

RCTs are widely regarded as the gold standard in clinical trials, particularly under the auspices of EBM. RCTs have the power to minimize bias because they randomly assign participants to the treatment or control arm such that the two groups are equal at baseline. Random allocation also maximizes the internal validity of the results, such that researchers have more confidence in making inferences about the effectiveness of the interventions. The methodological rigor of RCTs enables them to produce credible data to be utilized as the foundation for clinical guidelines and health policy. Moreover, by employing blinding methodologies, RCTs reduce placebo effects and establish the real effect of a treatment, enhancing the validity of their status as pillars in enhancing medical knowledge and practice. While their virtues have been cited, RCTs are far from perfect, and much debate has followed regarding their translatability to routine clinical practice. One of the failures of these studies is the tendentious process of inclusion and exclusion criteria, which can limit the generalizability of their findings to diverse patient populations. Consequently, interventions that have proven to be efficacious under trial conditions may not be able to replicate the same effects in more heterogeneous or more true clinical settings. In addition, the high financial burden and lengthy periods required in conducting RCTs may make them not feasible, particularly when researching new and emerging therapies.

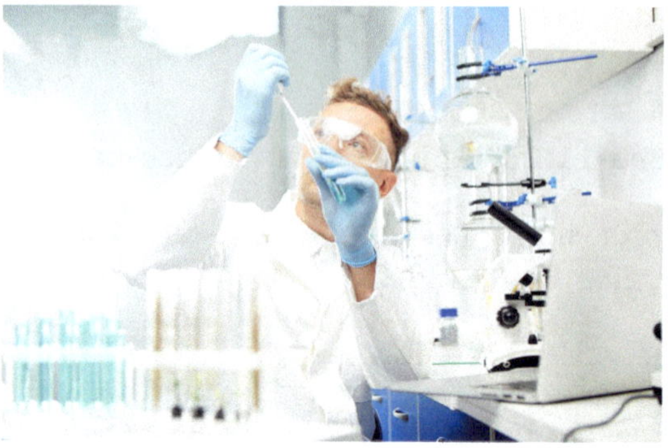

Figure 11.11. Randomized controlled trials.

Source: https://cdn-prod.medicalnewstoday.com/content/images/articles/280/280574/drug-trial.jpg.

Alternative research methods, such as comparative effectiveness research (CER), are therefore vital in bridging these gaps through emphasizing a holistic approach to the assessment of medical interventions (Paul, 2010). RCT results integration into practice remains the cornerstone of EBM, but the difficulty in meaningfully translating the evidence into practice still persists. For instance, while RCTs provide useful data about intervention effectiveness, they are not always complete regarding patient-reported outcomes or quality-of-life issues, which remain crucial for integral patient care. The need for more general measures of evaluation has arisen, particularly in fields such as supportive care for cancer patients, where emotional and psychological well-being are of significant concern. Evidence exists that Mindfulness-Based Stress Reduction benefits cancer patients, but the methodological deficits of current research highlight the ongoing need for well-designed RCTs adjusting for these variables (Altman et al., 2025). Lastly, continued growth of EBM will be based upon continued refinement of RCT protocols in conjunction with other modes of research to provide more comprehensive images of the complexities of patient care (Figure 11.11).

11.3.2. Cohort and Case-Control Studies

Cohort and case-control studies play an important role in the EBM environment by providing a framework for understanding exposure-outcome relationships. Cohort studies, where one cohort of individuals is tracked across time, quantify the effect of risk factors on health consequences. Temporal relationships can be established through longitudinal measurement, thereby making causal inferences more reliable. As an example, a cohort study in veterinary medicine of the impact of management changes on colic in horses has established some pertinent risk factors, thus guiding better prevention strategies (Burford et al., 2019). Through assessment of the quality of evidence from these studies, clinicians can make evidence-based decisions that close the gap between research and its practical application in patient care. Conversely, case-control studies offer an alternative approach by examining subjects with a specified condition (cases) and comparing them with subjects without the condition (controls). This design is particularly useful in rare disease or outcome situations since it is easy to find data with relative ease without even needing a high number of samples and a long follow-up period. These studies often illustrate correlations between disease outcomes and risk factors, illuminating potential avenues for future study. However, methodological limitations, such as recall bias and difficulties in establishing causality, are issues to be taken into account. For instance, a case-control study of medial patellofemoral ligament (MPFL) reconstruction assessed varied graft options, providing valuable insights, though limited due to the level of evidence, due to the absence of randomized controlled trials (Court et al., 2025). Ultimately, both cohort and case-control studies provide valuable evidence to EBM that impacts clinical practice as well as future research. Both have their own strengths and limitations that call for careful consideration in evidence synthesis for informing health care decision-making. While cohort studies may provide stronger evidence regarding temporal associations, case-control studies are best at generating hypotheses and identifying candidate risk factors to be further investigated. The integration of findings from the two types of studies enhances the collective understanding of disease processes and treatment results, upholding their worth in establishing standards for improved patient care and evidence-based interventions in fields of human and veterinary medicine (Figure 11.12).

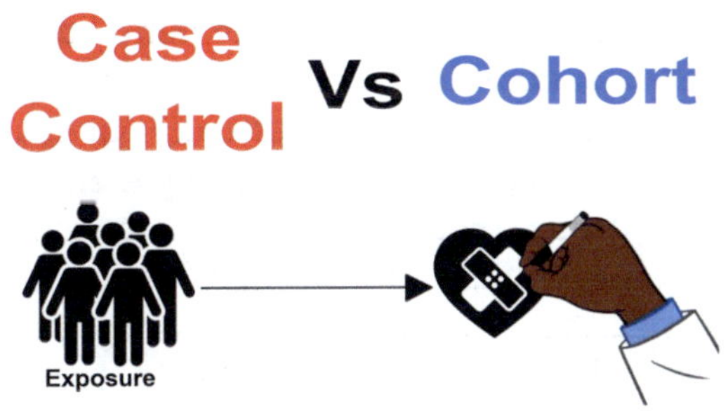

Figure 11.12. Cohort and case-control studies.

Source: https://i.ytimg.com/vi/CChBXiNXLhk/maxresdefault.jpg.

11.3.3. Expert Opinion and Clinical Guidelines

The addition of expert opinion to clinical

guidelines is an important aspect of EBM, especially in the absence of high-quality empirical evidence in certain areas. Clinical guidelines often need the use of expert opinion in order to answer some clinical questions, such as in psychiatric evaluations. A systematic approach to seeking expert opinion can offer valuable data that enhances the guideline, as demonstrated in a study employing a heterogeneous panel of psychiatric experts. Using a snowball sampling method, the researchers identified 1,738 experts with a good participation rate who provided insights into ratings relevant to first-line psychiatric assessments. The participation indicates the willingness of the experts to provide their expertise to help develop opinion-based recommendations that address best practice (Fochtmann et al., 2014). Expert opinion is invoked in certain medical disciplines due to complications and changing natures of conditions such as Mild Cognitive Impairment (MCI). Owing to the increasing burden of MCI in the elderly, timely and precise diagnosis is essential to improving patient outcomes. International panels of experts' guidelines cite the requirement for multimodal intervention by synthesizing lifestyle modification with nutrition interventions. Most notably, the effectiveness of Souvenaid as a dietary supplement has been proven by randomized trials, with the promise of offering an option to MCI patients, particularly those who are at risk of developing Alzheimer's disease. This is evidence of the merits of expert consensus in establishing clinical guidelines to point healthcare professionals towards making optimal decisions under real-life scenarios (Bertolucci et al., 2019). The incorporation of expert opinion within clinical guidelines is no problem either, given the need for open and reproducible methods to assess these opinions effectively. While expert opinions can potentially enhance the validity of clinical advice, they need to be systematically assessed to align with the tenets of EBM. Clinicians are faced with possible bias or differences in practice patterns that presumably skew expert opinions. Thus, clinical guidelines must be based on an equal combination of expert opinion and available evidence to optimize patient care. The success in engaging experts to develop guidelines for psychiatry and MCI presents an interactive process that is enriched by collective expertise without compromising the evidence-based limitations (Fochtmann et al., 2014; Bertolucci et al., 2019) (Figure 11.13).

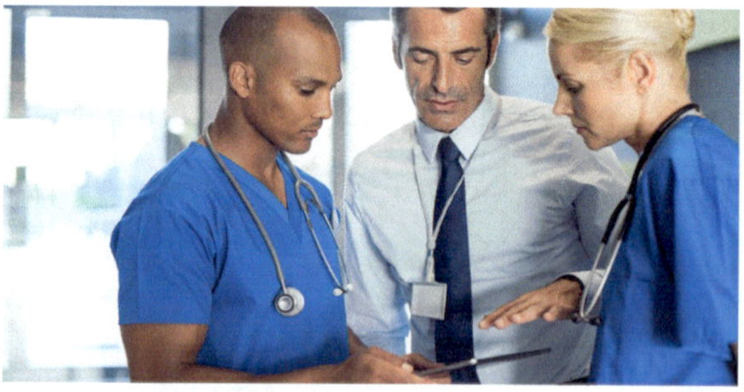

Figure 11.13. Expert opinion.

Source: https://trlaw.com/wp-content/uploads/2018/04/medical-conference-Facebook_1200x628.jpg.webp.

11.4. The Role of Technology in EBM

The integration of technology with EBM represents a paradigm shift in clinical practice that aims to enhance patient care by systematic application of the best evidence available. Electronic health records, for example, have become pivotal in managing patient data and hastening access to life-critical health information. EMR enables enhanced decision-making processes, resulting in improved patient outcomes. Most importantly, EMR systems enable better monitoring of patient histories, clinical guidelines, and treatment outcomes. But effective implementation of these technologies depends on repeated training and an evidence-based organizational culture. As exemplified in recent studies, while technology holds immense promise to maximize care coordination, the effectiveness of technology significantly depends on the attitude and style of healthcare administrators, and thus, a proper structure for technology use in EBM becomes essential (Morton et al., 2015). Moreover, technological developments extend beyond documentation systems to encompass several applications that can maximize patient engagement and education. Telemedicine consultation sites, as an example, not only increase medical service access but also create data amassing for analysis. Such innovations allow practitioners to monitor patient compliance and outcomes in real-time, further augmenting personalized medicine capabilities. Technology tools in this instance serve as patient enablers of participation in the care process, enabling informed decision-making and treatment protocol follow-through. In addition, such involvement can result in enhanced quality of life and fewer hospital readmissions, hence positively supporting system-wide health care efficiencies. With healthcare's ongoing development, the adoption of these digital tools serves to highlight the key function technology plays in achieving the concepts of EBM with a determination to manifest verifiable enhancements in the health of patients (Morton et al., 2015). With the optimistic promise of technology for EBM in mind, prudence is warranted because recent studies show equivocal evidence regarding the direct influence of technological innovations on health outcomes. For instance, while some hospitals are able to demonstrate improved quality of care with EMR system adoption, others are unable to establish any or minimal connection between these technologies and clinical performance. This inconsistency means that technology integration is far from a magic solution; rather, it completely depends on how institutions balance technology capability against strategic goals and care demands. Therefore, constant evaluation and improvisation are required in resolving any weaknesses experienced in healthcare provision systems. Achieving the potential optimum of technology in EBM relies on a collaborative effort by healthcare professionals, health organizations, and policymakers to ensure that digital innovation is utilized not only for the sake of efficiency but, instead, towards enhancing patient care (Avgar et al., 2009) (Figure 11.14).

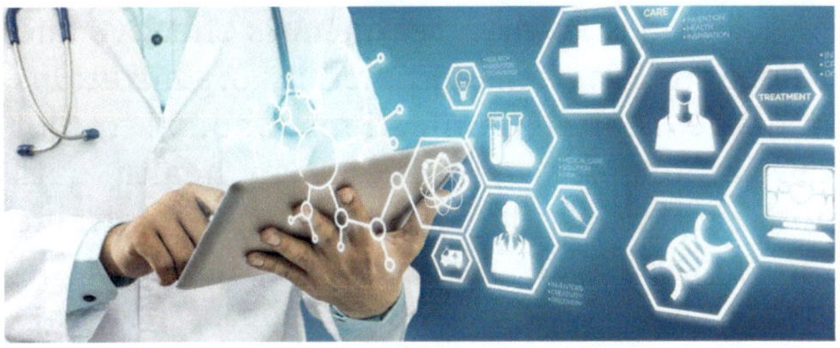

Figure 11.14. The role of technology in EBM.

Source: https://www.mlsgroupllc.com/hubfs/evidencebasedmedicine_mls_blog-1.jpg.

11.4.1. Electronic Health Records and Data Analysis

Integration of EHRs into contemporary healthcare systems allows the primary platform to seek EBM. EHRs make it possible to systematically collect, store, and compare patient data, thereby resulting in better clinical outcomes through informed decision-making. In countries such as Belgium, initiatives like the EBMPracticeNet work to enhance the quality of care through the provision of healthcare practitioners with access to a large database of guideline-validated data and clinical decision support incorporated in EHRs. The multi-stakeholder effort has exhibited potential, especially in the treatment of chronic conditions, as evidence availability has direct influence on treatment procedures and patient outcomes (Aertgeerts et al., 2013). Therefore, the sheer amount of information presented in EHRs not only bolsters the basis of EBM but also finds its meaning in the transition towards a patient-centered style of practice. Interpreting information drawn from EHRs can potentially change the course of healthcare provision, where clinicians can make conclusions that contribute to the improvement of clinical practices. The emerging trend of analytics in health information system data allows for systematic assessment of patient outcomes and treatment effectiveness by clinicians. Clinical trend analysis and patient population intelligence derived from EHR data can inform interventions by healthcare professionals so that treatment is effective and pertinent. Programs initiated by organizations like the Digital Connections Council target the importance of openness in health data and emphasize that accessible and editable information leads to innovation and patient safety (N/A, 2008). Such a process not only enhances the quality of personalized patient care but also assists in more comprehensive public health effects through evidence-based policymaking.

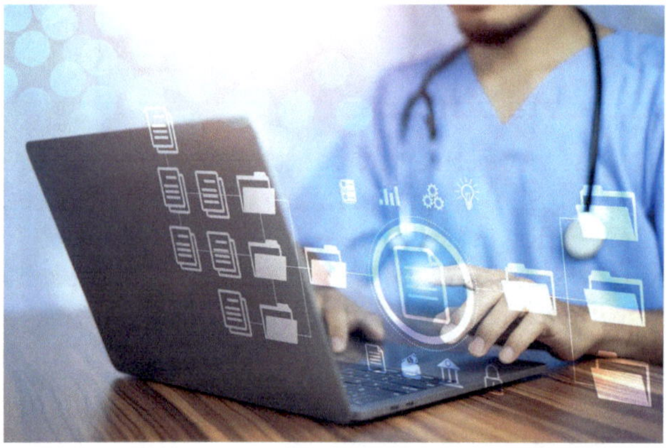

Figure 11.15. Electronic health records.

Source: https://hospitalsmagazine.com/wp-content/uploads/2023/08/Electronic-Health-Records.jpg.

But the successful adoption of EHRs and analytics relies on addressing a series of problems, primarily with data privacy and interoperability. While the advantages of improved clinical decision support are significant, safeguarding patient data is paramount in establishing confidence in healthcare systems. Facilitating regulatory environments should be established so that EHR systems fulfill stringent privacy requirements while allowing seamless data exchange between various systems. Moreover, interoperability among heterogeneous EHR systems remains a major stumbling block in realizing the full value of health data. These heterogeneous EHR systems need to be integrated with each other to fully leverage the benefits of EBM because such integration supports uniform analysis and application of clinical evidence across different healthcare settings. With the surmounting of these challenges, the integration of EHRs and sophisticated data analysis can be a starting point for improving the application of evidence-based medicine and consequently patient outcomes (Figure 11.15).

11.4.2. Decision Support Systems

Decision support systems (DSS) play a key role in the enhancement of EBM by offering clinicians tools that facilitate informed decision-making. Through the integration of vast amounts of patient and clinical information, these systems assist medical practitioners in disease diagnosis and treatment planning that is tailored to individual patient needs. Introduction of advanced technologies such as machine learning and artificial intelligence into DSS allows the integration of historical data as well as real-time data, thereby improving diagnostic accuracy and treatment effectiveness. Additionally, the use of such systems has been found to reduce human errors, allowing medical practitioners to do more patient care and less paperwork. As medicine becomes increasingly personalized, the requirement for robust decision support systems will only grow stronger, making them part and parcel of practice in the new modern healthcare. Artificial intelligence and machine learning employed within decision support systems are a significant advance in EBM. These make it possible to analyze large datasets, such as patient demographics, clinical outcomes, and even genetic information. Using analysis, AI-based DSS can provide recommendations based on the latest research and best evidence so that health care providers are able to have updated evidence at their fingertips while making clinical decisions. As emphasized by recent studies, the use of AI in clinical decision-making not only improves efficiency but also prompts a more systematic model for patient care. With the application of predictive analytics and natural language processing, DSS can manage the complexities of individual patient cases more effectively, leading to enhanced and accurate treatment decisions grounded in the practices of EBM, thereby enhancing the overall performance of the healthcare system (Fadare et al., 2025).

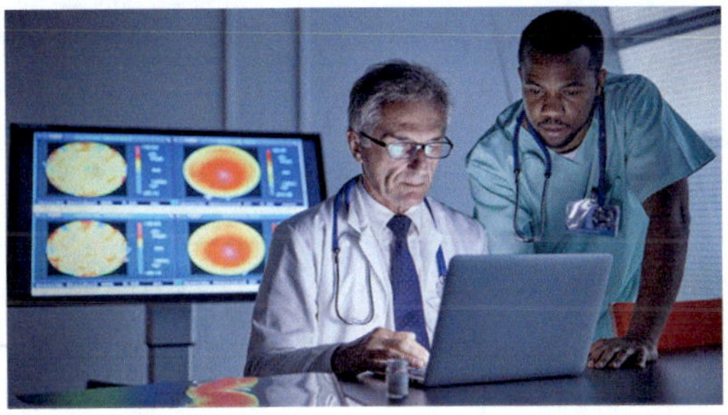

Figure 11.16. Clinical decision support systems.

Source: https://www.healthcareitnews.com/sites/hitn/files/082019%20Frost%20Sullivan%20Clinical%20Decision%20712.jpg.

Despite the huge benefits brought about by decision support systems, there are challenges, particularly in relation to ethical concerns and implementation barriers. Issues such as data privacy, bias in algorithms, and how the requirement for adequate regulatory frameworks would need to be addressed in order to unlock the full capability of these technologies. Additionally, health professionals must be trained to understand and use the insights that can be gleaned from DSS in order to utilize the tools in the right and effective way. As EBM continues to evolve, it will be critical to foster a collaborative relationship between technology developers and healthcare practitioners to overcome some of these challenges. Ultimately, the potential for future decision support systems in EBM is to advance clinical decision-making and patient outcomes, provided that ethical and practical considerations are carefully managed (Adriansjah et al., 2023) (Figure 11.16).

11.4.3. Telemedicine and Remote Patient Monitoring

The integration of telemedicine and remote patient monitoring is increasingly viewed as one of the cornerstones of successful EBM. These are technologies applied to enhance patient activation and enhance treatment plan implementation, resulting in better health outcomes. In primary care settings, clinicians' work is moving toward more intense patient management that depends on effective care monitoring and coordination. Telemedicine allows clinicians to overcome geography, extending specialist services directly into primary care practices, which is necessary for delivering comprehensive care to chronic patients. Enabling technologies, as described in the literature, offer potential to enhance communication and involve patients in their own care process, ultimately resulting in enhanced self-management of chronic disease as reported in Nesbitt et al. (2017). Yet telemedicine and remote patient monitoring are not free of challenges to their effective implementation. To be integrated smoothly into the health care system, the technology must harmonize with existing care procedures and workflows in primary care clinics. The literature suggests a set of hindrances, such as inappropriate reimbursement policies and the absence of infrastructure, that prevent telehealth solutions from being universally adopted. Furthermore, the debate on data security and privacy has continued to threaten patient trust, as well as the general ethics of telemedicine modalities. These concerns need to be resolved through collaborative efforts by stakeholders in healthcare, including policymakers and insurers, to establish frameworks that support the sustainability and affordability of telemedicine services, as noted in recent reviews examining telehealth policies (N/A, 2010). Moreover, the extent of telemedicine and remote patient monitoring is well beyond convenience; it is a healthcare revolution that centers on patient care. Evidence-based practice increasingly emphasizes the need for the inclusion of patient-reported data and real-time information in making decisions. Once patients are actively involved in their treatment via remote monitoring devices, clinicians can acquire immediate feedback regarding their health status so that they can make more accurate and targeted changes to treatment. This two-way process not only enhances clinical efficacy but also aligns with EBM principles, whereby practitioners apply evidence-based data alongside patient data to inform interventions. As telemedicine continues to evolve, its adherence to the principles of EBM will be crucial for maintaining effective, equitable, and responsive healthcare provision (Figure 11.17).

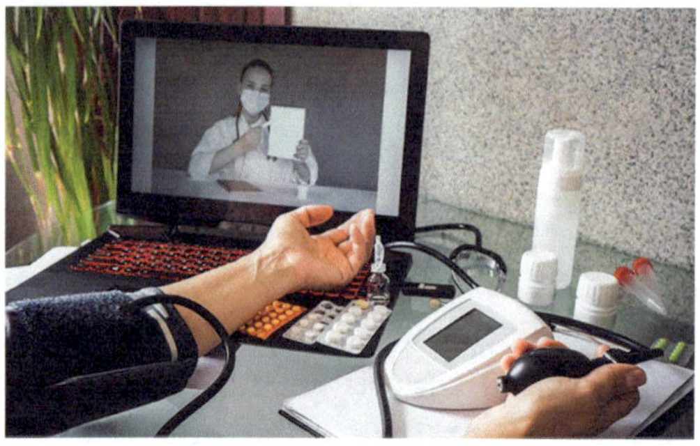

Figure 11.17. Remote patient monitoring.

Source: https://online.qmu.ac.uk/media/mageplaza/blog/post/0/5/05_remote_patient_monitoring.jpg.

11.5. Case Studies in Evidence-Based Medicine

The practice of EBM is solidly grounded in the analysis and synthesis of case studies that illustrate good clinical practice. Case studies serve as a bridge between theoretical models of evidence and practical applications in real-world healthcare settings. By close analysis of specific instances where clinical decision-making was grounded in high-quality evidence, practitioners are able to refine their techniques and enhance patient outcomes. Such case studies not only present research findings' application but also help to elucidate the complexities of evidence translation into practice. Case studies, for instance, can present discrepancies between what is usually prescribed as treatment and the response of patients, thus requiring a more tailored approach to care that reflects the complexity of practice in the real world. In addition, the usefulness of diverse research approaches in case studies cannot be overstated. Different types, such as qualitative research and quantitative datasets, are representative of different levels of rigor that are able to generate useful evidence of the impact of health interventions. This variety is evident by looking at case studies conducted in fields such as oncology, cardiology, or pediatrics. Each of these fields has particular requirements and concerns that govern the interpretation and use of evidence. Secondly, information generated through case studies is often not totally applicable to guidelines. Acknowledging the context of each case allows clinicians to appreciate the magnitude of factors that affect clinical decisions, thereby enhancing the generalizability of EBM across patient groups and specialties. In the long term, integrating case studies into EBM not only strengthens the science debate but also promotes continual healthcare delivery system improvement. As healthcare evolves, implications derived from varied case studies motivate practitioners toward ongoing learning and adapting their practice based on emerging evidence. This dynamism ensures EBM remains active and responsive to patient population demands. A compelling example of such progress can be seen in how some interventions have been revised in light of new evidence to lead to improved clinical guidelines for enhancing patient safety as well as treatment efficacy. Examples of EBM case studies are thus invaluable as they capture the cyclical nature of using evidence in the realities of day-to-day clinical practice to arrive at improved healthcare outcomes for each patient.

11.5.1. Successful Implementation in Chronic Disease Management

Effective implementation in chronic disease management is firmly rooted in an evidence-based approach prioritizing specific interventions to satisfy the individual patient's needs. The integration of technology and data analytics into care pathways plays a crucial role in facilitating personalized management protocols. For instance, disease management programs instituted in countries like Germany have proven that inclusion of information technology has the potential to enhance patient-provider communication, ultimately leading to enhanced health outcomes and satisfaction scores. Such initiatives allow for continuous monitoring and on-time interventions, which take care of the intricacies of chronic diseases. Experience of such programs attests to the necessity of robust evidence to make healthcare decision-making, ensuring approaches are effective and equally viable in the long run, ushering in the door to improved quality of care and patient experience for chronic disease management (Starke et al., 2011). A vital aspect of successfully implementing chronic disease management is the acknowledgment of the complexity of patients' healthcare needs. The heterogeneity produced by differences in vulnerability, age, and comorbidity can strongly influence both the cost and the quality of care provided. Working with these issues involves an evidence-based practice care management strategy that considers individual differences. The findings show that quality in care can be enhanced through chronic disease management while, at the same time, lowering related costs. Healthcare systems can optimize service delivery by tailoring interventions for the given individual differences. This adaptability not only finds expression in better patient outcomes but also in more efficient application of resources within the healthcare system, demonstrating the worth of evidence-based practice being introduced on all levels of chronic disease management (Berry-Millett et al., 2009). Secondly, no consideration of successful chronic disease management would be complete without reference to financial incentives. In interventions that offer financial incentives for achieving specific health gains, clinicians will be more inclined to emphasize evidence-based interventions. These incentives create the incentive for adhering to clinical guidelines and foster a climate in which quality improvement is prioritized.

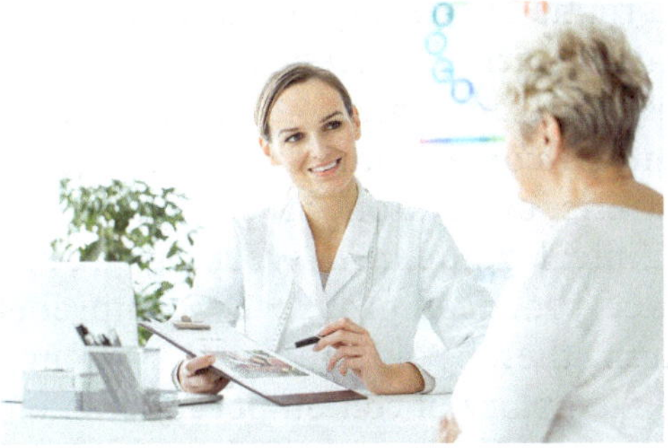

Figure 11.18. Chronic disease management.

Source: https://campmedicine.org/wp-content/uploads/chronic-disease-management-2107.jpg.

For instance, the introduction of quality assurance activities, coupled with sound financial arrangements, can significantly influence the treatment of chronic diseases in clinical practice. The achievement of such policies depends significantly on their ability to motivate healthcare professionals while maintaining the delivery of patient-centered care in the center. Thus, the alignment of economic incentives with evidence-based practice not only drives the effective management of chronic diseases but also brings into focus how strategic planning and implementation can provide long-term improvement in healthcare delivery (Starke et al., 2011) (Figure 11.18).

11.5.2. EBM in Surgical Practices

The application of EBM in surgical practice is a revolutionary method of care of the patient that significantly enhances the quality and results of surgical operations. Essentially, EBM is a process that aims to provide the most recent best evidence based on systematic research to inform clinical decision-making. This calibration of surgical procedures with solid empirical evidence ensures that surgeons are not just relying on traditional wisdom or anecdotal information, which could result in inconsistent outcomes. The application of EBM within the surgical community enables surgeons to determine the efficacy of surgical procedures, optimize patient selection, and quantify procedure-related risks, culminating in better patient outcomes and satisfaction. Through systematic evaluation of existing literature and clinical guidelines, working groups can embrace practices proven by comprehensive research, thereby advancing the science and being exemplary of contemporary standards in medicine. Furthermore, EBM enables surgery education and training improvements that are critical to preparing forthcoming generations of surgeons. As surgical training increasingly incorporates evidence-based principles, students improve their skills to critically evaluate research findings of studies, and subsequently apply them to clinical case scenarios. This emphasis on a systematic approach not only fosters a deeper appreciation of surgical practice but also inculcates future surgeons with the importance of ongoing learning in the health field. Teachers need to incorporate EBM into courses by emphasizing the scientific inquiry, data analysis, and clinician vigilance role. This approach not only enhances the technical skill of trainee surgeons but also equips them to be engaged patient advocates who can contest treatments and promote approaches based on sound evidence. Thus, the effect of EBM on surgical training is central to influencing informed, competent practitioners with the ability to meet evolving surgical care demands. Implementation of EBM also facilitates working in interprofessional teams, further enhancing the quality of patient care. The blending of various healthcare professionals, like surgeons, anesthesiologists, nurses, and rehabilitation experts, provides a multidisciplinary approach to handling patients. In this context, evidence-based practice may be formulated that extends beyond surgical techniques to postoperative care, rehabilitation, and overall patient outcomes. It is evidenced that interprofessional collaboration results in fewer errors, improved communication, and higher adherence to clinical guidelines (Kinnison et al., 2016). In a surgical team where EBM is adopted and utilized, it encourages a culture of valuing teamwork, leading to better and more complete interventions. Thus, this interdisciplinary setting enhances patient safety and satisfaction as well as a culture of ongoing improvement based on evidence, enhancing responsiveness of surgical procedures to patients' demands and enhancing healthcare quality as a whole (Frakes et al., 2015) (Figure 11.19).

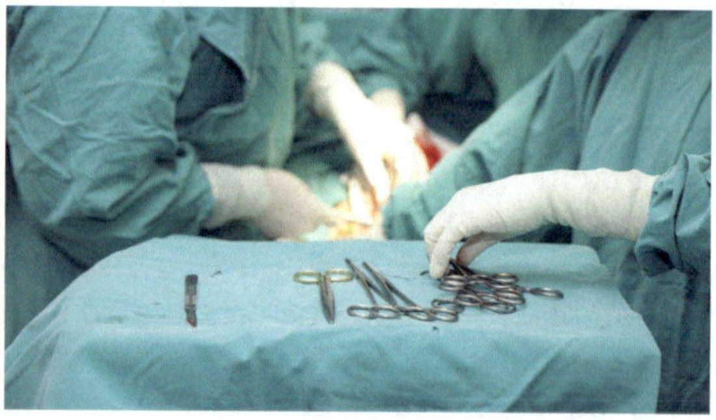

Figure 11.19. Evidence-based surgery.

Source: https://static.s4be.cochrane.org/app/uploads/2014/04/surgery.jpg.

11.5.3. EBM in Public Health Initiatives

Implementation of EBM in public health interventions plays a critical role in enhancing the effectiveness and efficiency of healthcare systems. EBM involves the careful use of best available evidence to inform decisions on patient care, as well as public health policies to control populations. Through the formulation of public health interventions on the basis of credible scientific evidence, stakeholders are in a position to identify priority areas and implement interventions that yield measurable results. The paradigm shift towards EBM enables a more science-approach-based reaction to health inequity and fosters a culture of accountability, whereby impacts are monitored and recorded in relation to defined benchmark standards. This is crucial in addressing new health problems, enabling public health practitioners to apply theoretically guided interventions that are also empirically grounded. Further, it takes an integrated system for collecting and analyzing data when making EBM available to public health programs. Quality measures, grounded on recognized best practices, are the major components employed for measuring the effectiveness of health interventions. For instance, the development, monitoring, and reporting of measure indicators are the gold standard to assess performance and patient outcomes in public health systems. Standard measures such as numerator, denominator, and risk adjustment not only assure local accountability but also global benchmarking against other healthcare systems. These markers will initiate dramatic shifts in the quality of care, eventually establishing a culture that enforces continuous improvement. Through collaborative application of EBM, public health programs can effectively utilize data to enhance practice, ensure quality, and improve health outcomes among populations. Finally, the intersection between EBM and public health programs calls for cross-stakeholder collaboration between researchers, clinicians, policymakers, and community members. The success of such efforts relies substantially on open lines of communication and shared accountability for data interpretation and decision-making. This type of collaboration promotes increased comprehensiveness in the understanding of determinants of health and guarantees that public health programs are responsive to the unique needs of different populations. Additionally, dedication to the practice of EBM principles in public health and ongoing education and training among healthcare professionals to ensure they remain proficient in applying the most current evidence from research. Finally, with the adoption of the tenets of EBM in public health programs, stakeholders are able to guarantee that interventions are not just scientifically valid but also specific to the demography, culture, and particular health issues that confront the populations that they serve, thus promoting greater overall public health outcomes (Figure 11.20).

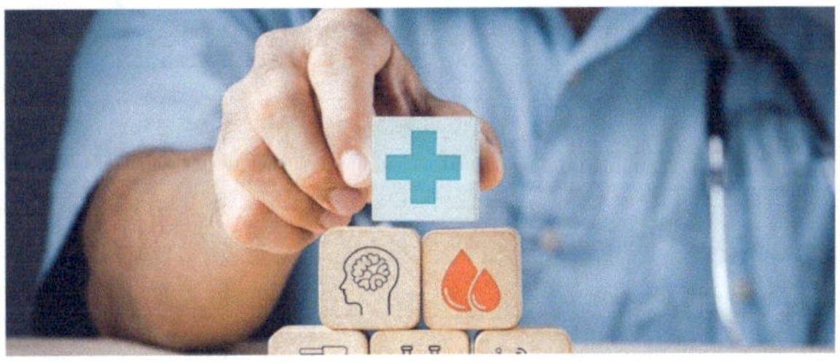

Figure 11.20. Public health initiatives.

Source: https://www.access16.tv/img/e573c5e0f6c63691a41183eea5c247ef.jpg?28.

Summary

Briefly, EBM is a revolution in medical practice because it entails the integration of the most up-to-date evidence from research with clinical practice. The controversy surrounding EBM touches on its fundamental role in the advancement of patient care and making sure that decisions within the clinical environment are based on sound scientific evidence. As the healthcare process becomes increasingly complex, the ability of clinicians to employ the principles of EBM becomes essential. This has been underlined by the shift towards statistical literacy among medical researchers, such that competencies in relation to understanding sources of bias and study design have been regarded as critical to the successful application of EBM principles within clinical settings (Benn et al., 2017). Moreover, the shift towards EBM necessitates a review of curricula in medical training courses. As pointed out in current research, integration of question-and-answer learning and EBM journal articles has been as effective, or even superior, to conventional textbook-based education in fostering both knowledge recall and resident satisfaction (Bove et al., 2020). These outcomes strengthen the calls for education methods alignment in order to better equip healthcare professionals, ultimately leading to enhanced interpretation of research and improved patient care. This overlap between learning styles and the day-to-day requirements of EBM is crucial to creating a workforce that is able to cope with the ever-evolving terrain of medical science. Lastly, the implications of adherence to EBM practice extend beyond individual clinicians to the realms of policy-making and healthcare systems as a whole. The dissemination of EBM not only improves clinicians' toolkits with a mechanistic strategy for decision-making but also optimizes accountability in healthcare provision. Consequently, the application of EBM is capable of providing dramatic improvement to clinical guidelines and public health policy, ultimately benefiting populations of patients. Accordingly, since the healthcare environment continues to evolve further, adherence to EBM is needed in order to continue providing high-quality care and to guarantee that medical practice is both evidence-based and patient-centered (Bove et al., 2020).

The implementation of EBM into practice has transformed clinical decision-making, with attention to the utilization of best available evidence to inform patient care. The central focus of this transformation is the requirement of rigorous needs assessments, which form the premise for tailoring interventions to address specific patient and population health needs. By mapping areas of knowledge and care gaps, health practitioners can develop customized strategies that promote better health outcomes. Additionally, ongoing monitoring and evaluation (M&E) are important components that not only enhance the ability of health programs to be flexible but also facilitate generations of evidence that attract further investments and partnerships. These key steps ensure that EBM practices are flexible and responsive to emerging healthcare problems, proving an affinity for ongoing improvement and accountability in the health system (Rinderle et al., 2012). Still another key aspect of EBM is the emphasis placed on bringing interventions into local health systems. . This maxim emphasizes the importance of leveraging existing infrastructure and assets to sustain health efforts beyond seed money periods. Measures instituted regardless of local contexts are typically unsustainable and, therefore, less effective. Through the institution of locally adapted curricula and supportive frameworks for supervision, health workers can ensure the highest retention of critical knowledge and skills, providing a platform on which evidence-based practice is fostered. Furthermore, establishment of robust communication channels for continuous learning among health workers fosters experience sharing and strategy sharing, thereby enriching the health community at the local level. This approach holds particular relevance to the lessons from global health programs, highlighting the urgency for integration of programs with domestic health agendas (Achee et al., 2012). Lastly, the relevance of innovative approaches to disease control within the EBM framework cannot be overstated. The quest for new paradigms in vector control, as in the case of public health, reflects the need for the incorporation of advanced techniques that emphasize evidence generation and deployment. The potential of sub-lethal products, such as spatial repellents, is not only reflective of the value of vector behavior modification but also speaks to the need for ongoing research and verification to determine their place effectively in disease control programs. As the evidence base for these interventions grows, so does the imperative to agitate for their integration into current health programs. This is all part of the grand agenda of EBM, in which the confluence of research evidence, clinical expertise, and patient values drives the pursuit of improved health outcomes (Achee et al., 2012).

CLOSER LOOK

FUTURE DIRECTIONS FOR EBM

With the help of advancing technological and philosophical developments, future directions of EBM are increasingly shaped by them. The convergence of digital health technologies in the form of data analytics and machine learning promises more customized treatment programs based on patient-specific data. With real-time health data, clinicians are better able to apply evidence in a way that refines outcomes through customized approaches. This personalized EBM practice not only refreshes clinical guidelines but also customizes them to different populations of patients, thereby enhancing the applicability and utility of medical evidence in day-to-day health decisions. Therefore, the future of EBM will most likely witness a shift from one size fits all to a personalized system accommodating unique patients' needs, hence optimizing healthcare delivery and efficiency in a dynamic medical setting. Furthermore, the evolving health care context requires greater consideration of the ethical implications of EBM practice. Ethical elements must become integral in creating and implementing evidence-based guidelines since guidelines play a huge role in influencing clinical decision-making and patients' outcomes. With increasing focus on social determinants of health, integrating equity and justice into EBM takes top priority. This involves not only the equitable distribution of medical evidence among various populations but also the involvement of underrepresented populations in research endeavors. In addition, through an interdisciplinary effort by teams of philosophers, bioethicists, and practitioners, the philosophical basis of EBM may be broadened to include questions about the obligation that comes with using evidence.

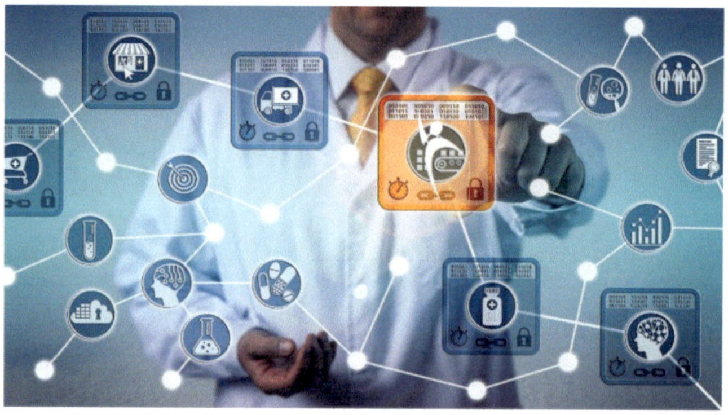

Figure 11.21. Conceptual representation of a healthcare professional interacting with interconnected digital health technologies and data networks.

Source: https://media.licdn.com/dms/image/v2/D4E12AQFg1oEvTBeVPg/article-cover_image-shrink_720_1280/article-cover_image-shrink_720_1280/0/1684265437755?e=2147483647&v=beta&t=gpVdvutmIiURjILppLRnveDZdFMEoG0V8Mf_paS1GlI.

This synergistic strategy will redefine the moral context of EBM, such that it responds to the complex problems faced by heterogeneous patient groups. Lastly, future directions for EBM can consider adopting interdisciplinary healthcare models emphasizing shared decision-making and patient-provider relationships. This evolution acknowledges the autonomy and dignity of patients as essential elements of clinical practice. By ensuring patients are empowered agents within their own care plans, clinicians can more effectively align medical interventions with patient expectations and desires, and thereby facilitate a more patient-centered approach. Furthermore, the inclusion of patient-reported outcomes within the EBM framework can facilitate the applicability of results while improving patient satisfaction. Such ongoing dialogue on such collaborative structures, like those addressing the opioid epidemic, as highlighted in the report from Johns Hopkins Bloomberg School of Public Health researchers, confirms the necessity for structured frameworks that educate practitioners on disseminating patient-focused care. With the coming together of these factors, the possibility of transforming EBM into a more representative and reactive structure emerges, ultimately enriching the practice of medicine in profound ways (Figure 11.21).

References

1. Aarons, G. A., Arch, J. J., Barnett, M., Best, A., et al. (2016). Proceedings of the 3rd Biennial Conference of the Society for Implementation Research Collaboration (SIRC) 2015: Advancing efficient methodologies through community partnerships and team science: Seattle, WA, USA. 24–26 September 2015. https://core.ac.uk/download/286729096.pdf (accessed on 25th June 2025).
2. Abdelfatah, S., Abu-Darwish, M. S., Banerjee, M., Bhakta-Guha, D., et al. (2019). Biopiracy *versus* one-world medicine–From colonial relicts to global collaborative concepts. https://core.ac.uk/download/228178415.pdf (accessed on 25th June 2025).
3. Achee, N. L., Bangs, M. J., Farlow, R., Grieco, J. P., et al. (2012). Spatial repellents: From discovery and development to evidence-based validation. https://core.ac.uk/download/9657620.pdf (accessed on 25th June 2025).
4. Adriansjah, R., Agarwal, A., Al-Hashimi, M., Alali, W., et al. (2023). Artificial intelligence in andrology: From semen analysis to image diagnostics. https://core.ac.uk/download/571213159.pdf (accessed on 25th June 2025).
5. Aertgeerts, B., Heselmans, A., Ramaekers, D., Van de Velde, S., et al. (2013). Feasibility and impact of an evidence-based electronic decision support system for diabetes care in family medicine: Protocol for a cluster randomized controlled trial. https://core.ac.uk/download/55889170.pdf (accessed on 25th June 2025).
6. Agarwal, A., Anonychuk, A., Barlow, J., Barth, W., et al. (2013). Adding value to laboratory medicine: A professional responsibility. https://core.ac.uk/download/9652177.pdf (accessed on 25th June 2025).
7. Alexander, G. C., & Frattaroli, S. (2015). The prescription opioid epidemic: An evidence-based approach. https://core.ac.uk/download/75783788.pdf (accessed on 25th June 2025).
8. Altman, K., Bishop, S. R., Centre for Reviews and Dissemination (CRD), Cochrane Cancer Network, Couzi, R. J., Kabat-Zinn, J., Lindley, C., et al. (2025). Mindfulness-based stress reduction as supportive therapy in cancer care: Systematic review. https://core.ac.uk/download/161115142.pdf (accessed on 25th June 2025).
9. Andrews, F., Coyle, D., Coyle, K., Crossfield, S., et al. (2014). EQUIPT: Protocol of a comparative effectiveness research study evaluating cross-context transferability of economic evidence on tobacco control. https://core.ac.uk/download/29139715.pdf (accessed on 25th June 2025).
10. Autrique, A., Broekaert, E., Colpaert, K., Vanderplasschen, W., et al. (2010). The human prerogative: A critical analysis of evidence-based and other paradigms of care in substance abuse treatment. https://core.ac.uk/download/55790687.pdf (accessed on 25th June 2025).
11. Avgar, A. C., Lamare, J. R., & Lipsky, D. B. (2009). Organizational strategies for the adoption of electronic medical records: Toward an understanding of outcome variation in nursing homes. https://core.ac.uk/download/19958902.pdf (accessed on 25th June 2025).
12. Barsky, C. K., & Glazek, S. D. (2014). 21st century ergonomic education, from little e to big E. http://arxiv.org/abs/1403.0281 (accessed on 25th June 2025).
13. Benmarhnia, T., Huang, J. Y., & Jones, C. M. (2017). Lost in translation: Piloting a novel framework to assess the challenges in translating scientific uncertainty from empirical

findings to WHO policy statements. https://core.ac.uk/download/323065046.pdf (accessed on 25th June 2025).

14. Benn, E. K. T., Carter, R. E., Enders, F. T., Grambow, S. C., et al. (2017). Statistical competencies for medical research learners: What is fundamental? https://core.ac.uk/download/323070500.pdf (accessed on 25th June 2025).
15. Berry-Millett, R., & Bodenheimer, T. (2009). Care management of patients with complex health care needs. https://core.ac.uk/download/71346306.pdf (accessed on 25th June 2025).
16. Bertolucci, P., Cappa, S., Chen, C., Chu, L., et al. (2019). Souvenir in the management of mild cognitive impairment: An expert consensus opinion. https://core.ac.uk/download/232208102.pdf (accessed on 25th June 2025).
17. Biega, B. (2024). *SCARES: A Clinician Guide to Spinal Cord Awareness, Response, And Emergency Support Creation and Implantation of SCARES Protocol Among Hospitalist Advanced Practice Providers*. https://core.ac.uk/download/619611492.pdf (accessed on 25th June 2025).
18. Bluhm, R., Jukola, S., Kennedy, A., Stegenga, J., et al. (2016). New directions in philosophy of medicine. https://core.ac.uk/download/131207236.pdf (accessed on 25th June 2025).
19. Blunt, C. (2015). Hierarchies of evidence in evidence-based medicine. https://core.ac.uk/download/46520039.pdf (accessed on 25th June 2025).
20. Bove, J., Hochman, S., & Ju, C. (2020). Does the removal of textbook reading from emergency medicine resident education negatively affect in-service scores? https://core.ac.uk/download/287621994.pdf (accessed on 25th June 2025).
21. Braun, W. von, & Karcz, W. K. (2016). Minimally invasive surgery for the treatment of colorectal cancer. https://core.ac.uk/download/211704631.pdf (accessed on 25th June 2025).
22. Brown, P. M. (2010). Personalized medicine and comparative effectiveness research in an era of fixed budgets. https://core.ac.uk/download/pdf/81790413.pdf (accessed on 25th June 2025).
23. Brownson, R. C., McKay, V. R., Morshed, A. B., Proctor, E. K., et al. (2018). Letting goes: Conceptualizing intervention de-implementation in public health and social service settings. https://core.ac.uk/download/287888057.pdf (accessed on 25th June 2025).
24. Budgen, A., Lonsdale, N., Penn, A., Sailer, K., et al. (2008). Evidence-based design: Theoretical and practical reflections of an emerging approach in office architecture. https://core.ac.uk/download/1682024.pdf (accessed on 25th June 2025).
25. Budgen, A., Lonsdale, N., Penn, A., Sailer, K., et al. (2009). Evidence-based design: Theoretical and practical reflections of an emerging approach in office architecture. https://core.ac.uk/download/100004.pdf (accessed on 25th June 2025).
26. Bukonda, N. K. Z., Chastonay, P., Kabengele Mpinga, E., Kandala, N., et al. (2013). Traditional/alternative medicines and the right to health: Key elements for a convention on global health. https://core.ac.uk/download/16663861.pdf (accessed on 25th June 2025).
27. Burford, J. H., Curtis, L., England, G. C. W., Freeman, J., et al. (2019). Risk factors for acute abdominal pain (colic) in the adult horse: A scoping review of risk factors, and a systematic review of the effect of management-related changes. https://core.ac.uk/download/223117254.pdf (accessed on 25th June 2025).
28. Campbell, F., Chechlinska, M., Colling, R., Craciun, O., Cree, I. A., Del Aguila, J., Didkowska, J.,

et al. (2024). A new hierarchy of research evidence for tumor pathology: A Delphi study to define levels of evidence in tumor pathology. https://core.ac.uk/download/599349887.pdf (accessed on 25th June 2025).

29. Campbell, F., Chechlińska, M., Colling, R., Craciun, O., et al. (2024). A new hierarchy of research evidence for tumor pathology: A Delphi study to define levels of evidence in tumor pathology. https://core.ac.uk/download/597466545.pdf (accessed on 25th June 2025).

30. Court, H., Doyle, J., Falzon, L., Fowler, B. L., et al. (2025). Graft choice for child and adolescent medial patellofemoral ligament reconstruction: A systematic review. https://core.ac.uk/download/639213498.pdf (accessed on 25th June 2025).

31. De Paepe, A., & Vanakker, O. (2013). Pharmacogenomics in children: Advantages and challenges of next generation sequencing applications. https://core.ac.uk/download/55848729.pdf (accessed on 25th June 2025).

32. Dreesens, D., Forland, F., Hulshof, C., Lukersmith, S., et al. (2018). Different knowledge, different styles of reasoning: A challenge for guideline development. https://core.ac.uk/download/158356171.pdf (accessed on 25th June 2025).

33. Engel, N. (2025). *Innovation Dynamics in Tuberculosis Control in India: The Shift to New Partnerships*. https://core.ac.uk/download/pdf/6371633.pdf (accessed on 25th June 2025).

34. Fadare, S. A., Faisal, S. M. W., Imran, M., Islam, R., et al. (2025). Transforming healthcare decision-making: The role of AI in evidence-based medicine. https://core.ac.uk/download/640070685.pdf (accessed on 25th June 2025).

35. Fochtmann, L. J., Kunkle, R., Nininger, J. E., Plovnick, R. M., et al. (2014). Who's your expert? Use of an expert opinion survey to inform development of American Psychiatric Association practice guidelines. https://core.ac.uk/download/213444916.pdf (accessed on 25th June 2025).

36. Frakes, M. D., Frank, M., & Seabury, S. (2015). Do physicians respond to liability standards? https://core.ac.uk/download/62571356.pdf (accessed on 25th June 2025).

37. Gaddi, A. V. (2010). Alcuni abstract di articoli che trattano argomenti relativi all'eHealth. https://core.ac.uk/download/11175501.pdf (accessed on 25th June 2025).

38. Gardiner, J. R. P. (2020). *Sport-Related Injuries in Canadian Interuniversity Athletics: A Descriptive Epidemiologic Analysis of Knee Injuries, 2014–2017*. https://core.ac.uk/download/322838013.pdf (accessed on 25th June 2025).

39. Gathoni, N. (2008). Evidence-based medicine: The role of the health information professional. https://core.ac.uk/download/47264708.pdf (accessed on 25th June 2025).

40. Georgiou, D. (2020). The research-practice gap in teacher education. https://core.ac.uk/download/395058940.pdf (accessed on 25th June 2025).

41. Geusens, P., Hosking, D. J., & Rizzoli, R. (2017). Osteoporosis therapy: An example of putting evidence-based medicine into clinical practice. https://core.ac.uk/download/85219429.pdf (accessed on 25th June 2025).

42. Haire-Joshu, D., Johnston, S., Mazzucca, S., Phad, A., et al. (2019). Developing priorities to achieve health equity through diabetes translation research: A concept mapping study. https://core.ac.uk/download/286537330.pdf (accessed on 25th June 2025).

43. Ioannidis, J. P. A., & Prasad, V. (2014). Evidence-based de-implementation for contradicted, unproven, and aspiring healthcare practices. https://core.ac.uk/download/pdf/81087152.pdf (accessed on 25th June 2025).
44. Jones, T. S. (2016). *Implementation of TeamSTEPPS*. https://core.ac.uk/download/129592699.pdf (accessed on 25th June 2025).
45. Kinnison, T., & May, S. A. (2016). Evidence-based healthcare: The importance of effective interprofessional working for high quality veterinary services, a UK example. https://core.ac.uk/download/76980966.pdf (accessed on 25th June 2025).
46. Lee, A., Vickers, A., MacLennan, A. H., Vickers, A. J., Vickers, A. J., Vickers, A., et al. (2001). *Systematic Reviews of Complementary Therapies–An Annotated Bibliography. Part 1: Acupuncture*. https://core.ac.uk/download/57903.pdf (accessed on 25th June 2025).
47. Liu, A. (2016). *Development of an Evidence-Based Medicine Mobile Application for The Use in Medical Education*. https://open.bu.edu/bitstream/2144/14690/1/Liu_bu_0017N_10523.pdf (accessed on 25th June 2025).
48. Lunet, N. (2025). Teaching meta-analysis using Stata. https://core.ac.uk/download/pdf/6314113.pdf (accessed on 25th June 2025).
49. M'charek, A., Prainsack, B., Butler, C., Cho, M. K., Cole, S., Dettlaff-Kakol, K., Fraser, H., et al. (2012). Bracketing off populations does not advance ethical reflection on EVCs: A reply to Kayser and Schneider. https://core.ac.uk/download/9986485.pdf (accessed on 25th June 2025).
50. Mamo, T. T., Seboka, B. T., Yawo, M. N., Yehualashet, T., et al. (2023). Perspective chapter: Evidence-based medicine–A new approach for medical education and practice. https://core.ac.uk/download/568373846.pdf (accessed on 25th June 2025).
51. Miller, C., & Miller, D. W. (2014). Medicine is not science. https://core.ac.uk/download/151210524.pdf (accessed on 25th June 2025).
52. Morrison, A., & O'Gorman, K. D. (2008). Hospitality studies and hospitality management: A symbiotic relationship. https://core.ac.uk/download/9018661.pdf (accessed on 25th June 2025).
53. Morton, S., & Dunn, W. (2015). Addressing the health needs of an aging America: New opportunities for evidence-based policy solutions. https://core.ac.uk/download/75783019.pdf (accessed on 25th June 2025).
54. Mungra, P. (2010). Teaching writing of scientific abstracts in English: CLIL methodology in an integrated English and medicine course. https://core.ac.uk/download/pdf/26847339.pdf (accessed on 25th June 2025).
55. N/A. (2008). Harnessing openness to transform American health care. https://core.ac.uk/download/71340559.pdf (accessed on 25th June 2025).
56. N/A. (2010). Staying connected: A progress report: Reimbursement under the Telemedicine Development Act of 1996. https://core.ac.uk/download/71355210.pdf (accessed on 25th June 2025).
57. Nesbitt, T. S., & Young, H. M. (2017). Increasing the capacity of primary care through enabling technology. https://core.ac.uk/download/323070127.pdf (accessed on 25th June 2025).
58. Rinderle, A., Hills, G., & Fiske, L. (2012). Boosting the immunization workforce: Lessons from

the Merck Vaccine Network–Africa. https://core.ac.uk/download/71360220.pdf (accessed on 25th June 2025).

59. Starke, D., Hansen, L., Altenhofen, L., & Stock, S. (2011). Disease-management programs can improve quality of care for the chronically ill, even in a weak primary care system: A case study from Germany. https://core.ac.uk/download/71358005.pdf (accessed on 25th June 2025).

60. Thornton, T. (2006). Tacit knowledge as the unifying factor in evidence-based medicine and clinical judgement. https://core.ac.uk/download/pdf/3966972.pdf (accessed on 25th June 2025).

61. Tolentino, S. (2009). *Perceptions of Nursing Students Regarding Evidence-Based Practice*. https://core.ac.uk/download/223074360.pdf (accessed on 25th June 2025).

62. Wagner, E., Sugarman, J. R., Phillips, K., Coleman, K., & Reid, R. J. (2012). Guiding transformation: How medical practices can become patient-centered medical homes. https://core.ac.uk/download/71358341.pdf (accessed on 25th June 2025).

63. Webb, W. (2018). Rationalism, empiricism, and evidence-based medicine: A call for a new Galenic synthesis. https://core.ac.uk/download/157697282.pdf (accessed on 25th June 2025).

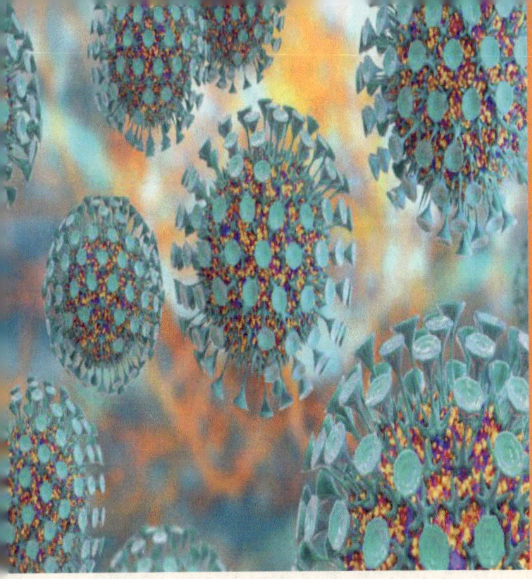

Chapter 12

EPIDEMIOLOGY OF INFECTIOUS DISEASES

Contents

Introduction

Epidemiology, as a science, provides critical data on the occurrence, reasons, and consequences of health and disease conditions in populations. Essentially, epidemiology is about learning about infectious disease transmission, determinants of such transmission, and its implications for public health in general. Using many study designs such as cohort, case-control, and cross-sectional studies, epidemiologists not only search for risk factors but also evaluate the efficiency of interventions used to contain outbreaks. Besides that, epidemiology plays a major role in the control of infectious diseases through the leadership of policy action and the control of resource deployment, particularly under unprecedented health crises. A complete understanding of the epidemiologic principles empowers healthcare practitioners to implement targeted interventions that markedly reduce infectious disease morbidity and mortality, ultimately leading to enhanced health outcomes at a population level. An emphasis on quantitative methodology is one of the most significant elements of the introduction to epidemiology, which serves as the basis for the analysis of disease incidence and prevalence data. This quantitative approach enables researchers to measure statistical relationships between exposure and health outcomes, hence better understanding the disease dynamics within populations. Epidemiological calculations such as attack rates and relative risks also provide helpful contextual information that aids in the assessment of emerging threats to health. For instance, Thin Plate Spline Regression (TPSR) has been applied in recent studies to model the spread of infectious diseases, such as Lumpy Skin Disease (LSD), gaining important information on infection spreading rates and possible hotspots. Applying strong data analysis, epidemiology bridges the gap between theory and practice, offering public health workers the tools necessary to combat infectious diseases more successfully. Moreover, the incorporation of epidemiological methods within healthcare institutions is the solution to the prevention of healthcare-associated infections (HAIs), an important problem with contemporary medicine. Recommendations developed through joint action, for example, those developed by organizations such as the Society for Healthcare Epidemiology of America, emphasize realistic means for coping with specific infections such as *Clostridium difficile*. By spreading such targeted prevention, health facilities stand a better chance of implementing evidence-based practices, hence reducing the incidence of HAIs as well as enhancing patient safety. Ongoing innovation in epidemiological study designs and guidelines not only facilitates establishing efficient public health interventions but also ensures that there is a continuous improvement culture within healthcare systems. Thus, epidemiology's contribution, in the case of infectious diseases, cannot be overstated since it is backed both by theoretical understanding and tangible health interventions (Figure 12.1).

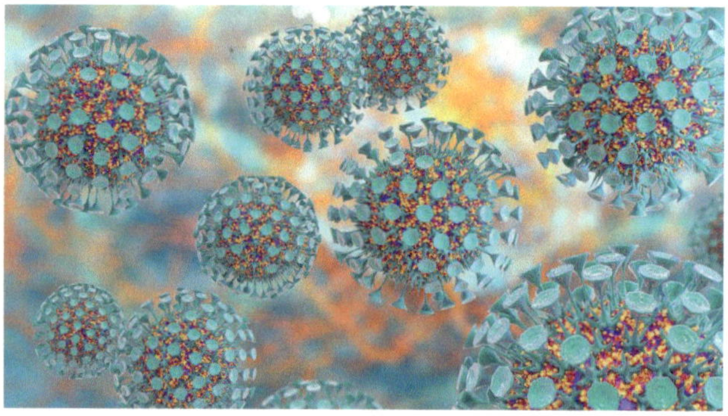

Figure 12.1. Epidemiology of infectious diseases.

Source: https://online.stanford.edu/sites/default/files/styles/widescreen_tiny/public/2020-08/Epidemiology-of-Infectious-Diseases_EPI231.jpg?itok=dHcJEqo-.

Definition of Epidemiology

Epidemiology forms the basis of public health because it studies the determinants and distribution of states or events related to health among given populations. In a structured manner, epidemiologists establish the patterns and rates of disease occurrence in populations, allowing for a greater understanding of how environment, lifestyle, and genetics combine to influence health outcomes. The domain encompasses many infectious illnesses with valuable knowledge regarding the transmission patterns and the risks involved. For instance, Infectious Disease Ontology (IDO) has been of great importance in classifying and annotating infections and, hence, enabling research activity in clinical and public health domains. IDO Core and its extensions enable a holistic understanding of infectious diseases, where researchers can investigate specific pathogens while concurrently monitoring disease interactions. This rigorous categorization is invaluable in creating successful intervention programs and successfully addressing outbreaks (Babcock et al., 2021). Further delineating disease transmission, epidemiology utilizes diverse statistical methods and models, most of which have been enhanced as network theory has evolved. Networks provide us with a means to research the interaction between infectious agents and hosts in populations and also key information about transmission pathways and the potential for outbreaks. This spawned network epidemiology, where human relationships are described as networks, allowing researchers to simulate disease spread and evaluate the effectiveness of public health measures. For example, understanding the social contacts that transmit diseases can give vital information on vaccination strategies and resource distribution amid epidemic outbreaks. Recent literature reports that network dynamics exploration assists in determining population weaknesses as well as response strategy maximization for combating infectious diseases (Danon et al., 2010). Finally, the title epidemiology transcends the simple gathering of facts; it is a holistic methodology that integrates multiple fields to address serious health problems. The interdisciplinary nature is particularly evident when dealing with infectious diseases, where biology, environment, and society all converge in important ways. Epidemiologists apply tools like the IDO framework and network analysis to study and mitigate the impact of infectious diseases. With the ongoing evolution of global health risk, the potential for epidemiology to innovate and implement new techniques will become increasingly important to establish our understanding of disease mechanisms and in informing public health policy. In this way, science is not only applied to direct response but to long-term planning to better anticipate future infectious disease outbreaks (Babcock et al., 2021; Danon et al., 2010).

Importance in Public Health

Understanding the role of public health is critical in infectious diseases since it is the foundation of shared health and disease prevention. Public health programs play a crucial function in monitoring and controlling outbreaks, thereby reducing morbidity and mortality from infectious diseases. By the use of epidemiological methods, disease vulnerability and transmission patterns within populations may be known by health officials, which informs the allocation of resources and intervention strategies. Secondly, public health campaigns sensitize the general population to protective habits, thus fostering proactive health-welfare action. This proactive effort is particularly relevant in the case of diseases like clonorchiasis, where there exists a disparity between disease prevalence and current research emphasis towards its cure. This imbalance highlights the need for increased investment in public health infrastructure and concerted efforts to combat the risks of infectious diseases (Yan et al., 2013). Yet another critical component of public health is the integration of cutting-edge technology and research techniques that support disease surveillance and response capabilities. Modern epidemiological modeling, having undergone development from its beginning, has revolutionized how public health policymakers forecast and respond to outbreaks of infectious diseases. In the wake of the COVID-19 pandemic, application of in-silico epidemiological models has increasingly been recognized for their ability to predict disease dynamics and inform public health policy. Such models are underpinned by advanced individual-based simulations to provide information on potential transmission patterns and the effectiveness of control interventions. As has been reported, major advances in machine learning have even strengthened these modeling activities further to allow for accurate model calibration that can inform the development and testing of interventions (Baydin et al., 2020). Through such technological improvements, public health interventions are based on scientific facts, thus optimizing their impact and penetration. Besides, public health is an important tool for addressing the social determinants of health that drive infectious disease burden. The understanding that the outcome of health is driven not only by individual behavior but also by socioeconomic factors widens the scope of public health interventions. Interventions addressing poverty, education, and health access can significantly lower the chance of infectious diseases. For instance, more educated and economically secure populations have manifested disease outbreak resilience through enhanced availability of healthcare services and health information. By promoting equitable health systems and addressing these determinants, population health as a whole can be enhanced, and vulnerable populations can be given the proper attention and support. This integrative approach is the bedrock of eliminating health disparities and the preserved capacity for controlling infectious diseases, securing the place of public health in the guarantee of global well-being (Figure 12.2).

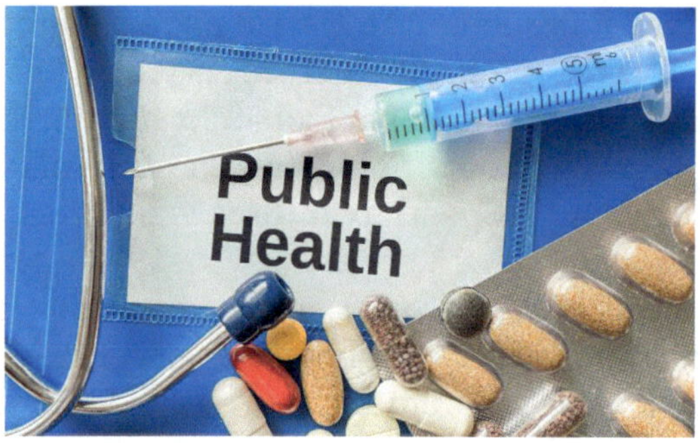

Figure 12.2. Importance of public health.

Source: https://www.tanner.org/upload/blogs/498/images/Public%20Health%20-%20784x488_202403051047361378.jpg.

Historical Context

The historical background of infectious diseases brings to light how the conditions and reactions in society determine epidemiological patterns. Public health responses can be traced as far back as great pandemics, like the Black Death of the 14th century, which fundamentally reshaped social and economic institutions. Such events illustrate the interrelation of disease, social behavior, and public policy. Through the observation of previous epidemics, scientists can identify trends in disease transmission, human patterns of behavior, and the effectiveness of interventions. The impact of these historical experiences remains a field of significance, with lessons learned that public health practice can apply today. The patterns of historical epidemics illustrate how culture and environment intertwine to influence health outcomes, thereby providing the basis for modern epidemiology. Again illustrating the importance of historical context, the HIV epidemic is a great case study. San Francisco was a focal point in early epidemic years, and social determinants, particularly housing, played a crucial role in shaping health outcomes. The city's strategy, as seen in efforts like the Getting to Zero campaign, is a move towards focused public health efforts that seek minimal rates of HIV infection, associated mortality, and stigma. Although the campaign is seen as innovative, it tends to ignore key socioeconomic factors, such as the interaction between housing instability and health. By considering the intersection of class, race, and public health, one can recognize the intricacies that have in the past impacted HIV transmission as well as the effectiveness of HIV-related interventions (Zaragoza et al., 2019). Historical public attitudes towards infectious diseases are also significant. The stigma surrounding diseases like HIV has its roots deep within public opinion as well as misinformation. Over the centuries, the public perception has occasionally responded to the narratives created around impacted populations, informing policy and population-level action. Public opinion regarding medical interventions illustrates how legacies shape stigma, adding to or diminishing it, with significant implications for health. By analyzing the path of public opinion regarding diseases like HIV, one can understand the ongoing implications for state and local health programs, a repeat of lessons learned from past experiences. Lastly, understanding the historical context of infectious diseases helps to better understand ongoing epidemiological challenges (Zaragoza et al., 2019) (Figure 12.3).

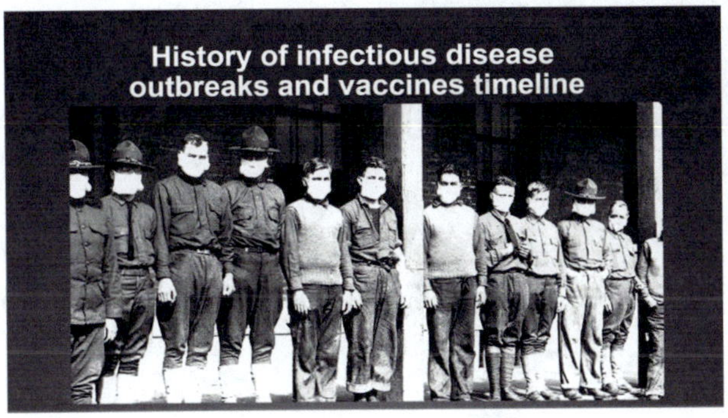

Figure 12.3. History of infectious disease outbreaks and vaccines.

Source: https://newsnetwork.mayoclinic.org/n7-mcnn/7bcc9724adf7b803/uploads/2022/01/History-16-x-9.jpg.

12.1. Types of Infectious Diseases

Infectious diseases can be classified into various classes based on their causative agent, transmission process, and host response. The four broad categories are bacterial, viral, fungal, and parasitic diseases. Bacterial diseases, such as tuberculosis and streptococcal pharyngitis, are caused by prokaryotic microorganisms that can grow very quickly in host tissues. Infections will cause a type of immune response that may lead to tolerance or exacerbation of the disease symptoms. On the other hand, viral infections, as in the case of influenza and HIV, are the result of smaller organisms that capture host cellular machinery to replicate, often causing cellular injury or immune evasion. A comprehension of the unique features of these pathogens is key, as such differences dictate prevention measures, therapeutic regimens, and public health interventions specific to fighting particular infectious diseases. Fungal infections, although frequently underappreciated, are serious threats, especially among immunocompromised individuals. Diseases such as candidiasis and histoplasmosis label the clinical subtleties of these eukaryotic pathogens, which can produce severe systemic disease. Fungal infections tend to favor warm, humid environments, and thus treatment protocols that must navigate their way through the infection, as well as the intricate host response, are more challenging. Parasitic infections such as malaria and Lyme disease also provide a different facet of infectious diseases where intricate life cycles and heterogeneous modes of transmission complicate epidemiological surveillance and control. Infections such as these require specialized interventions, i.e., vector control and education, as the parasites have a tendency to utilize intermediate hosts or vectors in the process of completing their life cycle, emphasizing the need for an integrated study and control of such infections. As the infectious disease topology evolves, so does the complexity of its classification. New mechanisms, such as the infectious disease ontology (IDO), have emerged to address the heterogeneity of these diseases by providing a consistent system for understanding their biomedical, clinical, and public health dimensions. IDO Core and extensions explain interactions between infectious disease agents and their epidemiological patterns, allowing better data management and research findings. Emerging developments in IDO, including the coronavirus infectious disease ontology (CIDO), identify the requirement for versatile and integrative frameworks in the face of emerging adversaries like COVID-19 and maximizing reproducibility in infectious disease research. Their further development is crucial to epidemiologists as they enable better identification, follow-up, and intervention for various infectious diseases, which eventually results in improved public health practices (Arthur et al., 2023; Babcock et al., 2021) (Figure 12.)4.

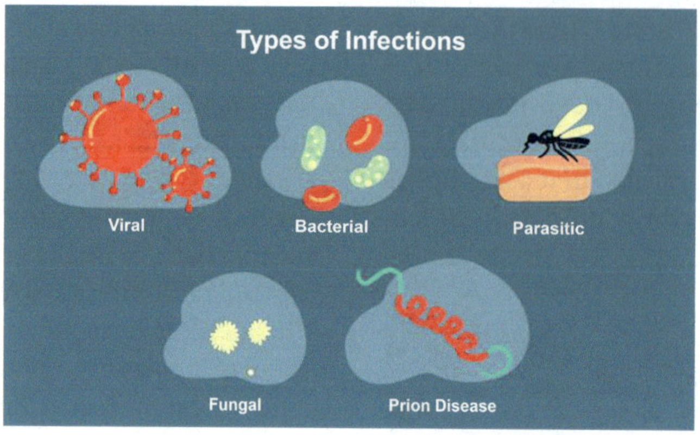

Figure 12.4. Types of infectious diseases.

Source: https://www.verywellhealth.com/thmb/HVLoB-Gfeddv1Zb1Wh67TKHi-Fo=/1500x0/filters:no_upscale():max_bytes(150000):strip_icc()/infection-5096014-Final-eaf7a90b39fd4eb69b3a1776b721d975.gif.

12.1.1. Bacterial Infections

Bacterial infections are a key field of infectious diseases whose epidemic risk threatens public health systems globally. The fact that bacteria have developed resistance to antibiotics, particularly carbapenemase-producing bacteria, gives added importance to surveillance and intervention. The infections are often caused by common bacteria such as *Escherichia coli* and *Klebsiella pneumoniae*, and the resulting poor health outcomes range from urinary tract infections to sepsis that can be fatal. Prevalence of such carbapenemase-producing organisms (CPOs) means the health care environment can be a reservoir for spreading, and thus infection control measures are required. More sophisticated detection procedures, such as nucleic acid-based tests, have evolved as crucial tools in the detection of such dangerous pathogens, enabling health care providers to initiate timely and efficient treatment actions to minimize their impact on public health (Bonomo et al., 2018). The epidemiology of bacterial infections has experienced sudden changes in recent history, largely due to globalization, urbanization, and excessive use of antibiotics. Greater population density and uncouth sanitation practices are causes contributing to the rapid spread of pathogenic bacteria. Furthermore, the cross-border spread of resistant strains can be facilitated by international travel. Such strategies need to be multi-pronged, as with public health education on the proper use of antibiotics and robust policy to avoid infection in healthcare settings. Active surveillance systems must also be a part of the effort, providing data to inform the allocation and resistance of CPOs. Multidrug-resistant organisms need coordinated action worldwide to deal with their spread and, in the long run, to enhance health outcomes while reducing the cost of treating multidrug-resistant organisms (N/A, 2025). The therapeutic choices for treating bacterial infections continue to evolve with the emergence of new agents and new combinations of antibiotics being added to clinical practice. The increasing prevalence of CPOs has necessitated reassessment of traditional therapeutic regimens since infections due to resistant pathogens are likely to result in a poor prognosis for patients and death. New therapeutic approaches, such as the utilization of currently available antibiotics in combination with novel drugs, are promising in overcoming resistance mechanisms and enhancing treatment efficacy. Studies are focused on clarifying genetic determinants of resistance and other non-conventional treatments such as phage therapy and immunomodulation strategies. Application of this information to practice will be important in countering alarming trends of bacterial infections, finally contributing to a more integrative strategy for infectious disease control in world populations (Bonomo et al., 2018) (Figure 12.5).

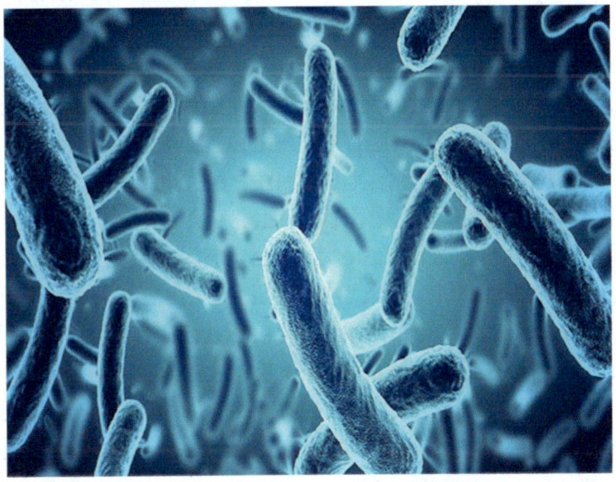

Figure 12.5. Bacterial infections.

Source: https://www.drpriyaskinandhairclinic.com/imageuploads/pages/2019/04/16/bacterial-infection-treatment-in-bangalore.jpg.

12.1.2. Viral Infections

Viral infections epidemiology is a key public health factor because the viruses impact the population worldwide significantly. The viruses that encompass influenza, human immunodeficiency virus (HIV), and hepatitis C virus (HCV) exhibit different transmission patterns that underscore the necessity of special epidemiologic interventions. For instance, understanding the modes of transmission of HCV in the risk groups, including individuals who inject drugs (PWID) and men who have sex with men (MSM), demonstrates the complex integration of behavior and viral spread. Utilization of harm reduction interventions, including counseling and education, can minimize such risks of transmission while considering socio-environmental contact that is responsible for high rates of post-treatment reinfection (Dalgard et al., 2016). These inputs are pivotal in creating effective public health interventions, and efforts should focus on adjusting the epidemiological approaches to align with the complexities of viral diseases. In addition, the emergence of new viral strains necessitates the requirement for constant surveillance and immediate response mechanisms to outbreaks. The need for functional and sustainable surveillance systems cannot be overstated, particularly in infectious diseases like influenza and hepatitis. As shown throughout the H1N1 influenza pandemic, timely data collection and analysis are imperative in order to respond to and contain outbreaks and control dissemination. New or new-fangled tests have the potential to enhance early capacity for detection, enabling the implementation of containment measures rapidly. There is a pressing need for robust laboratory infrastructure to provide good-quality diagnostics and surveillance, which are central to the understanding of viral transmission and vaccine development. It is only through comprehensive epidemiologic models that we can adequately combat the danger caused by re-emerging and emerging viral diseases (Conference I on Diseases EI, 2012: Atlanta et al., 2025). By addressing viral infections, we should also enhance the effectiveness of our preventive measures, treatments, and control strategies. Identifying the molecular epidemiology of such viruses adds a new component to public health measures, focusing on genetic as well as environmental determinants of viral transmission dynamics.

Such data can be applied to inform vaccination policy, particularly among high-risk groups who may have differential susceptibility to viral pathogens. Additionally, including policy implications in reactions to viral diseases is necessary, as seen in reactions to hepatitis and other sexually transmitted infections. Facilitating equal access to prevention and treatment will also help alleviate the burden on disproportionately hit populations for viral infections. With a combined approach by public health professionals, researchers, and communities, we can strive for comprehensive measures that address individual and community health needs in fighting viral infections (Dalgard et al., 2016) (Figure 12.6).

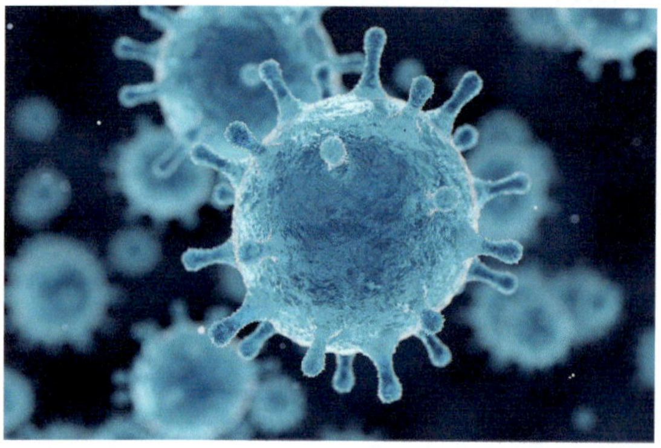

Figure 12.6. Viral infections.

Source: https://www.dzne.de/fileadmin/_processed_/4/7/csm_WEB-AdobeStock_333092093_a2a03c449d.jpg.

12.1.3. Parasitic Infections

Parasitic diseases form an important part of infectious disease epidemiology, accounting for millions of cases across the globe, particularly in the tropics and subtropics. Parasitic infections are caused by a large range of organisms, including protozoa, helminths, and ectoparasites. The World Health Organization has included a number of parasitic diseases, like malaria, schistosomiasis, and trichinosis, among the major public health problems due to their morbidity and mortality. The channels of transmission usually involve complex ecological interactions, such as vectors like mosquitoes and environmental elements favorable to the survival and reproduction of parasites. These trends are meant to sustain parasitic infections; thus, there is a need for particular surveillance and intervention strategies to assist in halting their spread, particularly in vulnerable communities whose health resources are limited. It is critical to appreciate the complex interactions of these parasites with the host and the environment to enable successful epidemiological control. Epidemiological patterns of parasitic infections are determined by variables such as geography, socio-economic status, and facilities for public health. Malaria, for instance, is prevalent in the majority of sub-Saharan African countries, spurred by socio-economic factors and poor health infrastructures. This disproportionately affects vulnerable groups like pregnant women and children, leading to wide health inequities. In addition, the resulting environmental changes due to climate variability could potentially expand the range of disease vector habitats, further exacerbating disease transmission risk. Together, therefore, comprehensive research into parasitic disease epidemiological trends is necessary in order to formulate viable public health intervention strategies. Enhanced surveillance systems, prevention measures including insecticide-treated bed nets, and education campaigns for community health are all integral components of an overall plan to avert such infections and the consequent health burdens in these affected regions. Effective control of parasitic infections calls for a multidimensional approach incorporating prevention, treatment, and education. Pharmacologic interventions, such as antiparasitic drugs, play a crucial role in eliminating infected humans but are not sufficient without flawless preventive strategies. Integrated vector control, sanitation facilities, and public education campaigns are necessary in reducing rates of transmission. Vaccination also comes into play, particularly with diseases such as malaria, where new vaccine candidates are underway. Moreover, social determinants of health knowledge are crucial in comprehending the contextual determinants responsible for the spread of such infections among poor segments of society. By the coordination of treatment, prevention, and health education interventions, public health agencies are able to combat parasitic diseases efficiently and enhance overall well-being for targeted groups so that interventions are sustained and equitable among different population groups (Conference I on Diseases EI (2008): Atlanta et al., 2025; Conference I on Diseases EI (2012): Atlanta et al., 2025) (Figure 12.7).

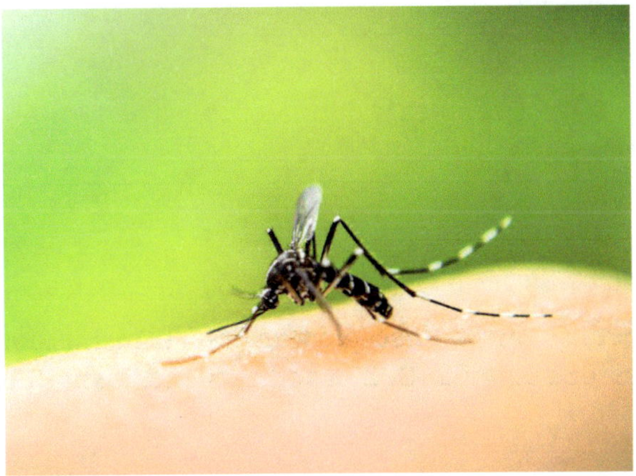

Figure 12.7. Parasitic infections.

Source: https://media.post.rvohealth.io/wp-content/uploads/2020/08/parasitic-infections_thumb.jpg.

12.2. Transmission of Infectious Diseases

It is necessary to understand infectious disease transmission in the development of effective public health interventions. Transmission dynamics may be classified into several broad categories with distinct mechanisms and implications for disease spread. Airborne transmission, for example, allows for pathogens to infect individuals through respiratory droplets or aerosols, which is problematic in densely populated settings. Conversely, waterborne and foodborne routes of transmission underscore the importance of hygiene and sanitation practices in stopping outbreaks. In addition, vector-borne diseases, which are spread through insects such as mosquitoes or ticks, draw attention to environmental processes in the epidemiology of disease. Such varied transmission modalities necessitate tailored public health responses that take into account the specific contexts in which they are occurring, justifying the need for the careful surveillance and focused interventions that help curtail the risks associated with infectious diseases (Fung et al., 2018). Zoonotic transmission is another essential domain in understanding infectious disease dynamics. These are diseases that cross the animal-human barrier, noting the intricate interconnectivity between wildlife, livestock, and humans. Zoonoses contribute to a significant proportion of emerging infectious diseases, often linked with land-use transitions, agriculture, and climate change. For instance, habitat encroachment can increase human-wildlife contact, augmenting the risk of transmission. To effectively manage zoonotic diseases, a One Health approach is required with the recognition of interlinkages in human, animal, and environmental health. Public health interventions to survey and control zoonotic reservoirs are critical in the prevention of potential outbreaks, particularly in zones where the pathogens are sustained by wildlife hosts (Fung et al., 2017). Finally, understanding the routes of infectious disease transmission underlies the successful use of control measures. These actions comprise a range of interventions, including vaccination, antimicrobial stewardship, and public health campaigns to modify risk factors. Population-targeted vaccination efforts are essential in reducing rates of transmission and encouraging herd immunity, both of which reduce disease incidence among populations. Infection control protocols, especially in healthcare settings, are also required to minimize nosocomial infection transmission that otherwise has broad implications for vulnerable populations. A firm understanding of modes of transmission not only guides such strategies but also enhances decision-making in times of outbreak. The ability to accurately utilize epidemiological tools is thus of paramount importance in controlling and preventing the outbreak of infectious disease, emphasizing the enduring value of research and public health education (Fung et al., 2018) (Figure 12.8).

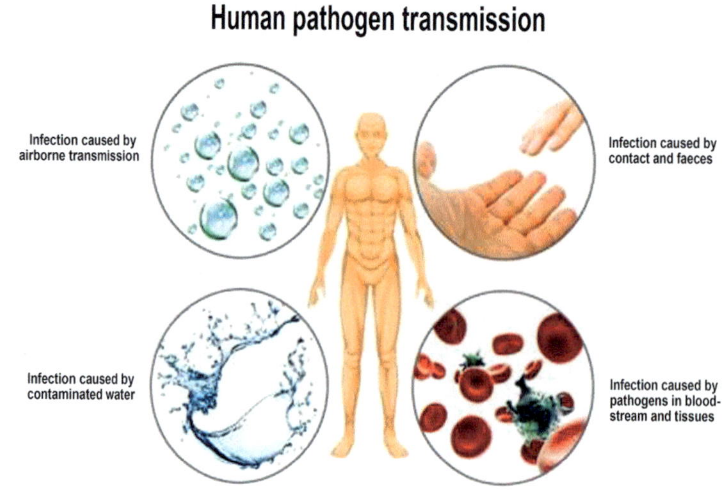

Figure 12.8. Transmission of pathogens.

Source: https://www.hartmann-science-center.com/-/media/country/hsc/glossary-s-v/transmission-paths_730x516.jpg?mw=840&rev=41d009ae8694496c9f052210e5248027&sc_lang=en&hash=8CFA31F192FA47A332CB3983E7BE8212.

12.2.1. Modes of Transmission

Understanding the modes of transmission of contagious diseases is most important in epidemiology because it provides the path a disease takes from its host to another host. Contagious agents are transmitted by various mechanisms and are primarily classified as either direct or indirect transmission. Direct transmission occurs when an infected individual transfers the pathogen to a potential host through direct physical contact, for example, by touching, kissing, or sexual contact. On the other hand, indirect transmission occurs through intermediary vectors such as the environment, vectors, or objects. For instance, airborne transmission occurs when pathogens are transferred through respiratory droplets or aerosols and are capable of infecting individuals breathing them from a distance. Such multifarious pathways being identified enables public health professionals to develop specific interventions that constrain outbreaks and inhibit disease transmission, thus fortifying community health measures (Fung et al., 2018). Among the various transmission modes, vector-borne disease is the most challenging since it relies on biological carriers such as insects. The vectors, in this case, like mosquitoes and ticks, transmit infectious agents and infect humans via biting, rendering control difficult. Since the vector-borne mode is complex, monitoring and prevention must be in a multimodal form. Surveillance systems play a crucial role in the detection of high-risk areas and the geographical location of individual vectors. Control measures such as insecticide spraying, habitat modification, and human and animal vaccination have also played an essential role in reducing the transmission rate. Control of these modes not only considers medical intervention but also emphasizes environmental control and education in order to minimize exposure (Fung et al., 2017). Food and waterborne transmission continues to be a major issue in infectious disease epidemiology, because contaminated supplies can lead to quick outbreaks. Bacteria, viruses, and parasites that carry diseases are some of the pathogens that might enter the water or food supply through different means, ranging from poor sanitation to incorrect handling of food or animal feces. The fact that the contaminants can multiply results in serious health threats, especially among weaker groups of people like children and older adults. Preventive measures, including stringent hygiene protocols, sanitation improvement, and food safety laws, are the most critical measures to break the transmission cycle. Public awareness campaigns also play a vital role in educating populations on how to handle food effectively and the advantages of access to clean water. Through food and waterborne transmission interventions, public health is able to significantly reduce morbidity rates and enhance overall population health (Fung et al., 2018) (Figure 12.9).

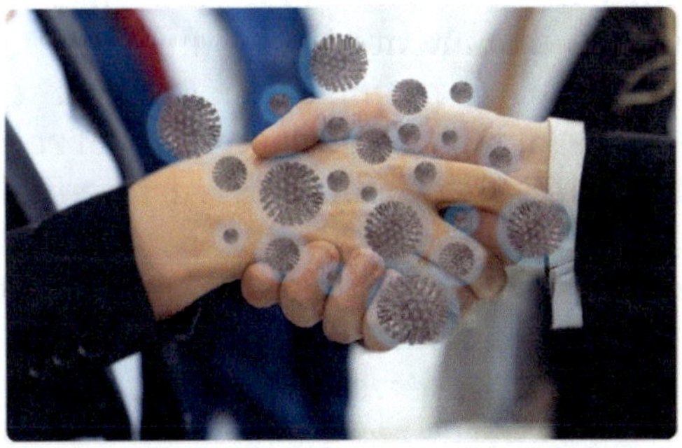

Figure 12.9. Modes of transmission.

Source: https://www.news-medical.net/image-handler/picture/2020/6/shutterstock_1628740948_(1).jpg.

12.2.2. Factors Influencing Transmission

The epidemiological spread of infectious disease is influenced by a multitude of factors that intersect the biological, environmental, and social domains. Genetic pathogen variability influencing the transmission pattern of pathogens is one of the biological factors. Hybrid strains in systems that involve multiple hosts have the potential to alter transmission patterns radically. In particular, studies of the Genus Schistosoma that produces schistosomiasis highlight how interspecific hybridization enhances the transmission potential through the broadening of the host range and response to treatment strategies. Given that these hybrids form in coexistence within the ecological niches of Africa's sub-Saharan region, they present additional challenges for disease and public health initiatives, a testament to the complex relationship between the evolution of the pathogen and the processes of transmission (Borlase et al., 2017). Understanding these factors is essential for developing effective intervention strategies that not only target the diseases themselves but also the systems in which they are situated. Environmental determinants also play a significant role in the transmission of infectious diseases as promoters for which the environment will facilitate or resist the spread of pathogens. For instance, biotic conditions such as temperature and rainfall condition vector species habitats, subsequently influencing disease transmission rates. Human alteration of the environment in endemic regions of schistosomiasis can enhance favorable conditions for the survival and reproduction of freshwater snails, which are intermediate hosts of Schistosoma parasites. Additionally, human-induced alteration of natural ecosystems, such as deforestation and urbanization, may alter endemic habitats, consequently resulting in heightened contact between hosts and pathogens. This implicit connection emphasizes the relevance of environmental issues in epidemiological modeling and demonstrates the ways in which the environment can exert a direct influence on disease transmission dynamics (Borlase et al., 2017). Consequently, public health actions for the management of infectious diseases call upon the inclusion of environmental aspects. Social determinants of health are crucial in the transmission of infectious diseases as they dictate individual and community behaviors regarding health routines and the availability of resources.

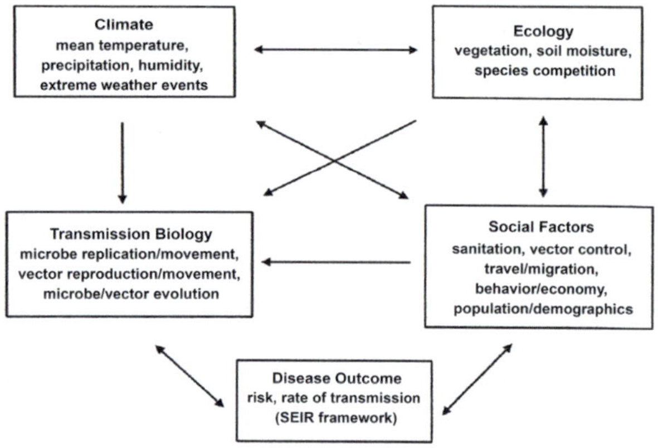

Figure 12.10. The Web of factors that influence the transmission of infectious disease agents.

Source: https://www.researchgate.net/profile/Linda-Mearns/publication/237288522/figure/fig1/AS:299309309415436@1448372308670/The-Web-of-factors-that-influence-transmission-of-infectious-disease-agents-Source.png.

Socioeconomic status, education, and cultural values could influence populations' response to disease threats. Incorporating social trends into epidemiological models allows for better characterization of disease dynamics with the recognition that infections are social phenomena in themselves. Hope then emerges as a significant emergent property that can shape collective actions during outbreaks and affect overall resilience when facing health emergencies. Such theoretical frameworks, which make use of emergent population variables, hold promise in elucidating human population transmission dynamics and creating more efficient public health programs. As scientists continue on the path of exploring interfaces between social variables and epidemiology, it is increasingly clear that fighting the human condition is central to controlling infectious disease (Figure 12.10).

12.2.3. Role of Reservoirs and Vectors

The role of reservoirs and vectors in infectious disease epidemiology plays a central role in understanding the dynamics of transmission of pathogens. Wild birds, for instance, are typically involved in carrying and transmitting infectious agents that can infect humans. Migrating birds actually have the potential to be long-distance vectors, facilitating the spread of pathogens across vast geographical distances. Although they could be potential agents of disease transmission, research indicates that disease-causing agent transmission by wild birds to humans is not frequent. A systematic review was employed in the identification of various pathogens associated with avian species, and it was discovered that while wild birds could be reservoirs of infectious agents like the influenza A virus and West Nile virus, there are limited documented cases involving direct transmission to humans (Bauchinger et al., 2008). This highlights the complexity of zoonotic transmissions and points towards the need for more research to establish these associations more clearly. Vectors play a crucial role in zoonotic disease transmission since they act as a link between reservoirs and human hosts. In many cases, these vectors, for example, insects including ticks and mosquitoes, facilitate indirect transmission by feeding on infected animals before infecting the human host. The interface of environmental changes and vector behavior has been proven to enhance disease emergence. For instance, intensification of agriculture can potentially change habitats and thereby expand the risk of zoonotic diseases by altering the way wildlife interacts with livestock and human society. Systematic review reported that climatic changes and land-use practices potentially raise the threat for zoonotic disease emergence by factors driven by changing ecological processes and human expansion into nature (Artois et al., 2013). Identification of the interaction between reservoirs, vectors, and their habitat is therefore crucial for predicting outbreaks and designing effective public health interventions. The idea of reservoirs and vectors extends beyond association with pathogens; it encompasses comprehending their ecological complexity. With increasing human populations and intensified agricultural production, the interaction between wildlife, livestock, and vectors becomes more complex. This necessitates holistic research into infectious diseases, whereby biological, environmental, and socio-economic factors are factored in. It is an emerging zoonosis that usually reflects the interconnectedness of ecosystems and human health and, therefore, requires that epidemiologic research embrace these processes as a whole. Secondly, studies that address the role played by changes in the environment in promoting the emergence of zoonotic disease show significant gaps within the study concerning the ecological and agricultural link. Sequencing these knowledge gaps will not only enlarge our understanding of the transmission of pathogens but will also facilitate focused interventions to diminish the risk posed by reservoirs and vectors in the fight against infectious diseases (Artois et al., 2013) (Figure 12.11).

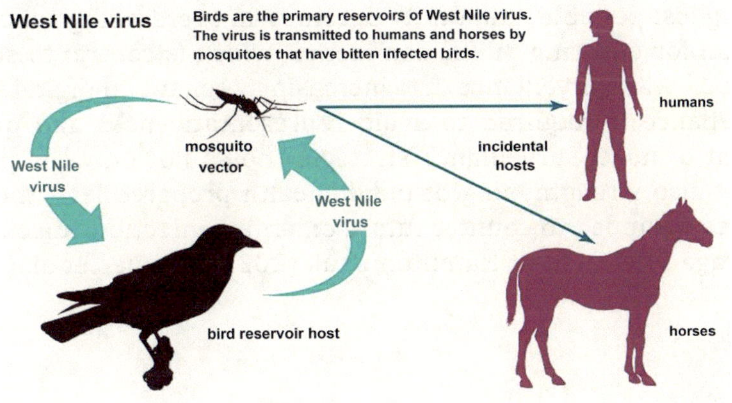

Figure 12.11. Birds are the primary reservoirs of West Nile virus. The virus is transmitted to humans and horses by mosquitoes that have bitten infected birds.

Source: https://cdn.britannica.com/96/78596-050-3FB7591F/virus-Birds-reservoirs-West-Nile-humans-birds.jpg.

12.3. Surveillance and Data Collection

The practice of epidemiology has been very far from the early days, particularly in how it leverages surveillance and data collection as the foundations for infectious disease control. The age-old surveillance systems have been in existence for years, monitoring health trends and providing information for the purpose of informing public health policy. The advent of digital technologies has transformed the game completely, with resources for tapping various sources of data that were yet to be leveraged for application in healthcare. The COVID-19 pandemic brought home the need for such innovations, with digital epidemiology demonstrating that it has the capacity to augment traditional surveillance methods by gathering real-time data from social media and other internet sources. Depending on this approach, public health professionals are able to derive important knowledge regarding the spread of diseases, which eventually allows for quicker response and management of infectious outbreaks. This blend of tried and true and new approaches could fortify public health infrastructure to endure current and future pandemics, as envisioned in Hamilton et al. (2021). Insight into the interdisciplinary nature of infectious diseases requires a new paradigm for data collection that emphasizes not just real-time monitoring but also intersectoral partnership. A key component of effective surveillance is the ability to link day-to-day health data with environmental factors, thereby creating a more complete picture of disease trends. Initiatives such as the national environmental public health tracking (EPHT) network are excellent examples of such an integrative approach, for they aim to connect existing environmental data with information on chronic diseases. The goal is simple but complex: to minimize health risks through acquiring knowledge of the role environmental exposures play in initiating health emergencies. Yet successful data amalgamation demands systematic updating by technological progress and collaboration, pointing to the dynamic nature of contemporary surveillance systems as noted in Balmes et al. (2004). Besides, the public health benefits and potential risks of such enormous data gathering must be examined closely to balance privacy and the latter. As digital epidemiology is highly reliant on data recovered through personal devices and web usage, ensuring privacy protection while achieving the highest possible data utility becomes an overarching concern. Addressing these ethical issues is pivotal for ensuring public confidence, which is central to successful surveillance campaigns. Furthermore, with surveillance data increasingly reliant on digital systems, technological infrastructure maintenance is required to avoid representativeness and quality issues of data. Successful deployment of novel surveillance strategies holds not only the promise of short-term control of disease but also strengthening of public health preparedness, thereby enabling health authorities to be better equipped to counter future emerging infectious disease threats, reiterating the overarching message presented in Hamilton et al. (2021), Balmes et al. (2004) (Figure 12.12).

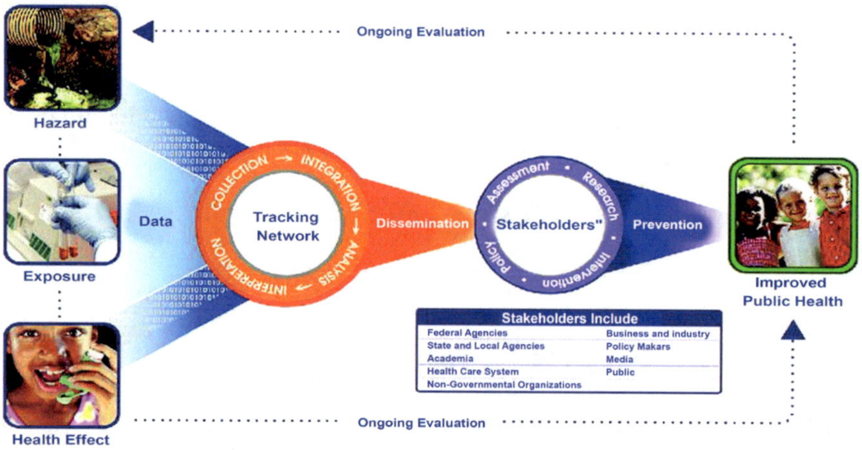

Figure 12.12. Environmental public health tracking.

Source: https://www.researchgate.net/publication/8243528/figure/fig3/AS:667201400999944@1536084618442/Environmental-public-health-tracking-Reproduced-from-CDC-http-wwwcdcgov-nceh.png.

12.3.1. Importance of Surveillance

Surveillance is a critical component in the discipline of epidemiology, and more so in the management of infectious diseases. Such a continuous process of data gathering, analyzing, and interpreting helps provide public health officials with information about the trends in disease occurrence as well as disease outbreaks. Surveillance systems act as critical early warning systems, facilitating timely action against potential public health threats. For instance, in the year 2015, as part of the EXPO Milan event, Italy launched an event-based surveillance (EBS) system that monitored infectious diseases. The installation of the system proved the worth of targeted surveillance within mass events, as varied communities meet and elevate the risk of disease transmission. Through prioritization of diseases and conditions, the EBS facilitated speedy identification and planning for response, ultimately working to safeguard public health during the event (Bastiampillai et al., 2016). Additionally, the significance of surveillance is not at the level of individual nations, but at the larger health environment globally, where coordination is required to control infectious diseases. Initiatives such as the DSN Initiative, presented by the Rockefeller Foundation, are characteristic of endeavors to enhance disease surveillance capacity in the developing world. The initiative aims at developing human resources committed to disease surveillance, and hence, assistance to national health systems to be able to monitor and respond effectively to outbreaks. Through cross-border cooperation through regional networks, the DSN encourages the mobilization of resources and information sharing across nations, which is critical in harmonizing cross-border health threats. Such collective actions highlight the importance of building resilience in disease surveillance systems, particularly in areas that may not be well-endowed with infrastructure and resources (Caridad et al., 2010). Focusing on the importance of surveillance underscores the fact that well-established systems can go a long way in shaping public health. Good surveillance, besides enabling detection of outbreaks, assists in making evidence-based policy and resource allocation decisions. The practices employed in surveillance, such as the EBS at EXPO Milan, point to the necessity of customizing interventions to specific contexts to ensure maximum efficacy. Furthermore, as travel and commerce between the globe continue to increase, the dynamics of interplay between local and global disease patterns emphasize the necessity of robust surveillance systems that transcend geographical space. Through constantly enhancing these frameworks and expenditure on labor skill creation, communities all over the world can enhance their capability to combat infectious ailments, leading eventually to a healthier global society (Bastiampillai et al., 2016; Caridad et al., 2010) (Figure 12.13).

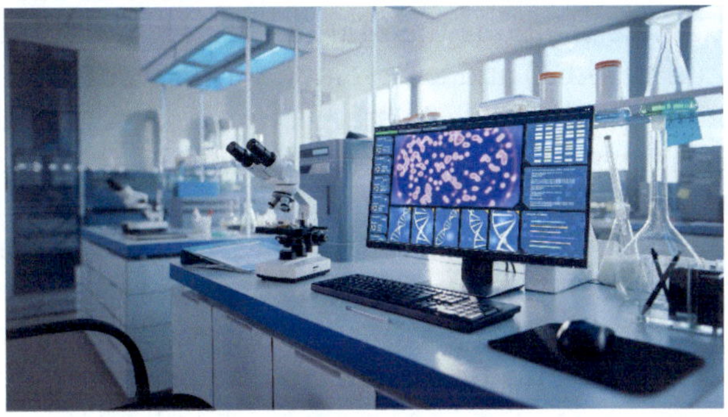

Figure 12.13. Establishing whole genome sequencing at the core of epidemiological surveillance.

Source: https://www.microbiologyresearch.org/upload/IMMEM.png.

12.3.2. Methods of Data Collection

In infectious disease epidemiology, methods for the collection of data are essential to understanding disease patterns and directing public health intervention. Standardized surveillance systems are one primary way of gathering data on the incidence and prevalence of diseases over time. Through such surveillance, public health authorities can identify early outbreaks, assess their transmission, and implement control effectively. For instance, the inclusion of environmental information in such systems of surveillance enhances knowledge regarding how environmental forces are involved in disease transmission. The Centers for Disease Control and Prevention's initiative towards the creation of a national environmental public health tracking network is an instance of such a holistic approach. By linking environmental and chronic disease data, stakeholders can recognize vulnerable populations more readily and react to emerging health risks, highlighting the dynamic nature of epidemiological data-collection methods (Balmes et al., 2004). Another essential data-collection method in infectious disease epidemiology involves cohort studies of tracking health outcomes among precisely defined cohorts of persons over time. One such example includes the Multicenter AIDS Cohort Study (MACS) and the Women's Interagency HIV Study (WIHS). These studies offer researchers a chance to assess the incidence of a number of respiratory infections among HIV-infected and uninfected individuals in various stages of treatment, i.e., prior to and subsequent to the initiation of highly active antiretroviral therapy (HAART). The data collected helps elucidate the chronic threats of respiratory infections in HIV-positive individuals, which indicates that constant monitoring is necessary. By using adjusted odds or hazards ratios, researchers can compare and achieve helpful conclusions that inform clinical protocols and public health strategies to complement reducing mortality and morbidity (Johannessen et al., 2013). Lastly, qualitative data collection methods such as interviews and focus groups are crucial in complementing quantitative data in infectious disease epidemiology. These methods provide deeper insights into the public's knowledge and beliefs concerning infectious diseases, for example, cultural beliefs and behavioral responses influencing disease transmission and prevention. Assembling this qualitative data allows epidemiologists to plan communication strategies that are properly customized, rendering interventions culturally suited and more effective. Secondly, combining qualitative and quantitative data enhances the overall efficiency of public health programs. Combining more than one methodology, researchers are capable of constructing combined models reflecting the complexities in disease processes more elaborately and guiding effective health interventions across various populations.

12.3.3. Challenges in Data Accuracy

In epidemiology, particularly in infectious disease settings, data precision is key to providing for the right public health interventions. One of the severe challenges to accuracy in obtaining this is the application of models that are specifically meant to predict trends such as influenza seasons. While enhanced modeling has improved over time, many have struggled to achieve accuracy in the past. For instance, the Centers for Disease Control and Prevention (CDC) attempted to estimate the accuracy of the predictions in the 2013–2014 flu season. The results showed that among 13 predictions, a few of them were able to predict significant milestones within a week's time frame, showing the ongoing challenge of producing reliable epidemiological predictions. This contradiction is indicative of a broader issue in which health administrators are confronted by predictive model uncertainties and tasked with accomplishing timely interventions to stem the outbreak of disease (Allen et al., 2016). Variable data quality derived from different populations and sites is the second primary challenge to data accuracy. Extensive epidemiological surveillance is hampered in most developing nations by their constrained infrastructure and resources. For instance, while novel bioinformatics approaches, such as in silico HLA typing from SNP data, have held much promise to advance genetic epidemiology research, their ability could be diminished in diverse populations due to genetic heterogeneity and local factors. A study evaluating predictions of HLA alleles in the Ethiopian Wolaita population showed high accuracy; however, the applicability of the approach to other African populations is not explored (Adeyemo et al., 2012).

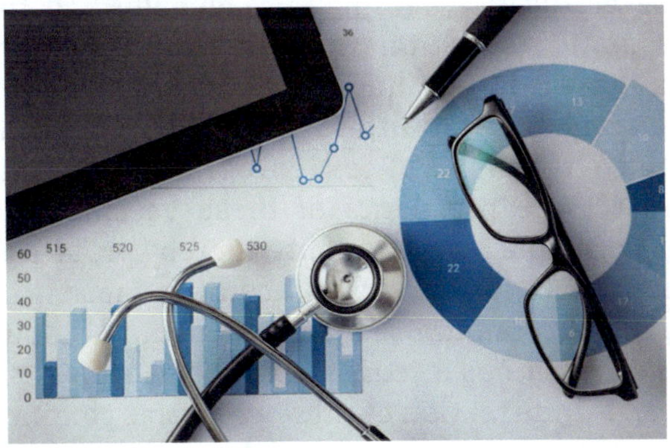

Figure 12.14. The accuracy limits of data-driven healthcare.

Source: https://specials-images.forbesimg.com/imageserve/620ad56ed042e09544bf109c/960x0.jpg.

This is a situation calling for continuous adaptation of data collection methods to meet local needs and variation, underscoring the fact that achieving data accuracy is not a technical task but also an exercise in logistical adaptability and cultural sensitivity. Lastly, the dynamic interplay between public health interventions and data accuracy makes for a recursive challenge that will impact the management of disease. Mistakes or lack of information can lead to bad policy-making, which may end up sustaining an outbreak or diverting resources from where they are needed most. For instance, misestimated predictions regarding the peak time of a flu season would lead either to over-preparation, straining healthcare facilities, or a lack of preparation that exposes populations to harm when a surge occurs. As noted in the above CDC challenge, learning from practice in forecasting is crucial to enhancing methodologies and developing predictive capacity over time. A robust feedback loop between analysis, data collection, and public health strategy must therefore exist to enhance the quality of epidemiological data. This interdependence illustrates that issues in data validity have to be solved comprehensively to create more robust public health systems in the context of infectious disease risks (Figure 12.14).

12.4. Control and Prevention Strategies

The infectious disease control and prevention policies are crucial in containing outbreaks and ensuring public health. One of the main policies is the implementation of vaccination programs, which have proved to be effective in disease control of such conditions as measles and influenza. Vaccination not only protects the individual who receives it, but it also contributes to the generation of herd immunity, thus reducing the prevalence of the disease within the population. Such herd immunity is able to prevent the spread of infectious pathogens, especially among high-risk populations that cannot be vaccinated due to health constraints. Vaccination promotion campaigns for vaccine take-up are also very important in addressing myths that typically inhibit participation, ultimately resulting in community resistance to infectious diseases. Utilization of epidemiological modeling to project disease patterns and help prevent disease is also a major strategy. Advanced computational techniques, such as in-silico epidemiological modeling, enable visualization of potential scenarios and outcomes of infectious disease transmission to be made by public health professionals. According to reports, breakthroughs in machine learning and simulation-based inference can potentially revolutionize the planning and execution of targeted interventions by enhancing models for optimization. These methods enhance public health interventions through facilitating focused control interventions based on specific population characteristics and patterns of disease transmissibility (Baydin et al., 2020). Thus, drawing from advancements in epidemiological modeling technology not only informs prompt responses but also makes societies responsive to future health emergencies. Surveillance platforms and data collection are also at the heart of control efforts through providing real-time monitoring of infectious disease transmission. Effective monitoring can detect outbreaks more quickly and implement necessary interventions, ranging from quarantine to the availability of resources for health care. Data analytics systems can identify trends rapidly and inform policy decisions regarding prevention and control (Tamás, 2025). By linking surveillance with community engagement, public health authorities can foster an educated public, effecting a response to emerging health threats that is active and cooperative. In the aggregate, these diverse prevention tactics provide a powerful system for control of infectious diseases and global health security (Figure 12.15).

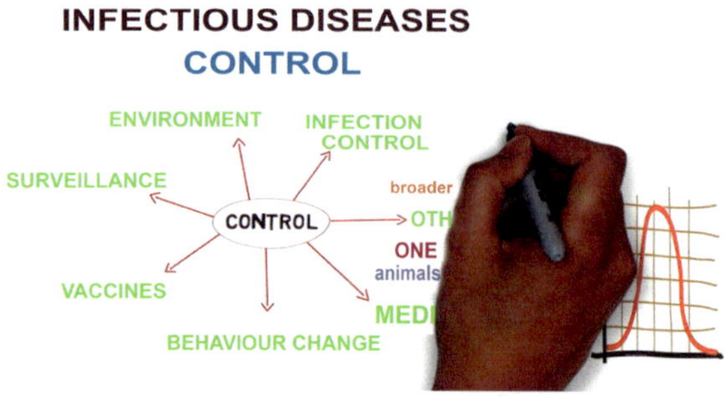

Figure 12.15. Infectious diseases control.

Source: https://i.ytimg.com/vi/2JWku3Kjpq0/maxresdefault.jpg.

12.4.1. Vaccination Programs

Vaccination campaign implementation is a cornerstone of infectious disease prevention and control and has a significant influence on public health. Vaccines stimulate the immune system to act and conquer pathogens and thus reduce the spread and disease outbreaks. The eradication of smallpox globally and the dramatic reduction in polio infections are an illustration of how concerted vaccination campaigns can initiate monumental public health triumphs. These programs not only protect the recipients of these vaccines but also promote herd immunity, thereby protecting the population at large, including those who cannot be immunized due to medical issues. Since infectious diseases continue to evolve, the design and creation of these programs continue to remain critical in responding to new health threats. As more evidence reveals the efficacy of vaccine administration to reduce disease incidence, public health programs must focus on such preventive care in a bid to benefit from long-term healthcare returns for the country (Lewnard et al., 2019). Furthermore, the health economic benefits of immunization programs extend beyond the advantages of enhanced healthcare, with them taking a central role in healthcare systems. Through the prevention of outbreaks of disease, vaccination programs can reduce financial burdens on governments and healthcare providers by reducing costs of treatment and lost productivity due to illness. For example, vaccination for controlling diseases such as Aujeszkys disease in animals not only offers animal health solutions but also significantly minimizes economic losses in agricultural production. The financial burden of direct costs of such outbreaks can be astronomical, covering the entire swine production chain, emphasizing the need to immediately undertake effective vaccination programs (Colomer et al., 2020). Integration of vaccination programs into overall public health economics offers a means of creating successful policies that can promote both economic stability and health security. Hence, investment in vaccination programs is both an effort in health care and an economic requirement. In addition, challenges associated with vaccination programs need ongoing research and development to maintain the pace with the dynamic situation of infectious diseases. Emerging new pathogens and strains of existing viruses depict the changing nature of epidemiology, necessitating vaccination programs to be constantly modified. For instance, integrating new molecular technologies and digital technology into disease surveillance can significantly enhance the effectiveness of such programs. As outlined in current studies, the analytical possibilities of the new technologies offer the potential to refine vaccination strategies and study their impact on infectious disease processes in detail (Lewnard et al., 2019). Continued follow-up and evaluation of the effects of vaccination are essential to account for factors such as vaccine efficacy and side effects, in order for vaccination to remain a cornerstone of infectious disease epidemiology. Therefore, future strategies must emphasize innovation and collaboration to address these challenges effectively (Figure 12.16).

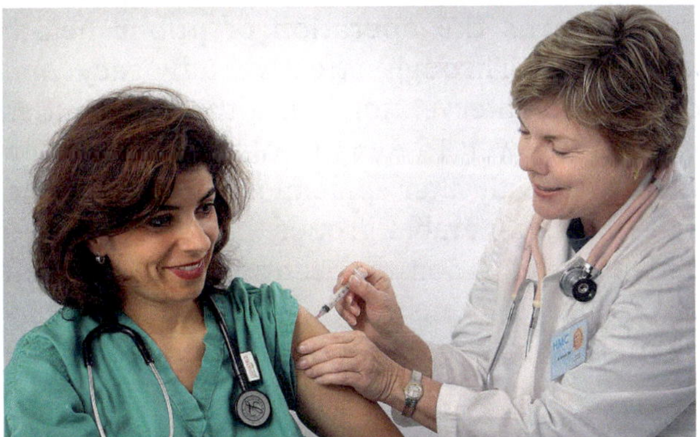

Figure 12.16. Health worker being vaccinated.

Source: https://miro.medium.com/v2/resize:fit:4800/format:webp/0*oeA7BYzHbGk5Welw.jpg.

12.4.2. Public Health Interventions

Public health intervention drives infectious disease control, as clearly demonstrated by the COVID-19 pandemic. Interventions entail vaccination drives and non-pharmaceutical interventions that are each tailored to what the population requires. Incorporation of in-silico epidemiological modeling has also become significantly relevant here. Not only does it forecast the dynamics of disease transmission, but it also assists policymakers in developing effective containment measures. Advances in machine learning, and particularly simulation-based inference, have opened new avenues for model calibration to allow more rigorous testing of proposed public health interventions. These advances mark a paradigm shift in the way public health authorities respond to outbreaks, adapting measures to real-time data and model outputs to diminish the contribution of infectious disease to communities (Baydin et al., 2020). The effectiveness of interventions in public health can be exemplified through several hypothetical situations mimicking real outcomes. ISTAM model studies have produced useful information on the effects of various non-pharmaceutical interventions. For instance, studies contrasting the effectiveness of interventions such as social distancing and quarantine of households during hypothetical influenza epidemics have established that the latter was the most effective intervention. Specifically, home quarantining led to a record decrease in peak and total numbers of cases, demonstrating the success of compliance with such measures. Such findings reiterate the importance of understanding the intricacies of human behavior and compliance in public health policy planning, as the timing and implementation of such measures can make a colossal difference in their overall effectiveness (Atkinson et al., 2011). Further, interaction between different public health interventions has the ability to provide synergistic benefits that, overall, enhance the effectiveness against infectious diseases. From the convergence of household quarantine and school closure, simulations reveal a substantial reduction in the dynamics of transmission, further defining the significance of collective intervention. The synergistic approach is useful in suppressing outbreaks, particularly in the vulnerable child groups, which are likely to act as drivers for disease spread. Use of such models to explore the spatial and temporal distribution of infections has the potential to reveal the most important points on how diseases disseminate through communities. Sensitivity analyses further indicate that there are higher returns with earlier implementation of control measures, adding the feeling of urgency with which public health interventions should be implemented in response to nascent infectious disease outbreaks (Atkinson et al., 2011) (Figure 12.17).

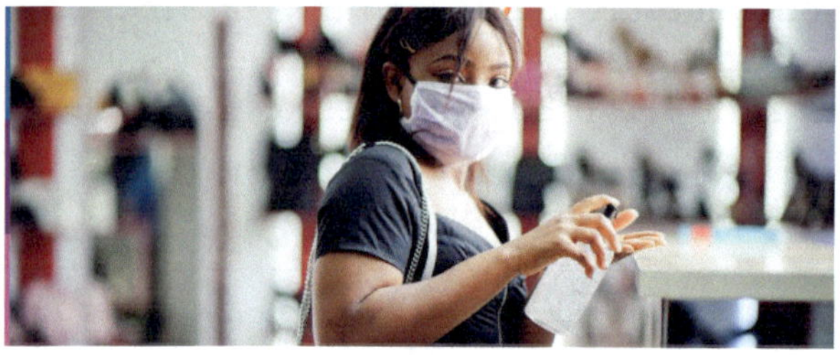

Figure 12.17. Public health interventions.

Source: https://media.licdn.com/dms/image/v2/D4E12AQFxEJoWzWr1VQ/article-cover_image-shrink_600_2000/article-cover_image-shrink_600_2000/0/1697026180966?e=2147483647&v=beta&t=Fqe4kX77xyKMr-JAaHlSTfmeSiJt30t4txSmDq-VTZw.

12.4.3. Role of Education and Awareness

The role of education and knowledge in the epidemiology of infectious diseases is key to their promotion of community well-being and effective containment of outbreaks. An educated public will be better able to understand the risks of disease, make informed decisions regarding immunization, and adopt preventive strategies. Educational programs specialized for specific communities can give them key information about transmission and prevention of infectious diseases. For instance, targeted promotion of awareness campaigns on sexually transmitted infections (STIs) has established the merits of testing recommendations by the Department of Health, among others to support chlamydia testing during antenatal care (Combs et al., 2008). By promoting knowledge on risk factors and testing processes, education can minimize stigma while encouraging people to take necessary health tests, ultimately resulting in early diagnosis and treatment. Besides, integration of awareness programs in public health initiatives significantly enhances community resistance to infectious disease struggles. Legislative support for compulsory vaccination is reflective of the paramount relationship between awareness and policy. For instance, efforts to implement a compulsory meningitis vaccination program in Alaska illustrate how education of the community can coordinate backing of public health policies (Hulstine et al., 2017). These initiatives not only educate members of the community regarding the perils of bacterial meningitis but also attempt to impart knowledge of the legislation that governs the operation of public health guidelines. Through effective advocacy and community intervention in health, communities gain the power to shape policy changes and thereby directly alter epidemiological trends and safeguard vulnerable groups. Lastly, continued active participation and continuous education are the keys to ensuring vigilance in an ever-changing public health environment. The ever-changing dynamics of infectious diseases, expressed in the form of newly emerging pathogens and shifting epidemiological patterns, necessitate ongoing educational interventions that inform populations of current risks and prevention strategies. Public health campaigns, fairs, and workshops have an important role to play in spreading appropriate resources to families and individuals to allow for continuous learning and compliance with health advisories. This preventive education ultimately empowers communities to be able to take care of their health themselves, resulting in enhanced health outcomes and reduced transmission of infectious diseases. By constructing robust networks for information exchange, the role of awareness and education becomes a fulcrum in the collaborative effort to stem the spread and impact of infectious disease.

12.5. Global Impact of Infectious Diseases

Infectious diseases continue to be a strong force worldwide, shaping public health programs and international relations. Disease emergence and re-emergence, such as HIV/AIDS and influenza, necessitate an international platform to improve health security extending beyond the borders of a country. Centers like the CDC have collaborated with countries like China, having program efforts in areas such as immunization, workforce capacity development, and global health security. These initiatives not only served to manage infectious diseases but also placed nations in a favorable position to deal with future outbreaks. From these collaborations, investments in surveillance for disease and capacity development are needed in order to increase health impact as well as decrease the infectious disease burden worldwide, maintaining the interdependence of health systems throughout the world (N/A, 2025). Indonesia has also benefited from increased partnership with the CDC, which has enhanced its capacity to fight infectious diseases like influenza and malaria. Technical support has, for over five decades, enhanced the Indonesian Ministry of Health's response to vaccine-preventable diseases and supported laboratory and surveillance systems. The alliance centers on the urgency of workforce training and the country's readiness in the event of emerging disease outbreaks. The global implications of such local actions highlight an evocative truth: the health security of a nation is inextricably linked to the health security of other nations. Thus, building strong public health programs in developing countries is vital in the battle against infectious disease spread and achieving sustainable health outcomes on a broader level (N/A, 2025). The global epidemiologic landscape of infectious diseases is also made complex due to emerging threats like antimicrobial resistance and zoonotic diseases. These issues underscore the need for a global appreciation of epidemiological patterns within different populations. Countries must exchange information, conduct collaborative research, and build diagnostic capacities in an effort to closely follow and contain diseases that ignore geographical boundaries. By making investments in global collaborations and applying technology to surveillance and response, the global community will be empowered to meet upcoming infectious disease crises. Thus, the collaborative efforts of these organizations not only aim to safeguard public health but also ensure economic stability, reflect collective responsibility in promoting the health equity, and collectively enhance resilience against the global impact of infectious diseases (Figure 12.18).

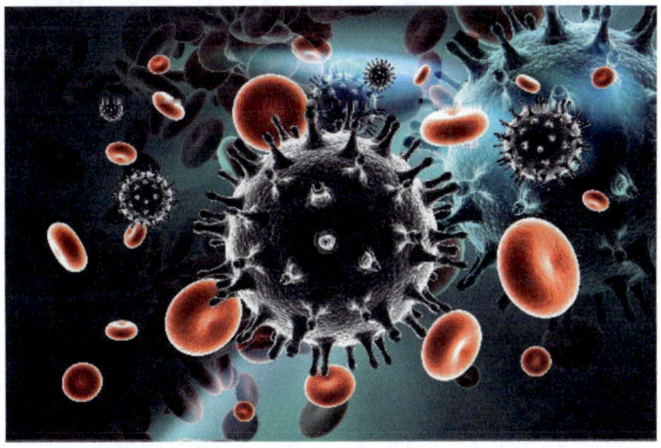

Figure 12.18. HIV and infections.

Source: https://medlineplus.gov/images/HIVAIDSandInfections_share.jpg.

12.5.1. Economic Consequences

The economic effects of disease outbreaks are profound and multifaceted, usually aggravating existing social inequalities and influencing public health systems. Recessions in the economy can potentially cause infectious disease outbreaks by compromising living standards and access to healthcare. For instance, when individuals are out of work and earn lower incomes, they are no longer able to pay for sanitation and medical services. This is reflected in several studies demonstrating a direct causality from economic recessions to increased levels of infectious diseases, particularly among marginalized groups such as migrants, homeless persons, and detainees (Abubakar et al., 2011). Given that these groups live in congested conditions and have limited access to healthcare services, they are fertile ground for the spread of diseases, and this may have ramifications for community health as well as economic stability. Moreover, the impact of economic crises on public expenditure in health cannot be overlooked. During economic downturns, governments cut spending on healthcare services, limiting prevention activities crucial in curbing infectious diseases. Tight budget conditions can hinder the execution of effective public health campaigns and swift intervention responses, which are fundamental to cutting outbreaks short. In tracing the interconnection between economic forces and infectious disease epidemiology, social epidemiology illuminates key factors in how population health is determined by factors of social origin, such as income inequality and outright poverty. By paying attention to these factors, researchers can better understand the patterns of disease transmission in times of economic hardship (Link et al., 2008). Such findings have significant implications, as they justify the need for robust healthcare financing, particularly during times of crisis. In the end, the reduction of the economic burden of infectious disease transmission requires an integrated approach involving economic policy and public health strategy. Governments must recognize the mutual dependence between economic stability and health outcomes, inducing resiliency against potential outbreaks through directed investment in healthcare infrastructure. However, the capacity to respond also depends on budgetary elasticity during times of crisis. The empirical evidence shows that well-programmed pre-emptive health interventions, despite economic recessions, can buffer long-term impacts of infectious diseases (Abubakar et al., 2011). It is therefore essential that policymakers prioritize health as a vital component of economic planning since population health directly mirrors economic recovery and resilience from crisis (Figure 12.19).

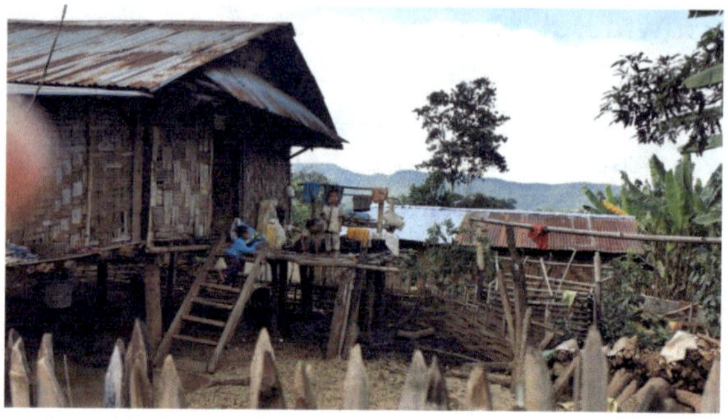

Figure 12.19. Economic impacts of infectious diseases of poverty.

Source: https://media.springernature.com/lw725/springer-cms/rest/v1/content/17667912/data/v2.

12.5.2. Social Implications

The social impact of infectious diseases extends far beyond the individual level, crossing into communities and reshaping societal trends. Because infectious diseases are contagious, they can exacerbate social inequalities, making disproportionately harder impacts on marginalized communities who may have extremely limited access to healthcare, resources, or information. The infection patterns have a lot to do with social routines, in which facets from the trust of public health facilities, accessibility of health services, and human interaction drive how diseases spread. It is important to know these social currents because Emile Durkheim argues that scientific research into society involves establishing 'social currents' that influence shared experiences and practices. Therefore, an examination of infectious disease epidemiology must include an examination of social dynamics in order to manage the broader societal circumstances of disease transmission and health consequences (Anderson et al., 2015). In addition, the interconnectivity of communities through social networks has a significant impact on infectious disease transmission patterns. The application of network theory to epidemiology shows that how people are interacting in social structures can facilitate or impede the transmission of pathogens. Networks are conduits of disease transmission, in which high-density relationships among individuals will result in quick outbreaks. But knowing the properties of these networks allows public health officials to create targeted interventions, taking into account the special social contexts of the infected populations. Through the identification of nodes or clusters of nodes that are apt to be influential in disease spread across networks, effective interventions may be used to contain infection while simultaneously addressing the social factors that make individuals vulnerable and resilient (Danon et al., 2010) Finally, the response to the social dimensions of infectious diseases involves the integration of both epidemiological data and socio-cultural perspectives. Public health messages, education campaigns, and community mobilization initiatives must be designed to be attractive to the heterogeneity of experience within populations affected. This involves the identification and use of the 'emergent properties' within communities, such as hope and collective efficacy, which have the capacity to influence public health significantly. By establishing a sense of resilience and agency in populations, public health programs can make the response to infectious disease a vehicle for empowerment and social cohesion. Through blending epidemiological insight with a deep sensibility about social context, policymakers can better address the complexities of prevention and disease response, and ultimately gain healthier communities (Anderson et al., 2015).

12.5.3. Case Studies of Epidemics

The analysis of case studies in epidemics provides significant data on the dynamics of infectious diseases and their spread. Data on the unique characteristics of various outbreaks helps researchers to know the influencing factors on disease spread. For instance, the 2014 Ebola outbreak in Bomi, Liberia, exhibited sub-exponential growth, which was indicative of slower growth regardless of the virulence of the agent. This case highlights the value of characterizing epidemiological profiles, which can serve to guide intervention policy in the future. Historical cases, in stark contrast, like the 1918 influenza pandemic, exhibit near-exponential growth, showing just how heterogeneous transmission dynamics can be from pathogen to pathogen and setting to setting. Comparing different outbreak scenarios allows for more nuanced epidemic behavior and provides crucial insight into controlling current and emerging public health threats (Lewnard et al., 2019). Careful analysis of case studies illustrates the impact of intervention strategies on epidemic growth patterns. A good case in point is the 1972 smallpox outbreak in Khulna, and how mass vaccination campaigns can speed up the containment of infectious diseases. Similarly, the Japanese HIV/AIDS epidemic exhibited a similarly linear pattern of growth, influenced by socio-behavioral determinants and targeted public health interventions. This heterogeneity emphasizes that epidemic dynamics cannot be attributed exclusively to pathogen attributes; human behavior, environmental factors, and the timeliness of interventions in appropriateness are major drivers of outbreak patterns. As revealed through varied patterns of growth, including the foot-and-mouth epidemic in Uruguay and heterogeneity in responses that occurred during the West African Ebola epidemic, setting context-specific strategies for response and surveillance epidemiologically is essential for effective control of disease (Chowell et al., 2016). The combination of new techniques in surveillance and advanced statistical models is imperative in having a better understanding of epidemic growth patterns. Application of a 2-parameter generalized-growth model to fit outbreak data is especially relevant in explaining initial epidemic phases. The capacity of such techniques to detect a wide range of growth behaviors highlights significant differences inherent in outbreaks of different infectious agents, which call for an adaptive response strategy. For instance, detection of sub-exponential growth behavior can indicate the necessity of altered public health interventions on the basis of alterations in contact patterns or risk groups. The inclusion of such analytical models in the training programs of epidemiology ensures that the future generation of researchers and practitioners possesses the ability to meet the challenges of infectious diseases in the ever-changing world (Lewnard et al., 2019) (Figure 12.20).

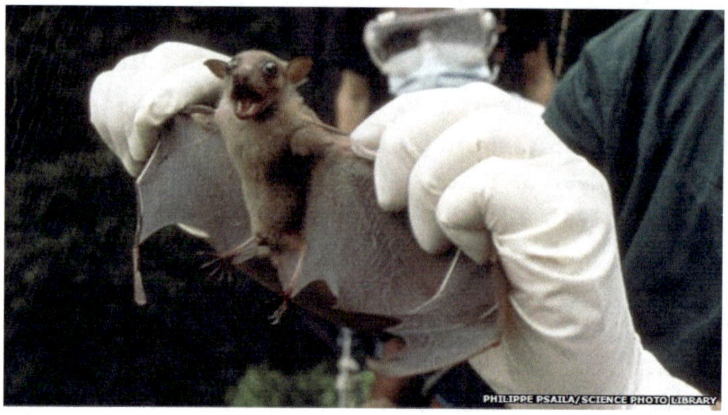

Figure 12.20. Bat — likely reservoir for the Ebola virus.

Source: https://miro.medium.com/v2/resize:fit:4800/format:webp/0*eZOHsoW3-ZBsWrZE.jpg.

Summary

In conclusion, the epidemiology of infectious diseases is an intricate interaction between environmental, biological, and socio-economic factors. As noted in recent research, biodiversity is a double-edged sword in infectious disease dynamics; it can serve as a source of pathogens and also contribute to the rate of zoonotic outbreaks. For instance, bird and mammal species richness correlates with the overall prevalence of infectious disease, whereas regions having higher threatened species exhibit more zoonotic outbreaks. The findings emphasize the importance of conservation studies, as maintaining biodiversity could be utilized as a defense mechanism against the emergence of new pathogens. This is particularly so in Southeast Asia, where the biodiversity hotspot has shown an alarming increase in disease emergence from activities that impact habitats and ecosystems (Morand et al., 2014). To this, the impact of climate change on the epidemiological landscape cannot be overstated. The observed changes in disease patterns, especially in targeted locations such as Thailand, indicate that climatic variability, i.e., events such as the El Niño Southern Oscillation (ENSO), directly results in the cases of diseases such as leptospirosis and scrub typhus. With climate change continually altering rainfall patterns and monsoon intensity, the risk of future heightened disease outbreaks is enhanced. This exchange underlines the necessity for inclusive surveillance designs that are sensitive to the fluidity of climate impact on host and pathogen interactions. Thus, with changes in epidemiological patterns, public health intervention must adapt towards being flexible by adopting models that are predictive and sensitive to climate-induced changes in disease patterns (Sabryla et al., 2014). Finally, the transition from infectious to chronic diseases, as observed in some regions, also poses additional challenges for epidemiologists and public health officials. With increasingly expanding societies and shifting populations, chronic diseases are destined to increase, typically aggravated by phenomena originally linked with infectious diseases, such as lifestyle issues and obesity. This epidemiologic transition calls for collective action on the part of health care workers to respond not only to infectious diseases but also to the rise in non-communicable disease burden. Effective public health interventions must now incorporate education and intervention on various levels, with a focus on changes in lifestyle and early detection to minimize the hazards presented by chronic diseases in response to previous infectious disease patterns. Such an integrated strategy is central to protecting the well-being and health of populations as they move through this complex world of evolving health threats (Sabryla et al., 2014).

Within the field of epidemiology, understanding the complexities of infectious diseases demands the use of sophisticated mathematical models as valuable analytical and predictive tools. Such models capture the underlying dynamics driving disease spread and transmission, providing insights into both population dynamics and individual behavior. For instance, the structure of individual-based models, used in programs such as SimpactCyan, permits HIV transmission dynamics simulation within sexual networks. The process underscores the significance of parameterizing over time, which is able to simulate various public health interventions. These models not only guide estimation of the impact of treatment eligibility criteria on HIV incidence but also give a data-generating tool for phylodynamic framework assessment, showcasing the diverse applications observed in epidemiological research (Delva et al., 2019). Epidemiological models are based on some important assumptions, which may have large impacts on their validity and predictability. One of the main issues arises from the widespread and often inaccurate assumption of infectious and latent period distribution in infectious disease transmission. It is known from research that neglect of the latent period or an exponential distribution assumption can lead to a serious underestimation of the basic reproduction number, a determining parameter in infectious disease outbreaks. By illustrating this with influenza outbreak data, researchers have revealed how such inaccuracies can propagate to inflated predictions of management interventions. This underscores the importance of rigorous model validation because assumptions always taint outcomes in disease control and prevention activities (Anon et al., 2005). The implications of these findings underscore the necessity for enhancing mathematical models to facilitate improved public health decision-making. Detection and elimination of biases inherent in the underlying assumptions will lead to more accurate epidemiological estimates required for effective policy formulation. As epidemiologists progress towards utilizing models to inform disease management strategies, they need to continuously examine and update underlying assumptions that inform these systems. A commitment to transparency in model structure not only improves the credibility of predictions but also allows for greater confidence in public health interventions. Therefore, guaranteeing models are congruent with the natural complexity of infectious disease spread is key to ensuring better health outcomes among populations (Anon et al., 2005).

CLOSER LOOK

OTHER TERMS USED IN INFECTIOUS DISEASE EPIDEMIOLOGY

Like all sciences, there are several commonly used terms in epidemiology that would be helpful to understand.

Infectivity: Infectivity is the ability of an infectious agent to infect a susceptible new host. By susceptible, I am referring to the host (think person) not being immune and therefore able to contract the disease. It is measured by the secondary attack rate, the proportion of susceptible contacts developing infection after contact with a primary case, calculated as a percentage of the number of such contacts who were at risk. Therefore, if a person with COVID-19 contacts 10 vulnerable people and 5 of them contract the disease, then the secondary attack rate is 50%.

Virulence*:* This is the ability of the causing agent to injure the host. One of the simple measures used is the case fatality rate, which is the number of deaths to the total cases of a disease during a specified time. That is, the case fatality rate is the number of disease deaths divided by the number of cases. It is usually expressed in percentage.

For COVID-19 this is very different from one country to another. For example, in Italy the case fatality rate currently is 10% and in Australia is about 0.5%. The denominator (lower half) of the formula for the case fatality rate is the number of cases of the illness that have been diagnosed. For COVID-19, this number is likely to be very under-estimated because in the majority of countries only a subset of the population has been tested. This means that the number of people actually suffering from the disease is much larger. So the current estimates of the case fatality rate are highly likely to be exaggerated, and globally, it is most likely to be between 1% (Figure 12.21).

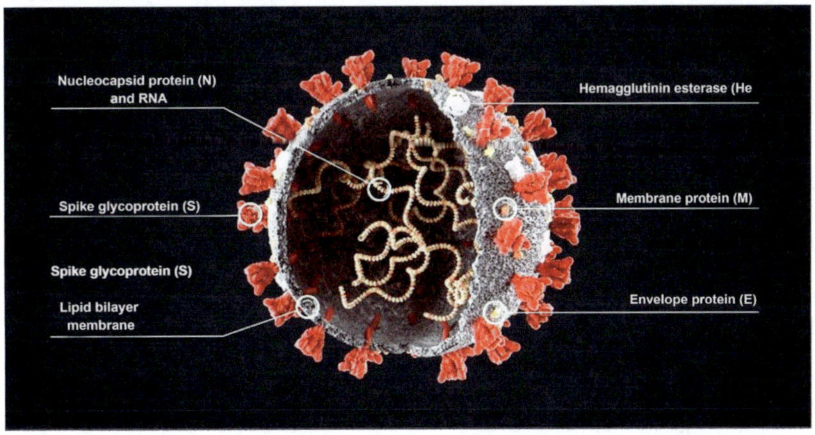

Figure 12.21. Realistic 3D illustration of COVID-19 virus structure diagram. Corona virus SARS-CoV-2, 2019 nCoV virus.

Source: https://www.news-medical.net/image-handler/ts/20240228074706/ri/950/src/images/Article_Images/ImageForArticle_19682_17091676251227888.jpg.

References

1. Abubakar, I., Basu, S., Desai, M., Hunter, P. R., et al. (2011). The impact of economic crises on communicable disease transmission and control: A systematic review of the evidence. https://core.ac.uk/download/13093583.pdf (accessed on 25th June 2025).
2. Adeyemo, A., Aseffa, A., Davey, G., Finan, C., et al. (2012). Prediction of HLA class II alleles using SNPs in an African population. https://core.ac.uk/download/9552150.pdf (accessed on 25th June 2025).
3. Akthar, M. S. (2019). Role of epidemiological studies in disease prevention. https://media.neliti.com/media/publications/301058-role-of-epidemiological-studies-in-disea-d4cd7a6e.pdf (accessed on 25th June 2025).
4. Allen, C., Alper, D., Aman, S., Kumar, A., et al. (2016). Results from the Centers for Disease Control and Prevention's Predict the 2013–2014 Influenza Season Challenge. https://core.ac.uk/download/98348865.pdf (accessed on 25th June 2025).
5. Ancheta, C. A., Perez, E. S., Richter, K., Tempongko, M. S. B., Sunpuwan, M., Mendoza, O. M., Pachuen, O., et al. (2010). *Disease Surveillance Networks Initiative Asia: Final Evaluation*. https://core.ac.uk/download/86445039.pdf (accessed on 25th June 2025).
6. Anderson, C., Cullingham, D. L., Horton, D. L., Dietzschold, B., Eng, K., Brunker, K., et al. (2012). Integrating the landscape epidemiology and genetics of RNA viruses: Rabies in domestic dogs as a model. https://core.ac.uk/download/9651666.pdf (accessed on 25th June 2025).
7. Anderson, D., Calfee, D. P., Harris, A. D., Kaye, K., et al. (2016). Which comorbid conditions should we be analyzing as risk factors for healthcare-associated infections? https://core.ac.uk/download/83100993.pdf (accessed on 25th June 2025).
8. Anderson, R. M., Aunger, R., Banaji, M., Barnett, T., Denton, D., et al. (2015). Some considerations concerning the challenge of incorporating social variables into epidemiological models of infectious disease transmission. https://core.ac.uk/download/36778292.pdf (accessed on 25th June 2025).
9. Arsevska, E., Bournez, L., Bronner, A., Calavas, D., et al. (2017). Modelling the spread of emerging infectious diseases in animal health: Case study of lumpy skin disease in the Balkans, 2015–2016. http://agritrop.cirad.fr/586538/1/ICAHS%20proceedings%20%282017%29%20-%20Modelling%20the%20spread%20of%20emerging%20infectious%20diseas.pdf (accessed on 25th June 2025).
10. Arthur, C., Banda, H., Chazya, R., Chijoka, M., et al. (2023). Epidemiological tools in focus: A comprehensive assessment of their role in addressing infectious disease challenges in Zambia. https://core.ac.uk/download/597862448.pdf (accessed on 25th June 2025).
11. Artois, M., Jones, B. A., Belotto, A., Boureau, E., Brown, D., Childs, J., Chomel, B., et al. (2013). Zoonosis emergence linked to agricultural intensification and environmental change. https://core.ac.uk/download/36776760.pdf (accessed on 25th June 2025).
12. Atkinson, P. M., Ettema, D., & Yang, Y. (2011). Analysis of CDC social control measures using an agent-based simulation of an influenza epidemic in a city. https://core.ac.uk/download/pdf/8603783.pdf (accessed on 25th June 2025).
13. Babcock, S., Beverley, J., Cowell, L. G., Smith, B., et al. (2021). The infectious disease ontology

in the age of COVID-19. https://core.ac.uk/download/305120399.pdf (accessed on 25th June 2025).

14. Baldacchino, G., Blome, S., Boinas, F., Costard, S., Davies, K., de Carvalho Ferreira, H., et al. (2016). Transmission routes of African swine fever virus to domestic pigs: Current knowledge and future research directions. https://core.ac.uk/download/45467769.pdf (accessed on 25th June 2025).
15. Balmes, J., Ritz, B., & Tager, I. (2004). Can lessons from public health disease surveillance be applied to environmental public health tracking? https://core.ac.uk/download/pdf/3775836.pdf (accessed on 25th June 2025).
16. Bastiampillai, A. J., Caporali, M. G., Costanzo, V., Declich, S., et al. (2016). Event-based surveillance during EXPO Milan 2015: Rationale, tools, procedures, and initial results. https://core.ac.uk/download/84928141.pdf (accessed on 25th June 2025).
17. Bauchinger, U., Falagas, M. E., Kelesidis, I., Kelesidis, T., et al. (2008). Human infections associated with wild birds. https://core.ac.uk/download/323062291.pdf (accessed on 25th June 2025).
18. Baydin, A. G., Darzi, A., de Witt, C. S., Dokania, R. K., et al. (2020). Simulation-based inference for global health decisions. https://core.ac.uk/download/396289157.pdf (accessed on 25th June 2025).
19. Boccia, D., Dowd, J. B., Fletcher, H., Hayward, A. C., et al. (2019). A systematic review of the impact of psychosocial factors on immunity: Implications for enhancing BCG response against tuberculosis. https://core.ac.uk/download/286270876.pdf (accessed on 25th June 2025).
20. Bonomo, R. A., Burd, E. M., Conly, J., Limbago, B. M., et al. (2018). Carbapenems-producing organisms: A global scourge. https://core.ac.uk/download/158611849.pdf (accessed on 25th June 2025).
21. Borlase, A., Rudge, J. W., & Webster, J. P. (2017). Opportunities and challenges for modelling epidemiological and evolutionary dynamics in a multihost, multiparasite system: Zoonotic hybrid schistosomiasis in West Africa. https://core.ac.uk/download/143477770.pdf (accessed on 25th June 2025).
22. Carling, P., Carrico, R., Donskey, C. J., Dubberke, E. R., et al. (2014). Strategies to prevent *Clostridium difficile* infections in acute care hospitals: 2014 update. https://core.ac.uk/download/70384907.pdf (accessed on 25th June 2025).
23. Chowell, G., Simonsen, L., & Viboud, C. (2016). A generalized-growth model to characterize the early ascending phase of infectious disease outbreaks. https://core.ac.uk/download/pdf/82033390.pdf (accessed on 25th June 2025).
24. Colomer, M. À., Sauce, L. J. F., & Margalida, A. (2020). Vaccination is a suitable tool in the control of Aujeszky's disease outbreaks in pigs using a population dynamics P systems model. https://core.ac.uk/download/323287755.pdf (accessed on 25th June 2025).
25. Combs, B. G., Giele, C. M., Kwan, K. S. H., Mak, D. B., et al. (2008). Audit of antenatal testing of sexually transmissible infections and blood borne viruses at Western Australian hospitals. https://core.ac.uk/download/61303469.pdf (accessed on 25th June 2025).
26. Dalgard, O., Lo Re III, V., Macias, J., Midgard, H., et al. (2016). HCV epidemiology in high-risk groups and the risk of reinfection. https://core.ac.uk/download/293881650.pdf (accessed on 25th June 2025).

27. Danon, L., Ford, A. P., House, T. A., Jewell, C. P., et al. (2010). Networks and the epidemiology of infectious disease. https://core.ac.uk/download/1381886.pdf (accessed on 25th June 2025).

28. Delva, W., Hendrickx, D. M., Hens, N., Kuylen, E., et al. (2019). *SimpactCyan 1.0*: An open-source simulator for individual-based models in HIV epidemiology with R and Python interfaces. https://core.ac.uk/download/286086461.pdf (accessed on 25th June 2025).

29. Freudenberg, N., Galea, S., & Vlahov, D. (2005). Cities and population health. https://core.ac.uk/download/323072008.pdf (accessed on 25th June 2025).

30. Fung, I. C. H. (2017). *EPID 7135A–Epidemiology of Infectious Disease*. https://core.ac.uk/download/229148076.pdf (accessed on 25th June 2025).

31. Hamilton, C., Borbolla, D., Novillo-Ortiz, D., Saigí-Rubió, F., Eguia, H., et al. (2021). Data and digital solutions to support surveillance strategies in the context of the COVID-19 pandemic. https://core.ac.uk/download/480394162.pdf (accessed on 25th June 2025).

32. Hulstine, A. (2017). Vaccine implementation: Alaska 2017. https://core.ac.uk/download/286607590.pdf (accessed on 25th June 2025).

33. International Conference on Emerging Infectious Diseases (2008: Atlanta, GA). (2025). *Emerging infectious diseases*. https://core.ac.uk/download/144197853.pdf (accessed on 25th June 2025).

34. Johannessen, A., Lindberg, A., Chaturvedi, A. K., Morris, A., Phillips, A. N., Balbi, B., Celli, B. R., et al. (2013). The impact of HAART on the respiratory complications of HIV infection: Longitudinal trends in the MACS and WIHS cohorts. https://core.ac.uk/download/12214715.pdf (accessed on 25th June 2025).

35. Koskella, B., & Lin, D. (2014). Friend and foe: Factors influencing the movement of the bacterium *Helicobacter pylori* along the parasitism-mutualism continuum. https://core.ac.uk/download/323080778.pdf (accessed on 25th June 2025).

36. Lewnard, J. A., & Reingold, A. L. (2019). Emerging challenges and opportunities in infectious disease epidemiology. https://core.ac.uk/download/323082106.pdf (accessed on 25th June 2025).

37. Link, B., Morroni, C., Myer, L., Susser, E., et al. (2008). Social epidemiology. https://core.ac.uk/download/1670083.pdf (accessed on 25th June 2025).

38. Morand, S. (2014). Climate, biodiversity, land use changes and zoonotic infectious diseases in Southeast Asia: O15. http://agritrop.cirad.fr/573884/1/document_573884.pdf (accessed on 25th June 2025).

39. N/A. (2025). *CDC in China*. https://core.ac.uk/download/153363517.pdf (accessed on 25th June 2025).

40. N/A. (2025). *CDC in Indonesia*. https://core.ac.uk/download/286647960.pdf (accessed on 25th June 2025).

41. N/A. (2025). *Clinical Infectious Diseases*. https://core.ac.uk/download/154402171.pdf (accessed on 25th June 2025).

42. Prisacari, V. (2013). Scientific activity of epidemiologists and microbiologists in the Republic of Moldova during 2008–2013. https://core.ac.uk/download/335258580.pdf (accessed on 25th June 2025).

43. Sabryla, A. (2014). Hypertension Grade I and prediabetic in woman, 56 years old and work as a teacher. https://media.neliti.com/media/publications/156248-ID-none.pdf (accessed on 25th June 2025).

44. Snow, M. (2011). The contribution of molecular epidemiology to the understanding and control of viral diseases of salmonid aquaculture. https://core.ac.uk/download/pdf/8555510.pdf (accessed on 25th June 2025).

45. Tekeli, T. (2025). Modelling and optimizing testing strategies for epidemic outbreaks. https://core.ac.uk/download/543227170.pdf (accessed on 25th June 2025).

46. Wearing, H. J., Keeling, M. J., Rohani, P., & Ellner, S. P. (2005). Appropriate models for the management of infectious diseases. https://core.ac.uk/download/44114.pdf (accessed on 25th June 2025).

47. Yan, F., Qian, M. B., & Chen, Y. D. (2013). Time to tackle Clonorchis's in China. https://core.ac.uk/download/pdf/81750184.pdf (accessed on 25th June 2025).

48. Zaragoza, G. (2019). Getting to zero HIV cases in San Francisco: Reconceptualizing housing as public health infrastructure in the framework of HIV prevention and treatment. https://core.ac.uk/download/287622090.pdf (accessed on 25th June 2025).

49. Zaragoza, G. (2019). Getting to zero HIV cases San Francisco: Reconceptualizing housing as HIV prevention and HIV treatment. https://core.ac.uk/download/287624137.pdf (accessed on 25th June 2025).

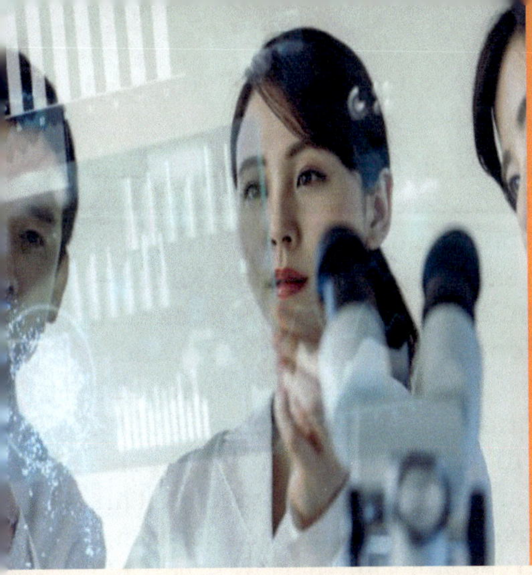

Chapter 13

CHRONIC DISEASE EPIDEMIOLOGY

Contents

Introduction

Chronic diseases, which are prevalent in modern populations, present significant public health issues due to their multifactorial aetiology and long-term effects. They are distinguishable from acute illnesses, which manifest quickly and respond within a short timeframe, as these present with a slow course of progression and usually require extended attention. Conditions such as diabetes, cardiovascular diseases, and chronic respiratory diseases illustrate the vast range of chronic diseases that can affect an individual's quality of life significantly. As has been covered by social epidemiology, health results are significantly determined by social and economic determinants that shape individuals' environments and possibilities for better health, and, as such, the necessity for a multi-faceted approach to comprehending the epidemiological aspects of such conditions is indicated (Link et al., 2008). The increasing rate of such diseases necessitates consideration of prevention, for instance, promoting healthy living and improving healthcare access, thus contributing to the broader debate on chronic disease epidemiology. The understanding of chronic disease epidemiology necessitates in-depth consideration of both the incidence and prevalence of such diseases. Epidemiologists use a variety of methods to study the spread of such diseases among populations to identify the risk factors and potential interventions. Of particular importance is the examination of comorbidities—those conditions that exist in conjunction with chronic disease and complicate treatment as well as prognosis. The Charlson Comorbidity Index, which is widely popular and applied everywhere globally, determines the burden of the comorbidities in diverse conditions using weights and thus provides useful data for risk estimation and resource allocation (Brusselaers et al., 2017). When analyzing these co-existing conditions, researchers are able to gain more insight into health inequalities and how the aggregation of multiple chronic diseases affects healthcare systems. This multifactorial perspective emphasizes the interaction of biological, environmental, and socioeconomic determinants, and therefore, it is vital to effective public health interventions. Furthermore, chronic diseases have significant implications for healthcare expenditure and resource utilization, both at the individual and system levels. Multidisciplinary care for chronic diseases is usually needed, involving more than one care provider, which can exert considerable pressure on healthcare systems globally. Being long-term in duration and necessitating extended treatment regimens, chronic diseases are likely to have greater healthcare expenses both to patients and to institutions. Consequently, identification of and reaction to the cost implications of such diseases is critical in formulating public health strategic policy. With the development of research, the incorporation of social epidemiology concepts and tools like the Charlson Comorbidity Index will enhance our ability to confront health inequities and optimize healthcare provision for patients with chronic disease (Link et al., 2008; Brusselaers et al., 2017). It emphasizes the need for collaboration between healthcare professionals, policymakers, and communities in order to promote chronic disease management and outcomes (Figure 13.1).

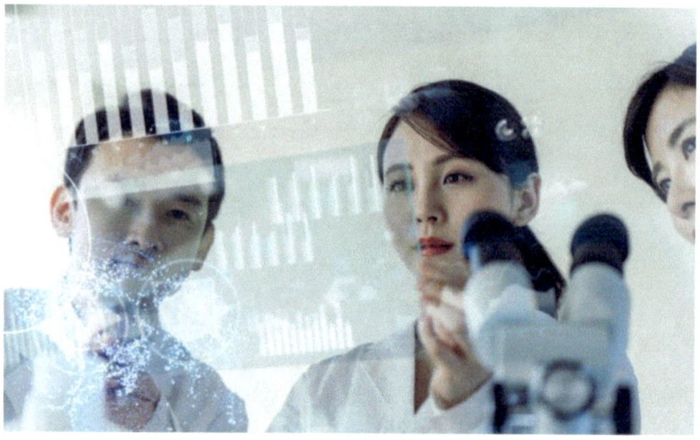

Figure 13.1. Chronic disease epidemiology.

Source: https://www.cdc.gov/populationhealth/statechronicepi/images_statechronicepi/EpidemiologyMicroscope_istock-medium.jpg.

Definition of Chronic Diseases

Chronic illnesses are an important focus of public health, and are conditions that persist over a long duration and normally worsen at a slow rate. Chronic illnesses are comprehensive and encompass diseases such as diabetes, cardiovascular disease, chronic respiratory disease, and cancer, among others. The World Health Organization emphasizes that those diseases are likely to emerge from an intermingling of genetic, physiological, environmental, and behavior-related causes, creating complex interactions, which stimulate and sustain them. Chronic diseases are not only defined by the degree of their prolongation but also by the high degree of their contribution towards morbidity and mortality worldwide, with increased healthcare costs and reduced quality of life in patients. Knowledge of these definitions forms the basis for consideration of the epidemiological trends and the health implications associated with chronic disease, the basis for creating successful public health interventions. Definition of chronic disease also suggests long-term illness that calls for care and management over a lifetime. Most often, patients with chronic illness must navigate through a healthcare system optimized for acute care and find it hard to access ongoing and full care. Proper management of such diseases, therefore, is largely dependent on lifestyle modifications, adherence to drug regimens, and frequent monitoring of health. Growing incidences of chronic disease place additional burdens on healthcare systems, particularly where resources are limited. Particularly, chronic kidney disease provides a good case study in understanding this burden, with morbidity and mortality associated with the condition having been methodically monitored. CKD reportedly had a huge disability-adjusted life years (DALYs) in 2017, highlighting the necessity for enhanced chronic disease prevention and management interventions (Abdoli et al., 2020). Furthermore, managing chronic diseases needs to consider a comprehensive approach that includes a deeper understanding of their epidemiological patterns. They do not manifest in all groups equally; there exist variations depending on socio-economic status, location, and access to healthcare services. As an example, there can be regions of the nation with varying prevalence rates that are related to ways of life, including dietary habits and levels of physical fitness. In addition, some chronic diseases, such as Q fever, possess different patterns of transmission in various ecosystems, depending on the high rate of *Coxiella burnetii* occurrence among diverse human and animal populations in African-based studies (Benkirane et al., 2014). This diversity underscores the necessity for sustained research on chronic disease epidemiology to facilitate targeted interventions and public health interventions that can neutralize their impact on vulnerable populations (Figure 13.2).

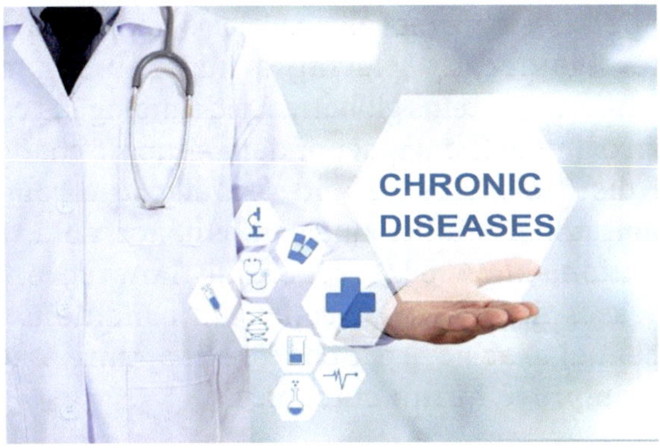

Figure 13.2. Chronic diseases.

Source: https://nutrition.org/wp-content/uploads/2022/08/CHRONIC-DISEASES-Healthcare-concept.jpg.

Importance of Studying Chronic Disease Epidemiology

The field of chronic disease epidemiology plays an important role in guiding public health interventions and policies that aim to reduce the burden of chronic diseases. By examining the distribution and determinants of diseases such as cancer, heart disease, and diabetes, researchers are able to establish risk factors underlying their causation and progression. This information is essential in the design of prevention interventions that are targeted to the particular needs of a given population. Further, chronic disease epidemiology emphasizes the importance of understanding health disparities, which may be influenced by a myriad of factors, including socioeconomic status, accessibility of health care, and environmental contexts. Such understanding is extremely critical for designing effective public health campaigns, not only to promote healthy practices but also to campaign for systemic changes that reduce health inequalities in targeted communities. Epidemiologic study of chronic disease further enables the identification of trends and patterns over time, which is critical to optimal healthcare planning and resource allocation. With population aging and urbanization set to persist, chronic diseases are expected to rise significantly, placing a huge burden on healthcare systems globally. Epidemiologists can approximate the impact of demographic change on disease incidence and prevalence through longitudinal studies and surveillance data. In addition, knowledge regarding how chronic diseases interact with comorbid conditions is essential to achieve patient care in optimal ways and improve health outcomes.

These intricacies are met by embracing a multi-dimensional strategy, thus the imperative for ongoing research in chronic disease epidemiology to inform public health programs and health care policy. The integration of principles of social epidemiology in studies of chronic diseases refines the understanding of determinants of health outcomes. The most recent studies place a focus on implicit racial and ethnic diversity and how it affects health disparities, thus becoming a necessity to explore within-population differences. As quoted in Ferraro et al. (2020), understanding the cumulative inequality related to unequal life course experiences is important in establishing the underlying cause of health inequities. Furthermore, examination of social determinants such as income inequality, discrimination, and access to health care is a sophisticated approach to the understanding of social determinants of chronic disease prevalence (Link et al., 2008). Through an integration of social epidemiology and chronic disease epidemiology, researchers can create equity-focused interventions that not only prevent disease but also foster health justice in diverse populations.

Overview of Common Chronic Diseases

Chronic illnesses are a significant public health problem, affecting millions of individuals across the world. Cardiovascular conditions, diabetes, and chronic respiratory illnesses are some of the most frequent conditions and have high morbidity and mortality. Cardiovascular illnesses, like heart attacks and strokes, are most frequently linked with risk elements like hypertension, being overweight, and inactivity. The International Society of Hypertension informs us that these conditions are preventable to a great extent through lifestyle modification and primary care management, emphasizing the urgency of early recognition and management regimens. With the increasing ageing of populations across the world, the prevalence of these conditions is expected to rise, necessitating a coordinated perspective on their epidemiology and risk patterns in different populations. The focus should thus extend beyond individual interventions in health but also towards the overall systemic change of healthcare delivery and policy. In addition to cardiovascular disease, diabetes is a prevailing chronic condition of significant public health relevance. Diabetes, particularly Type 2, is closely linked with obesity and lack of exercise, and poses a significant risk across all populations, but notably among the older population. It has been ascertained through research that almost 80% of older Australians are suffering from chronic ailments, including diabetes, which emphasizes the co-occurrence of chronic diseases among older people (Link et al., 2008). Diabetes treatment is composed of both medical treatment and lifestyle changes in the form of diet and physical activity, which would decelerate progression and complications. Moreover, socioeconomic determinants of diabetes prevalence have also been researched more so in recent years, calling for research into the impact of income inequality and access to healthcare resources on disease courses (Link et al., 2008). Chronic diseases often co-mingle and bring about a complex web of health consequences known as comorbidities. Synergies between chronic diseases can exacerbate health outcomes, complicating treatment regimens and fueling healthcare costs. For instance, individuals suffering from cardiovascular disease and diabetes have twice the risk of experiencing significant health outcomes compared to individuals with one condition. This is an idea that needs consideration while creating public health initiatives because peak chronic disease management needs to incorporate models with the ability to address comorbidity (Agnes et al., 2025). Prevention and education policy initiatives will need to account for these fields of overlap in health issues through systems thinking in creating holistic strategies that promote overall health among affected populations. As the paradigm of treating chronic disease shifts, information on such interplays will become key to optimizing patient outcomes and restraining healthcare expenditures (Figure 13.3).

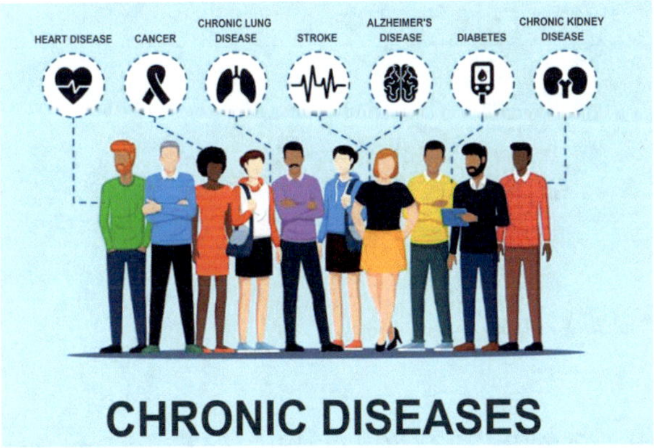

Figure 13.3. Common chronic diseases.

Source: https://mantracare.org/wp-content/uploads/2021/12/What-Is-Chronic-Illness.jpg.

13.1. Epidemiological Methods in Chronic Disease Research

Epidemiological methods are significant in the investigation of chronic disease because they provide a scientific approach to investigating patterns of disease, risk factors, and health outcomes among populations. Observational and experimental study designs are employed to examine the intricate relationship between biological, environmental, and behavioral determinants. By employing techniques such as cohort studies, case-control studies, and cross-sectional surveys, epidemiologists can account for the ways in which chronic diseases emerge and develop. For instance, social epidemiology—a leading field—addresses how socio-economic variables such as income disparity and race intersect with health outcomes and thereby expand traditional biomedical models of disease. These kinds of information are essential for the development of targeted interventions and public policies to decrease the chronic disease burden and improve population health outcomes (Link et al., 2008). Clinical trials, aside from observational studies, form the core of studies on chronic diseases, as they aid in determining causal inferences and evaluating the efficacy of various interventions. Randomized controlled trials (RCTs) are particularly valuable, as they eliminate bias and allow for a rigorous treatment versus control comparison. Outcomes derived from these trials can be utilized to establish evidence-based practice and guidelines that underpin the management of chronic diseases such as diabetes, cardiovascular diseases, and cancer. Moreover, future studies that longitudinally follow the participants are able to identify long-term consequences of exposures or interventions and are thus optimal in assessing chronic disease processes. Stringency of method in this form not only produces science but also has immediate implications for clinical practice and public health programs (Zanetti et al., 2015). Overall, integration of several epidemiological strategies allows a globalized understanding of patterns of chronic disease. By combining qualitative and quantitative approaches, the researchers can estimate various determinants of health, ranging from genetic tendencies to lifestyle choices, and their combined impact on chronic illnesses. Social epidemiology contributes significantly to this field by emphasizing social determinants, thereby highlighting health inequalities between population groups. Using such multidisciplinary perspectives is essential in dealing with the multidimensionality of chronic diseases, in order for researchers to recommend evidence-based interventions that are socially and culturally appropriate. Ultimately, the creation of epidemiological tools will continue to shape the course of chronic disease epidemiology, facilitating improved health outcomes at both population and individual levels (Link et al., 2008).

13.1.1. Study Designs Used in Chronic Disease Epidemiology

The field of chronic disease epidemiology employs a variety of study designs to examine the complex interaction between determinants of risk and disease outcomes. Among the most significant are cohort studies in which a group of people is followed longitudinally, tracking their exposure to suspected risk factors and resultant health impacts. By establishing temporal association, cohort studies provide strong evidence for causation. These studies tend to offer insightful data on the incidence and prevalence of chronic diseases, thereby allowing scientists to make patterns and correlations that can inform public health interventions. Moreover, the longitudinal nature of cohort studies allows it to be simple to examine how certain lifestyle elements or environmental exposures contribute to the causation of chronic diseases, thus allowing epidemiologic research to be multidimensional.

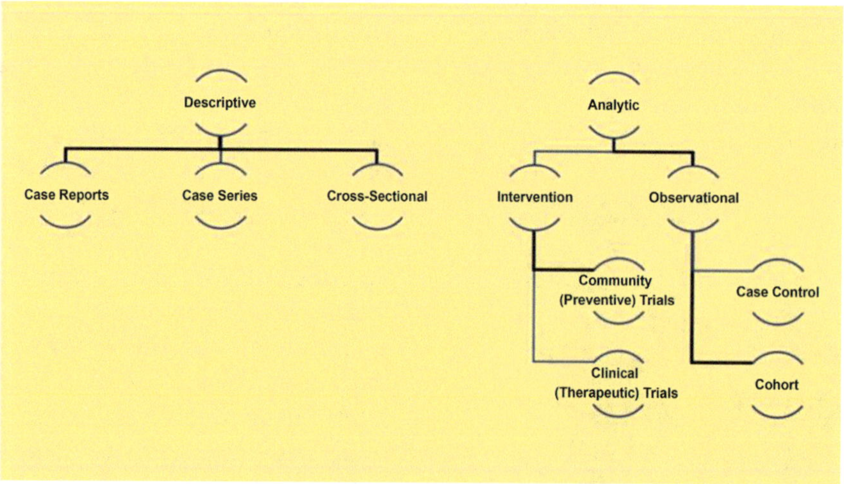

Figure 13.4. Types of epidemiological studies.

Source: https://minnstate.pressbooks.pub/app/uploads/sites/2/2021/08/Table-of-Study-Designs.-1024x686.jpg.

Case-control studies are also valuable in the epidemiology of chronic disease because they allow researchers to retrospectively compare exposure between individuals with a specific condition and control subjects who are disease-free. The technique is particularly valuable when researching those diseases that have lengthy latent periods, such as some types of cancer or cardiovascular disease, since it might be impossible to conduct long-term cohort studies. Through the identification of historical exposures, case-control studies are able to explain possible risk factors that can be involved in the development of chronic diseases. Nevertheless, the design is not without limitations, such as recall bias and the inability to establish a clear temporal association between exposure and the onset of disease. Case-control studies remain very useful and an important component in the epidemiologist's toolkit for research on chronic diseases. Cross-sectional studies also give a unique picture of chronic disease epidemiology in that they can capture the health status of the population at a single point in time. This study design can establish relationships between risk factors and health outcomes and can yield preliminary data that can be used to guide further research. Although cross-sectional research lacks the temporal relationship necessary to provide causal conclusions, it is extremely useful in investigating the prevalence of chronic disease and determinants in specific groups. Hence, it can inform public health policy decisions and resource allocation. With the evolution of chronic disease epidemiology, the incorporation of new study designs will be required to effectively come to terms with the challenges of chronic diseases in today's world and eventually end up with improved population health results (Lewnard et al., 2019; Rothman et al., 2011) (Figure 13.4).

13.1.2. Data Collection Techniques and Sources

Methods of data collection are crucial in chronic disease epidemiology, particularly because accurate data are required in order to inform disease pattern understanding and guide public health interventions. Data may be obtained through various methods, including population-based surveys, disease registries, and environmental monitoring systems. Population-based surveys, for instance, provide data on the prevalence and risk factors of chronic diseases among various populations. These surveys allow the collection of self-reported health data, behavior patterns, and lifestyle, and offer a complete view of the chronic disease situation. Registries also offer standard databases where individual health information is matched with diagnostic criteria, making it possible to analyze incidence and outcomes in a better way. Through these methods, researchers can detect targeted populations requiring contact and ensure that good intervention techniques are selected that are suitable for specific populations. Environmental data gathering is another essential element within the field of chronic disease epidemiology that provides holistic information on how external factors influence health outcomes. The process of creating the national environmental public health tracking (EPHT) network, according to literature, demonstrates the intersection of environmental and chronic disease information. Convergence is essential in comprehending how environmental exposures translate into risk factors for chronic disease prevalence. The EPHT will also involve the use of new technologies to enhance exposure and disease measurement and to make information available in order that it may inform public policy. Merging environmental data with health data not only allows for the evaluation of intervention effects but also allows for surveillance and research on a continuing basis. By continuously updating such systems, public health professionals are able to respond to emerging exposures and adapt strategies to avoid risks, leading to a more proactive approach in the combat against chronic diseases (Balmes et al., 2004). In a comparison of the merits and drawbacks of alternative data sources, no one method of data collection is sufficient in chronic disease epidemiology. For instance, while insurance claims provide big sample sizes, they are susceptible to selection bias, and the results can become distorted. Primary-care practice data, on the other hand, provide an excellent representation of the population at large but are often followed by challenges in data management or misclassification issues. Additionally, questionnaire surveys are efficient for collecting data but are susceptible to low response rates and recall bias, which compromise data validity. Notwithstanding these limitations, active surveillance systems based on secondary health data are able to maximize the surveillance and comprehension of chronic disease because they give more detailed information while reducing some of the biases that can be present with conventional approaches. Balanced data source selection is therefore critical to ensure sound chronic disease research (Brodbelt et al., 2014) (Figure 13.5).

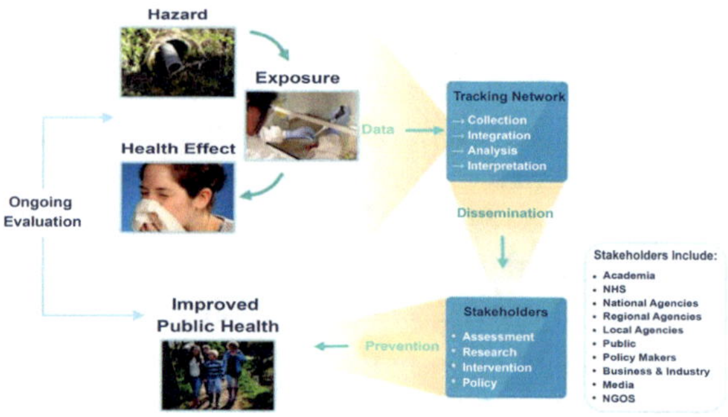

Figure 13.5. Environmental public health tracking components.

Source: https://www.mdpi.com/ijerph/ijerph-17-01976/article_deploy/html/images/ijerph-17-01976-g001.png.

13.1.3. Statistical Analysis in Chronic Disease Studies

Use of statistical modeling in studies of chronic diseases is crucial in understanding the complex determinants of population health status. Researchers are able to identify trends and associations that inform public health interventions through the use of various types of statistical analysis. For instance, time-series analysis allows one to investigate the occurrence of disease over various intervals of time, correlating with shifts in society, the environment, and the availability of healthcare. Such analytical techniques are at the heart of disease trajectory forecasting as models, which can guide health policy and resource allocation decisions in turn. Statistical interpretation of outcome is also at the heart of causal inference, enabling scientists to make inferences of association between risk factors and chronic disease, leading to more effective prevention interventions in the long run. The integration of socio-economic factors into statistical modeling also explains chronic disease knowledge better. It has been found in research that socio-economic position (SEP) strongly influences health-seeking behavior, particularly among vulnerable populations. For instance, disparities in gaining access to healthcare services are often allied with both economic and socio-cultural capital, and they affect maternal health-seeking behavior as evident from studies that examine antenatal care and facility delivery in various regions, including Egypt (Singh-Manoux et al., 2015). Through the lens of statistics, scientists can observe these factors and determine the mechanisms underpinning health inequalities, and the corresponding necessity for targeted interventions that address these socio-economic disparities. These results are required to develop tailor-made solutions to improve public health outcomes. In addition, the potential for integrating new sources of data and advanced statistical techniques has the potential to revolutionize chronic disease studies. Newer methods, such as big data analysis and machine learning, are promising to improve disease surveillance and facilitate real-time disease monitoring. As chronic disease epidemiology increasingly now tries to incorporate varied data—from social media use to clinical records—statistical analysis becomes crucial in aggregating these sorts of datasets into meaningful conclusions. This trend is in line with more traditional strategies that have always placed stress on long-term epidemiological trends (Lewnard et al., 2019). By embracing these new paradigms, researchers can address the challenges of chronic diseases more effectively through informed and proactive reactions, ultimately enhancing public health approaches and outcomes.

13.2. Risk Factors for Chronic Diseases

Chronic diseases are complex health conditions determined by a variety of risk factors that can differ greatly across populations and geographies. Age is an important one; as people age, their risk of developing conditions like CKD rises substantially. For instance, a study of CKD prevalence among rural Kenya and Uganda found that individuals 60 years and older had an adjusted prevalence ratio of 3.5 compared to young adults aged 18 to 29. This age group is especially relevant for describing disease patterns, particularly in areas like sub-Saharan Africa, where secondary conditions such as HIV infection contribute even more to the risk of CKD. The interaction of age and disease prevalence underlines the importance of age-specific public health interventions addressing older persons to mitigate the effect of these interlinked risk factors (Atukunda et al., 2020). Lifestyle determinants and socio-economic status present another dimension of complexity for chronic disease epidemiology. Smoking, sedentary lifestyles, and malnutrition are significant risk factors for the majority of chronic diseases like cancer, diabetes, and heart disease. Evidence shows that poorer socio-economic groups have less access to healthy foods and sporting facilities, thus extending health inequalities. For example, people who reside in places referred to as food deserts will experience obesity and chronic disease more often. Additionally, the impact of chronic conditions has the potential to create a cycle effect on socio-economic status, which can persist over generations. This contact highlights the need for strong public health policies that address both lifestyle and socio-economic determinants to reduce the burden of chronic disease among vulnerable populations (Bennett et al., 2014). Environmental determinants are also extremely crucial in chronic disease risk because chemical exposure and exposure to dangerous substances have long-term health effects. In urban and industrial settings, exposure to air and water pollution is possible, leading to respiratory disease and cardiovascular disease. In addition, the physical environment is a significant determinant of physical activity levels, with walkable environments facilitating the uptake of healthy lifestyles. More evidence is mounting that the incorporation of green space in urban design can reverse some of the chronic health risks by promoting outdoor living and reducing stress levels. Therefore, public policy and city planning must give utmost importance to environmental health strategies while acknowledging that changing these risk factors is essential to enhance the overall health of populations and minimize the prevalence of chronic diseases (Atukunda et al., 2020) (Figure 13.6).

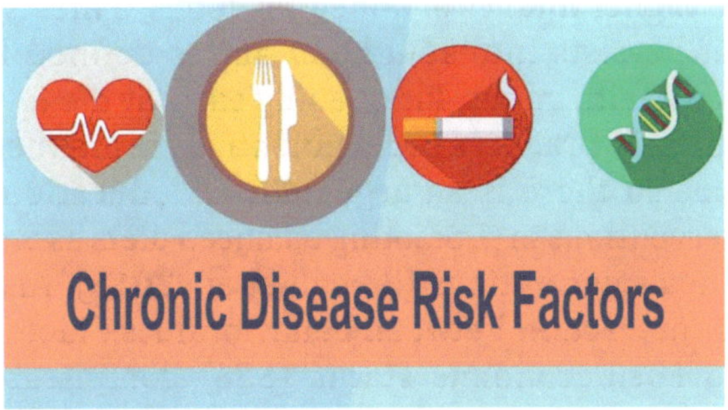

Figure 13.6. Chronic disease risk factors.

Source: https://i.ytimg.com/vi/236rfyMIGd0/maxresdefault.jpg.

13.2.1. Behavioral Risk Factors (e.g., Smoking, Diet)

Behavioral risk factors like diet and smoking play a focal point in the epidemiology of chronic diseases. Smoking is an established risk factor with significant contributions to cardiovascular disease (CVD) and a variety of other diseases. The harmful effects of smoking is evident in worldwide comparative risk estimates where smoking is credited with causing millions of deaths yearly. Through repression of oxygenation and promotion of inflammation, smoking exacerbates other risk factors such as high blood pressure and elevated cholesterol levels. The synergistic effect of smoking on these physiological conditions reinforces the necessity for special public health campaigns aimed at smoking cessation as a primary intervention for CVD mortality prevention, particularly in vulnerable populations (Elliott et al., 2016). Food selection also plays a central role in forecasting chronic disease-related health outcomes. According to studies, the consumption of energy-dense yet nutrient-poor food has substantial disease risk for obesity and metabolic syndrome. The association emphasizes increasing healthier food consumption, particularly among people of lower socioeconomic status with likely reduced access to healthy foods. There is evidence to suggest that adverse childhood experiences are related to reduced consumption of healthy foods and higher intakes of unhealthy foods, a lifestyle that persists into adulthood and is defined by poor health status. Intervening early at the level of dietary practices could potentially avoid these risks, so there is an argument for educational interventions in promoting balanced diets as well as healthier options (Boylan et al., 2018). Also, the interaction between behavioral risk factors and socioeconomic status (SES) complicates chronic disease epidemiology. SES determines adult health behavior in early life, influencing the amount of physical activity and eating habits. For instance, individuals from lower SES groups engage less in leisure-time physical activity, which is crucial to overall health. This disparity is particularly realized in comparing gender differences; low-SES women are much less likely to achieve healthy physical activity levels. These patterns of behavior then become associated with more instances of metabolic syndrome and unhealthy consequences. Breaking these behavioral risk factors using evidence-based interventions that consider SES-related barriers reduces chronic disease burdens in populations (Boylan et al., 2018) (Figure 13.7).

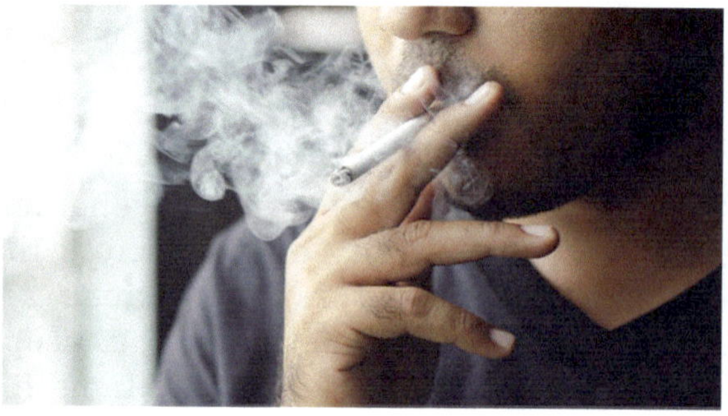

Figure 13.7. Smoking.

Source: https://daffodilcentre.org/wp-content/uploads/2022/04/Smoking_shutterstock_1811714497.jpg.

13.2.2. Environmental Risk Factors (e.g., Pollution, Occupational Hazards)

Understanding environmental risk factors such as pollution and occupational hazards is extremely critical in chronic disease epidemiology since they determine public health effects to a large extent. Pollution, air and water pollution, has been conventionally associated with different chronic conditions. For instance, exposure to particulate matter has been linked to respiratory disease, cardiovascular disease, and even cancer. The hazardous contaminants of industrial pollutants can pollute water sources, leading to drastic health implications for the exposed population. Besides, prolonged exposure to toxins, particularly among marginalized communities, amplifies health disparities and elevates the burden of chronic diseases. Hence, research on such environmental determinants proves an essential imperative for policy regulations to minimize exposure, underscoring the importance of environmental health programs within public policy. Occupational hazards also constitute another vast-scale environmental risk factor having a direct impact on the health of workers. Work environments often bring individuals into contact with all kinds of hazardous products, from chemical substances to toxic chemicals. Metalworking fluids, for instance, which are very prevalent in manufacturing sectors, have been found to increase the risk of ischemic heart disease (IHD) among some populations, as per recent studies. The study indicates that black males and white women have much higher risks associated with exposure to these fluids, which suggests that underlying factors such as socio-economic position and occupational safety practices are paramount to health outcomes. The complex interaction of these variables indicates that addressing occupational health is about more than just recognizing hazards; it requires a comprehensive understanding of how racial and gender categories might respond to such threats (Costello et al., 2014). Workplace interventions and health policy must then respond to not just eliminating environmental hazards, but also guaranteeing holistic approaches to health, considering mental and physical health. Interventions designed to improve working conditions can lead to worthwhile employee health benefits. Evidence shows that interventions such as ergonomic assessments, mental health interventions, and effective work-life balance can effectively reduce the occurrence of chronic diseases. Furthermore, promoting worker awareness of potential risks associated with occupational exposure is important. It contributes to an environment with a safety culture. As defined in numerous studies, the development of a congenial work culture is able to counteract the unfavorable impacts of occupational risks, backing the notion that preventive measures and holistic health strategies are critical in limiting the effects of environmental variables on the prevalence of chronic conditions (N/A, 2008) (Figure 13.8).

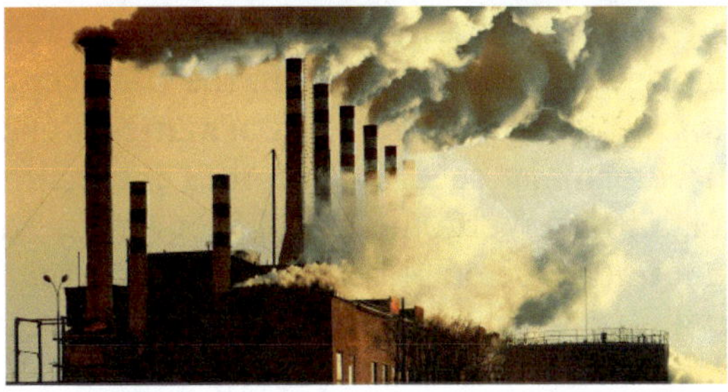

Figure 13.8. Environmental risk factors.

Source: https://cdn.cancercenter.com/-/media/ctca/images/others/blogs/2018/02-february/06-blog-enviromental-risks-l.jpg.

13.2.3. Genetic Predispositions and Their Role

In the epidemiology of chronic diseases, genetic predispositions play a pivotal role in identifying the susceptibility of an individual to various illnesses. Genetic predispositions inherited by an individual can determine how well they are going to respond to environmental exposure and lifestyles, thereby acting as a mediator to the development of chronic diseases such as heart disease, diabetes, and some cancers. As research continues to be conducted, it seems more and more that tracing the genetic origins of these diseases is the key to successful prevention and treatment strategies. Genetic screening, underutilized in the majority of populations, has the possibility of illuminating these susceptibilities. For example, patients with leukemia are not typically screened for hereditary vulnerabilities, yet research indicates that about 12 causal genes have been identified, which portrays an enormous divergence from current clinical procedures that can be addressed through enhanced awareness and adoption of genetic testing methodologies (Beecroft et al., 2018). Moreover, the example of individual breeds, the case of the German Shepherd Dog (GSD), highlights the importance of genetic predispositions in disease manifestation. In recent years, GSDs have been criticized for medical problems presumed to be due to breed-related genetic factors. In the face of declining breed populations in the UK, accurate demographic and disorder information derived from veterinary records becomes increasingly important. The VetCompassTM Program has also been found to be an effective tool in this regard, compiling clinical data regarding dogs presented for veterinary practice. Through the analysis of such data, researchers can determine the most prevalent health issues and guide breeding initiatives that counteract genetic susceptibility to certain long-term conditions in this breed (Agresti et al., 2017).

This approach not only enhances the health of the population of GSD but also offers a model for investigating the effects of genes on chronic diseases in humans. In addition, the inclusion of genetic susceptibilities in the overall paradigm of chronic disease epidemiology demonstrates the need for public health programs for personalized medicine. As better genomic technologies become widely available, they promise to make prevention and treatment strategies tailored to the individual's own genetic design. This change demands a collaboration among clinicians, genetic counselors, and public health professionals for effective integration of genetic data into practice. Education about genetic hazards and the benefits of early screening can lead to making informed health choices and, consequently, potentially decreasing the incidence of chronic diseases of genetic etiology. As the field evolves with an emphasis on genetic susceptibility and outcomes, it not only explains the nature of chronic illnesses but also paves the way for new and innovative public health interventions addressing the intricacies of the genetic factors in a diverse population (Figure 13.9).

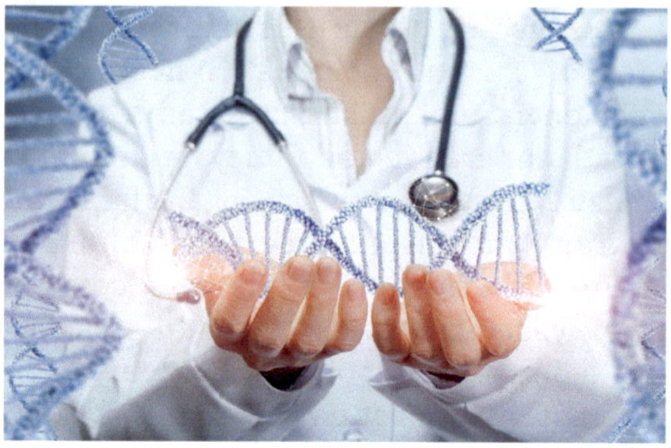

Figure 13.9. Genetic predisposition.

Source: https://centerforfamilymedicine.com/wp-content/uploads/2021/02/center-for-family-medicine-What-Does-It-Mean-To-Have-A-Genetic-Predisposition-Family-History-And-Your-Health.jpg.

13.3. Global Burden of Chronic Diseases

The impact of chronic diseases worldwide is a serious public health concern, characterized by complex epidemiological patterns in various populations. Chronic diseases such as cardiovascular conditions, diabetes, and chronic respiratory illnesses have become leading causes of morbidity and mortality worldwide, reshaping the health system at its foundation and causing economic burdens for the healthcare facility. For instance, in chronic kidney disease (CKD), the United States has had a worrying trend, as there was a reported substantial increase in disability-adjusted life years (DALYs) from 2002 to 2016. The rising burden, driven primarily by rising metabolic risk factors and population growth, underscores the urgent need for targeted interventions aimed at decreasing risks of chronic conditions (Al-Aly et al., 2018). Grateful that chronic diseases are not unique to the developed world, their growing prevalence in middle- and low-income countries necessitates a unified global response to this multifaceted challenge. There is proof that chronic diseases are affecting high proportions of populations all around the globe, with a significant percentage of these being older people. As an example, an estimated 80% of Australian elderly are affected by chronic diseases, which are the primary determinants of disability and premature death. Furthermore, the financial impact is enormous, with chronic diseases accounting for approximately 70% of total health expenditure in most countries (Agnes et al., 2025). As lifestyle and behavioral determinants are leading causes of the chronic disease burden, there is an urgent need to prioritize effective prevention and management in various populations. As chronic diseases spread, public health policymakers must reorganize their strategies in health education, lifestyle modification, and chronic disease control to make them culturally suitable and accessible. Along with this, insight into dynamic interactions between various risk factors, such as socioeconomic, demographic, and health-related variables, is also required to address the global burden of chronic diseases. The integration of microsimulation models with chronic disease progression models has been proposed as a sophisticated approach to predict the probable effects of intervention on costs and health outcomes. This type of modeling enables policymakers to forecast the long-run effects of a range of health interventions while taking into account the occurrence of comorbidities and the reduction in quality of life that results from disease progression. Through the establishment of strong analytical frameworks, researchers can offer insightful information on how specific interventions may decrease the burden of chronic diseases in the long run and improve the general well-being of people afflicted by them (Agnes et al., 2025). Thus, it is imperative that the research agenda in chronic disease epidemiology be moved forward in order to develop effective public health policies that can mitigate the world's burden of chronic diseases (Figure 13.10).

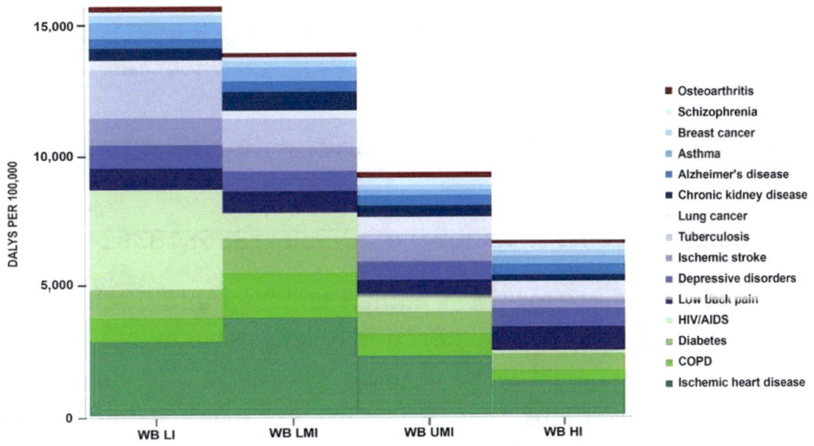

Figure 13.10. Age-standardized DALYs (rate per 100,000) for leading chronic diseases (1995–2015) for World Bank low-income (WB LI), low-middle-income (WB LMI), upper-middle-income (WB UMI), and high-income countries (WB HI).

Source: https://ars.els-cdn.com/content/image/1-s2.0-S2211335518302468-gr2_lrg.jpg.

13.3.1. Prevalence and Incidence Rates Worldwide

Global epidemiology of chronic diseases is noted for extensive variation in the range of incidence and prevalence rates, most of which are determined by socioeconomic, environmental, and lifestyle factors. An example of a classic nature is that of liver fluke infection, with high prevalence rates in certain low-income environments. Such an infection, supported by a complex combination of ecological, agricultural, and food preparation patterns, demonstrates how conditions at the local level may lead to extensive health issues, including high morbidity them. However, in affluent communities, these infections are relatively uncommon due to improved public health habits and access to healthcare. It is crucial to understand the epidemiology of such a disease since such parasites have also proven to be biological carcinogens. The wide gap in prevalence mirrors the significant role of socioeconomic factors in determining determinants of health outcomes in different populations, calling for targeted public health interventions closing the gap (Harrington et al., 2017). Yet another chronic condition that has increased in prevalence worldwide is obesity, which over the past few decades has risen dramatically. Currently, there are over 1.5 billion adults who are overweight and at least 500 million who are clinically obese, as per a Body Mass Index (BMI) of over 30 kg/m^2.

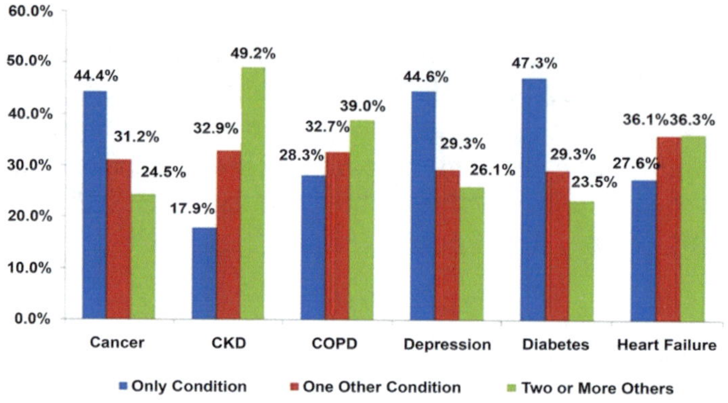

Figure 13.11. Proportion (%) of Medicare beneficiaries with MCC by selected chronic condition (2005).

Source: https://ars.els-cdn.com/content/image/1-s2.0-S2211335518302468-gr3_lrg.jpg.

This deplorable trend does not stop with adults; children and adolescents are experiencing record rates of obesity, paving the way for a generation of long-term health repercussions. The World Health Organization has classified obesity as a global epidemic, showing the urgency of dealing with the public health crisis. The rising rate of obesity is linked to lifestyle variables, including increased caloric intake and diminished physical activity, particularly in modern Western countries and developing nations. The fast-evolving epidemic calls for immediate action on the part of health policymakers to take steps to turn the trends around and mitigate their impact on world health (Kyrou et al., 2010). Chronic disease epidemiology is not just about numbers, since determinants of health underlying prevalence and incidence rates around the world are involved. Chronic diseases usually share risk factors, such as lifestyle practices, environmental exposures, and genetic factors, all of which have an influence on population health. For example, interaction among social determinants such as income and education strongly determines disease burden. Whereas in those regions with limited access to health care services, the incidence of avoidable chronic diseases may be elevated, resulting in increased morbidity and mortality. Measurement of incidence and prevalence rates thus provides valuable feedback about the health situation of populations, which will guide the planning of effective public health interventions. The reduction of these inequalities is essential in order to narrow the gap between population health outcomes and global burden of chronic diseases (Harrington et al., 2017; Kyrou et al., 2010) (Figure 13.11).

13.3.2. Economic Impact of Chronic Diseases

The economic impact of chronic disease extends beyond direct health expenditure, penetrating other spheres of social and economic life. Chronic illness such as diabetes and heart disease, besides taking the services of ongoing medical therapy, causes colossal losses in the workforce's productivity. When individuals become victims of the limitations imposed by these diseases, they may experience lower labor market activity, or their ability to perform at maximum levels could be lost. The impact is a ripple effect, especially in those economies that need a healthy workforce to control growth and development. Social epidemiology suggests that the impact of these health conditions is often aggravated by social determinants such as income inequality, which has a tendency to increase disparities in health status and economic security across groups (Link et al., 2008). Beyond their workforce implications, chronic conditions can be expensive for families, resulting in catastrophic health expenditures and draining savings and overall quality of life. Patients with chronic illness usually have high out-of-pocket costs for treatment, medication, and lifestyle modifications required, which may hamper their economic stability. The economic burden is particularly felt in families where workers are affected, reducing family income and increasing the demand for social help. It has been demonstrated that chronic illnesses, like chronic rhinosinusitis, cause definite impairment in the patient's quality of life and may be a factor in subsequent socioeconomic disadvantage (Anari et al., 2016). The relationship between chronic disease and economic resources is multifaceted and requires policy intervention on a comprehensive basis in both health and economic affairs. Mitigating the economic burden of chronic diseases requires inclusive strategies involving preventive health care, education, and equitable access to health care resources. Policymakers must address reducing the incidence of risk factors of these diseases through public health initiatives and community initiatives promoting healthy lifestyles. Enhancing access to health care, particularly in disadvantaged communities, can also serve to reduce the cost burden on individuals and families living with chronic disease. Investments in chronic disease management programs can also bring significant dividends in terms of decreased hospitalizations and utilization of expensive emergency services. Ultimately, the economic burden of chronic diseases is a complex problem that requires cooperation among multiple sectors, pointing to the urgent need for integrated strategies that tackle both health and economic disparities (Link et al., 2008).

13.3.3. Disparities in Chronic Disease Burden Across Populations

Chronic disease burden has significant inequalities across varied populations, following socioeconomic status, availability of healthcare resources, and cultural factors. Underprivileged populations, including racial and ethnic minorities, tend to experience obstacles that make their health conditions more complex. Recent studies indicate such populations are disproportionately affected by many chronic conditions (MCCs), both impairing their quality of life as well as imposing a significant burden on health systems. Understanding the multifaceted reality of these disparities takes more than a glimpse at the clinically defined conditions; it demands exploration of the social determinants of health that interact to shape results. Only by a concerted effort can we accurately measure the nuances of chronic disease burdens in these populations and develop successful interventions that account for both health care access and the underlying socioeconomic inequalities that produce these inequalities. Chronic liver disease is a tragic example of how inequalities manifest across populations, particularly among American Indian and Alaska Native (AI/AN) populations. A case study at an inner-city residential chemical dependency treatment center illustrates the egregious need for specifically targeted interventions to meet these disparities. Among the 928 analyzed AI/AN admissions, a significant percentage of individuals did not possess current immunity to vaccine-preventable diseases like hepatitis A and B, demonstrating severe deficiencies in preventative healthcare access. The findings underscore the importance of implementing prevention programs for high-risk groups, such as those treated for chemical dependency. By addressing their unique health issues, public health interventions can strongly reduce the burden of chronic liver disease and comorbid diseases in AI/AN communities, ultimately advancing health outcomes and closing disparities. Interventions to enhance the understanding of chronic disease burden among different groups must also consider the efficacy of interventions on MCCs among disadvantaged groups. It is evident that conventional strategies cannot bring to the limelight the intricacies involved in multifactorial diseases, leading to suboptimal care measures. As emphasized in the literature, MCCs are measured by a nuanced definition that identifies a wide range of health-related determinants in contrast to the mere aggregation of clinical conditions. Such measurement can detect crucial differences in health and access to healthcare among vulnerable groups and guide policy and practice for prevention and management. The U.S. Department of Health and Human Services has recognized addressing disparities between MCC populations as a priority area, with continued research and interventions being highlighted as necessary. Comprehensive approaches to improving the health of these groups are not only essential for personal health but for the resilience of the public health system as well (Figure 13.12).

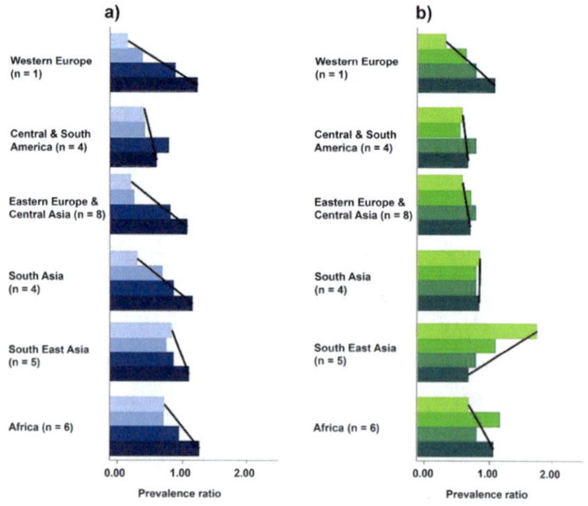

Figure 13.12. (a) Socioeconomic gradient of MCC prevalence (2003) by regions for age category 1 (<55); and (b) Socioeconomic gradient of MCC by regions for age category 2 (≥ 55) (2012).

Source: https://ars.els-cdn.com/content/image/1-s2.0-S2211335518302468-gr4_lrg.jpg.

13.4. Prevention and Control Strategies

The rapidly increasing prevalence of chronic diseases necessitates the use of comprehensive prevention and control strategies that target fundamental risk determinants. Obesity is a key factor that has increased to become the nation's second most preventable cause of illness and death, after smoking. Effective interventions targeting modifiable determinants such as weight control, diet change, and more physical activity play a central role in preventing chronic diseases associated with obesity, such as cancers. To combat the grim projections that obesity will emerge as the main modifiable cause of death, physicians must adopt a broad approach to prevention and management. This includes the inclusion of clinical guidelines, promotion of healthy lifestyle choices, and assistance in systemic initiatives in order to establish an enabling environment for healthier lifestyles (Brawer et al., 2009). The second most important aspect of effective prevention of chronic disease is to establish effective disease surveillance systems. Centers for Disease Control and Prevention's initiative to establish a national Environmental Public Health Tracking (EPHT) network serves as an illustration of the dedication to linking environmental data with chronic disease outcomes. Having a general surveillance framework enables the establishment of chronic disease risk factors and trends. While it is imperative to indicate that the link of information should extend beyond intermittent tracking to cover proactive systems that evolve with the technology changes and the rising health threats. By sequential updating of EPHT, public health professionals can improve the evaluation of the effectiveness of interventions for reducing exposure to harmful environmental conditions and thereby lower the risk for chronic diseases among the population. These preventive measures illustrate the significant environment and health interrelationships that form the basis of effective chronic disease prevention programs (Balmes et al., 2004). Public health action is made more effective by incorporating community participation in prevention and control programs. Public health action is made more effective by educating communities and individuals about their contribution to their own health. Education programs, accessible resources, and participatory interventions that address health can create a culture of resilience and health. Collaboration between policymakers, community groups, and health professionals can also yield more stable interventions tailored to local settings. Involving feedback from communities can support programs and increase their attractiveness to the target audience. This integrated method, the bringing together of clinical action and engagement with the community, is essential in addressing the complexities of chronic disease epidemiology and driving the public health agenda towards meaningful and lasting change (Figure 13.13).

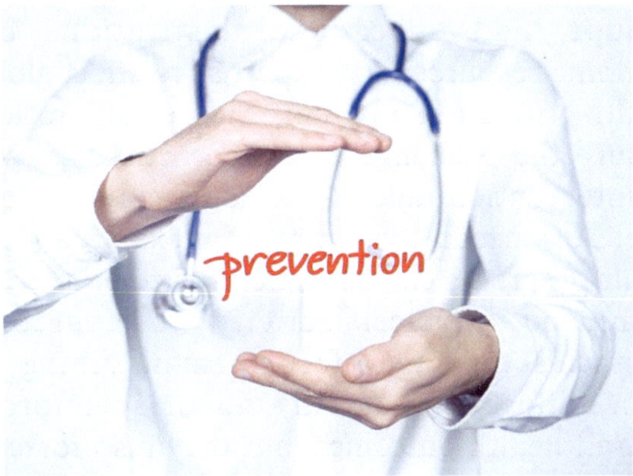

Figure 13.13. Prevention of chronic diseases.

Source: https://www.alcoa.ca/wp-content/uploads/2018/08/How-to-prevent-chronic-disease-at-an-old-age-880x660.jpg.

13.4.1. Public Health Initiatives for Chronic Disease Prevention

Public health interventions are likely to play a key role in the prevention of chronic diseases, imposing an immense burden on healthcare systems and society as a whole. Public health programs encompass various sorts of approaches for minimizing risk factors associated with chronic diseases such as diabetes, heart disease, and obesity. For instance, community programs aimed at adopting healthier lifestyles have the potential to significantly lower the incidence of these diseases. Through efforts aimed at education, access to healthy food, and promotion of physical exercise, public health programs have a targeted emphasis on lifestyle behaviors that result in the development of chronic diseases. Further, the 2010 healthcare reform act prioritizes the integration of preventive measures into the overall healthcare system, highlighting the need for long-term funding so that programs can be uniformly implemented and tracked over time (Barbara et al., 2011). Inter-agency collaboration among different stakeholders makes public health programs more effective in the prevention of chronic diseases. Cooperation between local health organizations, community groups, and educational institutions can combine resources and expertise to effect global health promotion programs. Such collaborations ensure the exchange of best practices as well as intervention tailoring to address the unique needs of various populations. For example, older adult programs can be structured to encourage increased physical activity, to overcome obstacles they may face in maintaining an active lifestyle. Not only do these improve overall health outcomes, but they also foster a support system and sense of community among participants. Hence, a collaborative approach involving multidimensional organizations and community members improves the potential for long-term behavioral change and prevention of disease (N/A, 2001). Assessment of public health program outcomes is critical to ensuring the validity and justification of ongoing investment in chronic disease prevention efforts. Systematic measurement of program results, such as the incidence of changing health behaviors and the prevalence of disease reductions, allows health departments to determine effective strategies and points of improvement. By using data-driven evidence, ongoing programs not only inform but also assist policymakers in making the case for needed resources and funding. Furthermore, through the dissemination of results to the broader public health community, successful models can be replicated or adapted in other regions of the world, and so the positive effect of such studies is enhanced. The evidence-based practice mandate is one aspect of a greater call for chronic disease epidemiology to clarify disease patterns and risk factors, eventually leading to more efficient and effective public health interventions (Figure 13.14).

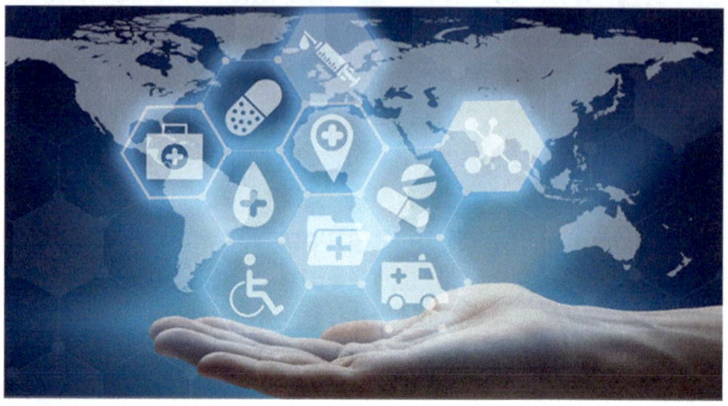

Figure 13.14. Public health initiatives.

Source: https://www.healthaffairs.org/do/10.1377/forefront.20200508.476872/full/HABlog_GlobalHealth.jpg.

13.4.2. Role of Healthcare Systems in Managing Chronic Diseases

Health systems' contribution to managing chronic disease is diverse and encompasses prevention and care through treatment to continuous care for the affected people. Effective health systems must use integrative mechanisms that tackle both the clinical determinants of chronic disease and the social determinants of health. This entails shifting from traditional models that focus on isolated conditions alone to expansive models that consider the nuances of multimorbidity. Broader operationalization of chronic disease care, as covering an array of health factors, is essential for effective assessment of the needs of various groups. This is particularly important for vulnerable populations, where health inequities in access to care and quality of care still dominate. Recent research indicates that being aware of the disparities is crucial in formulating targeted policies that can improve the health status of individuals with over one chronic condition, as documented by Shadmi et al. (2013). Health care systems also have a critical responsibility in establishing preventive guidelines for halting chronic diseases in diverse populations. Besides, the new technology landscape, particularly in machine learning and analyzing big data, introduces unprecedented opportunities for enhanced chronic disease epidemiology. Large data handling capabilities can make it possible to identify patterns and trends previously not perceivable. For instance, social media data can be utilized to analyze public attitudes towards health behavior or track disease outbreaks in real time. Joining such emerging data sources with traditional epidemiological methods has the potential to improve surveillance systems, allowing for prompt response to emerging public health crises. Further, as the chronic disease burden grows in low- and middle-income nations, technologically empowered options like mobile health apps have the potential to make epidemiological information accessible and democratic, enabling communities to embrace disease prevention initiatives. Lastly, the evolutionary history of pathogens and their host-parasite interactions calls for a longitudinal perspective in chronic disease epidemiology. The trajectories of evolution of certain bacteria, such as *Helicobacter pylori*, demonstrate the way the interactions between the pathogens and human health can evolve and how there would be a strong requirement for understanding such dynamics in order to effectively manage the condition. This evolutionary approach points to the fact that chronic diseases are not static but vary with dynamic host and environmental determinants. Future research endeavors should thus be focused on the influence of such interactions on disease severity and incidence. By discovering the evolutionary significance of microbial function in combination with host response, epidemiologists can inform evidence-based public health policy that optimizes long-term health benefits and disease control methods according to the intricate relationship between human hosts and their microbial communities (Koskella et al., 2014). Combining such findings with evidence-based counsel tailored to shifting health environments will be pivotal in further expanding the discipline of chronic disease epidemiology (Mayhew et al., 2009).

13.5.1. Emerging Trends in Chronic Disease Research

With the increasing prevalence of chronic diseases around the world, new trends in chronic disease research have become more central to the field of epidemiology. One such trend is the increased use of molecular and genomic technologies in public health efforts, through which researchers are able to decipher the complex genetic determinants of chronic disease. This trend marks the move away from classical models of epidemiology towards an appreciation of more complex disease pathways. For instance, research on human microbiota and its implications for health is transforming chronic disease models. By combining molecular data with well-tested epidemiological tools, scientists will be able to learn more about the mechanisms of chronic disease, and therefore allow more targeted prevention. This intersection of disciplines not only increases our understanding of chronic disease, but it also broaches the possibility of personalized medicine, revealing the necessity to tailor intervention to individualized genetic profiles as a solution to the management of the advent of chronic disease. Big data analytics is also a new and thrilling frontier in chronic disease research. With the presence of advanced computing machines, it is now possible for scientists to handle extensive data sets of various health markers, environmental factors, and behaviors. This shift in population enables deeper epidemiological studies taking into account multifactorial determinants of long-term conditions. By leveraging data from electronic health records, wearable medical devices, and social media platforms, epidemiologists can establish new patterns and trends that could not possibly be identified by other means. For instance, real-time data incorporation can significantly enhance disease surveillance systems to be able to respond to new public health dangers more quickly. Ultimately, the focus on big data is revolutionizing how chronic illness is studied, with an eye to the necessity of agility and responsiveness in research and practice. One of the main components of emerging chronic disease trends is the renewed emphasis on environmental health linkages, such as in the case of initiatives such as the Environmental Public Health Tracking (EPHT) network. The initiative aims to combine current environmental and chronic disease tracking data and highlight the significant role of environmental factors in shaping public health indicators.

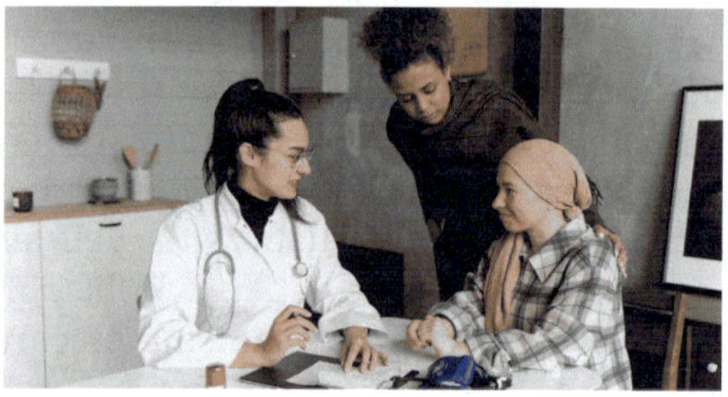

Figure 13.17. Emerging trends in chronic disease management.

Source: https://i0.wp.com/blog.medicai.io/wp-content/uploads/2024/09/611e2fe09205c4485f2de9cf_Frame-1508.png?resize=1920%2C1024&ssl=1.

The interface of environment, exposure, and chronic disease underscores the intricacy of the etiology of chronic disease, which necessitates combined actions by researchers and policymakers. By implementing a sound system capable of integrating environmental data with chronic disease information, public health practitioners will be better placed to identify vulnerable populations and develop effective interventions. Further, constant surveillance of these systems is critical, as it ensures they remain sensitive to new and developing public health threats. The dynamism in this topic speaks to not only the long-term complexity of sickness but the absolute priority of adaptive strategies in chronic disease epidemiology (Lewnard et al., 2019; Balmes et al., 2004) (Figure 13.17).

13.5.2. Technological Advancements and Their Implications

The rapidity of technological advancement is the foundation for drastic alterations in the field of chronic disease epidemiology, effectively redefining data collection, processing, and interpretation. Electronic health records (EHRs) have greatly transformed traditional practices by enabling quicker and more precise capture of patient health information. This transition from paper-based records to digital systems produces more stable datasets, enabling epidemiologists to track disease incidence, comorbidities, and outcomes across larger populations and longer periods. As increasingly common tools such as big data analytics and machine learning are present in healthcare environments, understanding the implications of these tools is vital. Innovative solutions have the promise of enhanced disease surveillance and control but come with a need to consider ethical concerns around patient privacy and data security (Conley et al., 2015). The question is, then, how to reconcile these emerging developments against the conventional foundations of public health ethics. In addition, as the health sciences evolve further, demands for interdisciplinary collaboration grow louder. New fields of study, such as health informatics, capitalize on technological innovation to not only facilitate research activities but also further refine educational methods for budding epidemiologists. Council for the Advancement of Nursing Science sees it as important to align PhD studies with current scientific research, pointing out that incorporating new technologies in research-focused doctoral programs is essential in preparing a skilled workforce for handling public health challenges of the time (Conley et al., 2015). By building the technological competencies and analysis skills of emerging generations of researchers, schools can better equip them to address such confounding issues as the treatment of chronic disease. The revitalized focus on technological literacies ensures that the next generation of epidemiologists will be prepared with the tools necessary to make sense of vast amounts of health information and improve health outcomes.

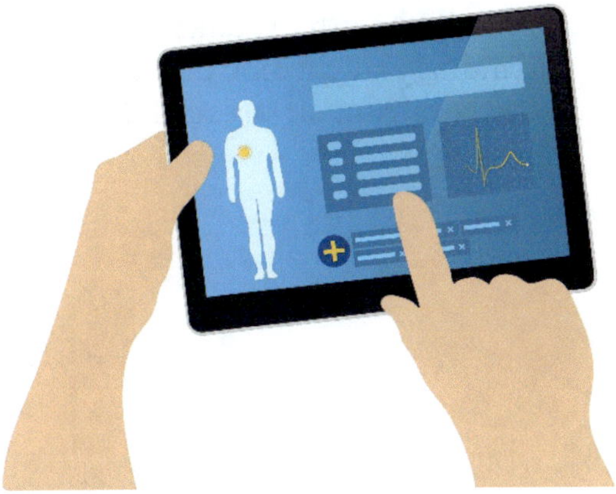

Figure 13.18. Monitoring chronic disease burden: Electronic health records can help meet a serious public health challenge.

Source: https://scx2.b-cdn.net/gfx/news/hires/2018/2-electroniche.jpg.

The intersection of technology with the epidemiology of chronic diseases also comes with new challenges, particularly with regard to interpreting and applying data. There is an abundance of electronic data that originates from diverse sources, including patient-entered health information and EHRs, which can impede correct analysis due to its complexity. Machine learning software, while effective, requires an advanced understanding of data characteristics, including the potential for implicit biases and errors incurred during data collection and processing (Arcuri et al., 2018). Therefore, if epidemiologists are embracing the advanced technology, they equally need to enhance their data literacy in a way that they can effectively apply the machine learning's potential. Strenuous testing protocols and the forging of best practices are essential to help ensure that knowledge gleaned from sophisticated data analysis is solid and implementable. Therefore, while technological innovation continues to spread, it is up to the epidemiological community to stay alert to the implications this transition has on research into chronic disease and public health interventions (Figure 13.18).

13.5.3. The Role of Policy in Shaping Future Research

Policy is a significant process that not only determines the path of research funding but also the priorities within chronic disease epidemiology. Resource allocation, as determined through government and organizational policy, has the ability either to advance knowledge in the field or to deter it. With academics traversing the landscape of chronic illness, their ability to secure funding is often made dependent on the appropriateness of their proposals to policy agendas. For instance, with funds available targeting specific health issues, such as HIV or HCV treatment, researchers are encouraged to tailor their research accordingly. This coordination ensures that there is a collective focus on high-priority health problems, and the findings of research are both timely and effective. Hence, an integrated understanding of policy is crucial for researchers seeking to successfully navigate funding contexts. In chronic disease epidemiology, policy interventions also guide the translation of research into public health practice. Regulations aimed at preventing diseases related to HIV and hepatitis C often rely on evidence derived from robust epidemiological research. A good example is the use of simulations such as those by SimpactCyan, which models dynamic epidemiological scenarios. This approach shows the potential for marrying evidence-informed policy-making with innovative research practices. Such tools enable policymakers to visualize what interventions could be like in practice before they become a reality, so that health resources are utilized efficiently. By this method, convergence of policy and research is important because it creates a feedback loop where research informs policy and policy dictates future research questions. The implications of policy also go beyond funding and implementation and influence ethical concerns and outcomes for population health. Recognition of chronic coinfections, such as the coaction of HCV and HBV, demonstrates the way in which policy decisions regarding vaccination and treatment procedures can shape long-term outcomes in health. The evidence that indicates previous HBV infection significantly increases risks of life-threatening liver disease in HCV sufferers, as revealed in more recent studies, indicates the need to ensure effective policies to support vaccination and treatment methods. Such decisions not only affect individual health but also have important bearings on public health systems and economic costs associated with chronic disease treatment. As the epidemiology of chronic diseases changes, the interplay between research and policy will remain at the forefront of areas that will drive sustainable health improvements.

Summary

In consideration of the complexity of chronic disease epidemiology, public health interventions must be able to address the co-morbid complexities of chronic disease. As demonstrated by the very high proportion of patients with respiratory complaints in the emergency room, the interplay between co-morbidities such as heart failure and COPD has a great effect on health outcomes. Specifically, the findings indicate that patients with shortness of breath transported by ambulance account not only for a high percentage of emergency services but also broader systemic health issues. Correspondingly, understanding about such interconnected health conditions can guide service planning and intervention processes, which emphasize the need for customized models of care considering each patient's entire medical history and existing health needs (Archer et al., 2016). In addition, the epidemiological profile of chronic disease, especially in diverse geographical settings, presents inequalities that call for focused research and resource utilization. Chronic kidney disease (CKD) in sub-Saharan Africa, as seen in a study among populations in rural Kenya and Uganda, highlights the need for localized interventions to address health issues. With the high prevalence of CKD among participants, particularly over the age of 60, it is critical to identify that conventional risk factors like diabetes and hypertension account for only part of the cases. This observation calls for a critical investigation into other risk factors, for instance, genetic susceptibility and the environment in these regions, which must be further investigated (Atukunda et al., 2020). Lastly, the conclusions drawn from these diverse studies not only report statistical results but also the sense of urgency of a holistic understanding of chronic disease dynamics. Efficient epidemiology studies must involve a more diverse array of variables, including socio-economic determinants, access to health care, and public health education. With the synergistic combination of results from diverse studies, health workers and policy makers can better respond to the needs of populations at risk. Such concerted approaches not only advance individual health impacts but also lower the overall burden of chronic diseases on the healthcare system. Enhancing further study and debate in chronic disease epidemiology is essential to improve and advance public health programs that are responsive and sustainable.

One of the valuable aspects of learning about chronic disease epidemiology is an understanding of the intricacies that inform the distribution and regulation of disease states such as HIV and obesity. A new instrument, such as SimpactCyan, offers a state-of-the-art platform for simulating individual-level approaches to HIV transmission in oscillating sexual networks. By discrete event simulation, researchers are able to measure the effects of a multitude of interventions over time and therefore develop a vital tool for the formulation of public health policy. With the ability to model the transmission of disease and the effects of interventions, HIV epidemiology is more clearly interpreted, and light is shed on future strategies regarding its containment in various populations (Delva et al., 2019). Another critical consideration of chronic disease epidemiology is the all-cause mortality association with body mass index (BMI). A systematic review and meta-analysis of cohort studies illustrates this association with a non-linear, subtle relationship. In fact, the findings have a J-shaped curve among never smokers, such that the risk is lowest at specific BMI levels. This research narrative highlights the importance of controlling for confounding factors such as smoking and preclinical disease that may skew results. By establishing the dose-response gradient between BMI and mortality, researchers can develop targeted interventions that are more sensitive to prevent the burden of obesity conditions and their associated mortality (Aune et al., 2016). This convergence of insights from mixed research in chronic disease epidemiology underscores the need for an interdisciplinary approach. Combining modeling tools like SimpactCyan with long-term cohort studies involving BMI and mortality, public health researchers can develop a more targeted path to effective disease control interventions. This holistic perspective leads to the potential importance of intervention tailoring on both behavioral and individual health indicators, thus potentially yielding better health outcomes. As long-term diseases continue to challenge public health systems, ongoing collaboration between researchers and practitioners will be key to alleviating their impact and promoting population well-being (Delva et al., 2019; Aune et al., 2016).

CLOSER LOOK

CHRONIC DISEASE CONTINUUM

For established infectious causes of disease, such as AIDS, measles, and influenza, one identified necessary cause (e.g., the microorganism) helps to focus epidemiologic study and intervention effort. For injury, the cause is often sudden and leads to immediate health effects, such as driving and drinking or a drowning child.

On the other hand, the wide variety of chronic diseases has no such common causative factors and is prone to develop across the life course. Research has demonstrated that many chronic diseases have their origins early in the life course (Felitti et al. 1998). These early life exposures and experiences to economic and social conditions increase the vulnerability to harmful behaviors in later life. Unhealthy lifestyles ultimately lead to diseases such as hypertension, obesity, or high blood cholesterol. Finally, individuals affected with such diseases are more likely to get chronic diseases, such as heart disease, cancer, or diabetes.

This chronic disease continuum framework is shown in Figure 1 and has been used to organize this document, with individual sections for chronic disease risk factors, chronic disease conditions, and chronic diseases. The chronic disease continuum also requires distinct methods of control of chronic disease and epidemiology. Because the causal process is long and often multifactorial, many small influences, rather than a single major cause, are implicated in the risk of developing disease. The long natural history of these diseases, with often a presymptomatic period and eventual development of chronic disease states, offers many overlapping opportunities for intervention. For most chronic disorders, the many small risk factors and the heterogeneity of opportunities for intervention make control difficult and typically require a multilateral strategy.

Because disease is the endpoint of a continuum, it is frequently difficult to determine whether "disease" even exists at all. For example, the common rise in mammography during the latter 1980s and 1990s has caused an enormous increase in the prevalence of an abnormal lesion known as ductal carcinoma *in situ* (DCIS). Although DCIS is not invasive breast cancer and the vast majority of women with DCIS will never develop invasive breast cancer, DCIS is typically treated as if it were invasive cancer—that is, surgically removed. The majority of women with DCIS describe themselves as having "breast cancer." Similarly, the majority of men with "prostate cancer" harbor a pathological lesion that never would have developed into clinical disease. In general, as our ability to detect earlier and earlier stages of the disease process improves, the point at which disease truly begins becomes increasingly unclear (Fryback et al. 2006).

One of the main considerations with chronic disease is the definition of "control" or what we are really trying to prevent. Chronic disease often strikes the quality of life years before it strikes the length of life, if it affects duration at all. Diabetic people, for example, do have higher mortality, but only years and years later. Meanwhile, however, they can grow blind, develop kidney failure, experience painful sores on their feet, have their leg amputated, receive a premature heart disease – all as a direct result of having diabetes. "Controlling" diabetes is not just about living longer, but, as much as anything, about improving the quality of one's life while one is living with diabetes. Disease-specific and generic quality of life measures have been developed and validated (McDowell and Newell 2006), and these are being used with increasing frequency to chart the course ("natural history") of disease and the effect of alternative methods of control.

Care must be taken with methodological norms in the majority of areas of the study and control of chronic disease. The need for accuracy of expression and idea is supported by developments which have taken place and by the expanding variety of alternatives available for dealing with chronic disease through public action for health. Here, we present some basic definitions and concepts which occur commonly in epidemiological literature on the causes, effects, and control of chronic diseases (Figure 13.19).

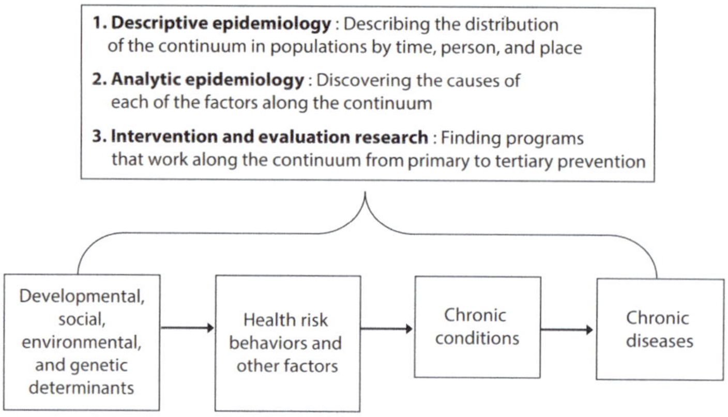

Figure 13.19. Methods used in chronic disease epidemiology, prevention, and control are applied along the chronic disease continuum.

Source: https://www.livingstonhealthcare.org/documents/Chronic-Disease-Epidemiology.pdf.

References

1. Abdoli, A., Abebe, M., Adebayo, O. M., Afarideh, M., et al. (2020). Global, regional, and national burden of chronic kidney disease, 1990–2017: A systematic analysis for the Global Burden of Disease Study 2017. https://core.ac.uk/download/287606258.pdf (accessed on 25th June 2025).

2. Agresti, A., Egenvall, A., Gough, A., Kathrani, A., Kyriazis, A., Peiravan, A., German, A. J., et al. (2017). Demography and disorders of German Shepherd Dogs under primary veterinary care in the UK. https://core.ac.uk/download/84659839.pdf (accessed on 25th June 2025).

3. Al-Aly, Z., Bowe, B., Li, T., Maddukuri, G., et al. (2018). Changes in the US burden of chronic kidney disease from 2002 to 2016: An analysis of the Global Burden of Disease study. https://core.ac.uk/download/288812793.pdf (accessed on 25th June 2025).

4. Allen, S., Barclay, S. T., Bhattacharyya, D., Dillon, J., et al. (2018). Impact of previous hepatitis B infection on the clinical outcomes from chronic hepatitis C? A population-level analysis. https://core.ac.uk/download/293863732.pdf (accessed on 25th June 2025).

5. Amutah, N., King, J., Leverett, C., Mahadevan, R., et al. (2015). Project THANKS: A socio-ecological framework for an intervention involving HIV-positive African American women with comorbidities. https://digitalscholarship.unlv.edu/cgi/viewcontent.cgi?article=1239&context=jhdrp (accessed on 25th June 2025).

6. Anari, S., Clark, A., Coombes, E., Erskine, S., et al. (2016). A case-control study of medical, psychological and socio-economic factors influencing the severity of chronic rhinosinusitis. https://core.ac.uk/download/41990799.pdf (accessed on 25th June 2025).

7. Archer, P., Asha, S. E., Bryant, M., Chalkley, D., et al. (2016). Epidemiology, prehospital care and outcomes of patients arriving by ambulance with dyspnea: An observational study. https://core.ac.uk/download/196603319.pdf (accessed on 25th June 2025).

8. Arcuri, A., Rector, A. L., Wood, A. M., Glas, A. S., Kulis, B., Cortes, C., Sammut, C., et al. (2018). Beyond volume: The impact of complex healthcare data on the machine learning pipeline. http://arxiv.org/abs/1706.01513 (accessed on 25th June 2025).

9. Atukunda, M., Balzer, L. B., Black, D., Charlebois, E., et al. (2020). The epidemiology of chronic kidney disease (CKD) in rural East Africa: A population-based study. https://core.ac.uk/download/323062882.pdf (accessed on 25th June 2025).

10. Aune, D., Janszky, I., Norat, T., Prasad, M., et al. (2016). BMI and all-cause mortality: Systematic review and non-linear dose-response meta-analysis of 230 cohort studies with 3.74 million deaths among 30.3 million participants. https://core.ac.uk/download/77011768.pdf (accessed on 25th June 2025).

11. Balmes, J., Ritz, B., & Tager, I. (2004). Can lessons from public health disease surveillance be applied to environmental public health tracking? https://core.ac.uk/download/pdf/3775836.pdf (accessed on 25th June 2025).

12. Beecroft, T. (2018). Patient attitudes toward genetic testing for inherited predispositions to hematologic malignancies. https://core.ac.uk/download/212897112.pdf (accessed on 25th June 2025).

13. Benkirane, A., Benslimani, A., Corwin, A., Omezzine-Letaief, A., Rekiki, A., Znazen, A., et al. (2014). Epidemiology of *Coxiella burnetii* infection in Africa: A One Health systematic review.

https://core.ac.uk/download/20480149.pdf (accessed on 25th June 2025).

14. Bennett, N., Blain, A., Briere, E., Clark, S., et al. (2014). Invasive *Haemophiles influenzae* disease in adults ≥65 years, United States, 2011. https://core.ac.uk/download/323062320.pdf (accessed on 25th June 2025).
15. Beratarrechea, A. G., Diez Canseco, F., Irazola, V., Miranda, J. J., et al. (2016). Use of m-Health technology for preventive interventions to tackle cardiometabolic conditions and other non-communicable diseases in Latin America—Challenges and opportunities. https://core.ac.uk/download/159285900.pdf (accessed on 25th June 2025).
16. Boylan, J. M., Lee, C., Ryff, C. D., Tsenkova, V., et al. (2018). Gender differences in the pathways from childhood disadvantage to metabolic syndrome in adulthood: An examination of health lifestyles. https://core.ac.uk/download/323067235.pdf (accessed on 25th June 2025).
17. Brawer, R., Brisbon, N., et al. (2009). Obesity and cancer. https://core.ac.uk/download/46966461.pdf (accessed on 25th June 2025).
18. Brodbelt, D. C., Church, D. B., McGreevy, P. D., O'Neill, D. G., et al. (2014). Approaches to canine health surveillance. https://core.ac.uk/download/36777547.pdf (accessed on 25th June 2025).
19. Brodbelt, D. C., Church, D. B., McGreevy, P. D., O'Neill, D. G., et al. (2015). Prevalence of disorders recorded in Cavalier King Charles Spaniels attending primary-care veterinary practices in England. https://core.ac.uk/download/36778636.pdf (accessed on 25th June 2025).
20. Brucker, R., Buffington, J., Castor, M. L., Forquera, R., et al. (2012). Integrating viral hepatitis screening and prevention services into an urban chemical dependency treatment facility for American Indians and Alaska Natives. https://digitalscholarship.unlv.edu/cgi/viewcontent.cgi?article=1013&context=jhdrp (accessed on 25th June 2025).
21. Brusselaers, N., & Lagergren, J. (2017). The Charlson comorbidity index in registry-based research: Which version to use?
22. Conley, Y. P., Dunbar-Jacob, J., Heitkemper, M. M., Henly, S., et al. (2015). Integrating emerging areas of nursing science into PhD programs. https://core.ac.uk/download/213079747.pdf (accessed on 25th June 2025).
23. Costello, S., Eisen, E. A., Picciotto, S., Rehkopf, D. H., et al. (2014). Social disparities in heart disease risk and survivor bias among autoworkers: An examination based on survival models and g-estimation. https://core.ac.uk/download/323081813.pdf (accessed on 25th June 2025).
24. Delva, W., Hendrickx, D. M., Hens, N., Kuylen, E., et al. (2019). *SimpactCyan 1.0*: An open-source simulator for individual-based models in HIV epidemiology with R and Python interfaces. https://core.ac.uk/download/286086461.pdf (accessed on 25th June 2025).
25. Elliott, P., Ezzati, M., Kontis, V., Tzoulaki, A., et al. (2016). Worldwide exposures to cardiovascular risk factors and associated health effects: Current knowledge and data gaps. https://core.ac.uk/download/77013626.pdf (accessed on 25th June 2025).
26. Ferraro, K. F., Kemp, B. R., & Williams, M. M. (2020). Diverse aging and health inequality by race and ethnicity. https://core.ac.uk/download/305123341.pdf (accessed on 25th June 2025).
27. Harrington, D., Lamberton, P. H. L., & McGregor, A. (2017). Human liver flukes. https://core.ac.uk/download/96882191.pdf (accessed on 25th June 2025).
28. Koskella, B., & Lin, D. (2014). Friend and foe: Factors influencing the movement of the

bacterium *Helicobacter pylori* along the parasitism-mutualism continuum. https://core.ac.uk/download/323080778.pdf (accessed on 25th June 2025).

29. Kyrou, I., & Weickert, M. O. (2010). Clinical problems caused by obesity. https://core.ac.uk/download/46324.pdf (accessed on 25th June 2025).
30. Lewnard, J. A., & Reingold, A. L. (2019). Emerging challenges and opportunities in infectious disease epidemiology. https://core.ac.uk/download/323082106.pdf (accessed on 25th June 2025).
31. Link, B., Morroni, C., Myer, L., Susser, E., et al. (2008). Social epidemiology. https://core.ac.uk/download/1670083.pdf (accessed on 25th June 2025).
32. Mayhew, L., Rasulo, D., & Rickayzen, B. D. (2009). The decomposition of disease and disability life expectancies in England 1992–2004. https://core.ac.uk/download/9983084.pdf (accessed on 25th June 2025).
33. N/A. (2001). *National Blueprint: Increasing Physical Activity Among Adults Age 50 and Older*. https://core.ac.uk/download/71346800.pdf (accessed on 25th June 2025).
34. N/A. (2008). *Work Matters for Health*. https://core.ac.uk/download/71347134.pdf (accessed on 25th June 2025).
35. N/A. (2009). *Deadly in Pink: Big Tobacco Steps Up Its Targeting of Women and Girls*. https://core.ac.uk/download/71350658.pdf (accessed on 25th June 2025).
36. Ormond, B. A., Bovbjerg, R. R., & Waidmann, T. (2011). What directions for public health under the Affordable Care Act? https://core.ac.uk/download/71357552.pdf (accessed on 25th June 2025).
37. Rothman, K. J. (2011). Methodological frontiers in environmental epidemiology. https://open.bu.edu/bitstream/2144/2603/1/envhper00381-0015.pdf (accessed on 25th June 2025).
38. Shadmi, E. (2013). Disparities in multiple chronic conditions within populations. https://core.ac.uk/download/pdf/29572286.pdf (accessed on 25th June 2025).
39. Singh-Manoux, A., Skrondal, A., Barros, A. J. D., Basu, A. M., Galobardes, B., Marston, C., Victora, C. G., et al. (2015). A mediation approach to understanding socio-economic inequalities in maternal health-seeking behaviors in Egypt. https://core.ac.uk/download/19747027.pdf (accessed on 25th June 2025).
40. Walker, A. E., & Colagiuri, S. (2025). Cost-benefit model system of chronic diseases in Australia to assess and rank prevention and treatment options. https://core.ac.uk/download/pdf/6428826.pdf (accessed on 25th June 2025).
41. Zanetti, A. R., Mele, A., Mariano, A., Galli, C., Spada, E., Taliani, G., Romanò, L., et al. (2015). Clinical, epidemiological and virological features of acute hepatitis B in Italy. https://core.ac.uk/download/153365546.pdf (accessed on 25th June 2025).

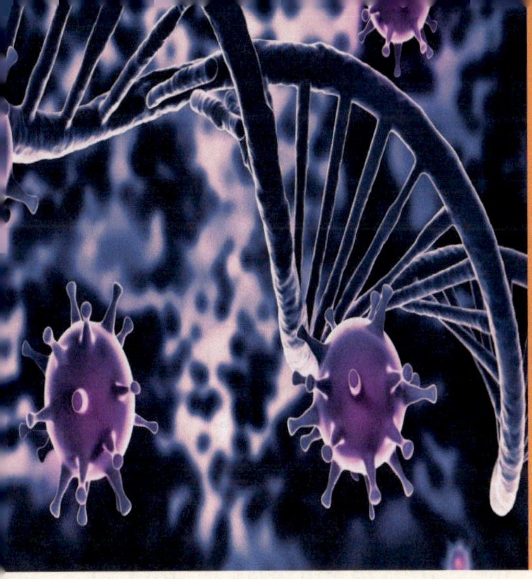

Chapter 14

GENETIC EPIDEMIOLOGY

Contents

Introduction

The field of genetic epidemiology sits at the central intersection of genetics and public health, illuminating the role of genetic contributions to disease and health in populations. Genetic epidemiology studies the heritable bases of diseases and, in doing so, enables researchers to untangle complex interactions among lifestyle, environment, and genes. Genetic epidemiology, by taking on a multidisciplinary approach, addresses the prevalence and patterning of genetic disease as well as investigating gene-environment interactions. Such subtle consciousness is required to draw up interventionist and prevention policies, ultimately optimizing public health outcomes. With the unfolding of science, integration of newer techniques and technologies only continues to enhance our consciousness of genetic susceptibility, leading to future personalized medicine. One of the breakthroughs transforming genetic epidemiology is the concept of exposome, which captures the life-long cumulative sum of environmental exposures from birth. The exposome approaches have repositioned traditional paradigms of epidemiological research by expanding the focus from isolated genetic factors to encompass the sophisticated interactions between genetic vulnerabilities and environmental exposures. The new course is appropriate for the growing recognition that outcomes of health are not dictated by individual genetic profiles but significantly shaped by extrinsic determinants. The exposome's conceptual and methodological innovations are the ongoing evolution of genetic epidemiology, compelling researchers to update established theories based on new information and technological innovation. Therefore, the knowledge of the exposome is key to enhancing public health interventions and promoting comprehensive disease prevention strategies (Canali et al., 2020). Furthermore, instrumental variable (IV) approaches, among other statistical methods, have been used in recent studies to transcend the challenge posed by unobserved confounding in observational studies. IV methods offer a technical solution for the estimation of causal effects and therefore illuminate the underlying genetic causes of observed health variation in populations. But one must be willing to recognize the complexities inherent with these methods, as they necessitate careful attention to assumptions and potential constraints. The need for sensitivity analysis signifies the importance of care in causal inference, particularly when confronted with the multi-factorial determinations of disease. Through the use of these sophisticated statistical frameworks, scientists are able to dissect the complexities of genetic data to ultimately develop a more insightful understanding of the interaction between genetics and health, as well as acknowledge the potential limitations that reside alongside methodological practice (Didelez et al., 2010) (Figure 14.1).

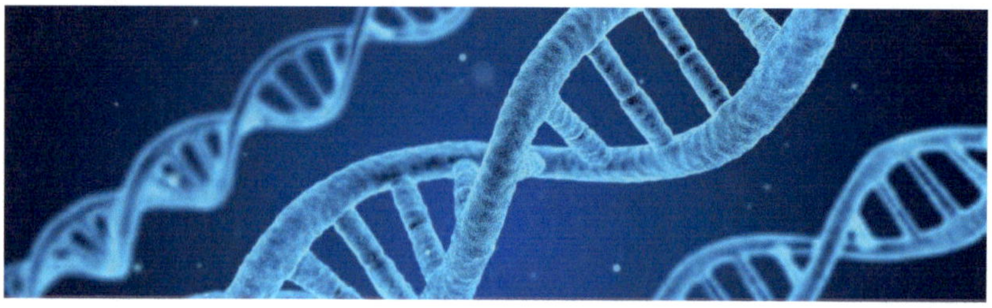

Figure 14.1. Genetic epidemiology.

Source: https://medicine.utah.edu/sites/g/files/zrelqx356/files/styles/billboard_tablet/public/media/images/2022/gen-epi-home.jpg?h=8eaef64c&itok=KbDMGE1w.

Definition of Genetic Epidemiology

Genetic epidemiology is an interdisciplinary field that investigates the interaction of environmental and genetic factors in the etiology of diseases. Genetic epidemiology utilizes concepts in genetics, molecular biology, and conventional epidemiology to address issues regarding the distribution, determinants, and control of disease in populations. Highlighting the role of genetic predisposition compounded by environmental exposure, genetic epidemiology aims to account for the complex routes that lead to health outcomes. The possible identification of specific genes associated with illness, and the interactions between genes and the environment, is fundamental to designing targeted treatments and prevention strategies. This comprehensive approach not only extends the scope of classical epidemiology but also presents us with a clearer overview of health disparities and disease susceptibility in different populations. Genetic epidemiology's scope extends beyond the sole detection of genetic markers for diseases; it also involves investigation into the heritability and population genetic correlations. For instance, investigations in large consortia like the Cohorts for Heart and Aging Research in Genomic Epidemiology (CHARGE) have shown large associations of genetic variants with various health conditions, i.e., relating to brain structure and function. Investigations into the heritability of traits like cortical thickness and neurodegenerative diseases illustrate the intricate biological processes at play. These findings are not just academic; they have practical uses for public health intervention and personal medicine.

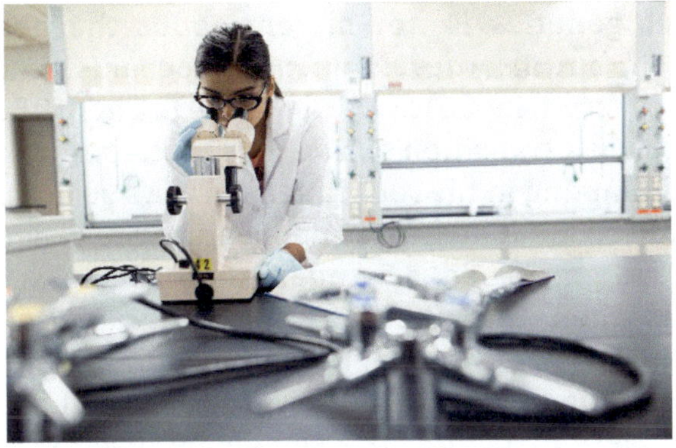

Figure 14.2. Definition of genetic epidemiology.

Source: https://onlinelibrary.wiley.com/pb-assets/assets/10982272/Stock_Image_Lab-1552957225323.jpg.

As the science evolves, with the addition of advanced computational tools and bioinformatics techniques, researchers can better understand the complexity of genetic contribution to complex diseases, ultimately leading to enhancing patient outcomes. Furthermore, genetic epidemiology is also about the broader contextual implications of genetic findings in disease and health. By examining the intersection of genetics and social, environmental, and behavioral factors, researchers can make inferences that guide health policies and interventions. As an example, developments in the study of melanoma identify the importance of knowledge of genetic susceptibility to consider environmental factors, such as exposure to the sun. Combining information from clinical studies of melanoma with fundamental pigment cell research has opened new avenues for prevention and therapy. Discussions ranging across the sciences of genomics and systems biology, genetic epidemiology not only enhances understanding of the causes of disease but also fuels advances in therapeutic approaches and public health interventions, opening up more scope for knowledge of health at the population level (Birlea et al., 2018; Adams et al., 2019) (Figure 14.2).

Importance in Public Health

The significance of genetic epidemiology in public health cannot be overstated since it provides valuable information about the interaction between genetics and environmental determinants of health effects. Information regarding how genetic predispositions are linked to the risk of diseases such as obesity and cardiovascular diseases is vital in developing effective prevention measures. The new study has cast light on the critical role of body-fat distribution, which emphasizes how genetic variations are capable of influencing this parameter and consequently influencing cardiovascular health. Identification of common and rare coding variants associated with body-fat distribution demonstrates the need for future research into genetic factors in health disparities. Through these correlations, public health programs can formulate interventions in populations that are genetically predisposed to specific diseases and thereby optimize the efficacy of disease prevention programs for the multicultural population (Abecasis et al., 2019). Advances in genomic and molecular data have also revolutionized public health strategies with new trends in early detection and intervention. Genetic epidemiology makes it possible to incorporate genetic information into conventional epidemiological systems, further elucidating disease causation and patterns of transmission. For example, the introduction of molecular surveillance has revolutionized our ability to respond to health threats within populations, especially the tracking of infectious diseases and foodborne pathogens. The interaction among genetic markers and epidemiological data not only assists in the detection of at-risk populations but also aids in public health policy design and resource planning strategies. Setting up standards to analyze the attributes of molecular surveillance systems will ensure an integrated strategy that taps the potential of both molecular innovations and traditional epidemiology (Dufour et al., 2015). Furthermore, the ability to conduct genetic research in populations with different diversity has general implications for health equity. Genetic epidemiology offers a tool for demarcating specific genetic determinants of health states among different population groups, which is an essential component in studying health disparities. Through the identification of genetic foundations of illnesses and their variable impacts among populations, public health programs can be more inclusive and equitable. For example, the understanding of some genetic factors that are most likely to predispose particular ethnic groups to more cases of chronic diseases grants power to health authorities to implement targeted educational programs and prevention programs. In this way, genetic epidemiology not only enhances the understanding of the determinants of health but also strengthens the rationale for particular public health interventions aimed at the elimination of health disparities and improving overall population health status.

14.1. Historical Background

The historical unfolding of genetic epidemiology is inextricably interwoven with the history of genetics and breakthroughs during the last 100 years. The genesis of genetic epidemiology lies in the major developments in molecular biology and genetics in the middle decades of the 20th century. Of particular significance are the contributions of researchers like Thomas Hunt Morgan and his research on heredity as a preparation for the comprehension of genetic inheritance and variation. These early enquiries constituted a vital debate between embryology and genetics, that is, in theorizing epigenesis. Conrad Hal Waddington's work in the 1940s still helped move the field at a much faster pace, fostering an understanding that genetics is not merely about the gene itself, but also developmental mechanisms, as uncovered in Costa et al. (2014). The 1950s marked a transition period for genetic research, culminating in the replication of DNA's structure and subsequent studies delineating the genetic paradigms used to understand sickness. It was then that methods first characterized genetics with the epidemiology of disease, combining genetic markers with population wellness dynamics. The significant discussions that occurred during the 1957 international conference in Gif-sur-Yvette clarified the changes of interest and interest among scientists. Scientists shifted from perceiving the view of genetics as pertaining to the whole organism only to emphasizing the significance of non-genetic factors in the expression of traits. These discussions prompted further research into the complexity of gene-environmental interactions that influence health outcomes, as validated by the newly developed field of epigenetics, as presented in Costa et al. (2014). In the later decades, genomic technologies and analysis improvements have significantly revolutionized the genetic epidemiology arena. Now that the Human Genome Project is complete, genetic components have been better elucidated, and one can make in-depth analyses of diseases like leishmaniasis. The epidemiology and genetic structure of *Leishmania donovani*, for instance, mirror such advancements, as uncovered through studies that explore genetic associations within populations. A cohort study, as in, yielded evidence of the genetic subgroups present in some geographical locations, which emphasized the function exercised by both genetic and environmental factors in disease susceptibility. This convergence of genetic data with epidemiological methods reinforces the integrative character of contemporary genetic epidemiology, where earlier contemplations regularly supply feedback to present actions and research methods (Figure 14.3).

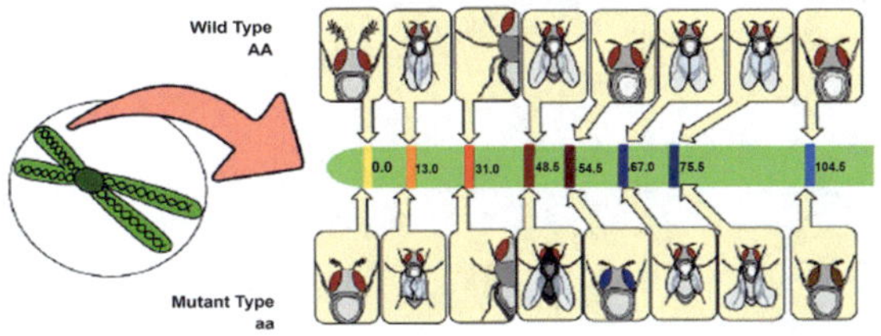

Figure 14.3. Thomas Hunt Morgan's Drosophila melanogaster genetic linkage map. This was the first successful gene mapping work and provides important evidence for the chromosome theory of inheritance. The map shows the relative positions of allelic characteristics on the second Drosophila chromosome. The distance between the genes (map units) is equal to the percentage of crossing-over events that occur between different alleles.

Source: https://upload.wikimedia.org/wikipedia/commons/4/46/Drosophila_Gene_Linkage_Map.svg.

14.1.1. Early Studies in Genetics

The early genetic research gave the fundamental outline of learning inherited principles for the transmission of traits through generations. Visionaries such as Gregor Mendel, through precise experimentation with pea plants, illustrated the segregation and independent assortment laws. These groundbreaking findings established the field of genetics, highlighting how certain traits may appear or disappear over generations as a result of interactions between dominant and recessive alleles. This early foundation played a critical role in laying the gene-based foundation for varying phenotypes, establishing an important link to modern genetic epidemiology, where studies on genetic variation enable the elucidation of disease susceptibility and population health patterns. The strategy used by early geneticists, particularly Mendel's systematic method, is crucial for the rigorous examination modern researchers employ in discerning genetic impacts on health outcomes. With the advent of science in the 20th century, advancements such as Watson and Crick's discovery of DNA's structure widened new horizons in genetics, permitting the genetic inheritance and mutation to be more readily understood. Molecular biological techniques incorporated into genetics allowed genetic markers for specific diseases to be studied, thereby transforming the discipline of genetic epidemiology. This time also saw the application of genetic mapping, employed to identify genes involved in inherited disease, demonstrating the way early genetic hypotheses were applied to real health issues. Knowledge gained from these advances not only shaped public health policy but also predated the emergence of genomic medicine and genetic counseling and underscored the applicability of genetics to disease prevention and control. During the last several decades, technological progress has rendered genomic sequencing technologies more accessible, thereby improving the field by enabling the gathering of gigantic data and the examination of genetic diversity in populations. All these advancements have better developed our understanding of genetic diversity and what it means for epidemiological studies. For instance, genetic research on *Trypanosoma cruzi*, the parasite causing Chagas disease, pointed out the dramatic impacts of genetic variation on disease transmission and severity (Acosta et al., 2009). Similarly, HIV genetic epidemiology research has employed phylogenetic methods to follow transmission and examine infection patterns within populations, indicating how genetics can be applied in guiding public health interventions and resource allocation (Leitner et al., 2018). The history of early genetic research reflects its catalytic contribution toward informing present-day strategies for comprehending illness by means of genetics, highlighting the interwoven nature of genetics and epidemiology in public health progression (Figure 14.4).

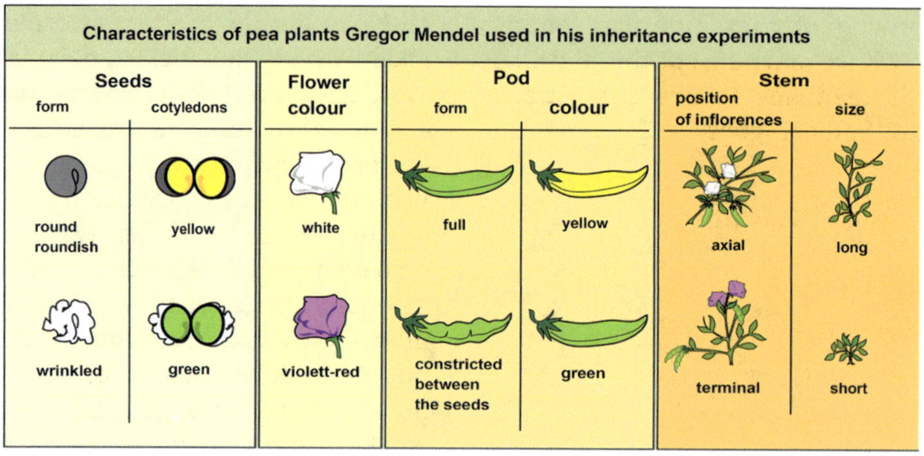

Figure 14.4. The seven characteristics of pea plants selected by Gregor Mendel.

Source: https://open.oregonstate.education/app/uploads/sites/28/2020/11/Fig-5-3-The-seven-characteristics-of-pea-plants.png.

14.1.2. Development of Epidemiological Methods

Advancements in epidemiological techniques have profoundly enhanced the knowledge of disease dynamics, especially for genetic epidemiology. Statistical modeling innovations and the integration of molecular methods have revolutionized the way researchers examine the transmission of diseases and their genetic components. There has been greater molecular epidemiology, which has enabled scientists to dig deeper into the genetic origins of disease, revealing information not available to earlier generations of epidemiologists. Information regarding genetics combined with demographic and environmental data is now utilized to track the multifactorial etiology of disease susceptibility and transmission, enabling the facilitation of enhanced public health interventions. Most significantly, viral metagenomics is a landmark change in epidemiological approaches. It is a culture-free method that enables extensive analysis of viral populations in given ecological niches, thereby extending the understanding of viral pathologies.

Through the use of high-throughput next-generation sequencing technologies, researchers gain high-resolution viral diversity information, which is crucial for the identification of novel viruses and the assessment of their effect on human health. This innovative method is especially helpful in the detection and monitoring of impending viral threats, and in carrying out high-throughput molecular epidemiology in an attempt to analyze patterns of viral spread and evolution, and ultimately inform improved disease monitoring and response activities (Albina et al., 2013). Additionally, molecular epidemiology has made it possible to explore complex disease patterns in various environments, for instance, sleeping sickness in humans caused by *Trypanosoma brucei spp.* Traditional microscopy cannot account for the complexity of this disease, which is characterized by single foci that result in epidemics and then endemicity. Application of molecular epidemiological techniques enables scientists to detect and identify genetic variants at several levels of taxonomy and thereby have information on the genetic heterogeneity of these parasites. This increased knowledge informs public health policy and focal interventions, since comprehension of genetic variation across subspecies is integral to controlling transmission patterns and reservoir hosts. The case of *Trypanosoma brucei* rhodesiense in Uganda shows how these methods have explained the causes and dynamics of sleeping sickness epidemics and have enabled more empowered and effective control (Tait et al., 2009).

14.1.3. Milestones in Genetic Epidemiology

The field of genetic epidemiology has witnessed several evolutionary milestones that have significantly enhanced our understanding of the interaction between genetics and the environment in the etiology of diseases. One of them was the successful completion of the Human Genome Project in 2003, which demonstrated a complete map of genes found in humans and their functions. This enormous endeavor not only expanded our understanding of genetic variations for many health conditions but also gave us a template for connecting particular genes to illness. The access to genomic sequences spurred the development of new strategies for conducting genetic epidemiologic studies, allowing researchers to examine complex traits and diseases at a nuanced level. Consequently, this milestone in history facilitated an intensifying revolution in the study of multifactorial diseases and placed greater emphasis on genetic factors towards health variation among different populations. Following the foundation established by the Human Genome Project, technological advancements in sequencing have yielded a tsunami of data rewriting genetic epidemiology. High-throughput technologies, such as next-generation sequencing, have enabled analyzing the genomic basis of disease more thoroughly, allowing for the identification of rare variants and their influence on health. Coupled with advances in bioinformatics, these technologies have transformed how epidemiologists screen genetic variants in populations. Notably, new informatics tools enable the integration of genomic information with phenotypic data, creating a setting in which subtle comprehension of the relationship between genes and the environment can develop. Moreover, technologies like Vision, which automate variation annotation in single-cell RNA-seq data, illustrate the capability of technology to minimize complex analyses and aid collaboration between scientists to expedite the identification of new genetic determinants that influence health outcomes (Ashuach et al., 2019).

Also, the research on model organisms has been key in genetic epidemiology, and this is best illustrated by the research of Arabidopsis thaliana in deciphering plant-microbe interactions and ecological genetics. This inconspicuous-looking wildflower has been an excellent model for understanding molecular processes that can guide conservation biology and ecological studies. The genetic data gained from the study of this organism has illuminated the intricate relationship between environmental factors and genetics, with significant information to further research of genetics in the animal kingdom. Consequently, the translation of results from model organisms to human health plays an essential role in bridging the divide between molecular biology and epidemiology. By synthesizing information from these multiple fields, researchers are better positioned to enhance their understanding of the influence of genetic variation on disease susceptibility and inform public health intervention policy (Falk et al., 2008) (Figure 14.5).

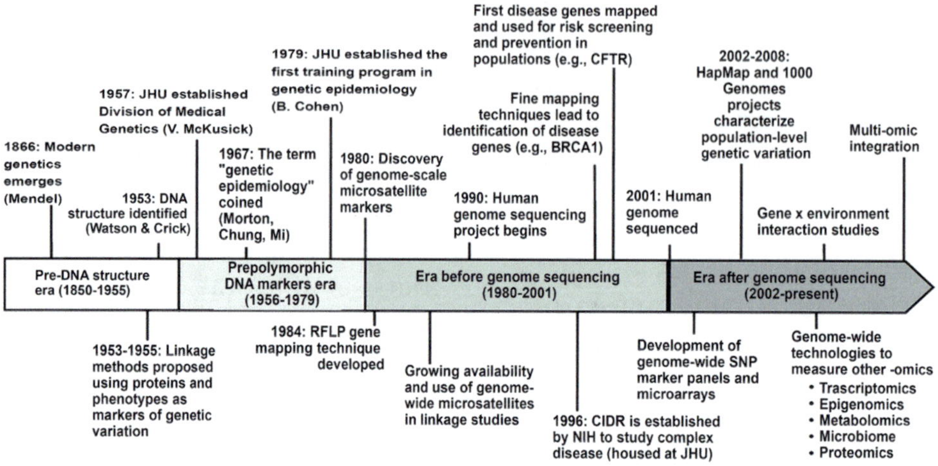

Figure 14.5. Timeline of the development of genetic epidemiology.

Source: https://www.researchgate.net/publication/335774754/figure/fig1/AS:869405143605252@1584293747773/Timeline-of-the-development-of-genetic-epidemiology-BRCA1-Breast-cancer-type-1.png.

14.2. Key Concepts in Genetic Epidemiology

In genetic epidemiology, there is a need for the interaction of environmental and genetic determinants. This is a field that crosses disciplines and explores the role genetics has in disease and health distribution and determinants among people. With the use of molecular surveillance as a tool, it is possible to know more about multigenic diseases, the specific genetic variants associated with various states of health. The application of molecular data in epidemiologic investigations provides valuable information, but keep in mind that such data are an addendum to traditional epidemiologic examinations and never a replacement. This is reiterated by more recent developments indicating the need for well-designed studies incorporating molecular data effectively (Dufour et al., 2015). This approach allows for a more comprehensive assessment of health risk and consequences, establishing a greater grasp of population health dynamics. Differentiation of genetic screening from similar terminology, particularly within prenatal settings, is another pillar of genetic epidemiology. Genetic screening refers to the use of tests to identify those at risk for specific genetic diseases, while prenatal screening is specifically used for the assessment of health in a fetus. Misunderstandings typically follow from practitioners conflating these terms, thereby misusing screening guidelines. Definite distinctions of these words are essential for policymakers and physicians since they facilitate informed decisions regarding genetic testing and its applicability in patient treatment (Alderson et al., 2001). Better communication of the unique strengths of every screening modality will maximize the good that accompanies genetic testing and ultimately benefit patients and their families. Finally, the new face of genetic epidemiology emphasizes the need for cross-disciplinary collaboration. As molecular biology and genomics continue to expand our understanding of disease, new paradigms for study design and analysis are required. Investment in an interdisciplinary skill set that cuts across molecular science and epidemiological principles is pivotal for the development of efficient surveillance mechanisms. This call for collaborative expertise reflects the interface of molecular and epidemiological information, expanding areas of research and public health program applicability. As indicated in recent publications, placing significance on the integration of these disciplines will facilitate comprehensive evaluations of genetic determinants of disease and health to guide public health policy and enhance healthcare provision (Dufour et al., 2015) (Figure 14.6).

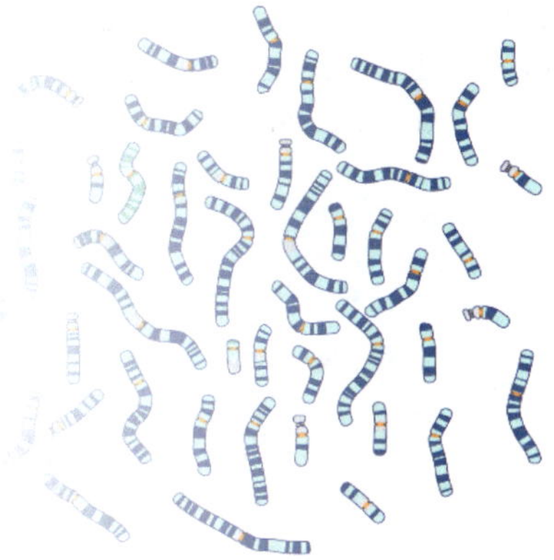

Figure 14.6. Understanding genetic epidemiology.

Source: https://www.genome.gov/sites/default/files/media/images/2022-04/Chromosome%20spread_hero.png.

14.2.1. Heritabillty and Genetic Variation

Heritability is a simple concept in genetic epidemiology and an index to quantify the proportion of phenotypic variation accounted for by genetic variance in a given population. More specifically, narrow-sense heritability (h^2) quantifies the proportion of measurable attributes that can be explained by additive genetic factors. Recent evidence has emerged to highlight the nuance of heritability estimates, particularly the disparity between genotyped SNP heritability (h^2g) and overall narrow-sense heritability (h^2). The divergence has been attributed to the effect of rare genetic variants, in addition to bias from common environment or epistatic gene-to-gene interactions. For instance, the novel h^2 estimation from unrelated individuals in admixed populations allows for a clearer understanding of heritability, free from these biases, and is essential to accurately portray the genetic architecture of traits and diseases in ethnically diverse populations (Assimes et al., 2014). Genetic variation is the cornerstone of heritability, which describes the variance in the genetic variation accounting for phenotypic variation among individuals. With advances in genomics technologies, genome-wide association analyses (GWAS) on a large scale have revealed significant associations between some genetic differences and diseases. For example, in a cohort of heart failure patients, research revealed that the heritability of AF could be explained partially by a genetic risk score for AF based on 97 SNPs. Amazingly, this genetic risk score accounted for 22.9% of AF's heritability. These findings underscore the importance of genetic influences on complex diseases and affirm the link between heritability and genetic diversity, presenting an even stronger image of how susceptibility to disease is influenced by genetics in diverse populations (Anker et al., 2020). It is important to debate heritability and genetic diversity to advance genetic epidemiology, particularly as it relates to public health and personalized medicine. Understanding the heritability of various traits helps researchers and clinicians better target vulnerable groups and intervene accordingly. Such data may facilitate the easier development of gene therapy, where interventions can be tailored individually according to genetic risk. Furthermore, as has been achieved by the integration of genetic risk scores into predictive models, genetic data helps enhance the predictiveness for conditions such as AF. This shift towards the application of genetic data in clinical care represents the promise of genetic epidemiology to transform healthcare outcomes and personalize treatment regimens, thus meeting the growing need for precision medicine in the management of complicated health conditions.

14.2.2. Gene-Environment Interactions

Gene-environment interactions. They form a crucial part of genetic epidemiology because they mediate health states. Gene-environment interactions are circumstances where specific genetic variation affects an individual's susceptibility to environmental insults, thus. They determine the trajectory of various states, such as respiratory diseases and obesity. For example, studies have indicated that genetic susceptibilities have the ability to modify the effect of environmental exposures, such as diet and air pollution, on obesity. As big cohort studies, for example, the National Children's Study (NCS), have developed, scientists are now able to perform these intricate interactions longitudinally. The longitudinal design of the NCS permits research on genetic effects intertwined with social, natural, and built environmental determinants, allowing for a solid platform for understanding the interaction of genes and environments to synergistically impact pediatric obesity (Carrel et al., 2009). Further, recent research on relationships between oxidative stress-related genes and environmental toxicants underlines the crucial role of gene-environment interactions in health. Genetic variants have been shown to modify the effect of harmful exposures, e.g., ambient air pollution or cigarette smoke, on lung function. For instance, some single-nucleotide polymorphisms (SNPs) are reported to have substantial interaction with particulate matter, influencing the rate of lung function decline in individuals. A study found that SNCA and PARK2 gene polymorphisms either accelerated or decelerated the deterioration of lung function with respect to exposure to pollution, suggesting that ignoring the gene-environment interactions would make it difficult to have an objective assessment of respiratory disease (Comandini et al., 2012). The finding supports the need for considering genetic susceptibility in addition to environmental exposures while examining disease epidemiology. The combination of gene-environment interactions with genetic epidemiology provides a systems viewpoint from which to look at public health problems. Genetic effect, as well as environmental issues, become clearly evident with conditions like obesity and respiratory illness, where causation is multifactorial. Such a range of scrutiny not only educates us more concerning disease mechanisms, but it also critically impacts intervention strategies.

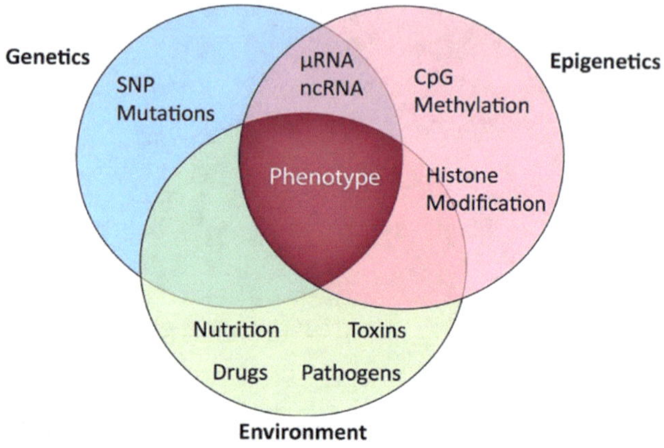

Figure 14.7. Schematic diagram representing the gene-environment interaction (genetic-epigenetic phenotype).

Source: https://www.researchgate.net/profile/Samuel-Uwaezuoke-2/publication/309274060/figure/fig1/AS:418894662651917@1476883678969/Schematic-diagram-representing-the-gene-environment-interaction-genetic-epigenetic.png.

By employing big longitudinal data assets like the NCS, researchers can systematically track the intricate routes through which some genetic variants intersect with environmental exposures. With progressive advancement in this field, monitoring these interactions will enlighten influential public health policies for minimizing risks from both genetic vulnerabilities and environmental threats, and towards a healthier population (Carrel et al., 2009; Comandini et al., 2012) (Figure 14.7).

14.2.3. Genetic Risk Factors

Genetic risk factors studied in genetic epidemiology present a multidimensional picture where the individual's genetic predisposition is accompanied by environmental determinants. Genome-wide association studies (GWAS) have proven to be efficient tools that have identified a number of genetic markers that are associated with a number of diseases. Nonetheless, one of the foremost limitations of such studies is that the majority of markers found confer proportionally small increments in risk and fail to account for most familial clustering observed in disease. To counter this obstacle, research initiatives such as the National Cancer Institute's workshop on Next Generation Analytic Tools for Large-Scale Genetic Epidemiology Studies of Complex Diseases have been established. This workshop concentrated on enhancing methodologies for the identification of genetic and environmental determinants for complicated diseases, eventually guiding the direction of future research in genetic epidemiology (Albert et al., 2012). For colorectal cancer (CRC), the genetic factors contributing to its pathogenesis underscore the necessity of uniting genetic epidemiology with clinical practice. In nations like Pakistan, the prevalence of CRC has been progressively increasing in the young adult population, calling for intensive research and preventive intervention. Risk determinants are more than lifestyle factors and include genetic determinants such as the CpG Island Methylator Phenotype (CIMP), Chromosomal Instability (CIN), and Microsatellite Instability (MSI). Identification of these molecular mechanisms is crucial to devising effective screening and treatment protocols, particularly for areas that have high rates of late-stage diagnoses due to the absence of proper screening programs. Therefore, an inter-disciplinary approach through genetic epidemiology can go a long way in improving health outcomes in CRC patients across various populations (Abbas et al., 2023). Greater incorporation of genetic risk factors in the realm of public health places more emphasis on prevention strategies that are individually modified to identify genetic predispositions as well as environmental factors. For instance, education about lifestyle modifications, coupled with genetic counseling, can be applied to enable individuals with proper information to minimize their risk for genetically conditioned illnesses. The creation of some genetic markers related to disease disorders will also raise screening activity and lead to more focused methods in treatment regimens. By incorporating geneticists, epidemiologists, and medical care providers, we will be maximizing the use of genetic information, thus translating into better disease prevention and intervention practices. As genetic epidemiology continues to advance, it is increasingly necessary to consider how these findings can be made realistic at the population level for healthcare systems to benefit populations globally, particularly in those with varied epidemiological profiles (Figure 14.8).

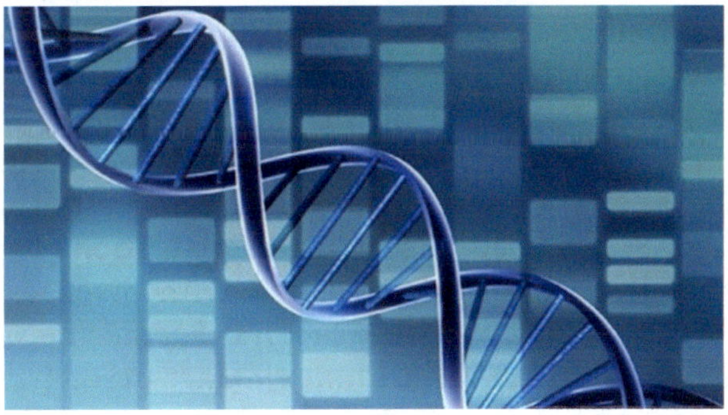

Figure 14.8. Genetics and the risk of colorectal cancer.

Source: https://coloncancerfoundation.org/wp-content/uploads/2016/09/CRCDNA-e1659804079288.jpg.

14.3. Methodologies Used

In genetic epidemiology, heterogeneous methods are essential for investigating the hereditary disease patterns and their complex interactions with environmental components. One of the central methods is multi-omics integration, including genomics, proteomics, metabolomics, and other forms of omics. This holistic method bypasses the limitation of single-omics research in not being able to view the entire biological landscape involved in disease development. By the use of multi-dimensional data, researchers are able to identify biomarkers directly associated with disease mechanisms and processes. This convergence has enhanced predictions of susceptibility and course of disease, ultimately toward the planning of individual treatment schemes. Consequently, the addition of multi-omics strategies enables genetic epidemiologists to explain the intricate weave of cardiometabolic diseases (CMD) as pointed out in the recognition of omics relationships of their pathophysiology (Argano et al., 2019). Another critical genetic epidemiology methodology is the application of advanced statistical models combined with machine learning techniques. These methods are well-equipped to handle large data sets that arise when genomic analysis is performed, and they enable scientists to identify genetic variations associated with specific health conditions. Genome-wide association studies (GWAS) are used to scan large populations for genetic differences associated with diseases, thereby identifying risk factors. Furthermore, machine learning algorithms enhance predictive modeling through the identification of patterns and relationships that may not be readily apparent using conventional statistical analysis. This methodological upgrade not only maximizes the use of existing data but also ensures that the resulting conclusions are evidence-based and reliable. Thus, the integration of novel statistical methods and machine learning is revolutionizing the realm of genetic epidemiology by providing deeper insights into disease mechanisms and susceptibility (Aas et al., 2016). Finally, how gender variation is addressed in genetic epidemiology is another required approach. The practice of gender medicine highlights how biological and sociocultural factors get interwoven to influence health outcomes. This approach emphasizes the significance of exploring genetic mechanisms leading to disease in the context of gender as a multifaceted factor influencing the disease process. Modifying research designs to account for sex differences in disease pathogenesis and response to therapy is feasible, and investigators can glean worthwhile information toward improved management by so doing. These approaches not only enrich the understanding of CMD mechanisms but also tackle broader social and cultural contexts, ultimately resulting in better health outcomes across varied populations. Hence, gender differences must be taken into account in order to advance the field of genetic epidemiology so that findings become generalizable and applicable to all (Argano et al., 2019).

14.3.1. Population-Based Studies

Population studies are a critical component of genetic epidemiology, providing a robust design to investigate the interaction of the environment and genetic factors in influencing health conditions. Population studies typically involve large representative cohorts from the general population so that researchers can quantify the incidence and prevalence of various diseases against some genetic markers. For instance, studies based on populations can elucidate the impact of HFE gene mutations on conditions such as liver diseases and diabetes. Heterogeneity in results among studies is typically because of differences in study design, case definition, and composition of populations, which underscores the value of standardizing methods for enhanced validity of evidence. Population-based research is thus important in arriving at meaningful conclusions that can inform public health policy and improve screening techniques for genetic predisposition to disease, ultimately translating to better health outcomes among different populations (Njajou et al., 2002). The incorporation of population-based health data with genetic information allows for the analysis of complex interactions between genetic variations and states of disease. A good example of this is the link between psychiatric disorders and gastrointestinal infections, as demonstrated in a sample study from Denmark. Researchers were able to study genetic factors that result in susceptibility to gastrointestinal infections within a population-based study, and also study correlations with mental health outcomes simultaneously to some extent. The findings were demonstrated to have high heritability estimates for infection susceptibility, as well as indicating high associations with disorders such as depression and autism. This approach demonstrates the power of population-based studies in determining genetic risk factors and their likely contributions to multifactorial diseases. This knowledge not only advances understanding of disease mechanisms but also leads towards integrative models, which can foster translational research in genetics and epidemiology (Appadurai et al., 2020). The knowledge derived through population-based studies is even utilized for clinical practice and public health interventions. By ascertaining specific genetic risk factors in large and heterogeneous cohorts, healthcare providers can tailor prevention strategies and intervention programs to better manage populations at higher risk. Personalization has ramifications for more effective disease management associated with genetic effects, as outlined in the hemochromatosis and resulting disorders study. The ability to quantify the impact of genetic mutations on disease manifestation enables public health personnel to develop unique screening and treatment programs based on consideration of genetic susceptibility. The population-based studies are therefore a bridge not only between epidemiology and genetics but also a foundation for setting appropriate public health policy that addresses the genetic etiology of prevalent disease (Njajou et al., 2002) (Figure 14.9).

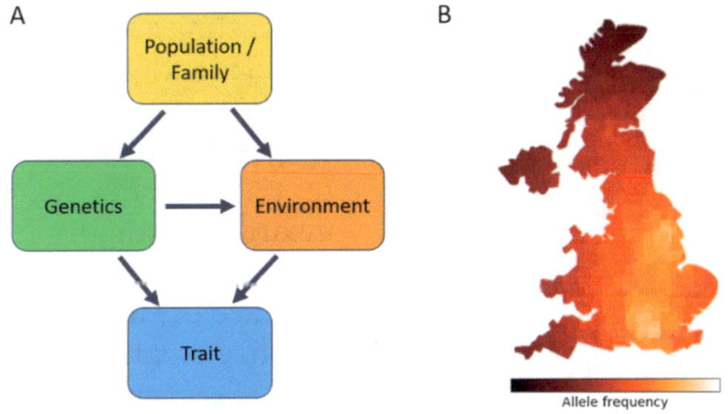

Figure 14.9. Population structure confounds human genetic studies. (A) The population that an individual is born into influences their genetics and their environment, which are the two components affecting traits; and (B) Even when considering a specific human group and controlling for the major axes of genetic variation in a cohort, the allele frequency of some variants can still vary across populations and exhibit clear geographic patterns, a problem known as "residual population structure."

Source: https://www.researchgate.net/publication/361432347/figure/fig1/AS:1169237854945281@1655779436433/Population-structure-confounds-human-genetic-studies-A-The-population-that-an-individual.png.

14.3.2. Family-Based Studies

Family-based research is crucial in the field of genetic epidemiology and has proved particularly helpful in the determination of how genetic characteristics are inherited. By acquiring data from families that have at least one affected member, researchers are able to analyze the passing of genetic variation from parents to offspring. This structure, besides facilitating closer examination of disease patterns within the family, also enhances the ability to control for shared environmental influences among relatives. Compared to population-based studies that may involve unrelated individuals, family-based structures offer a unique benefit in studying the operation of genetic susceptibility in a family context and, therefore, producing more precise insights into the heritability of complex disorders. These findings are critical for outlining the genetic architecture of conditions and guiding possible interventions targeting the reduction of disease risk over generations (Carlson et al., 2017). Aside from their methodological strengths, family-based research enables the investigation of phenotypic variability seen in complicated disorders. Different individuals within a family might show disparate expressions of a condition, based on an interaction of genetic and environmental influences. This heterogeneity can provide critical information regarding underlying biological pathways to disease expression. For instance, determining how certain genetic variants map onto phenotypes permits researchers to reveal pathways to disease, such as orofacial clefting. Consequently, family-based research not only deepens our understanding of the aetiology of diseases at a genetic level but also offers a system for synthesizing information regarding environmental effects, which is fundamental to the development of successful public health interventions and strategies (Laird et al., 2009). Synthesizing family-based data with other study designs, including case-control studies, is an important step in the field of genetic epidemiology. By combining multiple data structures, scientists can improve disease association estimates with fewer chances for bias—a problem particularly pertinent with the challenges of genetic interaction. Empirical Bayes-type shrinkage estimation procedures may be applied to combine varying types of data to generate a more powerful analytic platform. Integrated studies are also capable of finding genetic explanations for phenotypic heterogeneity, which single-method studies do not uncover. Lastly, the quiet understanding gained by family studies is essential in assisting to disentangle the intricate gene networks that underpin disorders of complexity, setting the stage for subsequent research efforts towards identifying targeted genetic and environmental interventions (Carlson et al., 2017).

14.3.3. Genome-Wide Association Studies (GWAS)

GWAS represent a breakthrough in the evolution of genetic epidemiology to examine complex genetic traits within various populations. By contrasting genetic variations across the genome, GWAS identify single-nucleotide polymorphisms (SNPs) linked with specific disorders or traits. Large-scale analysis has been especially helpful to uncover the genetic basis for numerous disorders, ranging from psychiatric illness to metabolic syndromes. GWAS findings not only enhance the understanding of disease pathology but also encourage the development of tailored risk assessment and individual therapies. As highlighted in discussions at large gatherings like the XXII World Congress of Psychiatric Genetics, the implications of these findings extend beyond mere identification, challenging traditional classifications of psychiatric disorders and providing a model for enhancing clinical nosology with genetic data (Andreassen et al., 2018). GWAS has further transformed psychiatric disorder research by enabling one to associate genetic variation and phenotypic expression. For instance, the inclusion of collaborative work such as that of the Psychiatric Genomics Consortium has shed strong evidence that there are genetic factors that play a role in the causation of a myriad of neuropsychiatric disorders. By correlating quantifiable traits with genetic data, researchers can discern patterns that could inform us about the nature of these disorders. This was one of the principal matters at recent conferences where the speakers not only accounted for what has been going on but also for the future implications of genetic epidemiology for mental health research. It raises important questions about the boundaries between normality and psychiatric disorder, and it could ultimately result in new diagnostic criteria on the basis of genetic results, which promises to disrupt traditional clinical practices (Aas et al., 2016).

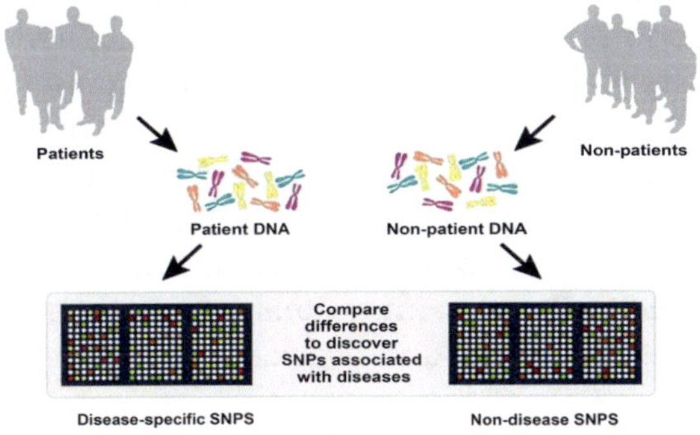

Figure 14.10. Genome-wide association studies (GWAS).

Source: https://www.researchgate.net/publication/328344689/figure/fig3/AS:682775615123476@1539797800304/Genome-wide-association-studies-GWAS.ppm.

The consequences of GWAS exceed the theoretical realm and enter the practical field, influencing clinical practice and public health interventions. Through the investigation of genetic predisposition to common diseases, GWAS provide critical data for risk stratification within populations. The study reinforces the coordination of environmental exposures with genetic determinants since it also underscores the need for an interdisciplinary approach to disease prevention. Further, as GWAS continue to progress, the use of heterogeneous ethnic populations is important in uncovering population-specific risk and ensuring discoveries are translatable on a larger scale. The presentation of these advances highlights potential as well as pitfalls in progressing from genetic discoveries to actionable healthcare solutions, promoting an enlightened perspective of genetic epidemiology in public health and patient care on an individualized basis (Andreassen et al., 2018) (Figure 14.10).

14.4. Applications in Disease Research

The integration of genetic epidemiology into disease studies has provided critical insights into the complex interactions between environmental determinants and genetic susceptibility. As a multidisciplinary area of study, it has enabled scientists to examine how genetic differences are involved in determining the risk of individuals to illnesses, primarily psychiatric conditions. There are new imaging genetics advances, as detailed in Hariri et al. (2006), that have allowed scientists to map the neurobiological signatures of genetic polymorphisms, advancing our understanding regarding how these differences may affect brain function and behavior. Employing neuroimaging techniques, scientists can visualize the biological processes underlying psychiatric disorders' causation, hence providing the foundation for selective treatment and enhanced therapeutic interventions. This focus on disease causality through genetics not only enriches our cognitive framework but also implies the possibility of personalized medicine interventions that tailor treatment to an individual's genetic makeup. Apart from psychiatric disorders, genetic epidemiology plays a key role in addressing the problems posed by overlooked zoonotic diseases (NZDs). According to Adamo et al. (2015), such diseases, which are often due to complex interactions between animal reservoirs and humans, accentuate the necessity to understand infectious agent dynamics in a multihost system. From the knowledge of population biology and transmission ecology of such pathogens, disease control strategies can be designed. An interdisciplinary approach that marries genetics with ecological and evolutionary theories is of utmost importance in the design of interventions, considering the interaction between animal and human hosts. Such integrated information facilitates the selection of key reservoirs and the tailoring of control measures, thus improving public health outcomes in developing as well as developed nations. In addition, genetic epidemiology's implications stretch to public health policy and practice, elevating disease prevention efforts to an entirely new level. The information learned from genetics informs targeted screening programs, enables early detection, and informs vaccine development. For example, understanding genetic susceptibility to a disease may enable more effective public health interventions among high-risk groups. The policy recommendations developed on the basis of genetic epidemiological research help policymakers direct resources more precisely and address problems of inequalities in health at the population level. Through integration of genetic information and socioeconomic and environmental data, researchers are able to better predict outbreaks of diseases and tailor interventions specifically, thereby promoting greater health outcomes overall. This synergistic integration highlights the revolutionary potential of genetic epidemiology in disease studies, affirming its significance for pushing public health initiatives forward.

14.4.1. Cancer Epidemiology

Epidemiology of cancer is a crucial field that explores causes, prevalence, and control of cancer in populations. An understanding of cancer's trend in epidemiology can provide information on probable genetic as well as environmental causes of risk. By analyzing various populations, scientists are able to identify incidence, prevalence, and mortality patterns that may be associated with particular genetic susceptibilities. For example, some populations will have a greater incidence of breast or colorectal cancer, implying both lifestyle and genetic determinants. Such emphasis on population data is essential in the planning of targeted preventive interventions as well as treatment algorithms. Secondly, findings from cancer epidemiological studies contribute to the broader health inequality debate as well as healthcare resource distribution, again emphasizing the efficacy of targeted intervention. Genetic interactions and cancer epidemiology are particularly relevant, since genetic tendencies exert a great influence on personal cancer risks. Genetic epidemiology tries to reveal how genetic diversity contributes to cancer susceptibility by inherited mutations as well as somatic changes that occur throughout the duration of one's life. For instance, BRCA1 and BRCA2 gene mutations are known risk factors for breast and ovarian cancers.

By identifying these genetic markers, epidemiologists can determine the true risk of an individual and provide customized surveillance and preventive measures. In addition, research combining genetic and epidemiologic data can characterize how environmental exposures interact with genetic predisposition, further elucidating the multifactorial nature of the majority of cancers. This convergence ultimately leads to a more comprehensive view of cancer prevention and treatment strategies. An important role for cancer epidemiology is to identify modifiable risk factors of the disease. Modifiable risk factors of the disease are diet, physical activity, and use of tobacco, and these have been shown to play an important role in cancer risk. Public health interventions could reduce the incidence of some cancers and hence alleviate some of the burden on healthcare systems. Furthermore, epidemiological evidence can identify the socioeconomic determinants that enhance cancer risk, highlight the importance of healthcare access, and inform policy interventions towards the reduction of disparities. Because cancer remains a leading cause of morbidity and mortality worldwide, integrating cancer epidemiology with genetic science will also further illuminate complex disease processes, giving rise to novel approaches in prevention, detection at an early stage, and treatments (Figure 14.11).

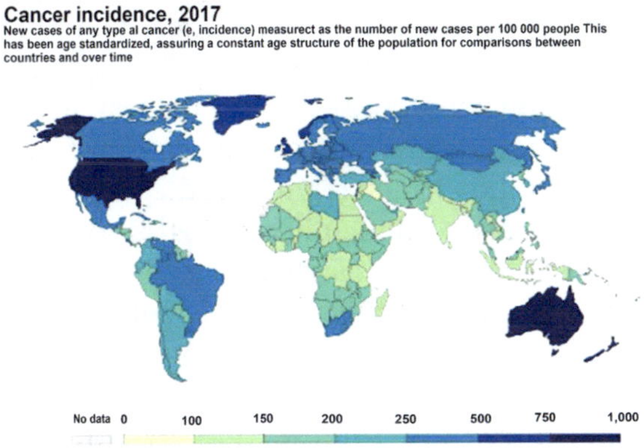

Figure 14.11. Age-adjusted, new cases of cancer, 2017.

Source: https://upload.wikimedia.org/wikipedia/commons/9/94/Cancer_incidence%2C_OWID.svg.

14.4.2. Cardiovascular Diseases (CVD)

The intricate interplay of genetics and CVD has been a significant domain of interest in the field of genetic epidemiology. As CVD remains a leading cause of death globally, it is vital to identify the genetic etiologies of such diseases. Recent advances in genome-wide association studies have identified numerous genetic variants that contribute to CVD by influencing various physiological processes. For example, some loci implicated in the QT interval—a critical element in cardiac repolarization—have been implicated in predisposing individuals to life-threatening arrhythmias and sudden death. Experiments identify that shared variations at NOS1AP and PLN positions are strongly associated with QT interval length, which suggests that genetic predispositions can cause clinically relevant electrophysiological changes that place individuals at heightened risk of cardiovascular events (Andrew et al., 2009). This illustrates the potential of genetic discoveries to guide prevention and treatment measures in cardiovascular disease in the future. With the exception of arrhythmias, coronary heart disease (CAD) has a well-established example wherein genetic factors contribute to cardiovascular risk. Meta-analysis of GWAS on a large population has revealed known and novel genetic loci associated with CAD. The research has confirmed established knowledge about common single-nucleotide polymorphisms (SNPs) and, in addition, has revealed new loci implicated in particular biological processes in the vascular system. The discovery of 10 novel loci, with some expressing additive and others of recessive inheritance models, is evidence of the complexity of CAD genetics and the significance of obtaining a clear view of fine genetic architecture (Alver et al., 2015). These findings not only advance the understanding of CAD etiology but also bring genetic screening into focus as a tool for risk assessment and targeted intervention. Furthermore, the impact of genetic research extends beyond the level of individual risk factors to promote a shift in the paradigm used to deal with cardiovascular disease from the public health perspective. Through determining genetic predisposition to CVD, medical professionals can implement more advanced prevention strategies tailored to one's genetic makeup. For example, recognition of the inherited nature of certain QT interval alterations can lead to increased monitoring of individuals with a family history of arrhythmias. Similarly, results for CAD genetic structure could help elucidate lifestyle and therapeutic interventions for individuals carrying high-risk alleles. With developments in genetic epidemiology, it has the potential to transform cardiovascular health practices, from predictive screening to customized treatment regimens, ultimately leading to healthier outcomes in populations at risk of cardiovascular disorders (Figure 14.12).

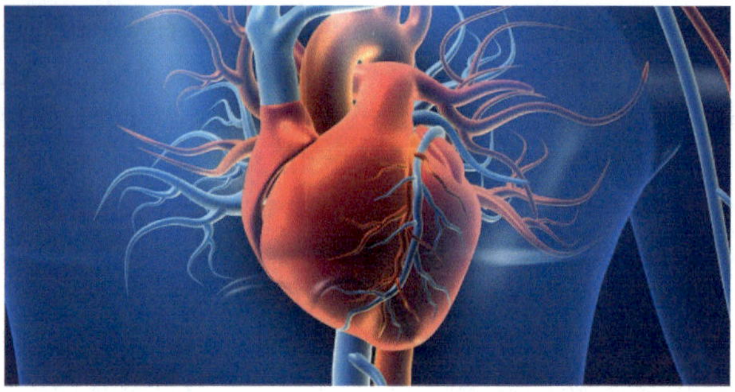

Figure 14.12. Cardiovascular diseases.

Source: https://dvl2h13awlxkt.cloudfront.net/assets/general-images/Knowledge/_1200x630_crop_center-center_82_none/CVD-iStock-1266230179.jpg?mtime=1653282867.

14.4.3. Infectious Diseases

The field of genetic epidemiology is an important science in the investigation of infectious diseases, as it unites the scientific fields of genetics, epidemiology, and microbiology to account for how genetic heterogeneity influences susceptibility and transmissibility to illness. Infectious diseases, being resultant from pathogens such as bacteria, viruses, and parasites, present unique challenges to public health. A close examination of their incidence and prevalence trends allows the detection of high-risk groups by health authorities, upon which they design targeted interventions. A specific perception of disease epidemiology guides the design of effective public health interventions. For example, while the developed world would be able to utilize better epidemiological data in combating outbreaks, underdeveloped and developing countries lack the ability to carry out sophisticated surveillance, something that could enhance the disease burden on vulnerable populations (Akthar et al., 2019). One key component of genetic epidemiology involves the use of molecular typing techniques to analyze the genetic heterogeneity of infectious agents. Understanding the genetic make-up of such microbes is central to effective disease management, as with #*Xanthomonas citri*# pv. #citri#, which is a virulent citrus plantation pest worldwide. Using techniques such as insertion sequence ligation-mediated PCR and multilocus variable-number tandem-repeat analysis, researchers have shown that such tools yield vital information regarding population dynamics and transmission modes of the pathogens. The findings determine substantial polymorphism rates in strains, which highlights the importance of genetic variation to epidemiological research. Possessing such extensive awareness is pivotal in formulating effective control measures and directing public health response to lower infectious disease burden (Ngoc et al., 2010). Furthermore, the intersection of infectious diseases and genetic epidemiology creates the necessity for interdisciplinary teams to enhance surveillance and response capacity. With the rise of new infectious diseases such as COVID-19, the importance of learning about genetic factors continues to grow. The virulence of pathogens in adapting to new environmental pressures and host dynamics underscores the necessity for genetic data to track evolution and resistance patterns. Deploying genetic epidemiological methods can enhance predictions of outbreaks and inform vaccine research and development, leading eventually to stronger public health systems. Methods based on solid genetic analysis can inform policy guidelines across the globe, so that preventative approaches are both effective and just. Such an integrative process not only tackles existing challenges in dealing with infectious disease but also positions societies for possible future pandemics (Akthar et al., 2019) (Figure 14.13).

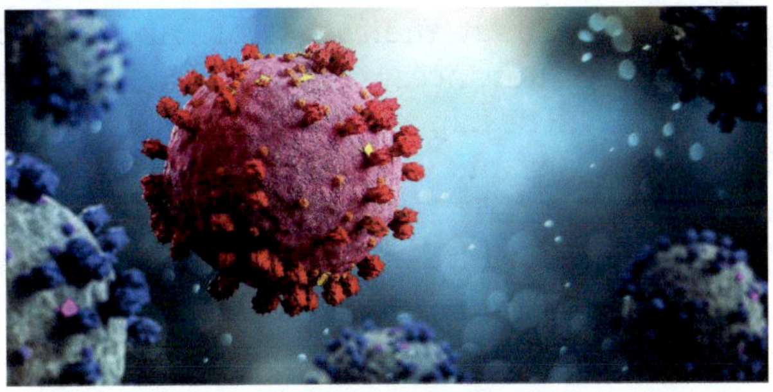

Figure 14.13. Infectious diseases.

Source: https://www.ctsu.ox.ac.uk/images/research/coronavirus/responsive_image?ratio=image&scale=w760.

14.5. Ethical Considerations

In genetic epidemiology, ethics become paramount because they dictate the behavior of researchers and clinicians as they navigate the complex arena of genetic information. The demarcation between prenatal screening and genetic screening demonstrates the need for precise definitions and ethical guidelines. Lack of clarity in terminology can generate disinformation in the public and among health professionals, which ultimately influences patient autonomy and informed consent. When genetic screening is equated with prenatal screening, the patient may misinterpret the nature and meaning of the tests available. Clarification of such semantic nuances helps mark the ethical ground, enabling stakeholders to make informed decisions on the basis of ascertainable facts as to screening choice and potential consequences (Alderson et al., 2001). Moreover, the consequence of genetic information extends to society in general from certain patients, leading to questions of privacy and discrimination. With the advancement in genetic epidemiology, there is a possibility for stigmatization of individuals on the basis of genetic risk factors. For instance, findings from trials like the SELECT trial indicate that it becomes simpler to identify the genetic risk factors for conditions like prostate cancer (Ahmed et al., 2020). But without strict codes of ethics, this information can be misused by employers or insurers, and thus, gene discrimination is made possible. Ethical guidelines must therefore ensure that genetic information is handled in the utmost confidentiality and precautionary measures to protect people from such stigmatization. Additionally, the ethical consideration of consent and use of genetic information must also address the inequality of access to genetic screening technologies. As developments in genetic epidemiology have a tendency to occur at a speed, disparities in access can increase existing health disparities. Among populations that have restricted access to healthcare, the ability to use genetic screening will probably be tremendously overextended, which raises issues about the equity of outcomes in health. Policymakers thus need to develop policies that maximize not just the appropriate utilization of genetic data, but also allow for equity and representation. By making ethical considerations a top priority in genetic epidemiology, the discipline can make a more equitable and inclusive healthcare system with benefits for all populations and not just a privileged few (Alderson et al., 2001).

14.5.1. Informed Consent in Genetic Research

Informed consent is one of the central principles in genetic studies to protect participants' autonomy while simultaneously addressing matters related to ethics in the application of genetic information. With growing genetic epidemiology, complex issues of informed consent also rise, particularly when working with vulnerable groups such as children. The ethical dilemma comes with balancing the inherent right of such subjects to gain access or withhold genetic information, often termed as the right not to know. As genetic testing increases, especially via direct-to-consumer interfaces and innovations in next-generation sequencing technologies, there is a need to respect this right while procuring adequate consent protocols. Incapacity to make well-informed decisions on one's genetic information has the capacity to lead to psychological distress or unwanted outcomes for children, thus requiring strong ethical frameworks for consent protocols among this vulnerable population (Borry et al., 2014). Furthermore, the role of biobanks in genetic research introduces new complexities to the issue of informed consent. Biobanks, which are stores of biological samples and associated information, are central to driving biomedical research forward, but the equitable availability of the material relies on well-coordinated consent procedures. While access to samples and data is typically provided by most biobanks, the conditions under which that access is granted constitute a balancing of economic and educational interests that can keep data from being freely shared. Scientists are usually requested to describe their intentions for using such resources, which creates barriers to the openness and cooperation that are needed for scientific progress. In this process, informed consent is to be modified to not only protect individual rights but also make biobank resources more universally accessible for the general welfare of society (Anagnostou et al., 2016). The increase in complexity relative to informed consent in genetic studies requires ongoing debates and streamlining of regulations. Legislatures, bioethicists, and scientists have to collaborate to balance methods that enhance transparency with preserving participant autonomy. This alliance is particularly vital in consideration of the implications of genetic information that may affect multiple family members, broadening the notion of consent from more than one individual to an understanding of genetic risk factors within a community. Furthermore, continuous education on the implications of genetic research, including the right not to know, should be integrated into the consent process to continue informing participants about their choices. As genetic epidemiology advances, reframing the consent discussion will be important in balancing respect for individual rights with maximizing scientific and social benefit from genetic discoveries (Borry et al., 2014; Anagnostou et al., 2016) (Figure 14.14).

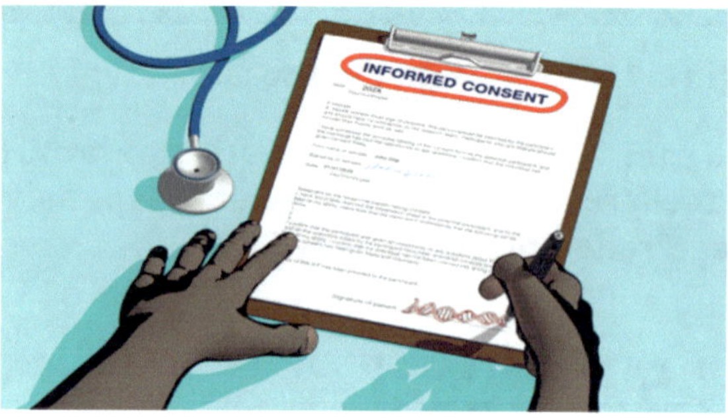

Figure 14.14. Informed consent in genetic research.

Source: https://www.genome.gov/sites/default/files/media/images/2022-01/patient-consent-dyn.jpg.

14.5.2. Privacy and Data Protection

With the still-young field of genetic epidemiology, the intersection of data protection and privacy is increasingly crucial. Because studies typically involve the collection and manipulation of sensitive data on individuals, researchers have been increasingly challenged about how they handle it. Genetic data, for instance, can have the ability to disclose not just an individual's risk for developing a particular disease, but also its implications for relatives, establishing ethical hurdles in consent and confidentiality. The fundamental privacy principles of keeping data collection to a minimum and storing and processing it safely must be followed with close consideration. The tension between scientific progress and the ethical obligation to protect people's rights is a dilemma, and privacy procedures thus become an integral part of any research plan in this sensitive area. Further, the multi-institutional and differential regulatory character of genetic epidemiology complicates data sharing and privacy enforcement. Extensive studies are greatly reliant on cross-institution data sharing that is derailed by the lack of uniform privacy safeguards in multiple jurisdictions. Increased data privacy issues have led to calls for robust privacy-preserving approaches. For instance, new advances in computational methodology attempt to seal off data in collaborative environments by way of solid cryptography and distributed computing infrastructure. By safeguarding models such as regularized logistic regression, researchers can examine sensitive data without infringing on privacy legislation or ethics. Such innovations reflect a paradigm shift in data protection in genetic epidemiology, driven by prioritizing composite solutions that enable collaboration and confidentiality (Li et al., 2015). The effects of adequate privacy and data protection are not limited to ethical considerations; they are part of accelerating genetic science and its integrity. If participants feel their genetic information is being threatened, this may create resistance to participation at the cost of validity and representativeness of research findings. Maintaining trust, hence, through transparency in data sharing and unambiguous communication of privacy controls is imperative. Furthermore, adopting best practices will not only elevate participation by respondents but also improve data quality through stronger participation from a wide range of populations. With the evolving genetic epidemiology scene, ethical seriousness in sensitivity to concerns of privacy will cultivate an environment that welcomes research ethics in regard to human dignity and rights, thereby creating space for scientific inquiry while guaranteeing the foundation of individual privacy (Beth et al., 2013) (Figure 14.15).

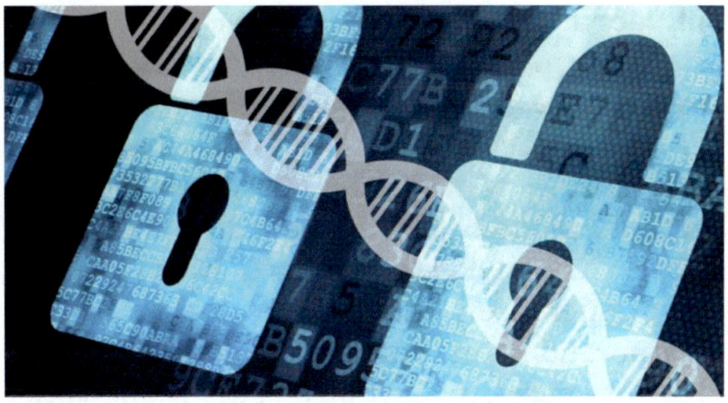

Figure 14.15. Privacy and data protection.

Source: https://geneticliteracyproject.org/wp-content/uploads/elementor/thumbs/privacy-pe4uw8hgsoyd9eery5ry9ysz8kv65ye8y31zbf1nns.jpg.

14.5.3. Implications of Genetic Testing

The uses of genetic testing in genetic epidemiology are multifaceted, and they influence not only individual disease outcomes but also public health policy. With its widespread use, it has the potential to identify individuals at risk of specific diseases, which would lead the way for early intervention, potentially altering the course of diseases significantly. For instance, improvements in genetic testing have been utilized to develop polygenic hazard scores to predict the age at onset for early-onset aggressive prostate cancer for early screening and preventive care. The ability to stratify risk based on genetic markers is transforming the future of controlling diseases like prostate cancer in clinical practice, underscoring the role of personalized medicine in optimizing survival and quality of life in patients. In addition, these technologies have the potential to optimize resource allocation in health systems by streamlining screening to high-risk populations, improving efficiency. Furthermore, the ethical and social concerns associated with genetic testing must be taken seriously as they relate to genetic epidemiology. Since genetic information can reveal personal details not only about the individual, but also his or her relatives, privacy as well as discrimination are at stake. Use of genetic information for predictive purposes raises issues around the responsibility of medical professionals to report such information and the potential psychological impact on individuals who are informed they are at increased risk for a certain disease. Incorporation of genetic testing into public health programs necessitates robust policy frameworks that resolve individual privacy issues while making beneficial screenings more accessible. As N/A (2018) argues, an understanding of the implications involves considering both the advantages of early detection and the ethical dilemmas of using genetic information. Balancing both will be fundamental to the effective application of genetic testing in society. Furthermore, the the public's perception of, and understanding of, genetic testing affects its application and effectiveness. Misinformation or lack of knowledge can stigmatize testes or raise unrealistic hopes regarding the power of genetic testing to provide.

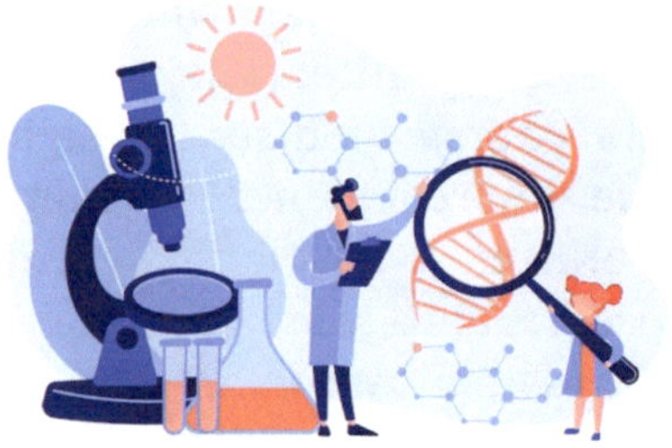

Figure 14.16. The legal and ethical implications of genetic testing.

Source: https://onlinelegaladvisor.in/wp-content/uploads/genetic-1-1.jpg.

Health literacy on genetic risk factors and test results is essential in facilitating informed decision-making among the population through educational interventions. Furthermore, as the genetic test environment continues to evolve, there is a need for healthcare professionals to learn how to guide patients through the complexity of interpreting genetic tests. Awareness programs, in the style of interventions used for other public health campaigns, could potentially promote understanding and acceptance and lead to more empowered health management. Emphasis on the scientific basis of genetic testing while addressing broader social concerns and ethical controversies will be pivotal to effective integration into public health practice (Figure 14.16).

14.6. Future Directions

As genetic epidemiology develops further, its future directions are highly likely to be shaped by technological advances and interdisciplinarity. Integration of genomic sequencing and bioinformatics with epidemiology has the potential to unravel complex genetic architectures and their interactions with environmental determinants. This paradigm shift will not only augment our understanding of disease processes but also simplify the identification of novel biomarkers for diseases such as melanoma. Continued research into melanocyte biology, as highlighted in recent reviews, reiterates the importance of giving high precedence to clinical melanoma and dermatological sciences in order to overcome emerging challenges in diagnosis and treatment. Specifically, by making use of genomics and systems biology advances, investigators will be capable of more effectively dealing with the varied presentations of melanocyte-related diseases and further enhance the design of personalized treatment protocols against the backdrop of specific genetic profiles (Birlea et al., 2018). A highly detailed statistical modeling will also find significance in subsequent genetic epidemiological research. Traditional methods of examining geographical variation in cancer occurrence, such as breast cancer, have provided a foundation for understanding disease patterns; yet they fall short in describing the determinants at play. In addressing such limitations, new models incorporating disparate sources of data are needed. The web-enabled and GIS-based system, as outlined in recent reports, exemplifies how technology can enhance the strength of statistical analysis in genetic epidemiology. These advancements enable scientists and policymakers to better visualize and comprehend complex data, ultimately contributing to a greater insight into why genetic and environmental factors lead to disease emergence (Adya et al., 2001). In the coming years, further emphasis on interdisciplinary collaboration research will undoubtedly enhance the landscape of genetic epidemiology. Opportunities that bring together clinical research, public health programs, and advanced computational approaches will be crucial to deal with the complexity of disease causation. Evaluation of the implications of genetic findings in epidemiology will not only augment the implementation of preventive methodologies but also initiate the formulation of targeted therapies. As the field grows, surmounting huge challenges — inequalities of access to genetic testing and the ethical complications of its use — will be of paramount concern. Lastly, the complementarity of strengths from a diversity of disciplines will provide us with a firm basis for understanding and managing the public health burden of genetic disease.

14.6.1. Advances in Genomic Technologies

The rapid evolution of technologies in genomics has tremendously enhanced our understanding of genetic epidemiology, particularly through the analysis of molecular data. The revolution has improved access to genomic information, which is paramount to advancing public health programs. Molecular surveillance has emerged as a complement to traditional epidemiological studies, with a call for genomic results to contain health problems. Through the conjunction of molecular and epidemiologic principles, researchers are able to design robust surveillance systems that better capture disease trends. This alignment focuses on making standards in study design while enhancing collaboration in interdisciplinary teams to advance the field of genetic epidemiology effectively (Dufour et al., 2015). Recent advances in nucleic acid sequencing and reverse genetics are revolutionizing infectious disease studies, specifically malaria. With the release of mass genomic data sets from Plasmodium species, human populations, and mosquitoes, it has become feasible to have a comprehensive understanding of the interactions during the lifecycle of malaria infections. This has enabled scientists to explore genetic evolution under selective pressure more comprehensively. For instance, identification of mutations in the kelch13 gene with artemisinin resistance has significant implications for treatment approaches. These observations indicate that the application of genomic technologies in genetic epidemiology has a profound influence on public health policy decisions and optimizes disease control measures (Kirchner et al., 2016). With continuing advancements in genomic technologies, their application in genetic epidemiology becomes increasingly vital in developing novel healthcare solutions. The insights of population genomics and genetic analysis guide the design of interventions to avoid drug resistance and enhance disease monitoring. Additionally, the realization of epigenetic regulation and how it controls gene expression has important implications for the dissection of disease etiology. With the field expanding, it is critical that there be a focus on remembering the importance of such technology to proximal healthcare issues. The concerted action of geneticists, epidemiologists, and public health professionals will be essential to bring this knowledge into effect in formulating effective policies and interventions for health that are relevant in different clinical practices (Dufour et al., 2015) (Figure 14.17).

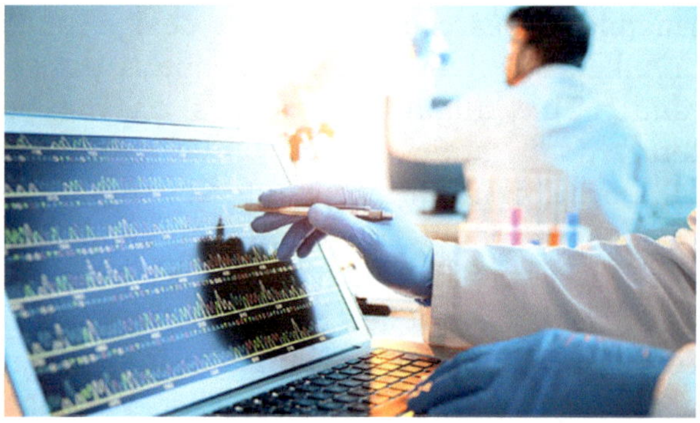

Figure 14.17. Using advanced genomic technologies to improve healthcare outcomes.

Source: https://www.nhcs.com.sg/sites/shcommonassets/Assets/DefiningMed/DefiningMed-2023/genomic-med-sddc-main.jpeg.

14.6.2. Integration of Big Data in Research

The use of Big Data in studies, and in the field of genetic epidemiology in particular, promises to better understand the dynamics of the disease. The use of Big Data facilitates the convergence of enormous amounts of data produced by genomic sequencing, patient medical history data, and the environment, hence giving epidemiological research a holistic perspective. The worth of Big Data is that it can reveal complex patterns and relationships that might go unnoticed by more conventional epidemiological tools. For instance, using molecular surveillance tools sheds light on the evolution of pathogen transmission and virulence by correlating genetic variation with epidemiological endpoints. As outlined in Dufour et al. (2015), interdisciplinarity through the combination of molecular information and established epidemiological practices is necessary, proposing that application of Big Data must complement rather than replace traditional techniques in disease surveillance and investigation. Additionally, the application of next-generation sequencing (NGS) is a classic example of the game-changing application of Big Data in public health research. As highlighted in Boon et al. (2019), NGS not only enhances outbreak investigations by making source tracing more precise but also enables tracing of drug resistance and dynamic transmission patterns of pathogens. This technology allows researchers to assess the development of pathogens based on public health interventions. The incorporation of these advanced genomic tools, however, necessitates an understanding of contextual data quality as well as sampling methods. Without such comprehension, conclusions drawn from Big Data analysis may be short of the level of rigor that can influence effective public health decision-making. An integration of Big Data into genetic epidemiology through strategic means is thus necessary to ensure that its full potential is achieved, as well as to address the challenges in data heterogeneity and complexity. The next direction of incorporating Big Data into genetic epidemiology is the formulation of cross-disciplinary research that synthesizes molecular biology, statistics, and epidemiology information. This is necessary for addressing the data integration and interpretation problem, where scientists balance high-dimensional genomic information with data of interest to clinicians and epidemiologists. As the literature suggests, the shift from research based on study-oriented approaches to the routine use of Big Data applications requires a collective effort towards uniform practice and formulating protocols for data collection and sharing. Global partnerships will be important in aligning across different healthcare settings with the vision of improved public health action. Cooperative efforts toward better data quality and methodological improvement will be key to unlocking the full potential of Big Data for the development of genetic epidemiology.

14.6.3. Potential for Personalized Medicine

The future of individualized medicine is heavily influenced by developments in genetic epidemiology, which examines the interplay between genetic predispositions and susceptibility to disease. Individualized medicine attempts to tailor medical intervention to particular traits, including genetic backgrounds, in an effort to enhance the efficacy of interventions. For instance, the understanding of host genetic markers can powerfully direct treatment, especially against such high-priority health issues as hepatitis C virus (HCV) infection. Where disease prevalence is high, e.g., in Latin America, such knowledge of genetic variants predictive of treatment response can be employed to assist clinicians in triaging individuals for DAAs even where access to the therapies remains restricted. Not only does this hold more promise of personalized outcomes, but it also optimizes healthcare resource use in settings where treatment costs are high and patient responses are variable. In addition, genetic knowledge in personalized medicine extends to infectious diseases alone and is utilized in various fields, including cardiology. One wonderful example is the identification of loci for QT-interval lengthening, a significant prognostic factor for cardiac potentially lethal diseases. It has been demonstrated by research that every 8–10% of QT-interval variance has an explanation by common genetic variants, reflecting the interweaving relationship between gene expression and cardiac repolarization processes. Identification of such variants not only enhances stratification of risk for diseases like long-QT syndrome (LQTS) but also informs treatment regimens that can reduce arrhythmia and sudden cardiac death (SCD) risk. Hence, awareness regarding genetic variation enables clinicians to initiate prophylactic measures and make therapeutic strategies patient-specific. In accordance with the expansion of genetic epidemiology, the integration of genetic information into practice is about to reshape customary treatment models. Personalized medicine becomes increasingly characterized by precision, with treatment decisions being led by an individual's unique genetic makeup. The promise for the application of pharmacogenomics, as evidenced in curing HCV and cardiovascular diseases, underscores the revolutionary potential of genetic data on patient care. This change needs a complete rethinking of existing healthcare systems to incorporate genetic testing and personalized interventions as part of standard practice. As more talk of personalized medicine and genetic epidemiology is being done, it is not just essential to learn the science behind it but also to offer reassurance for ethical concerns and proper access to these developments for all patient groups (Figure 14.18).

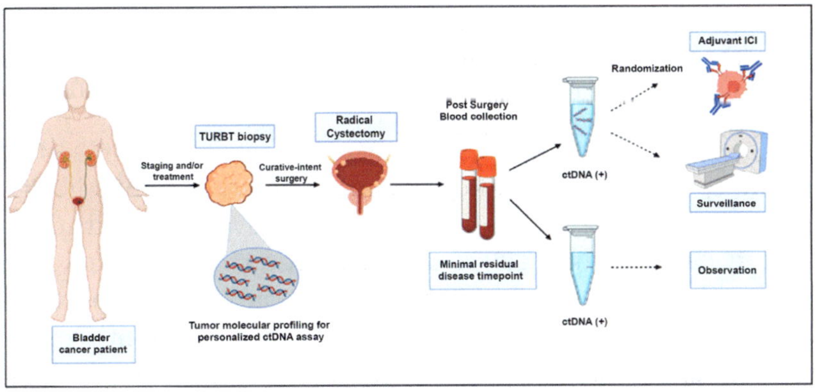

Figure 14.18. A figure showing the potential for personalized medicine.

Source: https://www.researchgate.net/publication/373628516/figure/fig1/AS:11431281203395078@1699297148938/A-figure-showing-the-potential-for-personalized-medicine.png.

Summary

The foray into the field of genetic epidemiology has greatly elucidated our knowledge of disease prevalence and the interaction of genetic and environmental contributions to the development of health outcomes. Studies have shown that hypertension, for instance, has different prevalence rates among various racial groups. The results showing that there is a variation in hypertension prevalence of 27 to 55% in white populations and 14 to 44% in black populations highlight the importance of taking into account both environmental and genetic predispositions in health disparities. Notably, even with the susceptibility that African-derived populations appear to have to hypertension, the evidence allows for the consideration that environmental factors, over mere differences in nature, could be accounting for such differences and necessitate an interdisciplinary approach to genetic epidemiology to inform public health interventions and policy development for improving health equity across different populations (Adeyemo et al., 2005). In addition, the relationship between B-type natriuretic peptide (BNP) concentration and type 2 diabetes (T2D) illustrates the complex interaction between genetic factors and metabolic disease. Studies reveal a potential inverse relationship between NT-pro-BNP concentration and susceptibility to T2D, thus hinting at the potential causal role of BNP in T2D pathogenesis. The findings that increased levels of NT-pro-BNP are linked with reduced risk of developing T2D provide further support for the importance of studying such genetic loci as rs198389. These types of studies not only enhance our understanding regarding the biochemical pathways to disease but also highlight the needfor more research studies to clarify the causative processes. The incorporation of genetic variables with environmental conditions provides a more understandable picture of disease development and prevention strategies in genetic epidemiology (Meirhaeghe et al., 2011). In summary, genetic epidemiology is an essential paradigm in the study of health determinants by acknowledging the complexity of the determinants of disease. The combination of genetic, environmental, and lifestyle determinants forms a more inclusive framework for understanding health differences and disease susceptibility. There is a need for further research that focuses on interdisciplinary collaborations to advance methodology and build on existing knowledge in this area. By considering the function of both genetic and non-genetic factors, public health interventions can be formulated in such a way that they better target specific population needs. Overall, the development of the field of genetic epidemiology has the massive potential for developing evidence-based targeted interventions in decreasing disease burdens among different populations and toward a healthier community (Adeyemo et al., 2005; Meirhaeghe et al., 2011).

The field of genetic epidemiology is a key boundary between public health and genetics that describes how genetic susceptibility plays a role in the prevalence and incidence of disease in populations. Through systematic analysis of the interaction between environmental exposures and genetic variations, researchers can understand the etiology of complex disorders. As science increasingly uses advanced genomic technologies, the capacity for identifying genetic markers for specific health outcomes has expanded significantly. This expansion emphasizes the importance of interdisciplinary strategies with a wide array of participants, as emphasized in recent workshops addressing the health of specific breeds among dogs. These collaborative efforts are aimed at optimal breeding practices, control of breed-specific disorders, and bringing about the necessary advances in genetic information within the purview of public health interest (Bartels et al., 2017). Further, integration of landscape epidemiology with genetics also provides a unique insight through the depiction of how disease processes are influenced by environmental factors. By integrating molecular approaches with spatial analyses, scientists are better able to understand infectious disease transmission, particularly in home environments such as dog rabies. Targeting human contact, mobility, and socio-cultural dimensions makes disease transmission more challenging to address. For instance, understanding how anthropogenic landscapes may act as barriers or facilitators to pathogen movement significantly enhances planning for disease control intervention. This perspective stresses intervention tailored to genetic susceptibility as well as to environmental exposures, and thus genetic epidemiology becomes an integrative model for dealing with public health issues (Anderson et al., 2012). Lastly, the dynamic character of genetic epidemiology underscores the necessity of continued data gathering and evidence-based policy-making. As results of genetic and epidemiologic studies inform public health initiatives, it is increasingly necessary to build continuity between research, clinicians, and policymakers. The International Dog Health Workshops are one such example of this collaborative spirit that is so desperately needed to develop implementable strategies addressing the genetics-driven health disparities. The dynamic interaction between extensive scientific inquiry and community engagement finally inspires a more robust public health approach, efficient in addressing and mitigating the impact of genetic and environmental health conditions that affect diverse populations (Bartels et al., 2017).

CLOSER LOOK

THE ROLE OF GENETIC EPIDEMIOLOGY IN FUTURE RESEARCH

The emergence of genetic epidemiology is of broad promise for the research of the future, and particularly so as it intersects across multiple areas of public health. As populations face an increasing number of illnesses—genetic, infectious, and metabolic diseases—there is a compelling necessity for learning about disease mechanisms. Genetic epidemiology offers a systematic approach to examining how genetic predisposition interacts with the environment to yield health outcomes. By including information from this field, researchers can develop targeted prevention schemes that address not only recognizable disease issues but also account for differences in disease prevalence among populations. Nevertheless, research work in the field must be boosted in underdeveloped and developing nations, where focus on disease epidemiology remains disproportionately low. Through the use of genetic epidemiological data, these regions can use targeted public health interventions, ultimately leading to lowering the disease burden and enhancing overall population health (Akthar et al., 2019).

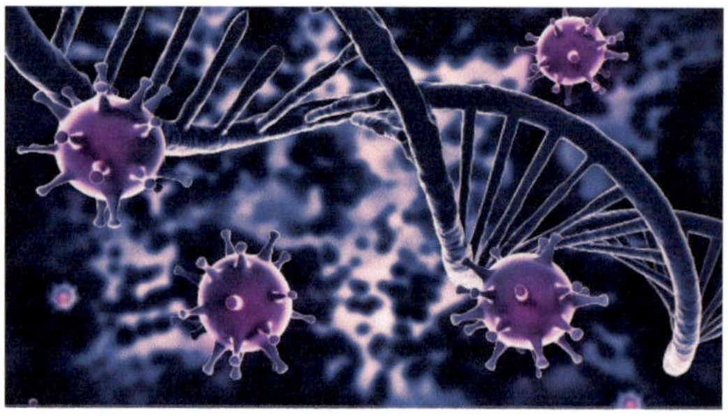

Figure 14.19. Illustration of viral particles interacting with DNA strands, representing molecular mechanisms of infection or gene therapy.

*So*urce: https://media.licdn.com/dms/image/v2/D5612AQHSUn_QTHDUiw/article-cover_image-shrink_720_1280/article-cover_image-shrink_720_1280/0/1731427544347?e=2147483647&v=beta&t=G729emPj5oojhKkJ2TrdPreWEmlvk_R7qefci6M6SCY.

Genetic epidemiology can potentially transcend merely identifying risk factors to understanding the complex interplay between the environment and genetics. Extensive cohort studies like the National Children's Study (NCS) are a perfect example of the proactive measures required to unravel these complexities. The NCS is tailored to study the environmental determinants of ill-health conditions such as obesity through a broad life-course research method tracing their effects from preconception to older adolescence. Gene-environment interaction studies, with such an approach, can locate both endogenous genetic susceptibility and exogenous factors that can exacerbate ill-health. The implications are immense; by establishing these relationships, subsequent research can inform public health efforts to address and mitigate risk for pediatric illness, paving the way for healthier generations to come (Carrel et al., 2009). With the evolving refinement of genetic epidemiology, its contribution toward understanding about chronic disease and prevention is of increasingly significant value. The integration of genomic data and traditional epidemiological methods will provide us with a better understanding of disease narratives. Future technological and computational biology advances will enable scientists to analyze vast amounts of data, uncovering complex gene-environment interactions that can significantly influence health outcomes. Future research initiatives must emphasize inter-disciplinary collaborations to make predictive models more precise and enhance the utilization of genetic information in public health. This cross-disciplinary approach will not only guide interventions on an individual basis but also guide policy development to optimize overall community health. While the science continues to evolve, making sure that genetic epidemiology is addressing health inequalities remains a central mission, driving future inquiry into the genetics of disease and health (Akthar et al., 2019) (Figure 14.19).

References

1. Aas, M., Blokland, G. A. M., Chawner, S. J. R. A., Choi, K., et al. (2016). Summaries of plenary, symposia, and oral sessions at the XXII World Congress of Psychiatric Genetics, Copenhagen, Denmark, 12–16 October 2014. https://core.ac.uk/download/227054289.pdf (accessed on 25th June 2025).
2. Abbas, A., Hameed, A., Khaliq, R. Z., Tahir, A., et al. (2023). Colorectal cancer in Pakistan: Genetic, molecular, and epidemiological perspectives. https://core.ac.uk/download/618235908.pdf (accessed on 25th June 2025).
3. Abecasis, G. R., Ackerman, M. J., Adamkova, V., Alonso, A., et al. (2013). Genetic association study of QT interval highlight's role for calcium signaling pathways in myocardial repolarization. https://core.ac.uk/download/29469527.pdf (accessed on 25th June 2025).
4. Abecasis, G., Alam, D. S., Alfred, T., Allison, M. A., et al. (2019). Protein-coding variants implicate novel genes related to lipid homeostasis contributing to body-fat distribution. https://core.ac.uk/download/323066646.pdf (accessed on 25th June 2025).
5. Acosta, N., Carrasco, H. J., Gaunt, M. W., Lewis, M. D., et al. (2009). *Trypanosoma cruzi* IIc: Phylogenetic and phylogeographic insights from sequence and microsatellite analysis and potential impact on emergent Chagas disease. https://core.ac.uk/download/13097915.pdf (accessed on 25th June 2025).
6. Adamo, A., Akopyants, N. S., Anderson, J. M., Antia, R., Azevedo, R., Berry, C., Betson, M., et al. (2015). One Health–An ecological and evolutionary framework for tackling neglected zoonotic diseases. https://core.ac.uk/download/36778696.pdf (accessed on 25th June 2025).
7. Adams, H., Ahmad, S., Ames, D., Amin, N., et al. (2019). Genetic determinants of cortical structure (thickness, surface area and volumes) among disease-free adults in the CHARGE Consortium. https://core.ac.uk/download/231719760.pdf (accessed on 25th June 2025).
8. Adeishvili, E., Babuadze, G., Carrillo, E., Chakhunashvili, G., et al. (2016). Sero epidemiology and molecular diversity of *Leishmania donovani* complex in Georgia. https://core.ac.uk/download/42372260.pdf (accessed on 25th June 2025).
9. Adeyemo, A., Luke, A., Stegmayr, B., Stegmayr, B., Agyemang, C., Grim, C. E., Lane, D., et al. (2005). An international comparative study of blood pressure in populations of European vs. African descent. https://core.ac.uk/download/1669190.pdf (accessed on 25th June 2025).
10. Adya, M., Forgionne, G. A., Gangopadhyay, A., Tan, Y. A., et al. (2001). BCAS: A web-enabled and GIS-based decision support system for the diagnosis and treatment of breast cancer. https://core.ac.uk/download/213082599.pdf (accessed on 25th June 2025).
11. Afaq, S., Afzal, S., Ahlqvist, E., Almgren, P., et al. (2018). Refining the accuracy of validated target identification through coding variant fine-mapping in type 2 diabetes. https://core.ac.uk/download/323077466.pdf (accessed on 25th June 2025).
12. Ahmed, M., Cieza-Borrella, C., Eeles, R., Goh, C., et al. (2020). Germline genetic variation in prostate susceptibility does not predict outcomes in the chemoprevention trials PCPT and SELECT. https://core.ac.uk/download/322366731.pdf (accessed on 25th June 2025).
13. Akthar, M. S. (Muhammad). (2019). Role of epidemiological studies in disease prevention. https://media.neliti.com/media/publications/301058-role-of-epidemiological-studies-in-disea-d4cd7a6e.pdf (accessed on 25th June 2025).

14. Albert, A., Andrieu, N., Bansal, A., Blot, W., Bochud, M., Breslow, R. A., Broeks, A., et al. (2012). Next generation analytic tools for large-scale genetic epidemiology studies of complex diseases. https://deepblue.lib.umich.edu/bitstream/2027.42/93578/1/gepi20652.pdf (accessed on 25th June 2025).

15. Albina, E., Bernardo, P., Eloit, M., Fernandez, M., et al. (2013). Pathology and viral metagenomics, a recent history. http://agritrop.cirad.fr/568021/1/document_568021.pdf (accessed on 25th June 2025).

16. Alderson, P., Aro, A., Dragonas, T., Ettorre, E., et al. (2001). *Prenatal Screening and Genetics*. https://core.ac.uk/download/pdf/83462.pdf (accessed on 25th June 2025).

17. Alver, M., Anand, S. S., Ardissino, D., Armasu, S. M., et al. (2015). A comprehensive 1000 Genomes-based genome-wide association meta-analysis of coronary artery disease. https://core.ac.uk/download/30664565.pdf (accessed on 25th June 2025).

18. Anagnostou, P., Bisol, G. D., Capocasa, M., D'Abramo, F., et al. (2016). Samples and data accessibility in research biobanks: An explorative survey. https://core.ac.uk/download/188827024.pdf (accessed on 25th June 2025).

19. Anderson, R., Cross, P., Cullingham, C. I., Horton, D. L., Dietzschold, B., Eng, T. R., Brunker, K., et al. (2012). Integrating the landscape epidemiology and genetics of RNA viruses: Rabies in domestic dogs as a model. https://core.ac.uk/download/9651666.pdf (accessed on 25th June 2025).

20. Andreassen, O. A., Edenberg, H. J., Faraone, S. V., Glatt, S. J., et al. (2018). Psychiatric genetics and the structure of psychopathology. https://core.ac.uk/download/161229734.pdf (accessed on 25th June 2025).

21. Anker, S. D., Artola, V. A., Benjamin, E. J., Dickstein, K., et al. (2020). Genetic risk and atrial fibrillation in patients with heart failure. https://core.ac.uk/download/286356101.pdf (accessed on 25th June 2025).

22. Appadurai, V., Benros, M. E., Buil, A., Bybjerg-Grauholm, J., et al. (2020). A large population-based investigation into the genetics of susceptibility to gastrointestinal infections and the link between gastrointestinal infections and mental illness. https://core.ac.uk/download/323065495.pdf (accessed on 25th June 2025).

23. Argano, V., Balistreri, C. R., Giarratana, R. M., Lio, A., et al. (2019). On the road to accurate biomarkers for cardiometabolic diseases by integrating precision and gender medicine approaches. https://core.ac.uk/download/268910274.pdf (accessed on 25th June 2025).

24. Ashuach, T., DeTomaso, D., Jones, M. G., Subramaniam, M., et al. (2019). Functional interpretation of single cell similarity maps. https://core.ac.uk/download/323081756.pdf (accessed on 25th June 2025).

25. Assimes, T. L., Berndt, S. I., Bhatia, G., Blot, W. J., et al. (2014). Leveraging population admixture to characterize the heritability of complex traits. https://core.ac.uk/download/323078760.pdf (accessed on 25th June 2025).

26. Bartels, A., AIDAP, Clarke, A. J., Greko, C., et al. (2017). Moving from information and collaboration to action: Report from the 3rd International Dog Health Workshop, Paris in April 2017. https://core.ac.uk/download/141439096.pdf (accessed on 25th June 2025).

27. Beth, A., Dandouras, I., Garnier, P., Mazelle, C., et al. (2013). "Whose data is it anyway?" The

implications of putting small area-level health and social data online. https://core.ac.uk/download/pdf/29026859.pdf (accessed on 25th June 2025).

28. Birlea, S., Bosenberg, M. W., Box, N. F., Brash, D. E., et al. (2018). Frontiers in pigment cell and melanoma research. http://arxiv.org/abs/1808.01869 (accessed on 25th June 2025).
29. Bis, J. C., Boerwinkle, E., Brody, J. A., Butler, J., et al. (2014). Associations of NINJ2 sequence variants with incident ischemic stroke in the Cohorts for Heart and Aging in Genomic Epidemiology (CHARGE) consortium. https://core.ac.uk/download/pdf/296165124.pdf (accessed on 25th June 2025).
30. Boon, N. A. M., Descamps, T., Devleesschauwer, B., Robert, A., et al. (2019). Status and potential of bacterial genomics for public health practice: A scoping review. https://core.ac.uk/download/227041617.pdf (accessed on 25th June 2025).
31. Borry, P., Howard, H., & Shabani, M. (2014). Is there a right time to know? The right not to know and genetic testing in children. https://core.ac.uk/download/237011214.pdf (accessed on 25th June 2025).
32. Bui Thi Ngoc, L., Pruvost, O., Vernière, C., Vital, K., et al. (2010). Investigating the population structure of *Xanthomonas citri* pv. *citri*. Which molecular markers to use to distinguish between low polymorphic bacterial populations? [P–96]. http://agritrop.cirad.fr/555770/1/document_555770.pdf (accessed on 25th June 2025).
33. Canali, S. (2020). What is new about the exposome? Exploring scientific change in contemporary epidemiology. https://core.ac.uk/download/323306328.pdf (accessed on 25th June 2025).
34. Caputo, M., Corach, D., Flichman, D. M., Hulaniuk, M., et al. (2017). Hepatitis C virus pharmacogenomics in Latin American populations: Implications in the era of direct-acting antivirals. https://core.ac.uk/download/159296291.pdf (accessed on 25th June 2025).
35. Carlson, J. C. (2017). Methods for family-based designs in genetic epidemiology studies. https://core.ac.uk/download/85137054.pdf (accessed on 25th June 2025).
36. Carrel, A. L., Cronk, C. E., Durkin, M. S., Gall, S., et al. (2009). Environment and obesity in the National Children's Study. https://core.ac.uk/download/213082314.pdf (accessed on 25th June 2025).
37. Comandini, A., Kumar, A., Fridley, B. L., Martin, B. W., Nickel, C., Tseng, C. F., Schindler, C., et al. (2012). Different genes interact with particulate matter and tobacco smoke exposure in affecting lung function decline in the general population. https://core.ac.uk/download/18261611.pdf (accessed on 25th June 2025).
38. Costa, R., & Frezza, G. (2014). Crossovers between epigenesis and epigenetics: A multicenter approach to the history of epigenetics (1901–1975). https://core.ac.uk/download/144472860.pdf (accessed on 25th June 2025).
39. Didelez, V., Meng, S., & Sheehan, N. A. (2010). Assumptions of IV methods for observational epidemiology. http://arxiv.org/abs/1011.0595 (accessed on 25th June 2025).
40. Dufour, S., Muellner, P., Stärk, K. D. C., Zadoks, R. N., et al. (2015). 'Next-generation' surveillance: An epidemiologists' perspective on the use of molecular information in food safety and animal health decision-making. https://core.ac.uk/download/46567794.pdf (accessed on 25th June 2025).

41. Falk, A., Ellingboe, A. H., Ellingboe, A. H., Slusarenko, A. J., Rehmany, A. P., Rehmany, A. P., Riethmüller, A., et al. (2008). Natural history of *Arabidopsis thaliana* and oomycete symbioses. https://core.ac.uk/download/105273.pdf (accessed on 25th June 2025).

42. Ghazal, T. M., Hasan, M. K., Alshurideh, M. T., Alzoubi, H. M., Ahmad, M., Akbar, S. S., Al Kurdi, B., et al. (2021). IoT for smart cities: Machine learning approaches in smart healthcare—A review. *Future Internet, 13*, 218–218. https://doi.org/10.3390/fi13080218 (accessed on 25th June 2025).

43. Hariri, A. R., Viding, E., & Williamson, D. E. (2006). Developmental imaging genetics: Challenges and promises for translational research. https://core.ac.uk/download/1674206.pdf (accessed on 25th June 2025).

44. Kirchner, S., Power, B. J., & Waters, A. P. (2016). Recent advances in malaria genomics and epigenomics. https://core.ac.uk/download/46580201.pdf (accessed on 25th June 2025).

45. Kitsiou, A., Caforio, A. L. P., Porta-Sanchez, A., Vahanian, A., Iung, B., Carrera, C., Szymanski, C., et al. (2013). ESC core curriculum for the general cardiologist (2013). https://core.ac.uk/download/55756305.pdf (accessed on 25th June 2025).

46. Laird, N. M., & Lange, C. (2009). The role of family-based designs in genome-wide association studies. http://arxiv.org/abs/1010.4629 (accessed on 25th June 2025).

47. Leitner, T., & Romero-Severson, E. (2018). Phylogenetic patterns recover known HIV epidemiological relationships and reveal common transmission of multiple variants. https://core.ac.uk/download/323062609.pdf (accessed on 25th June 2025).

48. Li, W., Liu, H., Xie, W., Yang, M., et al. (2015). Supporting regularized logistic regression privately and efficiently. http://arxiv.org/abs/1510.00095 (accessed on 25th June 2025).

49. Meirhaeghe, A., Ropero, A. B., Tabak, A. G., Meirhaeghe, A., Voight, B. F., Newton-Cheh, C., Sengenes, C., et al. (2011). Mendelian randomization study of B-type natriuretic peptide and type 2 diabetes: Evidence of causal association from population studies. https://core.ac.uk/download/1437139.pdf (accessed on 25th June 2025).

50. N/A. (2018). Polygenic hazard score to guide screening for aggressive prostate cancer: Development and validation in large scale cohorts. https://core.ac.uk/download/151178451.pdf (accessed on 25th June 2025).

51. Njajou, O. T. (Omer). (2002). A genetic epidemiologic study of hemochromatosis. https://core.ac.uk/download/18513610.pdf (accessed on 25th June 2025).

52. Paterson, A. D., Dominiczak, A., Pfeufer, A., Wallace, C., Newton-Cheh, C., Dalageorgou, C., Arking, D. E., et al. (2009). Common genetic variation near the phospholamban gene is associated with cardiac repolarization: Meta-analysis of three genome-wide association studies. https://core.ac.uk/download/6179341.pdf (accessed on 25th June 2025).

53. Smolarz, B., Szyłło, K., & Romanowicz, H. (2021). Endometriosis: Epidemiology, classification, pathogenesis, treatment and genetics (Review of literature). *International Journal of Molecular Sciences, 22*, 10554–10554. https://doi.org/10.3390/ijms221910554 (accessed on 25th June 2025).

54. Tait, A., Hide, G., Gibson, W., Mehlitz, D., & Morrison, L. (2009). Molecular epidemiology of African sleeping sickness. https://core.ac.uk/download/1662859.pdf (accessed on 25th June 2025).

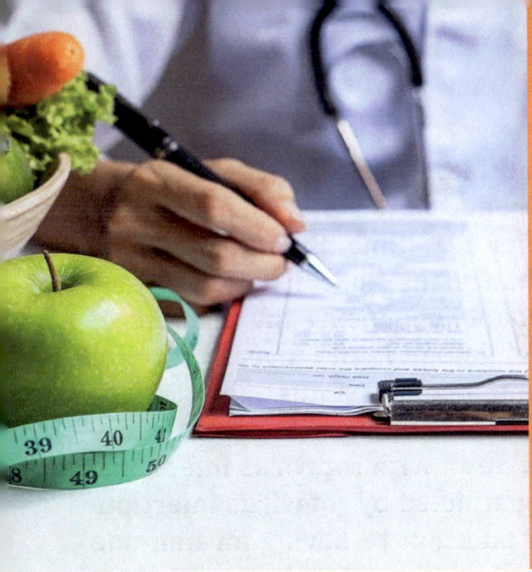

Chapter 15

NUTRITIONAL EPIDEMIOLOGY

Contents

Introduction

Nutritional epidemiology is an important subspecialty of epidemiology that investigates the relationship between dietary patterns and disease outcomes within human populations. By various study designs, including cohort, case-control, and cross-sectional studies, nutritional epidemiologists can assess the role of specific nutrients or food groups in the risk for chronic diseases such as obesity, diabetes, and cardiovascular disease. The field makes an important contribution to public health, as it shapes advice and policy intended to promote healthier eating and lower the incidence of diet-related diseases. Moreover, as diet is partly set by economic, social, and cultural determinants, nutritional epidemiology also illuminates the ways that such determinants interact and generate inequalities in health in populations. One of the more significant fields of interest in nutritional epidemiology is genetic susceptibility to obesity and body mass index (BMI). Emerging evidence indicates relationships between gene polymorphism, such as the fat mass and obesity-associated gene (FTO), and the traits of obesity. For instance, a study tracked the German GINI-plus and LISA-plus birth cohorts from birth through six years of age. It found that the impact of FTO genotype on BMI changes with age, suggesting that genetic effects may interact with eating habits over time. By studying such interactions between genes, nutritional epidemiologists can enhance the specificity of dietary interventions and recommendations to various population subgroups, enhancing the chances of effective weight reduction. A second key area of nutritional epidemiology is the investigation of infectious disease prevalence influenced by diet, as the interaction of nutritional status and rotavirus disease in children shows. In Mwanza, a study conducted discovered that children with acute watery diarrhea, an illness exacerbated by dehydration, had a strong correlation with rotavirus infections. In such children, malnutrition had increased the likelihood of being afflicted by rotavirus infection. This speaks to the importance of receiving the right nutrition in addition to having an immune system that will not be compromised by infectious diseases. By establishing these relationships between nutrition and health outcomes, nutritional epidemiology makes it essential to provide key information to guide effective public health interventions for the improvement of food consumption patterns, health equity, and reduction of disease burden (Figure 15.1).

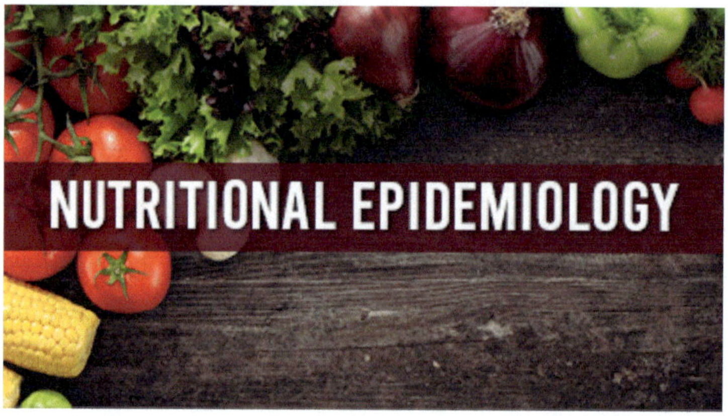

Figure 15.1. Nutritional epidemiology.

Source: https://www.alliedacademies.com/cms/track-images/1966-fsat-2022.jpg.

Definition and Scope of Nutritional Epidemiology

Nutritional epidemiology is a scientific field encompassing investigations of the contribution of diet and intake of single nutrients to the determination of health effects and disease risk in populations. This observational epidemiologic field aims to establish food consumption-related associations with health indicators and incidence of disease, whose data are important for public health action. It integrates epidemiologic and nutrition science methods to analyze data on observational studies, clinical trials, and diets. By monitoring dietary trends and identifying their impact on health outcomes, scientists can elucidate the multifaceted functions of nutrition in disease prevention and management. The ontology of nutritional epidemiology (ONE) activates this field by ensuring systematic frameworks of data combination and analysis, thereby facilitating improved comprehension of dietetic impacts on markers of health and disease patterns (Ambayo et al., 2019). Expanding from its etymology, nutritional epidemiology covers a wide range of human health and happiness. It looks beyond the direct impact of food choice on chronic conditions such as obesity, diabetes, and cardiovascular disease but also probes the role of dietary components as mediators within complex biobehavioral pathways. Researchers in this area are concerned with the relationship between nutrition, genetic vulnerabilities, environmental factors, and lifestyle factors. The analysis of targeted populations also adds to insights into how cultural, socio-economic, and demographic factors influence food habits and outcomes related to health. Central to these research is the linkage of all-around data resources, as evidenced by ONE, which supports navigating through the vast data universe to uncover realities regarding food-nutrient-disease relationships (Slee et al., 2012). Besides, nutritional epidemiology is also key in informing public health policy and nutrition recommendations. Nutritional epidemiologists generate evidence-based data on the associations between nutrition and health conditions, and this leads to the development of strategies that seek to stem the burden of diet-related disease. The best dietary recommendations are applied, and the combination of effective interventions tailored to populations and communities calls for ongoing research. With the evolving fields of nutritional epidemiology, it is all the more capable of addressing contemporary public health concerns, particularly in view of increasing global commitments to health and nutrition-related problems such as obesity and malnutrition. With the refinement of knowledge in the field, everyone can work together towards support for healthier diets that are more in line with scientific evidence, eventually realizing better health outcomes at a population level (Ambayo et al., 2019; Slee et al., 2012).

Importance of Studying Nutrition in Public Health

Recognition of the contribution of nutrition to public health is vital in constructing efficient intervention models to improve population health outcomes. Nutrition has a central role to play in the prevention of a myriad of chronic illnesses like obesity, diabetes, and cardiovascular conditions. Public health interventions focusing on dietary behaviors have the potential to open doors to healthier communities, reducing healthcare spending and improving quality of life. There is also a clear understanding of nutritional epidemiology that informs public health practitioners about the relationship between nutrition, lifestyle, and the determinants of good health and facilitates the application of evidence-based specific interventions. Additionally, with the aging population experiencing illnesses compounded by an inappropriate diet, understanding nutrition is imperative. It allows the determination of categorical nutritional needs among different populations, particularly vulnerable populations, thus ensuring equal progress in good health in society. Moreover, the inclusion of cutting-edge research on the nutrition-disease risk interface can enhance public health education and policy. Current evidence demonstrates how various nutrients and dietary patterns relate to disease prevention, suggesting a need for a holistic grasp of nutritional epidemiology. For instance, some dietary factors, such as antioxidants and fiber, have proven roles in reducing inflammation and metabolic health. This data is crucial because public health interventions aim to educate populations on food decision-making that reduces disease risk. Through the science of nutrition, public health policy can advance from immediate responses to preventive ones that encourage healthier eating patterns. The capability of influencing community health through carefully informed nutritional counsel makes interdisciplinary collaboration between nutritionists, epidemiologists, and public health professionals more critical. Finally, looking at nutrition in terms of public health fosters a wide conceptualization of health that extends beyond the level of individual choice. Several factors, such as socioeconomic status, cultural considerations, and access to healthy food, influence nutritional practice significantly. Public health professionals acknowledge that these determinants offer the channels through which they can advocate for policies that enhance food security, enhance access to healthy food, and foster nutritional awareness. For instance, initiatives like school nutrition education or community garden projects can establish healthier environments and support long-term nutritional change. Addressing disparities in nutrition health status is a key aspect of public health and nutrition. Such extensive research within nutritional epidemiology is thus vital in shaping the policies intended to bridge these gaps so that all can be accorded access to the potential of healthier living and, in the process, increase the commitment to public health equity (Figure 15.2).

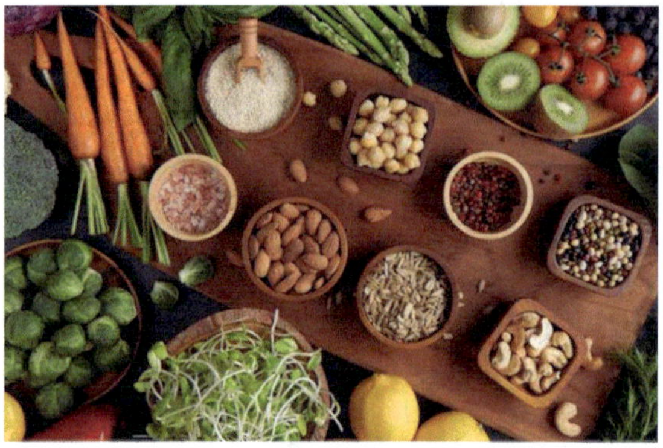

Figure 15.2. Importance of nutrition in maintaining a healthy lifestyle and preventing diseases.

Source: https://www.kemhospitalpune.org/wp-content/uploads/2023/10/importance-of-nutrition.jpg.

15.1. Methodologies in Nutritional Epidemiology

The approaches employed by nutritional epidemiology are at the core of explaining the complex interplay among diet, health, and disease in human populations. The approaches are more likely to include observational studies, and these include cross-sectional, cohort, or case-control studies. Cross-sectional surveys investigate dietary intake and health status at one point in time and provide a snapshot capable of raising associations but not causation. Cohort studies, in which populations are followed up longitudinally, enable investigators to determine the effect of long-term diet on health. Retrospective case-control studies examine dietary exposures in subjects with specified conditions versus those not having these conditions and can be used to identify potential risk factors. Each of these designs has unique strengths and limitations and, therefore, demands a judicious selection of design based on research questions and available resources.

The second most important field of nutritional epidemiology is the measurement of dietary intake, which is beset by numerous challenges and requires innovative strategies. Among the most frequent methods of measuring dietary intake are food frequency questionnaires (FFQs), 24-hour dietary recall, and food diaries. FFQs allow for the global estimation of typical dietary intake by measuring frequency of use during a specified period, while 24-hour recalls provide detailed information on food use over a day. However, such methods can be vulnerable to biases, such as underreporting or recall bias, that complicate the interpretation of findings. To address such constraints, researchers increasingly employ technology-based solutions, such as smartphone apps and web-based food diaries, that have the potential to reduce errors and engage participants maximally. With the expansion of the discipline, such methods must be continually refined to provide trustworthy data on the intricate relationship between diet and health. Moreover, the integration of ecological models of health behavior becomes increasingly relevant in nutritional epidemiology, particularly when evaluating macro-level diet patterns within groups. This is due to the fact that it considers that individual diets are shaped by a myriad of variables like societal norms, environmental cues, and socio-economic status. Schools, for example, are regarded as central sites where healthy eating habits need to be ingrained from childhood. School-based interventions to promote healthy eating often utilize ecological models that engage multiple stakeholders, including teachers, parents, and public health professionals. Understanding the dynamics between these players can assist researchers in designing improved interventions that consider cultural and contextual factors affecting eating habits. This integrated approach not only underscores the need for collaboration in program implementation but also suggests the need for constant research in order to evaluate the effectiveness and sustainability of such an endeavor in delivering enhanced health outcomes across different populations (Bishop et al., 2014).

15.1.1. Dietary Assessment Methods

In nutritional epidemiology, the validity and reliability of measures used to measure diet are essential in making sense of food intake patterns and their accompanying health consequences. A variety of techniques, such as 24-hour dietary recalls, food frequency questionnaires, and diet diaries, have their respective strengths and limitations. For instance, 24-hour dietary recalls provide detailed information on the pattern of eating in people but are prone to recall error and memory bias. In contrast, food frequency questionnaires enable scientists to measure usual diet over a long period, but can struggle with the accuracy of specific portion sizes. As such, a clear grasp of these methodologies enables scientists to choose the most appropriate assessment tool for their research design, with a significant effect on data quality and ensuing epidemiological evidence. New sets of methodologies in dietary assessment are now embracing technology to enhance data collection and analysis. Cellular health and wearable technology now make it possible to monitor in real-time what one is eating, providing a more fluid glimpse of individuals' consumption patterns. Not only do new techniques diminish some of the biases associated with traditional approaches, such as food consumption underreporting, but they also make it possible to incorporate contextual information like place and time of consumption. Moreover, advances in ontology-based data structures, such as the Ontology for Nutritional Epidemiology (ONE), enable the integration of data collected through various methods. With standardized vocabulary and categorization of reporting instructions, ONE enables improved consistency in dietary assessment between studies, enabling researchers to make more informed comparisons and inferences about dietary practices and health outcomes (Ambayo et al., 2019).

Moreover, the intricacy of diet evaluation is even more highlighted by the need to evaluate the food production chain and the impact it has on the pattern of diets. Emergence of new research has shown that building predictive models that integrate food intake information with broader consumption and production patterns can overcome the limitations encountered in applying traditional evaluation. By adopting a risk-benefit framework, scientists are able to examine how various factors, such as socio-economic status and cultural determinants, affect food selection and diet-related risks. This combined strategy not only enhances the science of nutritional epidemiology but also facilitates public health interventions towards the promotion of improved dietary habits. Therefore, the integration of new measurement techniques and predictive modeling is a significant step in the understanding of diet versus health interaction (Dekker et al., 2002) (Figure 15.3).

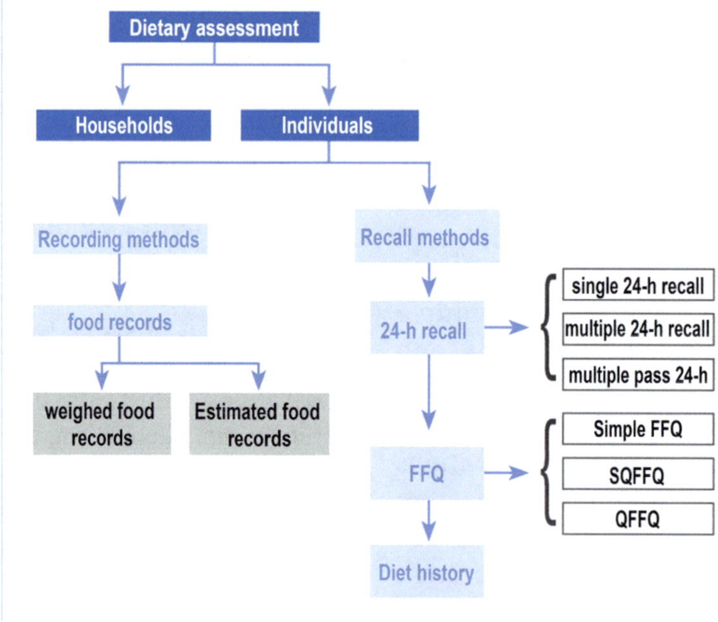

Figure 15.3. Dietary assessment methods: FFQ: food frequency questionnaire, SQFFQ: semi-quantitative food frequency questionnaire, QFFQ: quantitative food frequency questionnaire.

Source: https://www.researchgate.net/profile/Una-Macintyre/publication/277838884/figure/fig1/AS:668999549456394@1536513330362/Dietary-assessment-methods-FFQ-food-frequency-questionnaire-SQFFQ-semi-quantitative.png.

15.1.2. Observational Study Designs

Observational study designs are valuable in nutritional epidemiology since they enable scientists to investigate the food consumption patterns and their health associations without the interference of experimental manipulation. The design is convenient for assessing the proper eating habits and their effect on populations. Cohort, case-control, and cross-sectional study designs afford the convenience of viewing foods consumed, lifestyle factors, and health conditions over time. By considering the complexity of human behavior when it comes to nutrition, such designs allow for the identification of potential correlations and causations to help direct public health policy and nutrition interventions. Another significant advance in observational studies is the development of methods to create ontologies to enhance the analysis of nutritional data. For instance, the Ontology for Nutritional Epidemiology (ONE) facilitates improved data integration and harmonization by elucidating the connections among various taxonomic terms of relevance to nutritional inquiry. Through the use of ontological frameworks, investigators can improve report consistency and accuracy, which is essential when taking into account the evaluation of study evidence and drawing meaningful conclusions from observational data." This structured data approach makes it easier to identify research gaps and apply standard vocabulary, thereby improving the level of observational studies in the field. Also, the inclusion of predictive modeling in observational studies addresses complex food-diet issues that are present in nutritional epidemiology. By combining food intake data, dynamic consumption patterns, and risk-benefit analysis, scientists can create models that better reflect real-world environments. These predictive models allow for the investigation of the impact of diet on health outcomes while adjusting for the multifaceted nature of nutrition and its inherent implications. As the field develops, emphasis on systematic structuring of data and predictive analysis in observational research will enhance researchers' capacity for evidence-based decision-making, which will lead to improved public health policy tailored to the nutritional needs of the population (Ambayo et al., 2019; Dekker et al., 2002).

15.1.3. Statistical Analysis Techniques Used in Research

Statistical analysis techniques play an important part in nutritional epidemiology since, besides making it feasible to identify associations between dietary factors and health outcomes, they also increase the strength of findings. Techniques such as regression analysis are frequently employed for summarizing the association between nutritional factors and disease prevalence to enable researchers to control for confounding variables. For instance, with multivariate regression, researchers can establish the effect on long-term disease risk that different diets may have, holding other factors constant, such as age, sex, and socio-economic status. Additionally, large data sets can provide more generalizable results, particularly beneficial in population-level nutritional effects. Such statistical techniques have a key function in obtaining evidence-based dietary guideline advice, ultimately aimed at improving public health. The application of advanced statistical modeling techniques has also become increasingly applicable in study design within nutritional epidemiology. Predictive modeling, for instance, is an effective ability to forecast how eating habits are most likely to evolve with respect to various endpoints of health. This has been underscored in research that developed a prediction model which incorporated food intake data with dynamic consumption patterns, hence overcoming the challenges inherent with dietary measures. Incorporation of the predictive models allows researchers to assess risk-benefit scenarios in nutritional therapy, as delineated in Dekker et al. (2002). All food behaviors must be analyzed with a statistical perspective to understand their unique health outcomes, with more attention being given to different populations having different food cultures. Thus, statistical analysis skill not only increases the validity of the research findings but also facilitate improved public health intervention planning for specific nutritional needs. Where data may be sparse or in doubt, statistical analysis can cast significant illumination upon nutritional health disparities.

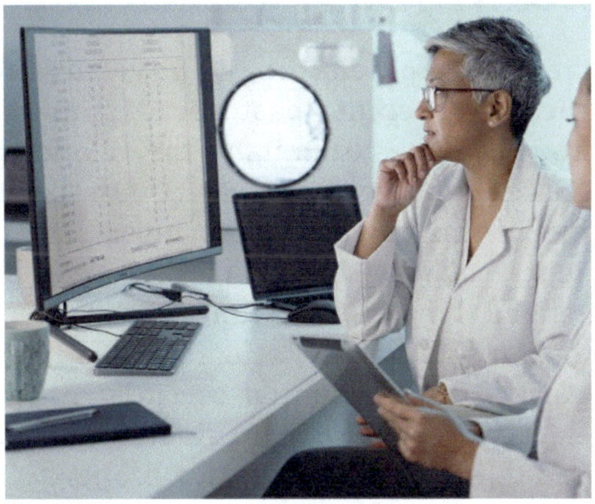

Figure 15.4. Statistical analysis techniques.

Source: https://ugc.futurelearn.com/uploads/images/f6/73/header_f67368a5-9494-4f6d-a881-22037f0ecbb2.jpg.

Such was the case when examining childhood morbidity in the Democratic Republic of Congo, where geographic mapping identified significant health disparities that were inclusive of nutrition. By using spatial analysis methods on information from more than one indicator, analysts would be able to map patterns of disease prevalence and blame them on food-related dimensions, as seen in Ahiadeke et al. (2009). Awareness of such patterns can assist policymakers in focusing on those places that have the greatest need and budget for interventions that will yield results. In addition, spatial residual mapping would explain how various socio-economic indicators interact with health indicators in the long run and ultimately influence better policy-making and strategic planning for nutritional public health. Statistical methods are hence worthy tools in not only analyzing historical information but also predicting future trends in nutritional epidemiology (Figure 15.4).

15.2. Key Nutritional Epidemiology Studies

Nutritional epidemiology has advanced significantly over the past decades, much of it through studies examining the relationship between diet and chronic disease. One fascinating avenue of this research is to investigate key nutrients such as selenium, which has been challenged for its dual function in disease and health. Historically, selenium was initially categorized as a potential carcinogen in the 1940s; however, subsequent studies eventually pointed to its cancer-preventive property. This was followed by more recent randomized controlled trials, which gave mixed results, including no significant cancer protective effect and suggested low-dose toxicity effects.

The complexities of selenium may be attributed to the differential biological activity of its chemical forms, emphasizing the necessity of a multifaceted understanding in dietary counseling and public health advice. Thus, understanding these complex relationships can direct our public health policy and dietary intake in terms of micronutrient intake (Ammar et al., 2013). Another key area of concentration for nutritional epidemiology concerns the role that eating habits have in neurological health. There is research that has come to increasingly examine links between diet and neurological illness, as scientists study illnesses such as epilepsy and konzo. These illnesses highlight the need to understand how different foods interact with one another to influence neurological function and health status. Further, there is an urgent requirement to enlighten the public regarding such interactions, ranging from policymakers to parents, as extensive brain research would assist in the identification of the cause of such diseases. Raising awareness can lead to interventions that would ensure a rise in the quality of diet, which might reduce the severity of symptoms or even prevent the development of some neurological diseases. Therefore, the encouragement of the debate on nutritional contribution to neurological health is crucial in shaping informed public policies and effective health actions (Ngudi et al., 2014). Further, technological incorporation into nutritional epidemiology has changed the process of data collection and analysis, offering more detailed information about dietary patterns as well as health status.

The employment of mobile diet apps and online questionnaires allows researchers to obtain more precise and up-to-date dietary data, thereby enhancing the validity of their findings. This technology provides intensive longitudinal studies that can track changes in eating patterns across diverse populations. With scientists studying complex interactions between diet, genes, and environment, this evidence-based method uncovers targeted nutritional interventions. Lastly, these studies indicate how tailored nutritional interventions can turn back the tide of disease risk and foster overall health, further substantiating the relevance of nutritional epidemiology in contemporary public health debates. Where these fields overlap, the potential for improving population health through mindful eating habits grows exponentially (Figure 15.5).

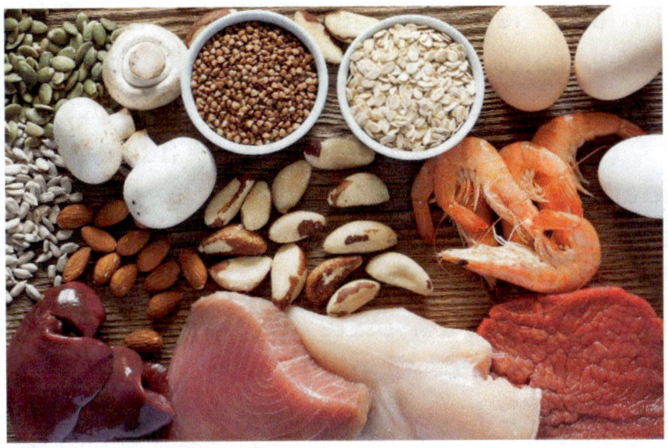

Figure 15.5. Selenium.

Source: https://nutritionsource.hsph.harvard.edu/wp-content/uploads/2024/11/AdobeStock_209980251.jpeg.

15.2.1. Landmark Studies and Their Findings

Landmark studies in nutritional epidemiology have greatly influenced our understanding of the diet-health outcome relationship. An example is the association between grip strength and diabetes, as studied in a large cohort study with the UK Biobank. The investigation found that diabetic subjects had a significantly increased risk of all-cause and cardiovascular disease (CVD) mortality, particularly among individuals with low grip strength. In particular, the research cited hazard ratios with evidence of a four-fold increase in risk of CVD mortality among the patients with diabetes and low grip strength over their counterparts with higher grip strength. These findings suggest that grip strength can be a significant indicator for identifying high-risk individuals among diabetics and demonstrate the value of physical strength as a protective factor against adverse health outcomes in nutritional epidemiology (Anderson et al., 2017). Another important area in nutritional epidemiology includes intricate interactions between genetic susceptibility and dietary modification. Research has underlined the need for people to receive personalized nutritional guidance based on their individual genetic makeup, paving the way for more effective public health interventions. The growing body of evidence suggests that genetics will play a role in explaining the heterogeneity of diets and the efficacy of various interventions. As pointed out in the debate concerning strong classifications of psychological disorder, the incorporation of genetic and biological information into nutritional epidemiology represents a shift toward an integrated understanding of health. By accepting the interaction between genomics, environmental exposure, and diet, researchers can develop more precise designs for persons' unique health needs, further establishing the importance of genetics to informing dietary policy (Bracha et al., 2006). To that end, milestone studies have emphasized the importance of long-term studies in explaining long-term eating patterns and their roles in chronic disease development. Recent studies highlight the fact that long-term eating habits over extended periods create more definite health effects than short-term dietary tests on shorter timescales. For instance, studies assessing diet changes across decades are likely to correlate with instances of conditions such as obesity, diabetes, and cardiovascular disease. These findings underline the significance of having a longitudinal perspective to understand the impact of diet cumulatively so that one can establish trends and causality in an effective way. Integrating the outcomes of these studies, it is evident that specific dietary analysis considering genetic susceptibilities, as well as trends in the long term are significant if nutritional epidemiology and public health policy are to progress (Anderson et al., 2017).

15.2.2. Impact of Cohort Studies on Dietary Guidelines

Cohort studies are especially valuable in making dietary recommendations, as they provide longitudinal data on the health impact of a given diet. They track health outcomes over a period in a defined population, typically leading to knowing the associations between chronic disease, lifestyle, and diet. For example, findings of various cohort studies have indicated that increased consumption of particular groups of foods, such as fruits and vegetables, is associated with lower risks of chronic disease, including cardiovascular disease and certain cancers. Moreover, the majority of these studies included heterogeneous populations, allowing researchers to explore how genes, environment, and socio-economic status interact with diets to influence health outcomes. As a result, the data provided by cohort studies is at the forefront of developing evidence-based dietary recommendations for use in supporting public health interventions to reduce disease incidence and improve nutritional status as a whole. Cohort studies extend their influence beyond influencing just dietary recommendations; they inform the behavioral aspects of food consumption, too.

For instance, studies of food eating habits have demonstrated that higher diet quality is correlated with better psychological health in children and that the eating pattern can impact mental health as well. Evidence drawn from longitudinal studies, such as those contained in recent research, has established that specific eating habits can exacerbate or alleviate behavioral issues. These findings can be helpful in formulating dietary guidelines that are not only directed towards physical health outcomes but also consider the mental health impact of nutrition. Thus, such comprehensive guidelines would promote more holistic dietary advice, leading to the overall well-being of various segments of society, especially vulnerable segments, such as children. Furthermore, cohort studies are best placed to deliver the critical evidence of long-term diet effects in clinical populations, like those who are at risk of metabolic disease. For example, research in patients who have had a liver transplant indicated significant weight gain and metabolic deterioration during the first year after transplantation, associated with Western-type dietary intakes high in saturated fats (Campbell et al., 2016). These results underscore the importance of targeted dietary treatment in some patient groups to minimize adverse effects. By measuring dietary intake and its impact on state of health over time, cohort studies determine the most important nutritional issues for each group, facilitating personalized recommendations. Therefore, it is essential to interpret the cohort study evidence to develop dynamic diet guidelines that not only serve the needs of the general population but also target the needs of risk groups and further advance nutritional epidemiology in humans (Figure 15.6).

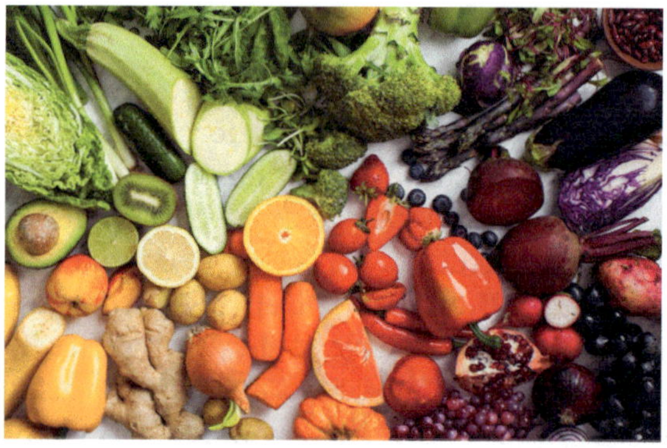

Figure 15.6. Increasing fruit and vegetable variety helps to lower disease risk.

Source: https://nutrition.org/wp-content/uploads/2023/08/Increasing-fruit-and-vegetable-variety-helps-to-lower-disease-risk-1030x687.png.

15.2.3. Role of Meta-Analyses in Synthesizing Research

The discipline of nutritional epidemiology has been greatly enhanced by the application of meta-analyses, powerful tools for synthesizing a wide body of research evidence. By formally combining results from multiple studies, meta-analyses enable investigators to draw stronger conclusions than single studies can provide. This is particularly important in nutritional epidemiology, where dietary determinations are typically composed of heterogeneous approaches and populations, yielding incomparable results. With the use of statistical tools, meta-analyses can identify patterns and resolve inconsistencies and thereby provide a clearer picture of the impact of diet on health outcomes. The ability to pool results enables a more sophisticated interpretation of complex interactions between diet and illness, and that is required in the design of public health guidance and clinical practice. For chronic diseases, the role of meta-analyses becomes even more important. Several reviews have identified associations between dietary factors and long-term diseases such as cardiovascular disease and colorectal cancer. For instance, there is evidence that intake of processed meat is linked to increased risk of colorectal cancer, and excess risk estimates vary significantly across high intakes compared to non-consumption behaviors, implying a potential risk increment of 20 to 50% (Corpet et al., 2008). Meta-analyses can pool such epidemiological findings to assign a figure to the combined risk and identify threads shared across multiple studies, which can be useful to policy-makers and healthcare professionals who are interested in designing effective dietary interventions and advice. Meta-analyses also serve to unveil the complexities of the pathophysiology of disease for examining underlying determinants that can influence health outcomes in nutrition. For example, chronic kidney disease (CKD) is an illness that involves multiple physiological derangements associated with dietary habits and potentially accounts for the contribution of numerous nutritional interventions to patient outcomes (Slee et al., 2012). By synthesizing data related to hormonal, inflammatory, and metabolic determinants associated with nutritional intake, meta-analyses have the ability to shed light on multifactorial mechanisms for disease and ultimately impact future research agendas and clinical practice. This integrated approach underscores the importance of comprehending the effects of diet in overall health situations, fundamental to progressive nutritional epidemiology and optimizing population health strategies (Figure 15.7).

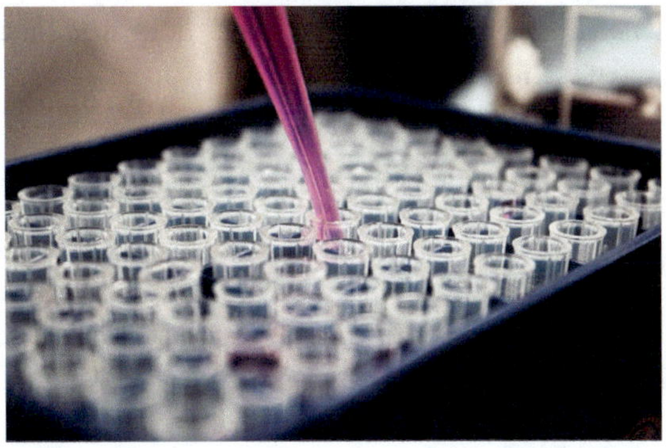

Figure 15.7. Meta-analysis in nutritional epidemiology.

Source: https://images.unsplash.com/photo-1532187863486-abf9dbad1b69?crop=entropy&cs=tinysrgb&fit=max&fm=jpg&ixid=M3w3MDgyMDR8MHwxfHNlYXJjaHwxfHxtZXRhLWFuYWx5c2lzJTJDJTIwbnV0cml0aW9-&ixlib=rb-4.1.0&q=80&w=700&utm_source=numberanalytics&utm_medium=referral.

15.3. Nutritional Epidemiology and Chronic Diseases

The association between nutritional epidemiology and chronic diseases is one that cannot be overstated because eating habits can potentially have an effect on the occurrence and progression of conditions such as diabetes, obesity, and cardiovascular diseases. Research in this field emphasizes the importance of understanding how specific nutrients and general dietary patterns influence health outcomes across various populations. For instance, epidemiological studies repeatedly incriminate that high consumption of fruits and vegetables is associated with reduced risk of chronic diseases, and saturated fat and sugar consumption are associated with increased disease prevalence. This literature puts forward the potentiality of certain nutritional interventions that would neutralize these risks, and thus it is necessary to ensure that there is a coherent policy for diet trends in public health programs. Yet, as noted in more recent reviews, mathematical modeling is seldom applied in research on global health indicators due to the fact that intervention studies are lacking, and consequently, fewer definitive statements can be made (Joffe et al., 2005). Another important area of research in nutritional epidemiology is the socio-economic determinants of dietary habits and conditions of ill health. Early childhood, being an early critical developmental stage, has been found to have long-term effects on the future health pathway and learning ability of an individual. Socio-economic disadvantage and nutrition tend to overlap particularly, and studies have found that children in poor socio-economic households often suffer from a lack of access to healthy food intake. Disadvantage has the potential to lead to nutritional inadequacies and obesity, and hence provide a pathway for a range of multiple chronic conditions later in life. Consequently, early childhood nutrition programs become a priority, suggesting a policy shift directed at these years of development specifically. In interventions, this can be invaluable not only in improving health in the short term but also in creating lifelong habits of healthy living, thereby shaping the chronic disease profile (Sweeny, 2025). As well, the evolution of nutritional epidemiology as an area of research requires multi-method evidence that spans numerous populations and reflects the heterogeneity of dietary behavior. This strategy must incorporate multiple methodological frameworks, such as qualitative research that considers cultural, social, and environmental determinants of dietary habits. Integrating epidemiological evidence with information from behavioral sciences will enable researchers to appreciate the complex ways in which nutritional determinants converge with individual and community well-being. The investigation of intervention strategies must also involve consideration of stakeholders' perspectives to ensure that they are contextually based on real-world realities. Ultimately, closing the gap between practice and research will be essential in designing effective public health campaigns to stem the tide of chronic disease burden. This calls for increased emphasis on ongoing research and interdisciplinary work to create more effective strategies in nutritional epidemiology (Figure 15.8).

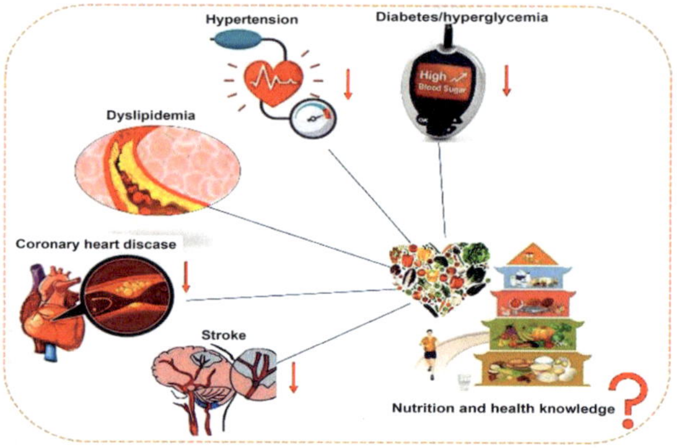

Figure 15.8. Association between nutrition and health knowledge and multiple chronic diseases.

Source: https://pub.mdpi-res.com/nutrients/nutrients-15-02096/article_deploy/html/images/nutrients-15-02096-ag.png?1682559947.

15.3.1. Relationship Between Diet and Cardiovascular Diseases

The diet-cardiovascular disease (CVD) connection has been of significant importance in nutritional epidemiology, and evidence that several dietary patterns can significantly impact cardiovascular health has been demonstrated. Those diets characterized by high intake of fruits, vegetables, whole grains, and healthy fats, such as those in the Mediterranean dietary pattern, have consistently been linked with reduced CVD incidence. By contrast, intake of highly processed food, red meat, and sweetened beverages has been shown to be associated with cardiovascular risk. This verifies the importance of dietary composition, as specific nutrients may either promote cardiac health or complicate existing conditions. Growing research emphasizes not just the intake of calories but also the caloric quality consumed. Accordingly, the relationship between some dietary factors and cardiovascular disease is of primary significance in working to develop proper public health recommendations to avoid the development of CVD. Moreover, chronic illnesses such as CKD significantly complicate the relationship between diet and cardiovascular health. CKD tends to accompany metabolic and physiological diseases, including hypertension and dyslipidemia, which are CVD risk factors. Specific dietary changes are critical for managing these complications. For instance, the inclusion of anti-inflammatory nutrients and micronutrients could reverse the detrimental effects of excessive proinflammatory cytokines, which are typical in CKD patients. Studies show that dietary changes, particularly reduction in protein intake and protein source quality improvement, can reduce CVD risk with CKD progression (Iacobini et al., 2017). The emphasis on diet not only regulates kidney function but also has an international effect on cardiovascular health, illustrating the interconnected nature of these systems. In addition, the influence of diet on cardiovascular health is compounded when considering the influence of inflammation and metabolic activities. Elevation in inflammatory markers like C-reactive protein has been associated with both CKD and increased CVD risk (Slee et al., 2012). Nutritional therapies aimed at these inflammatory processes have been shown to enhance patient outcomes. Foods that are high in antioxidants and omega-3 fatty acids, for example, can reduce inflammation and enhance endothelial function, all of which are critical in cardiovascular health. Additionally, lifestyle modifications, such as regular exercise combined with a balanced diet, can significantly optimize overall metabolic profiles. Thus, adopting an integrated approach to nutrition and health care management among populations at risk of both CVD and CKD can reverse these interrelated conditions of health, making the case for person-centric dietary interventions for disease prevention and control (Figure 15.9).

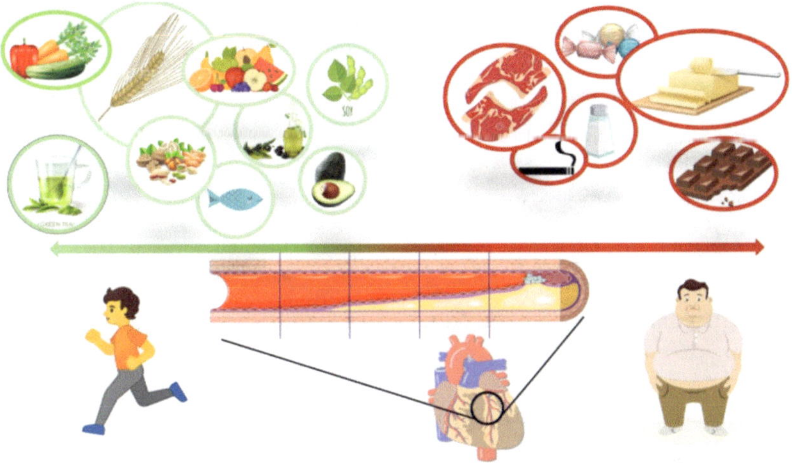

Figure 15.9. The role of nutrition in cardiovascular disease.

Source: https://pub.mdpi-res.com/nutrients/nutrients-15-01064/article_deploy/html/images/nutrients-15-01064-ag.png?1676958319.

15.3.2. Impact of Nutrition on Diabetes Prevalence

The relationship between nutrition and diabetes prevalence is multifaceted, with food intake playing a crucial role in type 1 and type 2 diabetes risk. Diets that consist of high intakes of processed food, added sugars, and saturated fats are the cause of weight gain and insulin resistance, the leading risk factors for type 2 diabetes. Results from epidemiological research suggest that populations with diets composed of high intakes of whole grains, lean protein, and healthier fats have lower incidence rates of diabetes. Such an association highlights the need for public health initiatives that will be able to enhance dietary intake, particularly among risk groups. Additionally, the elimination of nutritional deficiencies is also critical in that inadequate intake of essential vitamins and minerals could worsen metabolic dysregulations and consequently prevent or impede diabetes control. Nutritional interventions, in the form of individualized dietary counsel, not only prevent diabetes but also enhance general health outcomes in high-risk groups. Understanding nutrition's impact within the framework of chronic disease recognizes the role specific nutrients play in avoiding diabetes. Omega-3 fatty acids found in fish and certain plant oils, for instance, are associated with increased insulin sensitivity and reduced inflammation, which are welcome when managing risk from diabetes. In addition, dietary fiber plays a significant role in carbohydrate metabolism; increasing dietary fiber helps to regulate blood sugar and promote satiety, ultimately contributing to weight control. In contrast, excessive consumption of refined carbohydrates may lead to spiking of blood sugar and perpetuate insulin resistance in the long term. As studies learn more about these interconnections, it is apparent that a holistic approach to nutrition education can yield better health results and a reduction of the prevalence of diabetes among diverse populations (Bordoni et al., 2015).

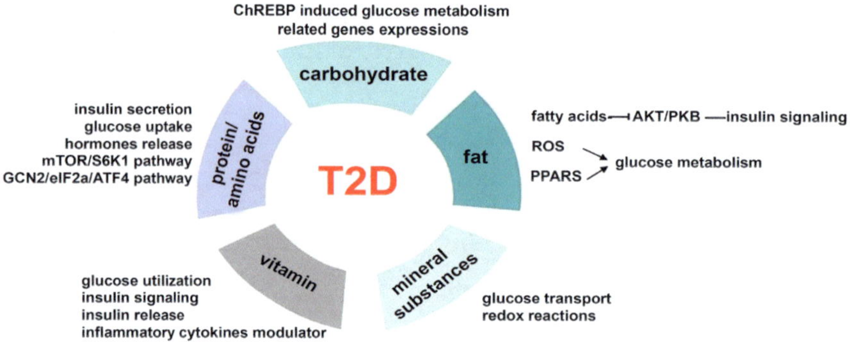

Figure 15.10. The role of nutrients in type 2 diabetes.

Source: https://www.frontiersin.org/files/Articles/575442/fbioe-08-575442-HTML/image_m/fbioe-08-575442-g003.jpg.

In addition, studying the overlap of aging and nutrition further explains the prevalence of diabetes. Aging individuals tend to experience changes in appetite, digestion, and nutrient absorption due to physiological changes in the gastrointestinal tract. These changes with age can limit access to such essential nutrients, leading to malnutrition, a risk factor for most chronic diseases, such as diabetes. Even deficiencies of vitamins like vitamin D and certain minerals have been causally linked with increased risks of diabetes in older age. Also, the inflammatory processes involved in malnutrition can cause insulin resistance, which can lead to a self-perpetuating cycle of inadequate nutrition contributing to greater susceptibility to diabetes complications. Thus, it is important to make better sense of aging and its nutritional implications for the design of effective interventions to reduce the prevalence of diabetes among the elderly (Slee et al., 2012) (Figure 15.10).

15.3.3. Role of Diet in Cancer Risk and Prevention

The influence of diet on cancer risk and prevention is an emerging area of study in nutritional epidemiology. Increasing evidence indicates that the etiology of various cancers has a significant relationship with dietary patterns, and thus, a balanced, nutrient-dense diet becomes imperative. Major food constituents, including fruits, vegetables, whole grains, and lean meat, have been reported to be associated with reduced cancer risk. They have a rich source of phytochemicals and antioxidants with the potential to protect cells from oxidative stress and inflammation—two etiologic mechanisms in carcinogenesis. Conversely, consumption of processed foods and foods rich in saturated fats and sugar has been linked with increased cancer risk. Epidemiological studies have shown that individuals on a Mediterranean-type diet with high intake of fruits and vegetables and healthy fats have lower incidences of cancer, highlighting the potential of diet in preventing cancer. Evidence has focused on individual dietary factors such as red and processed meat intake, which has been identified as linked with the risk of colorectal cancer. Epidemiologic studies consistently demonstrate that heavy consumers of processed meats may have a 20 to 50% higher risk of colorectal cancer compared with non-consumers. Such an association is thought to be attributed to several mechanisms, like the formation of carcinogenic chemicals during cooking processes and the inclusion of heme iron in red meat, which enable carcinogenesis. The mechanisms by which processed meat is involved in cancer risk, such as the formation of N-nitroso compounds and increased insulin resistance through fat-rich consumption, point to the complexity of diet in causing cancer. Intervention of such dietary practices, particularly in affluent countries, may be critical in minimizing the threat of colorectal cancer in the population and further encouraging public health intervention towards dietary modification (Corpet et al., 2008). Recent work has also examined the role of micronutrients and their complex interactions with cancer risk. Of the micronutrients, one that has been a source of considerable controversy is selenium, which has been shown to have carcinogenic as well as cancer-preventive potential depending on the dose and chemical form. While earlier theories proposed selenium supplementation to lower cancer risk, recent randomized controlled trials evidenced no preventive action and questioned possible adverse effects at higher intakes.

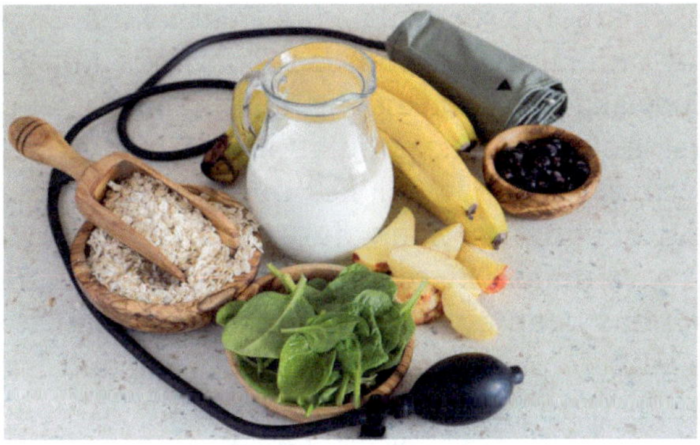

Figure 15.11. Diet for cancer prevention.

Source: https://www.careinsurance.com/upload_master/media/posts/April2020/vq5v3a82CVaSs2xNqWEa.jpg.

The variable outcomes of selenium's impact on cancer illustrate the need for personalized dietary advice according to nutritional condition and the forms of nutrients consumed. This covert approach highlights the complexity of the subject in nutritional epidemiology when the complex nature of diet-health relationships can empower individuals and health professionals to make intelligent food choices for cancer prevention (Ammar et al., 2013) (Figure 15.11).

15.4. Socioeconomic Factors in Nutritional Epidemiology

Socioeconomic status has powerful influences on food habits and nutritional status, dictating the population's health under varying conditions. Populations with higher socioeconomic status (SES) are more likely to have better access to a diverse range of foodstuffs, fresh vegetables and fruits, lean proteins and meats, and whole grains. By contrast, lower SES individuals face challenges such as food deserts, limited means of transportation, and financial constraints, which lead to a reliance on cheaper, processed foods with high sugar and unhealthy fat content. This inequality is especially prevalent among marginalized groups, such as indigenous populations, who have been discovered to have higher obesity and related health complications due to socioeconomic disadvantage. The correlation between SES and BMI has been established in studies conducted on adult populations, such as the Wichí and Toba people of Argentina, to highlight socioeconomic disparity as a contributing factor toward poor nutritional health among these groups (Burke et al., 2009). Compounded to these issues is the intersection of culture and nutrition. People of varying cultural backgrounds may follow traditional foodways that conflict with foods available in contemporary marketplaces. For Aboriginal people, foods gathered from the wild have been supplanted by food from stores to a significant extent, which not only has limited nutritional content but also plays a key role in changes in eating habits that impact public health. As they urbanize, communities are deprived of access to their long-standing nutrient-rich diets, leading to higher rates of obesity and other metabolic disorders. This population trend makes it imperative that interventions include focused nutrition that is sensitive to cultural preferences while promoting healthier dietary practices. Ultimately, understanding the cultural nuances of the socioeconomic setting can be employed to construct more adaptive public health policy to consider nutrition disparities and health inequities (Burke et al., 2009). As nutritional epidemiology develops, its emphasis increasingly emphasizes the importance of dietetic practices in mental well-being, particularly for older adults. Recent evidence suggests that lifestyle modification, including diet, has a positive influence on cognitive patterns, offering an intervention window. In a systematic review, many dietary interventions aimed at enhancing cognition were reported to have statistically significant neuropsychological test score improvements. It should be mentioned that there are controversies concerning the clinical significance of these effects and the need for larger studies. While there is some evidence to show that certain dietary patterns play a protective role in preventing cognitive decline, current evidence remains inconclusive and necessitates further research about how socioeconomic determinants influence access to such protective diets. Therefore, comprehending in a nuanced manner how both socioeconomic determinants and nutrition interact can inform public health interventions to encourage cognitive health throughout the life course.

15.4.1. Influence of Income on Dietary Choices

The relationship between income level and food choice is a significant area of study in nutritional epidemiology, as financial resources have a direct impact on food accessibility and consumption. Individuals and families with higher incomes tend to enjoy easier access to nutrient-rich food diversity, including fresh fruits, lean meat, and whole grains. This access enables them to choose healthier foods, guided by counsel emphasizing the intake of fruits and vegetables for the avoidance of chronic disease. However, the poorer have restrictions that force them to consume cheaper, calorie-dense, and lower-quality food options. Such variations in food choice emphasize the complex association between socioeconomic status and nutritional health, in relation to the need for policy action that increases food access among low-income groups (Cash et al., 2025). Furthermore, income affects not only the nutritional quality of food consumption but also dietary variety, which is crucially important for nutritional health. There is evidence that dietary diversity, in terms of food variety consumed, has a positive relationship with levels of income. Affluent households have been observed to have increased demand for diet diversity, reflecting more varieties of food groups such as fruits, vegetables, dairy products, and meat, which is significant for proper nutrient intake. For instance, it was found that in a Canadian eating behavior study, income, household size, and age all play significant roles in allocating food diversity, and with higher income comes more risk for consuming a more diversified and balanced diet (Drescher et al., 2025). Conversely, low-income families have fewer food choices, leading to imbalanced diets and nutrition-related chronic disease risk. The effects of income on food choices are also evident in nutritional policies and public health initiatives aimed at addressing dietary deficiencies across different socioeconomic levels. Policymakers are responsible for creating environments that facilitate equitable access to healthy foods, particularly in low-income communities where poor households reside. Initiatives that have worked include subsidies for fruits and vegetables, enhanced funding for food assistance programs, and nutrition education at the community level. With the implementation of such interventions, it is possible to offset the adverse effects of constricted income on food decisions and thereby improve health equity in the overall population (Cash et al., 2025). Intervention within the connection between income and food selection can thus go a long way in improving public health outcomes and reducing levels of diet-related illness among vulnerable groups (Figure 15.12).

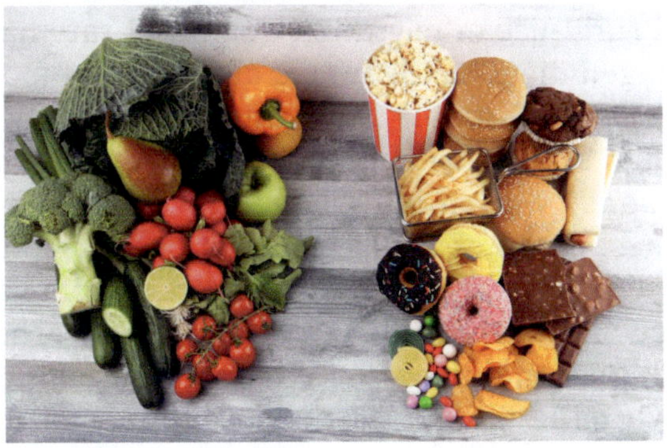

Figure 15.12. Income influences food choices.

Source: https://competitions-app.datacamp.com/1.53/food-wealth-wellness/food-wealth-wellness.jpg.

15.4.2. Access to Healthy Foods in Different Communities

Healthy food availability is among the most significant determinants of nutrition and general well-being in various communities, especially urban communities. The concept of food deserts identifies a rather alarming fact where residents lack easy access to grocery stores and fresh vegetables and fruits, leading to increased degrees of food insecurity. Inner-city dwellers are typically particularly vulnerable because the absence of supermarkets and abundance of fast-food outlets mean fewer nutritional options. Food insecurity in such populations is closely linked to rising obesity levels, type 2 diabetes, and cardiovascular disease, which underscores the direct impact poor access to quality foods has on public health. Therefore, it is of paramount importance to address food environments and ensure that healthy food is accessible and affordable in order to prevent such adverse effects on health, which ultimately contributes to improving community well-being and protection against diet-related diseases (Ilochi et al., 2011). The nutrition transition, characterized by a double burden of disease, exacerbates the complexity of food supply in urban settings. Most noticeably in Southern Africa, urbanization and rural-urban migration at a rapid rate have changed diets, as the intake of processed foods that are affordable but nutritionally poor is higher. The transition most affects low-income persons, who most frequently possess the highest rates of food insecurity. Urban policy makers have the imperative responsibility to act on such populations' dietary environments since both undernourishment and over-nourishment are public health issues of concern. The acknowledgment of the broader implications of food availability beyond its impact on physical well-being also informs policies for building sustainable urban food systems that promote comprehensive health equity and increase access to healthy food for all communities (Crush et al., 2011). Community involvement is paramount in providing access to healthy food, particularly in the food deserts that have been labeled as such. Strategic initiatives, such as the Mobilizing for Action through Planning and Partnerships (MAPP), are effectively able to involve residents in exploring their food surroundings and advocating for change to enhance access. Through the development of alliances among neighborhood governments, healthcare providers, and community organizations, such initiatives can develop customized solutions that specifically remove barriers to access to healthy food. The approach is holistic, involving not just availability but also education on labeling of food and nutrition, laying the ground for well-informed consumer choices. Increased awareness and access among urban populations are capable of eradicating epidemiological correlates of health inequalities related to food insecurity, ultimately contributing towards a healthier population and confirming the central interface between nutrition and epidemiology in intricate human environments (Ilochi et al., 2011) (Figure 15.13).

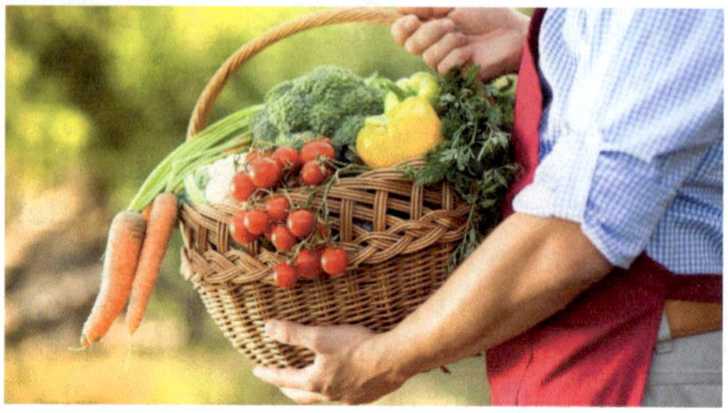

Figure 15.13. Access to healthy foods in different communities.

Source: https://commongroundpg.com/wp-content/uploads/2022/08/Untitled-design-57-4-1024x576.jpg.

15.4.3. Cultural Factors Affecting Nutrition and Health

Cultural determinants significantly affect food habits and nutrition status, as they shape beliefs, customs, and food choices among various groups of people. The relationship between culture and health is most evident in the manner by which indigenous food traditions are maintained, modified, or dissipated in the face of globalization. For example, when communities are increasingly exposed to processed foods, traditional diets, which can include whole grain bread, locally produced fruits and vegetables, and organic livestock, are usually replaced with convenience foods containing high sugar and saturated fats. This change has disquieting implications for public health since a model of prediction combining food intake data and risk-benefit calculations reveals a link between changing dietary habits and increasing rates of obesity and metabolic diseases (Dekker et al., 2002). In particular, these alterations make culturally sensitive health interventions that are culturally aware and appreciative of traditional food customs all the more imperative in an attempt to promote sustainable nutrition. In addition, cultural perceptions of health, illness, and food play an important role in dietary practice and nutritional well-being. In certain cultures, for example, among Tanzania's pastoral people, indigenous understanding of diseases, including zoonoses, is firmly established in traditional livelihood and cultural practices. Despite a few recognized health risks associated with animal products, the majority of pastoralists embrace these risks due to their cultural significance in social affiliation and rituals (Catley et al., 2017). This aspect highlights the intricacies of health education and intervention models, as neglecting beliefs and practices rooted in culture can result in ineffective health outreach initiatives. A solid grasp of such cultural frameworks is necessary for planning nutrition interventions that are effective within given communities, thus advocating for healthier outcomes and triggering diet changes that are in line with local traditions. Finally, addressing cultural factors affecting health and nutrition requires an interdisciplinary approach with input from sociology, anthropology, and nutritional science. Public health practitioners can use diet choices occurring within social contexts to create effective campaigns intervening between traditional practices and modern nutritional needs. For example, educational courses that highlight the health advantages of traditional food, along with contemporary health risks, could lead to improved compliance and acceptance among target groups. Furthermore, collaborations between local leaders and community members in planning nutrition programs may render them culturally specific and more effective in the long run. Finally, the recognition and incorporation of cultural determinants within nutritional epidemiology led to an enhanced appreciation of dietary patterns and health, creating a state of well-being within heterogeneous groups while valuing their respective cultural identities (Figure 15.14).

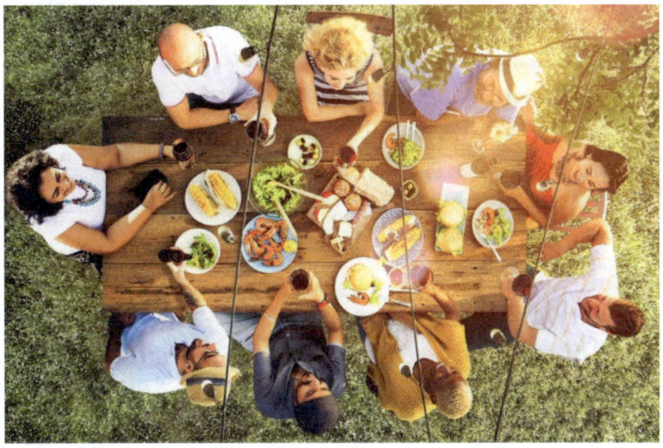

Figure 15.14. Culture and society influence healthy eating.

Source: https://cdn.shopify.com/s/files/1/0539/5621/4984/files/how-society-influences-diet.jpg.

15.5. Global Perspectives in Nutritional Epidemiology

In nutritional epidemiology, global perspectives are key to developing our understanding of food intake and its health implications in diverse populations. A mix of a variety of cultural, socio-economic, and environmental determinants must be included, as nutrition is highly relevant to worldwide public health issues. Comparing food habits in various national settings will allow researchers to identify global trends and unique regional issues. Specifically, such global evidence informs public health policy and stimulates the development of culturally relevant interventions and hence more effective interventions. In addition, the mixture of local data and global information assists in combating nutritional diseases like obesity and diabetes, which have recorded a record surge worldwide. The holistic nature of nutritional epidemiology thus necessitates an all-inclusive approach that pays homage to our globalized world. One of the most important aspects of global nutritional epidemiology is the employment of innovative frameworks such as the Ontology for Nutritional Epidemiology (ONE). The ONE ontology is a formal representation to enhance the integration and interpretation of data from several studies, thereby providing an overall vision of nutritional outcomes. Through establishing uniform logical relations between taxonomic terms, ONE not only standardizes nutritional study terminology but also improves databases to enable simple sharing and analysis of data worldwide. Case studies incorporated into ONE development further demonstrate its practical uses, such as manuscript annotation and completeness reporting evaluation.

This new approach is a classic example of how technology can strengthen the field of nutritional epidemiology, ultimately contributing to improved public health outcomes and evidence-based policy-making (Ambayo et al., 2019). Additionally, nutrition being a convergence field with other areas, such as Water, Sanitation, and Hygiene (WASH), reflects the interdisciplinary nature of international nutritional epidemiology. Evidence has indicated that WASH conditions can have significant effects on nutritional status, especially among vulnerable groups. School attendance, dietary hygiene practices, and maternal and newborn health are all importantly affected by WASH intervention.

By expanding the scope of WASH to include these intersectoral elements, public health interventions could deal with a number of determinants of health simultaneously. Approaches that integrate nutritional education and WASH improvements can enhance health outcomes, demonstrating the importance of an integrated response to global health problems (Mills et al., 2016). Thus, nutritional epidemiology must evolve to consider these linkages in order to design comprehensive and effective interventions.

15.5.1. Nutritional Challenges in Developing Countries

The nutritional issues of developing countries are strongly associated with the socio-economic development of the countries. Food insecurity is the prime cause of such issues and affects millions of people due to the combined effects of poverty, adverse agriculture, and climatic shocks. When food availability to healthy diets decreases, populations become reliant on energy-dense, nutrient-poor diets, leading to both undernutrition and obesity—a condition that is referred to as the double burden of malnutrition. It is compounded by unfavorable healthcare access, where there is underutilization of healthcare services that drains the potential for nutritional education and interventions. Removal of these economic and systemic barriers is central to reducing the nutritional deficits and fostering sustainable health improvements in these populations. Outside of socio-economic status, cultural beliefs and practices significantly influence food consumption in developing nations. Traditional diets do not always promote modern nutritional concepts and are likely to lead to micronutrient deficiencies, especially among susceptible groups such as children and women. For example, the consumption of some basic foods, such as cassava or maize, may be so predominant in local diets that more diversified and nutritious ones are not used as much because they are not available or because people have a cultural preference. Thus, activities aimed at improving nutrition need to be oriented not only toward food availability but also toward cultural acceptability and knowledge concerning balanced diets. Interventions that incorporate planning by local communities for nutrition interventions have been promising in promoting better food consumption patterns and addressing some deficiencies prevalent in these environments. The recent pandemics of health, including the COVID-19 pandemic, have further increased the nutritional problem in developing countries. The pandemic has disrupted food supply chains, resulting in increased prices for food and reduced access to staple foods. Simultaneously, it has strained healthcare systems, diminishing access to nutrition care and prevention services. Mental health impact at such times can easily propel eating behavior into further decline, further increasing risk of diet-related disease and malnutrition.

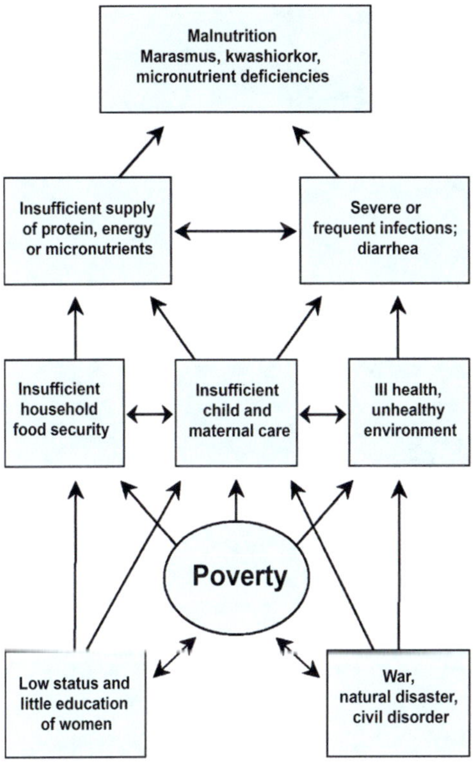

Figure 15.15. Direct and indirect causes of malnutrition.

Source: https://www.cmaj.ca/content/cmaj/173/3/279/F2.large.jpg?width=800&height=600&carousel=1.

Public health interventions, therefore, have to make resilience against such breakdowns a central aspect, ensuring nutrition is maintained as a priority even in emergency times. Long-term strategies that include nutrition within models of overall health, and tailored interventions in high-risk groups, will be vital in minimizing both the impact of current and new health conditions on overall nutrition (Bray et al., 2024; Singhal, 2020) (Figure 15.15).

15.5.2. Global Trends in Obesity and Malnutrition

The nutritional health world is now more and more defined by the simultaneous rise in malnutrition and obesity, a phenomenon often referred to as the double burden of disease. This is a complex phenomenon caused by a number of drivers, including urbanization, economic change, and lifestyle change. For instance, in Southern Africa, rapid rural-to-urban migration has led to significant shifts in food culture and increased food insecurity among the urban poor. As documented, the change impacts the most vulnerable, erasing previous gains in health and driving the public health burden of malnutrition and obesity. Those contradictory trends in nutritional epidemiology complicate policy-making and demand integrated strategies that address the unique needs of different populations vulnerable to these twin problems (Crush et al., 2011). In nations such as Iran, studies have indicated that undernutrition trends among children differed significantly between ethnic groups, and this indicates the extreme effect of socioeconomic status on nutritional levels. For example, evidence has suggested that while stunting rates decreased generally among children under five years old belonging to various ethnic groups, rates of underweight status progressed differently, increasing in a few groups. The imbalance in diet emphasizes the importance of examining economic determinants since undernutrition is more prevalent among children in low-income households, worsened by ethnic disparities. It is an indicator of the covert complexities of malnutrition, even with rising obesity rates across the world, that present a specific public health risk that needs targeted interventions addressed to group communities (Veghari et al., 2015). With the increasing prevalence of obesity globally, its relationship with malnutrition provokes some fundamental questions regarding public health and nutrition policy. Obesity, described as an epidemic, is often encountered in conjunction with undernutrition in the same population, particularly in low- and middle-income settings where good food access is weak. This occurrence lessens the effectiveness of single traditional public health interventions for obesity or undernutrition individually, as both diseases are capable of impacting health outcomes concurrently. To this end, understanding the global trends in these interrelated issues is essential in formulating uniform strategies that capture the nuance of nutritional health. Policies must respond not only to increasing access to healthy food but also to developing educational programs that support sustainable consumption patterns among different population groups (Crush et al., 2011; Veghari et al., 2015) (Figure 15.16).

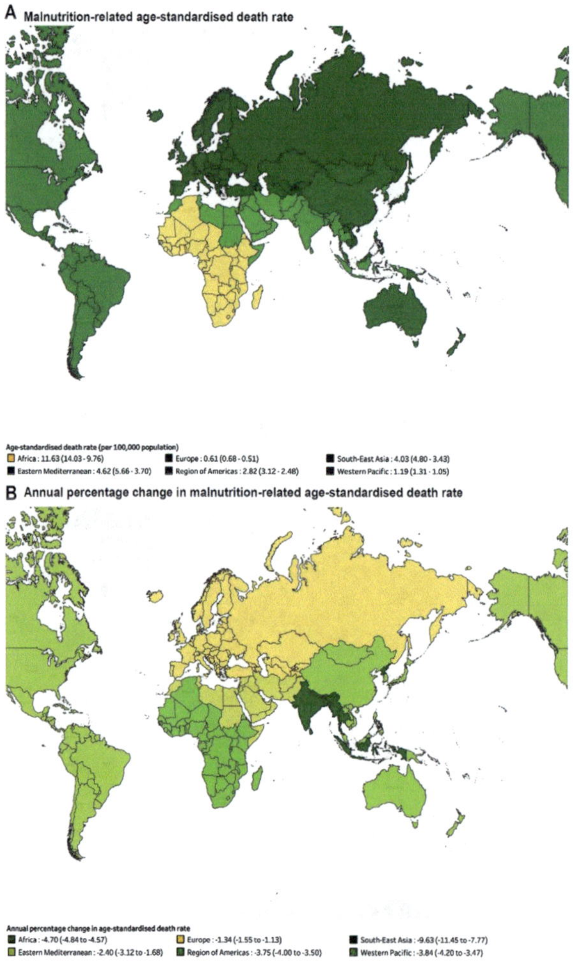

Figure 15.16. The global trends of (A) obesity related age-standardized mortality; and (B) annual percentage change in malnutrition-related age-standardized death rate.

Source: https://www.thelancet.com/cms/10.1016/j.eclinm.2023.101850/asset/8c40c37e-5edd-4e43-8d90-f5fe7f896fb1/main.assets/gr3_lrg.jpg.

15.5.3. International Collaborations and Research Initiatives

Global research partnerships are required in the pursuit of the field of nutritional epidemiology, which analyzes the intersection of nutrition and health outcomes across different populations. Partnerships can enhance the sharing of best practices, methodologies, and data, hence leading to enhanced knowledge of nutritional issues that transcend borders. For instance, multi-country studies provide a snapshot of dietary habits and prevalent diseases in different regions, allowing researchers to identify risk factors that may be overlooked in single-country studies. Additionally, collaborative research can support surveillance systems, which are critical for monitoring food trends and the associated impact on public health. Through the implementation of collaborations among government agencies, non-government organizations, and academic institutions, researchers can target common health issues while leveraging the salience of each participating organization to achieve mutually rewarding goals. One of the greatest values of global collaborations is the potential to overcome domineering health problems like malnutrition, obesity, and infectious diseases driven by poor diets. With the sharing of resources and expertise, research activities can establish targeted interventions and education for health programs for specific identified communities. For example, from the conduct of successful public health interventions in developed nations, there may be extremely valuable lessons on effective strategies in developing nations with malnutrition issues. The exchange of information streamlines intervention efficiency and guarantees cultural appropriateness in program development. These collaborative approaches highlight the importance of international thinking in nutritional epidemiology, whereby diverse populations can inform locally responsive and adaptive public health interventions that lead to better health for everyone. Global partnerships can also play a key role in addressing complex health issues such as antibiotic resistance and its intersection with nutrition. As the example of tuberculosis demonstrates, effective global health initiatives require well-balanced approaches that account for the multidimensionality of nutrition and disease. Countries that bear the dual burden of infectious and non-communicable diseases, such as India, can be assisted by common knowledge and ideas to improve their public health systems. The development of rapid diagnostic tests and enhanced treatment interventions, as suggested in tuberculosis debates, can similarly be made available for different nutritional disorders. Besides, the exchange of information about dietary trends and their effects on health, countries can join forces to identify and counteract the effects of malnutrition, enhancing the collective response to priority global health issues. This shared commitment to research and intervention is a critical step toward the achievement of global health equity in nutritional epidemiology.

Summary

On the whole, nutritional epidemiology science holds vast potential to elucidate the complex interactions among diet, disease risk, and health outcomes. As can be seen through the development of the ontology for nutritional epidemiology (ONE), applying standardized structures to data collection and reporting can significantly improve research capacity in this area. By creating a systematic ontology that brings together many of the data points related to nutrition and health, researchers are able to automate data integration, make it more searchable, and improve the completeness of dietary intake assessment. Through such a systematized approach, not only is improved analysis possible, but transparency and reproducibility also enter the domain, allowing results to loop back into the broader body of knowledge encompassing nutritional epidemiology (Ambayo et al., 2019). Furthermore, the examination of specific eating habits and their link with diseases illustrates the intricacy of nutrition-related health issues. The example of research on the causes of risk for esophageal cancer among Iranian Turkmens is a case in point to illustrate how lifestyle choices and genetic factors get intertwined as causes of health. The study highlights the significance of certain dietary patterns, such as the consumption of stale food and butter, which were found to have a positive correlation with increased cancer risk. Such findings indicate the need for radical epidemiological studies considering a variety of determinants of health, such as genetic determinants, environmental determinants, and cultural determinants. Continued research on such interactions will be of first-order significance in informing public health programs and dietary advice aimed at reducing rates of disease (Besharat et al., 2007). Lastly, as the science matures, the need for interdisciplinary collaboration becomes increasingly clear. Nutritional epidemiology is a complex field requiring input from a broad spectrum of disciplines, from microbiology, through public health to behavioral science, in order to fully describe the dynamic interaction between diet and health. This cooperative approach can provide stronger and more inclusive interventions that promote optimal nutrition and reduce disease risk. With these aspects in mind, the future of research must aim to develop holistic methodologies and models for tackling the multifaceted issues of human nutrition and health. By embracing such strategies, the field of nutritional epidemiology can contribute more meaningfully to global health and lead major changes in dietary practices (Ambayo et al., 2019).

Nutritional epidemiology has yielded important evidence on diet and health outcomes, particularly for chronic diseases. The evaluation of dietary patterns has been inclined to reveal the protective roles of some food patterns, such as fruits and vegetables, in relation to diseases like cardiovascular disease and certain forms of cancer. But nutritional epidemiology is not free of its complexities, as the effects of individual nutrients can be highly variable based on their sources and conditions of total dietary intake. For example, recent findings have pointed towards the divergent effects of different types of selenium on health, proving that while some may have protective effects, others could also facilitate other risk factors in health, thereby rendering it increasingly difficult to determine dietary requirements within the general population (Ammar et al., 2013). The variability of this scenario reflects the significance of embracing a personalized approach to diet that considers personal profiles of health as well as environmental factors. Again, another notable discovery in the field of research regarding micronutrients and how crucial they are to influencing outcomes on health is that poor micronutrient status has the potential to predispose an individual to infections such as visceral leishmaniasis. Systematic reviews have demonstrated that deficiencies in vitamins have the potential to exacerbate the severity of such infections and complicate treatment outcomes (Nandy et al., 2010). Alternatively, adequate micronutrient intake has been shown to improve immune function and general health and therefore the importance of dietary variety. This fact highlights the importance of nutritional epidemiology beyond surveillance of macronutrients also to put great emphasis on micronutrient status, particularly in high-risk populations where malnutrition is the norm. Furthermore, the interrelation between nutrition and socio-economic determinants has been a research area of keen interest in nutritional epidemiology. It is increasingly recognized today that poverty and resource access significantly influence food choices, which in turn affect health. Evidence indicates that poor individuals have poor access to healthy food and resort to consuming cheaper, energy-dense foods, which can have adverse effects on their health in the form of obesity and related non-communicable diseases. Furthermore, the complexity of risk factors—i.e., housing conditions and living conditions—only reinforces this link, as noted in disease studies, such as the case of kala-azar, where the quality of housing affects the risk of infection (Nandy et al., 2010). To achieve nutritional health, this means having an integrated approach combining both food culture as well as socio-economic determinants.

CLOSER LOOK

IMPORTANCE OF CONTINUED RESEARCH IN NUTRITIONAL EPIDEMIOLOGY

Nutritional epidemiology studies are crucial to the continued insight into how genetic factors and the environment interact with each other to support healthy outcomes. For instance, studies of the fat mass and obesity-associated gene (FTO) demonstrate the complex interaction of genetic susceptibilities and characteristics involved with obesity. Research findings demonstrate that while early childhood BMI appears unaffected by certain FTO genotypes, significant associations emerge by age four, pointing to a critical developmental window where intervention may be most effective (Bauer et al., 2010). This underscores the necessity for ongoing investigations into how dietary patterns, lifestyle factors, and genetic variations contribute to obesity, subsequently informing preventive strategies and public health policies. Through the probing of these intricate dynamics, scientists can produce personalized nutritional guidelines that respond to individual genetic differences, ultimately contributing to better population health outcomes. Another area in which continued research is still vital is the resolution of psychological and behavioral issues related to nutrition. As modern diets evolve, identifying their impact on mental health is increasingly becoming essential. Emerging evidence suggests that nutritional deficiencies can hasten psychological disease or mental deterioration.

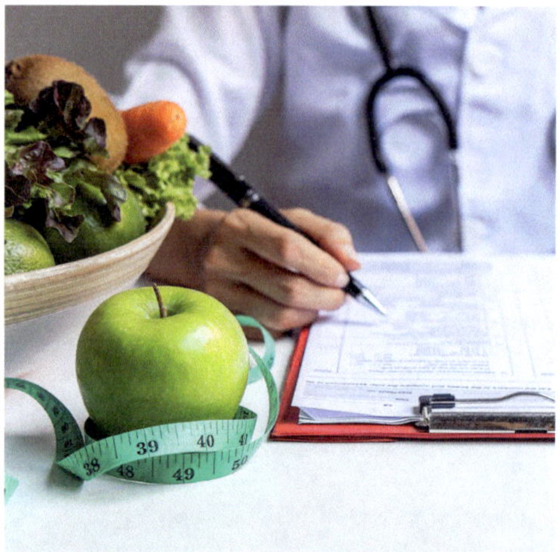

Figure 15.17. Nutritionist documenting dietary information with a focus on healthy eating and weight management.

Source: https://peterattiamd.com/wp-content/uploads/2022/02/Nutritional-epidemiology-1x1-1.jpg.

By emphasizing research on the linkages between mental health, gut health, and diet, we are better able to understand the way in which nutritional interventions may be employed as therapeutic measures for mental illness. For instance, nutrient-dense diets can be protective against diseases such as depression and anxiety, suggesting an application of nutritional epidemiology towards developing inclusive treatment measures (Hokororo et al., 2012). More studies in this field will consolidate our knowledge of such connections and help individuals make informed food choices that not only foster physical but also psychological well-being. Moreover, the world of nutrition is dynamically changing at global, national, and local levels due to factors such as globalization, urbanization, and technological advancements in food. In this regard, nutritional epidemiology research assists in assessing the consumption patterns and health implications of different populations globally. The estimation of the prevalence of specific dietary habits and their influence on health will be employed in creating public policy to combat malnutrition and diet-related disorders. With the numerous health ailments confronting the world today, including obesity and micronutrient deficiency, a good research agenda will provide culture-specific diet recommendations. Therefore, the ongoing emphasis on nutritional epidemiologic studies is essential for addressing the varied range of nutritional needs across populations and supporting health equity at the global level (Figure 15.17).

References

1. Ahiadeke, C., Boerma, T., Dunyo, S., Einterz, E., Ezzati, M., Fahrmeir, L., et al. (2009). Diarrhoea, acute respiratory infection, and fever among children in the Democratic Republic of Congo. https://core.ac.uk/download/47394.pdf (accessed on 25th June 2025).
2. Alexieva, I., Krastanov, A., Lante, A., Mihaylova, D., et al. (2018). Polyphenols as suitable control for obesity and diabetes. https://core.ac.uk/download/168405564.pdf (accessed on 25th June 2025).
3. Ambayo, H., Bouwman, J., Bronselaer, A., De Baets, B., et al. (2019). An ontology to standardize research output of nutritional epidemiology: From paper-based standards to linked content. https://core.ac.uk/download/222452585.pdf (accessed on 25th June 2025).
4. Ammar, E. M., Bhattacharya, A., Bjelakovic, G., Blot, W. J., Buntzel, J., Malagoli, C., Crespi, C. M., et al. (2013). Friend or foe? The current epidemiologic evidence on selenium and human cancer risk. https://core.ac.uk/download/323076133.pdf (accessed on 25th June 2025).
5. Anderson, J., Celis-Morales, C. A., Gill, J. M. R., Gray, S. R., et al. (2017). Associations between diabetes and both cardiovascular disease and all-cause mortality are modified by grip strength: Evidence from UK Biobank, a prospective population-based cohort study. https://core.ac.uk/download/96884272.pdf (accessed on 25th June 2025).
6. Baba, B., Häsler, B., Rushton, J., Lightowlers, M., Bruce, M., Pradère, J. P., et al. (2017). Using a One Health approach to assess the impact of parasitic disease in livestock: How does it add value? https://core.ac.uk/download/45467978.pdf (accessed on 25th June 2025).
7. Backhouse, S. H., Brissonneau, C., Christensen, A., Collins, R., et al. (2014). *Study on Doping Prevention: A Map of Legal, Regulatory and Prevention Practice Provisions in EU 28*. https://core.ac.uk/download/29018868.pdf (accessed on 25th June 2025).
8. Bauer, C. P., Berdel, D., von Berg, A., Borte, M., et al. (2010). Associations between BMI and the FTO gene are age dependent: Results from the GINI and LISA birth cohort studies up to age 6 years. https://core.ac.uk/download/16432421.pdf (accessed on 25th June 2025).
9. Bauer, C. P., Berdel, D., von Berg, A., Heinrich, J., et al. (2012). Food intake, diet quality and behavioral problems in children: Results from the GINI-plus/LISA-plus studies. https://core.ac.uk/download/16432923.pdf (accessed on 25th June 2025).
10. Besharat, S., Kalavi, K., Moradi, A., Qujeq, D., et al. (2007). Risk factors of esophageal cancer in Turkmen Sahra of Iran. https://core.ac.uk/download/52205105.pdf (accessed on 25th June 2025).
11. Bishop, D., Evans, A. B., Evans, D., Keegan, R., et al. (2014). The importance of parents and teachers as stakeholders in school-based healthy eating programs. https://core.ac.uk/download/17171089.pdf (accessed on 25th June 2025).
12. Bordoni, A., Dupont, D., Gille, D., Kachal, J., et al. (2015). Understanding the gastrointestinal tract of the elderly to develop dietary solutions that prevent malnutrition. https://core.ac.uk/download/286575279.pdf (accessed on 25th June 2025).
13. Bracha, H. S. (2006). Human brain evolution and the "Neuroevolutionary Time-depth Principle:" Implications for the reclassification of fear-circuitry-related traits in DSM-V and for studying

resilience to warzone-related posttraumatic stress disorder. https://core.ac.uk/download/pdf/86611.pdf (accessed on 25th June 2025).

14. Bray, F., Laversanne, M., Sung, H., Ferlay, J., Siegel, R. L., Soerjomataram, I., & Jemal, A. (2024). Global cancer statistics 2022: GLOBOCAN estimates of incidence and mortality worldwide for 36 cancers in 185 countries. *CA: A Cancer Journal for Clinicians, 74*, 229–263. https://doi.org/10.3322/caac.21834 (accessed on 25th June 2025).

15. Brennan, L., & de Roos, B. (2017). Personalized interventions–A precision approach for the next generation of dietary intervention studies. https://core.ac.uk/download/131024429.pdf (accessed on 25th June 2025).

16. Bruno, G., Canevelli, M., Cesari, M., Lucchini, F., et al. (2016). Nutrition and dementia: Evidence for preventive approaches? https://core.ac.uk/download/98338858.pdf (accessed on 25th June 2025).

17. Burke, K. M., Fernandez Duque, E., & Valeggia, C. R. (2009). Nutritional status and socioeconomic change among Toba and Wichí populations of the Argentinean Chaco. https://core.ac.uk/download/287881909.pdf (accessed on 25th June 2025).

18. Butler, G., Cooper, J. M., Leifert, C., Lueck, L., et al. (2007). Effects of organic and 'low input' production methods on food quality and safety. https://core.ac.uk/download/10925455.pdf (accessed on 25th June 2025).

19. Caesar, M., Crush, J., Drimie, S., Frayne, B., et al. (2011). *No. 05: The HIV and Urban Food Security Nexus*. https://core.ac.uk/download/157834898.pdf (accessed on 25th June 2025).

20. Campbell, K. L., Fawcett, J., Hickman, I. J., Jarrett, P., et al. (2016). Changes in dietary patterns and body composition within 12 months of liver transplantation. https://core.ac.uk/download/196605093.pdf (accessed on 25th June 2025).

21. Cash, S. B., Cortus, B., Goddard, E. W., Han, D., et al. (2025). Integrating food policy with growing health and wellness concerns: An analytical literature review of the issues affecting government, industry, and civil society. https://core.ac.uk/download/pdf/6522474.pdf (accessed on 25th June 2025).

22. Castle, D. (2007). Genomic nutritional profiling: Innovation and regulation in nutrigenomics. https://core.ac.uk/download/28966982.pdf (accessed on 25th June 2025).

23. Catley, A., Catley, A., Roug, A., Chengula, A. A., Majule, A. E., Kilale, A. M., Kiwara, A., et al. (2017). Exploring local knowledge and perceptions on zoonoses among pastoralists in northern and eastern Tanzania. https://core.ac.uk/download/76981015.pdf (accessed on 25th June 2025).

24. Corpet, D. E., Pierre, F., & Santarelli, R. L. (2008). Processed meat and colorectal cancer: A review of epidemiologic and experimental evidence. https://core.ac.uk/download/12039008.pdf (accessed on 25th June 2025).

25. Crush, J., Frayne, B., & McLachlan, M. (2011). *No. 07: Rapid Urbanization and The Nutrition Transition in Southern Africa*. https://core.ac.uk/download/159478647.pdf (accessed on 25th June 2025).

26. Dekker, M., Jongen, W. M. F., & Plaami, S. P. (2002). Functional foods: A conceptual model for assessing their safety and effectiveness. https://core.ac.uk/download/pdf/29295489.pdf (accessed on 25th June 2025).

27. Ngudi Diasolua, D. (2014). *KONZO: The IBRO Africa Regional Committee (ARC) Organizes its First Global Advocacy Workshop for Neuroscience in Kinshasa*. https://core.ac.uk/download/55767487.pdf (accessed on 25th June 2025).
28. Dowler, E., & O'Connor, D. (2012). Rights based approaches to addressing food poverty and food insecurity in Ireland and UK. https://core.ac.uk/download/1384858.pdf (accessed on 25th June 2025).
29. Drescher, L. S., & Goddard, E. W. (2025). Observing changes in Canadian demand for food diversity over time. https://core.ac.uk/download/pdf/6449386.pdf (accessed on 25th June 2025).
30. Mills Esteves, J., & Cumming, O. (2016). The impact of water, sanitation, and hygiene on key health and social outcomes: Review of evidence. https://core.ac.uk/download/75761114.pdf (accessed on 25th June 2025).
31. Ezekiel, L., Kivuyo, S. L., Mfinanga, S. G. M., Ngadaya, E., et al. (2011). Public health concern and initiatives on the priority action towards non-communicable diseases in Tanzania. https://core.ac.uk/download/pdf/11307332.pdf (accessed on 25th June 2025).
32. Gamon, M. (2013). *Multidrug-Resistant Tuberculosis in India: Solving A Problem by Reconstructing The Public Health Infrastructure*. https://core.ac.uk/download/67755957.pdf (accessed on 25th June 2025).
33. Hokororo, A., Kamugisha, E., Mshana, S. E., Mwizamholya, D. L., et al. (2012). Prevalence and factors associated with Group A rotavirus infection among children with acute diarrhea in Mwanza, Tanzania. https://core.ac.uk/download/pdf/11307761.pdf (accessed on 25th June 2025).
34. Iacobini, C., Menini, S., Pesce, C., Pugliese, G., et al. (2017). Dietary interventions to contrast the onset and progression of diabetic nephropathy: A critical survey of new data. https://core.ac.uk/download/80314820.pdf (accessed on 25th June 2025).
35. Illner, A. K., Lachat, C., & Slimani, N. (2014). Assessing food intake through a chest-worn camera device. https://core.ac.uk/download/55814362.pdf (accessed on 25th June 2025).
36. Ilochi, P. I. (2011). Factors that impact access to quality food in the inner city. https://core.ac.uk/download/12206451.pdf (accessed on 25th June 2025).
37. Joffe, M., & Mindell, J. (2005). Mathematical modelling of health impacts. https://core.ac.uk/download/1669570.pdf (accessed on 25th June 2025).
38. Lampugnale, C. A. (2017). Surgical assessment of the geriatric oncology patient. https://open.bu.edu/bitstream/2144/26707/5/Lampugnale_bu_0017N_13146.pdf (accessed on 25th June 2025).
39. Maulder, P. S., & McDonald, K. (2018). The effects of morning preconditioning protocols on testosterone, cortisol and afternoon sprint cycling performance [Conference presentation]. https://core.ac.uk/download/187724674.pdf (accessed on 25th June 2025).
40. Nandy, A., Palit, A., Palit, A., Ranjan, A., Chakravarty, A. K., Mukhopadhyay, A. K., Mukhopadhyay, A. K., et al. (2010). Of cattle, sand flies and men: A systematic review of risk factor analyses for South Asian visceral leishmaniasis and implications for elimination. https://core.ac.uk/download/46495.pdf (accessed on 25th June 2025).

41. Roberts, E., & Inwood, K. (2025). Longitudinal studies of human growth and health: A review of recent historical research. https://core.ac.uk/download/pdf/6314865.pdf (accessed on 25th June 2025).

42. Singhal, T. (2020). A review of coronavirus disease-2019 (COVID-19). *The Indian Journal of Pediatrics, 87*, 281–286. https://doi.org/10.1007/s12098-020-03263-6 (accessed on 25th June 2025).

43. Slee, A. D. (2012). Exploring metabolic dysfunction in chronic kidney disease. https://core.ac.uk/download/17352998.pdf (accessed on 25th June 2025).

44. Sweeny, K. (2025). The influence of childhood circumstances on adult health. https://core.ac.uk/download/pdf/30672978.pdf (accessed on 25th June 2025).

45. Tymicki, K. (2025). The correlates of infant and childhood mortality. https://core.ac.uk/download/pdf/7127213.pdf (accessed on 25th June 2025).

46. Veghari, G. (2015). The comparison of under-five children's nutrition status among ethnic groups in North of Iran, 1998–2013: Results of a three stages cross-sectional study. https://core.ac.uk/download/52205730.pdf (accessed on 25th June 2025).

INDEX